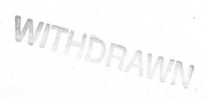
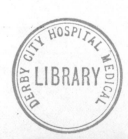

Oxford University Press makes no representation, express or implied, that the drug dosages in this book are correct. Readers must therefore always check the product information and clinical procedures with the most up-to-date published product information and data sheets provided by the manufacturers and the most recent codes of conduct and safety regulations. The authors and the publishers do not accept responsibility or legal liability for any errors in the text or for the misuse or misapplication of material in this work.

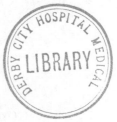

Child Psychiatry

A DEVELOPMENTAL APPROACH

THIRD EDITION

Philip Graham

Emeritus Professor of Child Psychiatry
Institute of Child Health, London

Jeremy Turk

Senior Lecturer in Child and Adolescent Psychiatry
St George's Hospital Medical School, London

And

Frank C. Verhulst

Professor of Child and Adolescent Psychiatry
Sophia Children's Hospital, Rotterdam
The Netherlands

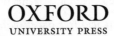

OXFORD

UNIVERSITY PRESS

OXFORD

UNIVERSITY PRESS

Great Clarendon Street, Oxford OX2 6DP

Oxford University Press is a department of the University of Oxford
and furthers the University's aim of excellence in research, scholarship,
and education by publishing worldwide in
Oxford New York
Athens Auckland Bangkok Bogota Buenos Aires Calcutta
Cape Town Chennai Dar es Salaam Delhi Florence Hong Kong Istanbul
Karachi Kuala Lumpur Madrid Melbourne Mexico City Mumbai
Nairobi Paris São Paulo Singapore Taipei Tokyo Toronto Warsaw
and associated companies in
Berlin Ibadan

Oxford is a trade mark of Oxford University Press

Published in the United States
by Oxford University Press, Inc., New York

© P. J. Graham, J. Turk, F. C. Verhulst, 1999

The moral rights of the author have been asserted

First published 1987
Second edition published 1991
Third edition published 1999

British Library Cataloguing in Publication Data

Library of Congress Cataloging in Publication Data
1 3 5 7 9 10 8 6 4 2

ISBN 0 19 262864 X

Typeset by Newgen Imaging Systems (P) Ltd., Chennai, India

Printed in Great Britain on acid free paper by Biddles Ltd., Guildford, Surrey

Preface to the third edition

For this edition, Philip Graham, the sole author of the first two editions of this book, has been joined by Jeremy Turk and Frank Verhulst. As well as substantial revision of the whole text, this has made possible significant expansion of some sections, especially those relating to neurodevelopment, neuropsychiatry, and the psychiatry of adolescence.

We would like to thank all those with whom we have discussed our ideas and who have influenced our thinking, especially our trainees and the children and families we have seen in clinical practice. We would also particularly like to thank those who have commented on sections of the book, Peter Fuggle, Anna Graham, Helen Martyn, Mike Patton, Cathy Taylor, and Vicky Turk.

London	P.G.
London	J.T.
Rotterdam	F.V.
October, 1998	

Preface to the first edition

This book is intended to be of use to all doctors dealing with children and their families, but especially to paediatricians and psychiatrists in training. I hope that a number of others, such as medical students, clinical medical officers, general practitioners, medical and psychiatric social workers, nurses, psychologists, general and child psychiatrists, will also find it helpful. The level of the book is intended to be suitable for those with an elementary as well as a somewhat more advanced knowledge of paediatrics, and I have tried to bear in mind the very different settings in which professionals dealing with children and families may carry out their work.

Throughout the book, with few exceptions, I have referred to both children and professionals as if they were all male. The exceptions consist of children suffering from conditions with a heavy female preponderance (such as anorexia nervosa) and when reference is made to professionals such as nurses who, at least in the children's field, are nearly all women. I realize this is unsatisfactory, but the alternatives seemed even more so.

In the section on physical conditions, I was aware that, especially with less common disorders, many clinicians such as family doctors, clinical medical officers, and child psychiatrists (as well as non-physicians such as psychologists and social workers) might find it helpful to have available an introductory résumé of the physical aspects of the condition before psychosocial aspects were discussed. I have therefore included a certain amount of such information, but it should be emphasized that this book is in no way a substitute for a textbook of paediatrics. I hope it will be seen as complementary to such a textbook, filling out in more detail an aspect of paediatric care which has so far received less attention than the prevalence of psychosocial disorders in childhood suggests it should.

London   P.G.
June, 1986

Preface to the second edition

Encouraged by the response to the first edition of this book, I have prepared the second edition with the same intention, namely, to provide a book that is helpful to a wide variety of professionals dealing with disturbed children, but particularly those working in paediatrics, psychiatry, general practice, psychology, and social work, as well as those training to enter these fields. I hope that readers who find themselves expected at times to take a perspective of the subject from an unfamiliar professional vantage-point will find this an enriching as well as a disconcerting experience.

I should once again like to thank my colleagues at the Hospital for Sick Children, Great Ormond Street, and the Institute of Child Health, London, for the opportunities they provide for stimulating discussion. Michael Rutter's work at the Institute of Psychiatry, London, has continued to be a rich source of intellectual inspiration.

I owe particular thanks to those who have read and commented on sections of the book, particularly Arnon Bentovim, Roger Freeman, Roy Howarth, Richard Lansdown, Bryan Lask, Tessa Leverton, Stuart Logan, Jeanne Magagna, Tony McShane, Celia Mostyn, David Skuse, Jeremy Turk, and Dieter Wolke.

Finally, my thanks are due to Jackie Moore, whose secretarial assistance has once again been invaluable.

London   P.G.
July, 1990

Contents

1 Introduction

1.1	Overview	1
1.2	Theories of development and its disorders	2
1.3	Family influences	12
1.4	Classification and prevalence of psychiatric disorders	17
1.5	Assessment and diagnosis of psychiatric disorders	24
1.6	Psychological assessment	35

2 Maltreatment in the family

2.1	Physical abuse	43
2.2	Munchausen syndrome by proxy	48
2.3	Neglect	50
2.4	Emotional abuse	51
2.5	Sexual abuse	54
2.6	Outcome following child maltreatment	59

3 Neurodevelopment and neuropsychiatric disorders

3.1	Motor development and disorders of movement	61
3.2	Normal language and speech development	68
3.3	Intelligence and learning disorders	84
3.4	Attention and attention deficit hyperactivity (hyperkinetic) disorder	110
3.5	Pervasive developmental disorders	120
3.6	Sensory development	132
3.7	Chromosomal abnormalities	138
3.8	Disorders of the central nervous system and muscle	149
3.9	Metabolic disorders	169

4 Development and developmental psychopathology

4.1	Fetal and infant development	172
4.2	Feeding and eating control disorders	186
4.3	Sleep and its disorders	201
4.4	Emotional development and disorders of mood	207

4.5   Social development and antisocial behaviour   235
4.6   Bowel and bladder control   251
4.7   Prepubertal sexual development   262

5   Adolescence and psychiatric disorders often beginning in adolescence

5.1   Adolescence   267
5.2   Sexual development in adolescence   269
5.3   Early pregnancy   272
5.4   Anorexia nervosa   273
5.5   Adult-type psychiatric disorders   280
5.6   Psychoses   295
5.7   Drug use and abuse   304
5.8   Personality disorders   313

6   Child–adult continuities in psychiatric disorders

6.1   Introduction and definitions   314
6.2   Findings   315

7   Psychosocial aspects of physical disorders: general

7.1   Psychosocial causes of chronic physical disease   318
7.2   Impact on parents   319
7.3   Impact on the child   322
7.4   Impact on the sibs   326
7.5   Principles of psychosocial management of physically
        handicapped children and their families   326
7.6   Hospitalization   330
7.7   Care of the dying child   334
      Further reading   337

8   Psychosocial aspects of specific physical non-neurological conditions

8.1   Stillbirth and neonatal death   338
8.2   Sudden infant death syndrome (cot death)   339
8.3   Malformations   341
8.4   Injuries to children   344
8.5   Infectious diseases   349
8.6   Metabolic disorders   356

8.7   Endocrine disorders   359
8.8   Blood disorders   364
8.9   Respiratory disorders   370
8.10   Genitourinary disorders   378
8.11   Organic gastrointestinal disorders   382
8.12   Congenital heart disease   383
8.13   Skin disorders   386
8.14   Immunodeficiency disorders   389
8.15   Juvenile chronic arthritis   390

9   Prevention and treatment

9.1   Preventive approaches   392
9.2   Treatment   400

10   Services

10.1   The estimation of service needs   455
10.2   Health services for children with mental health problems   455
10.3   Social services and child protection   466
10.4   School influences and special education   479

References   487

Index   541

1

Introduction

1.1 Overview

What is paediatric or child psychiatry? More than most branches of medical practice, the field is difficult to define. The central foci of the subject are the behavioural and emotional disorders of childhood and adolescence, but many would include those 'psychosomatic' physical symptoms, such as non-organic headache and stomach pains in which stress or other environmental factors appear to play an important causative role. Delays and deviations in development, as well as general and specific learning problems, lie in the borderland of child psychiatric practice. Environmental factors are often important in their causation, and they are often, but by no means always, accompanied or followed by significant emotional and/or behavioural disturbance.

Because children's development is so closely bound up with the quality of care given by parents, failures of parenting and the fostering of parental skills are often seen as an integral part of child psychiatric practice. There are indeed some child psychiatrists who prefer to see themselves as family psychiatrists. This can often be a helpful approach, but it is important to remember that, although usually children's problems can best be seen as arising from an interaction between the child, the family, and the wider environment, in a significant number of cases (as in childhood autism, for example) a serious primary disturbance does indeed lie in the child.

Defining the territory of child psychiatry in this way makes it clear that most professional assessment and treatment of child psychiatric disorder is carried out by non-psychiatrists and indeed by professionals not medically qualified. These include family doctors, paediatricians, and clinical medical officers, as well as psychologists, nurses, social workers, and teachers. The situations which call for the particular skills of a child psychiatrist (Graham 1984) will vary, but, in general, psychiatrists are most likely to be appropriately involved where a disorder is severely handicapping and persistent. With training, other medical and non-medical professionals can, of course, be effective in assessing and treating problems in this field of work.

Finally, an important characteristic of child psychiatric disorders lies in the degree to which they affect different aspects of the life of the child and the family. The family of a seriously disturbed child will require the services of many different types of professional, drawn especially from the health, education, and social welfare services. An important principle of practice involves the need for all practitioners, no matter to which discipline they belong, to respect the contribution that other disciplines may make, to be aware of the point at which another discipline may need to be involved, and to maintain as close communication with other disciplines as is compatible with professional confidentiality.

1.2 Theories of development and its disorders

1.2.1 INTRODUCTION

Mrs Brown brings her 10 year old son, Kevin, who suffers with headaches, to the family doctor, then to a specialist paediatrician and finally to a psychologist. She has been asked to take Kevin to the doctor by his teacher, who 'knows' that Kevin gets headaches because his parents do not get on and are constantly quarrelling and occasionally separating. On the other hand, Mrs Brown 'knows' that the headaches are inherited because her brother had exactly the same symptoms when he was in school. Kevin's father has not come to the consultation because he 'knows' that the headaches are manufactured because Kevin finds school difficult and his mother fusses over him thus making them worse. By contrast, Kevin's 17 year old sister is a believer in astrology, and 'knows' that her brother's birth sign, Aries, is an infallible indication of explosive temperament of which the headaches are but one manifestation. Finally, Kevin 'knows' that he has meningitis, a topic much in the newspapers recently.

The family doctor, paediatrician, and clinical psychologist also have theories.

- The *family doctor* believes, on the basis of an unfortunate experience of a missed brain tumour several years ago, that headaches can be an ominous symptom of physical illness and always refers such problems to a paediatrician for further investigation.
- The *paediatrician* has a theory that headaches in childhood commonly respond to medication for migraine even when the cardinal symptoms are not present. But the tablets are ineffective and Kevin is referred to the psychologist.
- After an assessment of the whole family, the *psychologist* comes to the conclusion that Kevin's symptoms are the result of what family therapists call 'triangulation', a process in which a child becomes symptomatic when there is a problem between the parents. He recommends family therapy. However, as there is not a single member of the family who agrees with him, and as he fails to 'hold' them in therapy, the family drops out of treatment and Kevin's headaches persist.

Does this mean that one theory is as good as another, and that the theories held by health professionals are on a par with those held by family members? In one sense, they are. The ideas are equally meaningful to those holding them. But meaningfulness is not the only criterion by which to judge the value of a theory. Ideas can also be judged by their helpfulness, by their value in leading to positive change in both the external world and in the internal world of individuals.

1.2.2 EVIDENCE-BASED CHILD PSYCHIATRY

Let us suppose that a theory exists that can provide understanding of Kevin's non-organic headaches that leads to a form of psychological treatment with a scientifically demonstrated, better than chance possibility of improving his symptoms. Let us also suppose that this is an outcome that Kevin would actually prefer. This assumes, for example, that he would really like to attend school on a regular basis. The possession of such a theory, together with the skills to apply the techniques arising from it, would allow the health professionals to offer an effective form of treatment. This would not mean that Kevin and his family would necessarily want or be able to accept the treatment. The health professionals would need to have the skills to negotiate successfully with the family members to put their own theories 'on hold' for the time being, while they gave a chance to the treatment that was on offer.

What health professionals therefore need is a set of theories from which forms of treatment scientifically demonstrated to be effective have been derived. In fact, a number of such theories and techniques do now exist, and these are often complementary to each other rather than in competition.

1.2.3 THEORIES OF CHILDHOOD BEHAVIOUR:
A BRIEF HISTORICAL ACCOUNT

There is no point at which one can say that the history of childhood begins. At least since classical times, the importance of childhood as a preparation for adult life has been recognized. Despite views to the contrary (e.g. Aries 1973), childhood has always been recognized as a separate phase of life, and indeed it would be amazing if this were not so.

For our purposes, it seems sufficient to begin 200 years ago with the famous and often quoted words of a French philosopher and an English poet. Jean-Jacques Rousseau believed the infant was born infinitely malleable and with a potential for moral goodness that experience of life corrupted. 'Everything is good' he wrote in 1762 'that leaves the Creator's hands: everything degenerates in the hands of man'. In the sexist language acceptable in his day, William Wordsworth's 'The child is father of the man' asserts the continuity of behaviour over the life span.

Since the end of the eighteenth century, the concept of childhood as a time of extreme impressionability and therefore of crucial significance for the development of personality has been a powerful force in political and social thought, as well as in fiction. The introduction of universal compulsory education, and the special protection afforded children in employment and in the juvenile justice system have stemmed from this influence. The descriptions by Charles Dickens of the terrible living conditions of the poor were meant to move politicians and they did. Fagin's kitchen bred delinquent children, and only social reform could solve the problem.

But in the mid nineteenth century a new set of ideas emerged that led to different conclusions. Evolutionary theory, as proposed by Charles Darwin, led to interest in the biology of childhood and particularly into the way the genetic constitution of children, developed for adaptive purposes, affected their growth, intelligence, and behaviour. The growth of the eugenics movement in the second half of the nineteenth century was associated with the idea of selective breeding. Treatment of genetic deviations was then inconceivable, and the only way to improve the health of the population was thought to be by the selective propagation of 'good' genes. These ideas were largely discredited by their brutal application in Hitler's Germany in the 1930s and 1940s, but selective breeding with compulsory sterilization of people with mental retardation continued well into the second half of the twentieth century in Sweden and Norway.

Up to the late 1950s, the development of these two strands of thought concerning the influences on intelligence and behaviour continued more or less independently. Behavioural scientists usually took either a genetic or a behavioural stance. Social reformers would take a strongly environmentalist stance, while biological theorists would place emphasis on genetic inheritance. Those who were knowledgeable in both fields would make statements like 'The contribution to intelligence is about 60% genetic and 40% environmental'.

At this time, John Bowlby, a child psychiatrist influenced by relatively new ethological studies, began to bring together these two areas in a more meaningful way (Bowlby 1971, 1975, 1980). He pointed to the way attachment of infants to their mothers and of mothers to their infants was a biological phenomenon, affected by the way mothers behaved towards their babies. Biological processes were influenced by environmental factors such as separation and deprivation. At the same time, it was rediscovered that individual differences in the temperament and personality of children were by no means always caused by different forms of upbringing. Genetic factors were also significant in determining whether, for example, a baby was 'difficult' or 'easy' to bring up (Thomas, Chess and Birch 1968).

A further important theoretical development in the understanding of psychological disorders occurred in the 1980s. Biological, social, psychological, and developmental factors were encompassed in one overarching scientific endeavour, the field of developmental psychopathology (Sroufe and Rutter 1984). The characteristic mode of explanation in this relatively new theoretical approach is its emphasis on two-way interaction between different influences and outcomes. For example, Plomin and Daniels (1987) have pointed out, mainly on the basis of studies of twins, that our genes do not merely influence our behaviour, they may 'create' our environment. A baby born to be 'difficult' may upset his parents so much that a reasonably equable couple may turn hostile to the baby and even to each other. Their hostile behaviour may then negatively influence that of the baby.

Although the science of developmental psychopathology is relatively new, it seems likely that it is here to stay for several decades before it is superseded. Advances in all the neurosciences, for example in genetics, neuroimaging, neurochemistry, and neuropsychology (especially cognitive psychology) will ensure that our knowledge of the processes of brain–behaviour interactions will continue to grow. It will also become more complex. In order not to confuse the reader, the different approaches outlined above will be discussed in isolation from each other. But it should not be forgotten that the understanding of difficult behaviour and emotional problems in children nearly always involves an understanding of the interaction of different branches of knowledge derived from different theories. All experienced practitioners in this field recognize that the multiplicity of theories available means that none is totally satisfactory and that different models can be helpful in different situations. It is not surprising that there is no one theory capable of explaining all child and family behaviour, and one of the skills of the practitioner lies in selecting a way of looking at a child's problems that helps the family understand it better and relieves the distress associated with it.

1.2.4 BIOLOGICAL THEORIES

Strictly speaking, biology is the study of living organisms and includes the investigation of environmental as well as physical influences but, by convention, in psychiatry, the use of the term 'biological' usually refers only to physical or physiological influences. There is a variety of ways in which such influences contribute to the development of psychiatric disorders and learning disabilities. These include:

- *Genetic factors.* The development of the brain and other neural structures is largely under genetic control. Twin studies have demonstrated that many aspects of learning as well as some features of temperament and personality are influenced by multiple genes, and occasionally by the effects of single genes. Genetic anomalies are also probably responsible for a small number of child psychiatric disorders such as autism. In others such as the hyperkinetic syndrome (attention deficit hyperactivity disorder) there is a significant genetic influence, but environmental factors such as the quality of parental care may, in some cases, play a significant part. Most psychiatric disorders of childhood, are produced by an interaction of genes and environment (Eaves *et al.* 1997).
- *Brain damage or dysfunction.* This may occur before, at, or after birth. Damage to the fetus may be caused by physical illness in the mother, such as rubella or maternal phenylketonuria, or by toxins such as alcohol or illicit drugs. Damage to the brain at birth may arise as a result of a traumatic delivery. It is often difficult to know whether pre-existing abnormalities in the fetus have been, at least in part, responsible for a prolonged or otherwise abnormal delivery, or whether the birth itself is solely responsible for subsequent brain dysfunction. After birth, damage to the brain may occur as a result of various insults such as trauma to the head or a cerebral infection. The presence of brain damage or dysfunction in a child may give rise to physical symptomatology such as a hemiplegia or epilepsy, or to learning disabilities, sometimes of a specific nature. In addition, it has a non-specific effect on liability to show emotional or behaviour problems.

- *Other physical influences.* These include metabolic abnormalities, such as hypo- or hyperglycaemia, anaemia, or chronic infections such as that caused by the human immuno-deficiency virus.

Biological influences are of particular importance in the development of neuro-psychiatric disorders described in Chapter 3.

1.2.5 BEHAVIOUR OR LEARNING THEORIES

Early learning theories, such as those put forward by John Watson (1878–1958), suggested that all forms of behaviour and emotional expression were learned as a result of experience. The role of internal mental processes could thus be ignored. One could understand behaviour simply by studying the stimuli to which the organism was exposed, and noting the responses. Two main mechanisms for learning were described:

- *Classical conditioning.* In this form of conditioning a stimulus was paired or associated with a response a number of times, until the mere presence of part of the stimulus would elicit the response. Thus Pavlov sounded a bell at the same time as he produced food for his dogs. After several repetitions of this experience, the sound of the bell alone was sufficient to produce salivation. Children who develop fears of places where they have previously been frightened by dogs show a similar phenomenon.
- *Operant conditioning.* This form of learning occurs as a result of a process whereby a positive outcome following a particular behaviour leads to its repetition so as to reproduce the same desirable outcome. B. F. Skinner (1904–90) demonstrated this phenomenon with pigeons who learned to peck at a button because they had previously been given grain for this behaviour. Positive reinforcement (usually a reward) occurs when behaviour is followed by an event that tends to make the behaviour more likely to occur in the future. Negative reinforcement occurs when a behaviour is followed by the removal of an unpleasant stimulus. Intermittent positive reinforcement is said to occur when there is only occasional 'reward' following an event; such reinforcement is often more powerful than if it is continuous.

1.2.6 COGNITIVE AND COGNITIVE BEHAVIOUR THEORIES

The main contributor to early cognitive theory was Jean Piaget (1896–1980). He carried out countless observational experiments on children of different ages. He described four major phases of cognitive development:

- *Sensorimotor phase.* Below 2 years the infant understands the world directly through perception and action. He learns directly from what he can see, hear, feel, and taste, as well as from the results of his own activity impinging on the external world.
- *Pre-operational phase.* From 2–6 years the child is now able to make mental representation of objects, and imagine actions related to them, but he is still

completely egocentric, unable to imagine the world from the perspective of other people.

- *Concrete operational phase.* From 7–11 years the child is able to think logically, but only in concrete terms. The perspective of others is now fully appreciated.
- *Formal operational phase.* From 12 years the child is able to think in abstract terms and develop concepts of, for example, the relativity of man-made rules.

Piaget's ideas have needed considerable modification since he first formulated them. It is clear that his emphasis on laboratory observation and on the results of formal experiment led Piaget to underestimate what children can do in real life. Piaget's ideas have, however, cast light on the egocentricity of the young child, and on the process of moral development in the child with a conduct disorder. An awareness of Piaget's concepts can alert the child health professional to take into account a child's level of understanding, when, for example, communicating with a child about his chronic illness.

Piaget's work, largely conducted before the Second World War, has had a major influence on educational practice and stimulated numerous studies of children's thought processes, but it has had relatively little impact on our understanding of child psychiatric disorders.

In the last 40 years, however, arising from studies of information processing in the 1950s, there has been a very significant growth in cognitive psychology. For example, theoretical advances and empirical studies have been carried out in language processing, problem solving, reasoning, and decision making, and the complex interactions between emotions and cognition (Eysenck and Keane 1990). The science of cognitive psychology has, so far, been relatively poorly integrated into our ways of looking at the psychiatric disorders of childhood, although cognitive neuropsychology has had a much greater impact in our understanding of neuropsychiatric disorders.

The development of cognitive behaviour theory and various forms of therapy derived from it has been well described by Rachman (1997). It occurred as a result of the merging of behaviour theory (described above) and cognitive theory. Cognitive theorists propose that disturbances arise from faulty cognitions or faulty cognitive processing. Albert Ellis (1962) argued that emotional or psychological disturbances are largely a result of thinking illogically or irrationally, and that one can rid oneself of most of one's emotional or mental unhappiness if one learns to maximize rational or minimize irrational thinking.

Aaron Beck developed a form of cognitive therapy based on the rationale that an individual's affect and behaviour are largely determined by the way in which he structures the world (Beck 1976). The development of basic cognitive science over the last 40 years has given further impetus to this approach. These ideas merged with those of behaviour theory and therapy with their emphasis on the need for objective outcome measures and empirical validation of techniques. The result has been a form of therapy with very wide application to the behaviour and emotional problems of children and their families (Graham 1998a). Perhaps their most satisfactorily validated use is in depressive disorders (Harrington *et al.* 1998) and obsessive–compulsive disorders (March 1995). Their potential value is much wider, but, at this stage, more controlled trials need to be carried out before more general use can be recommended.

Early behavioural theories were useful in explaining some aspects of child behaviour such as the acquisition of simple habits, and the development of monosymptomatic phobias. Later elaboration of learning theory by the introduction of cognitive concepts and processes such as imitation and observation has widened the possible applications very considerably.

1.2.7 FAMILY THEORIES

Although the classification systems in child psychiatry refer exclusively to pathology within the individual child, many clinicians regard the problems they see as better understood by considering the family as the unit in question. Family theories provide ways of conceptualizing the processes that go on within families that may result in one family member, especially a child, being presented as a problem or a patient. Such theories include the following:

- *Systems theory*. A family system is conceived as a functional unit operating according to its own rules, and with certain special characteristics. Such a concept can be applied to systems of family functioning that would not be applicable to the functioning of individuals. In particular, those who use systems theory often also borrow from the science of cybernetics to explain how a family system regulates itself. Every change in the relationship between two family members is likely to result in changes in other relationships within the family, before the system reaches equilibrium again. Some family systems are dysfunctional and work badly, especially those that are rigid and inflexible and cannot react to changing demands of children.
- *Communication theory*. For a family to function well, messages between family members need to be transmitted and received unambiguously. Family life consists of a constant series of demands, requests, and injunctions to do or not do this or that. There is also a flow of factual information not requiring immediate action but perhaps important for the future. Finally, there is a need for the communication of feelings. Children need to know when their parents feel warm and approving, as well as when they are upset and condemnatory. In dysfunctional families, one or more types of communication are often transmitted poorly or ambiguously. One characteristic type of dysfunction involves passing double messages—for example a parent might laugh at a child's naughtiness as if it were trivial or even a lovable fault, but moments later shout at the child for the same behaviour as though bitterly disapproving of it. The 'double bind' theory of schizophrenia involves a suggestion that such double messages are important in the causation of schizophrenia. This has now been discredited as a cause of schizophrenia (Leff 1978), but the transmission of ambivalent messages from parents to children (and sometimes vice versa) certainly causes confused feelings in family members, who may then suffer significant symptoms.

- *Structural theory*. The relationships in a family can be regarded as organized or 'structured' in a characteristic way. Minuchin (1974) describes a variety of ways in which family organization or structure can be dysfunctional. The intergenerational boundaries may be blurred, and parents behave like the brothers and sisters of the children. Conversely children may take care-taking roles in relation to their parents. Parents and children may be overinvolved or emotionally 'enmeshed' with each other, or they may be too uninvolved emotionally, disengaged, or detached. There may be alliances or coalitions between family members—a mother and son ganging up against a father, for example. Finally, structure may be impaired by 'detouring' of conflicts rather than dealing with them directly. Characteristically, disputes between the parents are not settled by open and honest disagreement, argument, and negotiation between them. Instead, when for example a mother feels angry with her husband for sexual inadequacy, she may aggressively focus instead on her son's shortcomings which otherwise would have passed unnoticed.

Family theories have been directly applied in therapeutic work. They are particularly useful in situations where the primary pathology almost certainly lies in family interaction rather than in the individual child.

1.2.8 PSYCHOANALYTIC THEORIES

For a period of about 50 years from the 1930s to the 1980s, psychoanalytic theories dominated the field of child psychiatry. Although, quite appropriately, they continue to exert an influence on many practitioners, their contribution is now widely seen as much more limited and many of the claims made on behalf of psychoanalytic theory are now thought to lack empirical validation.

It is quite impossible to do justice to the richness and diversity of psycho-analytic theory in a brief summary. The works of the founder of psychoanalysis, Sigmund Freud (1856–1939) alone fill 15 volumes in the original standard edition. The elaboration of his theories by his daughter, Anna, and by numerous other followers, especially Melanie Klein and Donald Winnicott, have ensured that the theory is in a state of constant evolution. For a comprehensive, recent review of psychoanalytic theory, including more recent developments, and its relevance to our understanding of child development and pathology, the reader is referred to Fonagy *et al.* (1995). This review will concentrate on those features of psychoanalytic theory of most relevance to the non-specialist reader.

Psychoanalysis can be regarded as having made three main types of contribution to child psychiatry:

- A theory of the development of personality in childhood, with the following components:
  - Children are born with basic instinctual drives which govern their behaviour. A characteristic mental structure exists consisting of the source of the drives (*id*), the conscious part of the mind mediating between the drives and the environment (*ego*), and a moralizing or conscience-driven part of the mind (*superego*).

As they develop, children go through characteristic phases in which different parts of the body (the mouth, anus, and phallus) are primary sources of pleasure. For various reasons, children can become stuck or 'fixated' at one of these levels, and this can give rise to serious psychiatric pathology.

— During childhood, characteristic patterns of family relationships emerge. These are different for boys and girls. Boys, for example, develop an '*Oedipus complex*', in which they are closely attached to their mothers and have a fear or even a hatred of their fathers.

This theory of child development has failed to stand the test of time, and is now largely only of historical interest (Rutter 1995). However, it is still influential in some specialist centres.

- A theory of mental function with the following components:
  — An *active unconscious*. It is considered that a considerable part of mental activity that has influence on our behaviour is unconscious or only partly conscious. Some of our unconscious thoughts, fantasies, and feelings are only with difficulty made available to our conscious mind, because they are unacceptable to it.
  — *Defence mechanisms*. These, it is suggested, enable us to deal with real or imagined threats and the unacceptable content of our unconscious mind. An extended account of these was provided by Anna Freud (1966). They include *regression* (reverting to an earlier phase of life), *projection* (putting one's own unacceptable thoughts, feelings etc. into someone else, and *denial* (refusing to accept the facts at their face value). Some psychiatric disorders can be seen to arise partially or completely as forms of defence. Analysts speak of *obsessional*, *schizoid*, and *hysterical* (splitting) defences to explain the development of these disorders.

  In adapting to adverse situations, these mechanisms can be helpful or harmful. For example, denial of the life-threatening nature of a child's illness can help a parent cope with the rest of life, but such denial might prevent the parent from seeking the best form of help for the child.

  An understanding of these mental mechanisms and their operation is often found extremely valuable by counsellors, non-analytic psychotherapists, and indeed all other professionals engaged in trying to help disturbed or physically ill children and their families.

- An intensive form of psychological treatment classically characterized by:
  — A focus on the '*transference*' relationship between the therapist and the client, especially on those aspects of the relationship carried (transferred) into it from previous family and other relationships.
  — Emphasis on the recapitulation of unconscious thoughts, feelings, etc., especially those experienced in early childhood.
  — Treatment for 50 minutes, 4 or 5 times a week for 3 or more years by a psychoanalyst who has himself or herself had a similar, prolonged, personal experience of the therapy.

There is little evidence to justify the use of classical analytic therapy as summarized above, although it is still practised in some specialist centres and in private practice. Nevertheless there is some evidence of the value of less intensive forms of analytically or dynamically orientated psychotherapy. Awareness of the different types of mental mechanism is helpful to all practitioners. The importance of the quality of the relationship between the patient, client, or carer and the professional trying to help by offering a service is now very widely acknowledged, even by many of those with a strong behavioural bias to their work. This issue and others related to different forms of psychotherapy are discussed in Section 9.2.

1.2.9 ATTACHMENT THEORY

Attachment theory was developed by John Bowlby (1908–90) and elaborated in a trilogy describing psychological processes related to attachment, separation, and loss (Bowlby 1971, 1975, 1980).

Bowlby describes attachment as a complex two-way process in which the child becomes emotionally linked to members of his or her family, usually the mother, father, and sibs in diminishing order of intensity. Bowlby described attachment, especially to the mother, as an adaptive, biological process serving the needs of the child for protection and nurture. He suggested that it can best be understood as a 'control system' in which proximity to the mother is maintained through a series of signals emitted by both mother and child. The later capacity of the child to develop social relationships is considered to be based on the way with which attachment behaviour is established. Bowlby put particular emphasis on the central importance of both the biological and social ties with the mother.

Although the infant's tendency to form an attachment to its mother is genetically determined, the behaviour of those around the child will influence the security of the attachment. According to Mary Ainsworth and her co-workers (Ainsworth *et al.* 1978) there are three main patterns of attachment that can be characterized by observation of the toddler's behaviour with the mother. These observations are based on an experimental situation artificially set up in a laboratory. The focus is on the reactions of the child to being separated from the mother and left with a stranger, following which his behaviour is observed when he is reunited with his mother.

- *Secure attachment.* The mother initially provides a secure base for exploration, and the child is readily comforted if distressed. When reunited with his mother, if he has been distressed, he will immediately seek and maintain contact.
- *Anxious/resistant attachment.* The child is initially too anxious to leave his mother to explore, and is wary of new situations and people. When reunited after a separation he may be aggressive, cry, and refuse to be comforted or show considerable passivity.

- *Anxious/avoidant attachment.* The child explores readily away from his mother, and indeed is unduly friendly with the stranger. After a period of separation he will ignore or avoid his mother.

Subsequently a further pattern was recognized:

- *Disorganized/disorientated attachment.* When reunited with his mother, the child appears to have conflicting feelings of anger, fear, and a wish to be with her. He may seem confused and show stereotypies.

In recent years, it has been possible to link the early childhood experience of parents with the attachment patterns of their children as described above (Fonagy *et al.* 1991).

Theories of attachment are particularly useful in increasing our understanding of disorders of social relationships, of anxiety states (both generalized and specific) and of situations such as admission to hospital or placement in day care when brief or prolonged separations are in question.

1.2.10   CHILD DEVELOPMENT AND LIFE EXPERIENCES

These theories of child development that have been described all emphasize processes that unfold within the child. As the theories have been subjected to critical evaluation, it has become clear that each of them is capable, at best, of only telling part of the story. They have all needed to be modified to take account of children's life experiences in all their variety. The practitioner seeing a child with a problem must ask not just 'How has this child developed?', but also 'What has happened to this child?' The ways in which experience makes and is made by individual personality is a fascinating one (Goodyer 1990). In the clinical situation, understanding this interaction with the help of one or more of the theories described here is often the key to success.

1.3 Family influences

1.3.1 FAMILY STRUCTURE

Fortunately, healthy psychosocial development is compatible with a wide range of types of family structure. Although family structure can have an indirect influence on development, that influence is not as great as the quality of relationships, or the way the family functions. There were marked changes in family structure in western European families during the second half of the twentieth century. However, it is still true to say that most children experience what might be regarded as a traditional childhood in which they are brought up by both their two biological parents in an unbroken relationship. All the same, there is now much greater diversity than used to be the case (Central Statistical Office 1995).

Some types of family structure are *risk factors* for behaviour and learning problems. This means that their presence is an indicator of an increased likelihood of such problems being present. However, it does not mean that the type of family is itself a cause of problems. In fact, most evidence suggests that family structure itself is relatively unimportant in causing problems. Much more significant is the quality of family relationships and of child rearing. If a child is living with a single or stepparent in a family, this is quite likely to mean that he has experienced a period of disharmonious family relationships when child care was impaired. But some parents manage to achieve transitions in their relationships without long-lasting rancour.

About one-third of children in the UK are now born outside marriage, and the rates are only somewhat lower in many other western European countries. However, three-quarters of those born outside marriage are registered jointly in the names of both the father and the mother. Of those children with married parents, about 1 in 4 will experience the divorce of their parents by the age of 16 years. The rate of breakdown of parental cohabitations is not known, but cohabitation is less stable than marriage, so the breakdown rate must be considerable.

- *Single parents*. About 90% of single parent families are headed by mothers and the rest mainly by fathers. Only a minority of single mothers have never married or cohabited during the lives of their children. Most are separated or divorced from their husbands, and single parenthood may only be a temporary state. Children living in single parent families are slightly more likely to be showing a range of behaviour and learning problems than those living in conventional families. This is partly related to the fact that single parents are financially less well off than are two parents, and financial stress may lead to less than satisfactory child care.
- *Extended families*. Children living in societies where there is a pattern of extended family care (with much reliance on grandparents, aunts and uncles, etc. for child care) have about the same rate of psychological disorders as do children living in nuclear families with two parents and a small number of children (Cederblad 1968). The strains and stresses of living in an extended family are probably different in nature, but no less severe than those occurring in nuclear families.
- *Anomalous or unusual family structures* are not, in general, harmful to children unless the quality of relationships within the family is poor. Thus, for example, children brought up by two homosexual women do not, at least in their prepubertal years, appear to have an unduly high rate of problems (Golombok *et al.* 1983). Some anomalous family structures, such as communes, are almost inevitably unstable, and thus are likely to be unsettling for children brought up in them.
- *Large family size* is associated with somewhat delayed development and lowered intelligence, and with higher rates of educational and behavioural problems (Davie *et al.* 1972), especially in later born children. Having a large number of brothers and sisters is, of course, quite compatible with normal development, but a large sibship does predispose to psychological difficulties. Large families are more likely to suffer economic hardship, and parental stimulation is likely to be less easily available. As expected therefore, only

children appear to have a small advantage as far as intellectual development is concerned.

- *Ordinal position* or position in the family is of little psychological significance as far as risk of behaviour disturbance is concerned, though oldest and only children have a slight advantage in intellectual development (Davie *et al.* 1972). Twins are somewhat slower to develop language, and this is probably because of a mixture of divided parental attention and a reduced need for communication in twins who have each other for company.

1.3.2 FAMILY FUNCTIONING

Parental marital relationship

The quality of the parental marriage is an important factor in whether a child develops an emotional or behavioural disorder. Children of parents whose marriages are characterized by quarrelling, tension, mutual dissatisfaction, criticism, hostility, and lack of warmth are more likely to become disturbed. The fact that children of divorced parents have a distinctly higher rate of disturbance (Hetherington *et al.* 1982), whereas children of parents separated by death, although suffering initial bereavement reactions (van Eerdewegh *et al.* 1985), have only a slightly raised rate of disturbance later on, suggests that it is parental disharmony rather than separation from parents that is the crucial factor. This is not to say that children are unaffected by the death of a parent. Of course they are, often very profoundly. They may grieve for months and be especially susceptible to loss in the future. But they do not show higher rates of psychiatric disorder as do children of separated and divorced parents.

In fact, although their rate of disorder is distinctly higher than children in an intact family, only a minority of children of divorced parents become disturbed. Protective factors include the degree to which parents can make amicable arrangements for access, the quality of their own relationship with the child, the availability of other good relationships within the home (with sibs), and the child's temperament. The protective effect of a good relationship with an adult (usually a grandparent) outside the nuclear family has also been demonstrated in children whose parents have disharmonious marriages (Jenkins and Smith 1990).

Parental care

Emotionally warm, continuous, sensitive care from parents or their substitutes is the main, but by no means the only necessary precondition for healthy psychological development. Its presence goes far to ensure the development of secure 'attachment' of the child to the parent. This quality to the parent–child relationship results in the young child developing a whole range of adaptive forms of behaviour, including confident exploration of the environment and the appropriate seeking of parental protection when danger threatens.

Linked to this need for parental warmth and sensitivity is a requirement for parents to provide adequate consistent control and structure to the child's life. As the child gets older, so he will achieve greater autonomy, and parental capacity to allow the child independence in decision-making becomes important. The forms of reward and punishment (e.g. whether or not there is smacking or material rewards are given) are less important than the consistency of parental behaviour, agreement between parents, and maintenance of acceptance and responsiveness to the child's needs even when the child is being difficult. Children reared by authoritative parents who are nurturant, responsive, and able to reason with them, are less likely to show disturbance than children of authoritarian parents who are harsh and rigid in enforcing rules (Baumrind 1967).

Parental stimulation

The quality of verbal and non-verbal stimulation provided by parents has a significant influence on intellectual development and academic attainment. The amount that parents talk to their children may be less important than the degree to which they succeed in maintaining two-way conversation (Tizard and Hughes 1984). The availability of toys is probably less important than the degree to which the child, with parental help, can be encouraged to explore objects and spatial relationships in his natural environment. The availability of books in the home, and the degree to which parents are able to help their children learn to read by listening to their efforts are factors of importance in the speed with which skill in reading is acquired (Hewison and Tizard 1980). Parental stimulation of these various types will be more effective if it takes place in the context of a warm, loving relationship.

Parental mental illness

As in the rest of the adult population, mental health problems in parents are common. Mostly the disorders they experience are characterized by depression and anxiety, and are related to adverse social circumstances (poor marital relationships, inadequate housing, financial hardship, etc.). However, a significant number of parents show other disorders such as schizophrenia, alcoholism, and aggressive personality disorders. The impact of mental ill health in parents on children has been extensively studied (Rutter and Quinton 1984).

A significant number of parents involved in non-accidental injury or sexual abuse have mental health problems, although serious mental disorder is uncommon among them. All types of mental disorders are linked to a raised rate of behaviour and emotional problems in children. Children of parents with psychoses such as schizophrenia and manic-depressive psychosis are less prone to show such problems than children of parents with depressive and anxiety states, alcoholism, and personality disorders.

Except in the children of parents with schizophrenia and possibly major depressive disorder, genetic factors are probably of minor importance in the transmission of mental health problems; other mechanisms are probably of more relevance. Many forms of mental ill health directly impair the quality of parental care. In particular, a depressed mother is likely to be less responsive to the needs of her child, less able to provide consistent discipline, and less likely to initiate interaction (Weissman and Paykel 1974; Mills *et al.* 1984). Morbidly anxious mothers often transmit their anxieties to their children by example. For example, a mother who is frightened of lifts or of travelling on trains will often communicate fear of travelling to her children. Less usual forms of direct impact of illness occur when a child is involved in obsessional rituals or implicated in paranoid delusions.

Factors frequently associated with parental mental disorder are probably of greater importance than psychiatric symptoms themselves. It has been shown (Rutter and Quinton 1984) that childhood disturbance is more closely linked to parental marital discord and generally disharmonious marital relationships than to parental mental ill health. Parents with chronically aggressive personalities are particularly likely to have marital difficulties, so that their children are especially predisposed to develop behaviour and emotional problems themselves. Various processes are involved in the production of childhood disturbance in this situation:

• The child may imitate or identify with violent behaviour.
• Impulsive parents are likely to be inconsistent and frustrating to their children.
• Both parental separations and deprivation will occur frequently.
• Actual violence or threats of violence within the family will provoke anxiety.

All these factors will predispose the child to serious disturbance. Factors modifying the child's risk of developing disturbance if a parent has a psychiatric disorder include the mental health of the other parent, the quality of the relationship with the other parent, and the temperament of the child.

Parental physical illness

There is a slight but definite tendency for the children of parents with chronic physical ill health to have a raised rate of psychiatric problems. Such children may be involved in looking after the sick parent to a degree that isolates them from other children of their own age, and imposes responsibilities they are too immature to face. There may be poor communication within the family about the illness, so that the child is more uncertain and anxious about the future than is necessary. Alternatively, as is often the case, when the mother, for example, develops a condition such as breast cancer, the child may be completely shielded from information until an advanced stage of the disease has been reached. Finally, illness may cause or be associated with disturbed family relationships that are upsetting for the child.

Sib relationships

Until relatively recently sib relationships have been rather little studied. Such relationships may be ambivalent and marked by both strong positive protective feelings and a sense of rivalry. The reactions of older children to the birth of younger siblings depend, for example, on the temperament of the older child, on whether the younger child is of the same or different sex, on the behaviour of the mother with the new baby, and on the quality of the mother–older child relationship before the younger child is born (Dunn 1988).

Family social circumstances

The link between social adversity and the presence of psychological problems in children and adolescents is complicated, but recent work has done much to clarify them (Rutter and Smith 1995).

There is little connection between the material prosperity of a population and the levels of psychiatric disorder. For example, what evidence we have of rates of disorder in children living in large poverty-ridden cities such as Bombay and Calcutta does not suggest that rates of disorder are especially high there. Further, though prosperity increased in western nations in the 50 years after the Second World War, so did rates of conduct and possibly depressive disorder.

When one looks at individuals rather than populations, a very different picture emerges. Socially deprived children, those exposed to poverty, high rates of parental unemployment, homelessness, or crowded living conditions, do show high rates of disorders, especially conduct problems. This is particularly the case if social adversities are multiple (Kolvin *et al.* 1988). Thus overcrowded housing circumstances, parental unemployment, and financial hardship may, if present singly, not act as risk factors, but if present in combination as they often are, their negative effect may be considerable.

The social status of a family is usually assessed in population surveys according to the employment of the father or the main breadwinner in the home. Intelligence and educational attainment are related to social class assessed in this way, with children of professional and other middle-class parents performing better than the skilled working-class and much better than children with unskilled working-class parents. Behavioural and emotional disorders are, however, found to be only weakly related to these measures of social class (Rutter *et al.* 1970*a*).

About a third of UK and about a half of US mothers of pre-school children go out to work. Whether a mother works or not has a major influence on the life of her children (Graham 1990). However, there is little evidence that maternal employment is, in itself, a significant advantage or disadvantage for children as far as their behavioural or cognitive development is concerned. Of greater importance is the quality of substitute care available, and whether the mother feels comfortable and satisfied with her decision about work. The quality of mother–child attachment is closely related to whether a mother is satisfied with her employment status whatever decision about work she has made.

1.4 Classification and prevalence of psychiatric disorders

The grouping of cases according to their distinguishing features is called classification, and the defining characteristics of disorders are specified in classification systems such as the Diagnostic and Statistical Manual of Mental Disorders (DSM-IV; American Psychiatric Association 1994), or the International

Classification of Diseases (ICD-10; World Health Organization 1992). The DSM system is used particularly in the USA, whereas the ICD is used in much of the rest of the world. The USA is under treaty obligation to maintain a terminology which is compatible with the ICD. Therefore, the newest editions of both systems, the DSM-IV and the ICD-10, are compatible (Table 1.1).

Both systems allow the classification of different facets of a condition on five axes that differ somewhat between the two systems. The official ICD-10, which contains the essential core, does not describe multiple axes. However, it was designed in such a way that it is possible to put the section on psychiatric conditions in a multiaxial format (Rutter 1989). The official DSM-IV describes which areas of the child's functioning should be coded on each axis. There are axes for clinical psychiatric syndromes, developmental disorders, physical disorders, psychosocial and environmental problems, and the child's level of adaptive functioning. On each axis there must be a coding in all cases. There is also the provision of a 'no abnormality' code. Multiple codings per axis are allowed.

The greatest difference between the two systems is the way the diagnostic criteria are specified. The ICD employs descriptions of disorders supplemented by global guidelines that read like a clinical text and offers a comprehensive picture of the core clinical concept, whereas the DSM offers operationalized criteria that must be met before the diagnosis can be made. The ICD system uses a prototypical approach in which the clinician decides whether or not the child's problems fit the conceptual picture. This approach involves to some degree arbitrary decisions, but it should be realised that many of the DSM-IV diagnostic criteria have also been determined through arbitrary decisions.

The advantage of the use of classification systems is the comparability of an individual's problems with those diagnosed earlier by the same clinician or with those diagnosed by others. The coding of ICD or DSM axes also has the advantage that information can readily be stored and communicated. This can be

Table 1.1   Comparison of the ICD-10 and DSM-IV classifications

Axis no.	ICD-10 (modified)[a]	DSM-IV[b]
1	Behavioural and emotional disorders with onset usually occurring in childhood and adolescence	Clinical disorders
2	Developmental disorders	Personality disorders, Mental retardation
3	Intellectual level	General medical conditions
4	Medical condition	Psychosocial and environmental problems
5	Associated abnormal psychosocial situations	Global assessment of functioning

[a] Rutter (1989).
[b] American Psychiatric Association (1994).

useful for clinicians as well as for policy makers. However, as argued earlier, classification should be incorporated in the final diagnosis in the broader sense including possible aetiological, consequential, and background features in addition to the description of the disorder in ICD or DSM terms.

1.4.1 CLASSIFICATION OF PSYCHIATRIC SYNDROMES

In both the classifications mentioned above, the first axis concerns psychiatric disorders, and this is the axis most likely to be employed by physicians. Most disorders can be classified in the scheme shown in Table 1.2, an abbreviation of the two most relevant sections of ICD-10. Each of these categories has, to some degree, been validated, i.e. there is evidence available that the type of disorder mentioned has a characteristic presentation, aetiology, and course.

Table 1.2   Abbreviated ICD-10 classification

F90–99		*Behavioural and emotional disorders with onset usually occurring in childhood or adolescence (abbreviated)*
F90		Hyperkinetic disorder
	.0	Disorder of activity and attention
	.1	Hyperkinetic conduct disorder
F91		Conduct disorders
	.0	Conduct disorder confined to the family context
	.1	Unsocialized conduct disorder
	.2	Socialized conduct disorder
	.3	Oppositional defiant disorder
F92		Mixed disorders of conduct and emotions
	.0	Depressive conduct disorder
F93		Emotional disorders with onset specific to childhood
	.0	Separation anxiety disorder
	.1	Phobic disorder of childhood
	.2	Social sensitivity disorder
	.3	Sibling rivalry disorder
F94		Disorders of social functioning with onset specific to childhood or adolescence
	.0	Elective mutism
	.1	Reactive attachment disorder of childhood
	.2	Disinhibition attachment disorder of childhood
F95		Tic disorders
	.0	Transient tic disorder
	.1	Chronic motor or vocal tic disorder
	.2	Combined vocal and multiple motor tic (Tourette syndrome)
F98		Other emotional and behavioural disorders with onset usually occurring during childhood
	.0	Enuresis
	.1	Encopresis
	.2	Feeding disorder of infancy or childhood
	.3	Pica

.4   Stereotyped movement disorder
.5   Stuttering
.6   Cluttering

F80–89   *Developmental disorders (abbreviated)*
F80   Specific developmental disorders of speech and language
.0   Specific speech articulation disorder
.1   Expressive language disorder
.2   Receptive language disorder
.3   Acquired aphasia with epilepsy
F81   Specific developmental disorders of scholastic skills
.0   Specific reading disorder
.1   Specific spelling disorder
.2   Specific disorder of arithmetical skills
.3   Mixed disorder of scholastic skills
F82   Specific developmental disorders of motor function
F83   Mixed specific developmental disorders
F84   Pervasive developmental disorders
.0   Childhood autism
.1   Atypical autism
.2   Rett syndrome
.3   Other childhood disintegrative disorders
.4   Overactive disorder associated with mental retardation and stereotyped
     movements
.5   Asperger syndrome

1.4.2 DRAWBACKS OF EXISTING CLASSIFICATION SCHEMES

There are various problems with the existing schemes which make them less than satisfactory (Graham 1982) and indeed discourage some practitioners from using them at all.

- They necessarily involve a judgement of the nature of the problem 'within the child'. For many practitioners the essential nature of the disturbance is usually seen elsewhere—within the family, or within the interaction between the child and family members, or the child and wider society.
- The existing diagnostic categories, although reasonably well validated, provide only a very rough guide to aetiology, treatment, and prognosis. They generally need to be amplified by a formulation giving a more extended account of the child's condition and background features before action can be taken.
- Many of the situations of psychiatric concern with which family practitioners and paediatricians quite frequently deal cannot readily be categorized within this classification system. Non-accidental injury and monosymptomatic abdominal pain of psychogenic or uncertain origin are examples.
- The positioning of some of the categories is occasionally arbitrary and might be misleading. For example, the introductory section to Developmental Disorders in ICD-10 defines such disorders in terms of their early onset, delay in functions strongly related to biological maturation, and steady course; yet

enuresis, which often fills all these criteria, is classified as a behavioural or emotional disorder. The problem is that some symptoms, like enuresis and perhaps hyperactivity, may occur either as developmental disorders or as signs of emotional disorder, and consequently their place in the classification is inevitably somewhat arbitrary.

Nevertheless, the framework of these new classification systems in child psychiatry does represent a real advance on previous attempts, and the organization of much of this book is based upon them.

1.4.3 PREVALENCE OF PSYCHIATRIC DISORDERS

Epidemiology is the study of disorders in populations, rather than in individuals. Information about the *incidence* (number of new cases) and *prevalence* (number of cases in the population over a defined period of time) of child psychiatric disorders has accumulated rapidly over the last three decades. Prevalence studies can provide helpful information on the need for services. Epidemiological studies of background factors and of rates of disorder in different population groups can point to possible causes of disorders and thus make rational prevention more feasible.

The design and methods used in an early study of the prevalence of disorders on the Isle of Wight has set the pattern for a large number of subsequent studies carried out in different parts of the world (Rutter *et al.* 1970a; Rutter 1989). The entire population of 10 and 11 year olds was screened using teacher and parent behaviour questionnaires. On the basis of their scores on the questionnaires, children were selected as at risk for psychiatric disorder, and they, together with a control group, were seen for individual semi-structured interviews and psychological testing. Parents and teachers were also interviewed.

An overview of 49 studies, involving over 240 000 children in many different countries, in which the prevalence of the overall level of psychiatric disorder had been determined, revealed that the median prevalence over a period of a year was 12.3% (Verhulst 1995). Different researchers use different methods to calculate rates of disorder. Those who calculate simply on the basis of symptom frequency arrive at much higher rates, sometimes as high as 49% (Bird *et al.* 1988), than those who only consider disorder is present if there is a significant degree of social impairment present, where the figure arrived at in a Dutch national sample (7.9%) is much more typical (Verhulst *et al.* 1997).

Information about the background factors and prevalence of different disorders is provided below in the relevant sections. In this section we will limit discussion to factors related to overall prevalence.

Age

Measuring the rate of disorders in babies and infants is problematic, though attempts have been made at classification (National Center for clinical Infant Programs 1994). Around 10–15% of older pre-school children show significant psychiatric disorders (Campbell 1995). Rates remain relatively steady during the rest of childhood and adolescence, although there are some suggestions of a rise during adolescence. However, the types of disorder found vary considerably during this age period. So-called *externalizing disorders* (those characterized by aggressive and other types of antisocial disorder such as stealing, truancy, and lying) are stable during childhood and then decline after early adolescence, while so-called *internalizing disorders* (those involving especially depression and anxiety) rise slowly during childhood but much more sharply during and after puberty (Crijnen *et al.* 1997).

Social factors

Using a relatively weak indicator of social advantage and disadvantage, such as social class measured by parental occupation, there is only a slight association with overall prevalence. However, with stronger measures of social variables including parental education, income and housing conditions, the associations become much greater. This is particularly the case for conduct disorders, and is much less marked for internalizing disorders.

Gender

Prepubertal boys are much more frequently referred to child psychiatric clinics than are girls, and this occurs because of their much higher rate of conduct disorders. In contrast, during adolescence the proportion of girls referred increases because of their greater tendency to develop depressive and anxiety disorders.

Urbanization

Early studies reported higher overall rates of disorder in children living in cities than those living in rural areas (Rutter *et al.* 1975). These findings have been generally confirmed (e.g. by Offord *et al.* 1987), but have not been universally found (Achenbach *et al.* 1991). They are thought to be related to the increased stress involved in city living, with higher levels of social and family disorganization.

Ethnicity

Great caution has to be exercised in comparing rates of disorder in different ethnic groups. Concepts of unacceptable behaviour and ways of showing distress may vary from group to group. In general, few differences have been found between ethnic groups (Achenbach *et al.* 1991; Bird *et al.* 1989; Earls and Richman 1980), although in the UK, rates may be somewhat lower in Asian minorities (Kallarackal and Herbert 1976). This does not mean that referral rates are similar. For example, it is common for referred children to come much less frequently from minority than majority indigenous groups. A Muslim father is more likely to consult an Islamic priest than a mental health professional if his child is showing problems.

Migrant groups

Immigrant children are often under special stress, because of disruption to family ties, racism, and other stresses. On the other hand, community support and family cohesion is often greater in these groups. Some studies have shown higher rates of overall disorder in these groups. A study of Turkish migrant children living in the Netherlands (Bengi-Arslan *et al.* 1997) revealed somewhat higher rates of parent-rated disorder than in the indigenous population. This might have been a reflection of higher standards of behaviour in the migrant parents, or a true difference in prevalence.

Secular trends

It is widely believed that rates of psychiatric disorder in children and young people increased considerably in the second half of the twentieth century. The evidence for changes over time in rates of different disorders in European countries has been reviewed by Rutter and Smith (1995), and there is indeed evidence for an increase in some disorders such as depression and conduct disorder, although the changes are not nearly as dramatic as some have suggested. Indeed, some have not found any changes at all. A study in the Netherlands using exactly the same methods 10 years apart in samples of 4–16 year old children found very small and inconsistent changes over this period (Verhulst *et al.* 1997). On the other hand, a study of changes in prevalence of disorder in an area of Khartoum, Sudan, that underwent rapid urbanization, found quite a marked reduction in problem-free children (Cederblad and Rahmin 1986).

Family circumstances

Unsurprisingly, family circumstances are strongly associated with overall rates of child psychiatric disorder. Disharmonious family relationships are those most significantly linked, and the fact that rates of disorder are higher in children from families broken by separation and divorce, and not higher in families broken by parental death, is a reflection of this fact. There are various other family risk factors (variables that increase vulnerability to disorder). These include physical and mental illness in one or both parents or in a sibling. Child rearing practices that involve inconsistent or harsh physical punishment, critical or hostile attitudes of parents towards their children, lack of affection, and poor parental supervision also increase overall risk of disorder.

Factors within the child

Different disorders vary in which personal factors increase the risk of occurrence, and this issue is discussed in the relevant sections. However, genetic vulnerability, often shown in the early years by adverse temperamental characteristics, is often relevant. Chronic physical disability (especially if this arises from brain dysfunction) and educational failure are other risk factors. Intelligence is also of relevance with brighter children showing lower rates of overall disorder at all levels. Children with mild mental retardation have a slightly raised risk of disorder, but those with severe retardation have much higher rates.

Life events

Life events that have an adverse impact on a child's life generally increase the risk of disorder, so that groups of children living in disadvantaged circumstances may be expected to have higher rates (Goodyer 1990). High rates of loss of or separation from loved relatives, friends, or pets—as occurs in areas plagued by armed conflict—will increase overall rates of disorder.

1.5 Assessment and diagnosis of psychiatric disorders

Although the specialized skills of a child and adolescent psychiatrist are necessary for complex problems, most appraisals of behaviour and emotional disorders are carried out by non-psychiatrists—family practitioners, nurses, psychologists, social workers, and other professional groups. This section aims to provide guidance to all professionals carrying out such assessments.

The aims of a psychiatric assessment of a child with a psychosocial problem or with physical symptoms having psychosocial implications are to:

- appraise the nature and severity of the problem
- identify likely causes, be they social, familial, individual, physical, or, as is commonly the case, a combination of these
- plan with the child and family members a form of effective treatment and management.

Most psychiatric appraisal occurs because a family wants help with a problem in their child. However, increasingly psychiatrists and other professionals are requested to undertake assessments for other reasons, for example as part of a statement of a child's special educational needs, to assist a juvenile court in coming to a decision concerning a child charged with an offence, or as part of a child protection investigation.

A secondary but important set of aims relates to the need to communicate sympathy and support for the child and other family members, to convey an understanding of their problems, and to provide for them some meaning and significance to their predicament.

Finally, for administrative purposes, the clinician increasingly needs to make a diagnosis using a recognized multiaxial classificatory system such as ICD-10 (World Health Organization 1992) or DSM-IV (American Psychiatric Association 1994).

1.5.1 FACTORS INFLUENCING THE ASSESSMENT PROCEDURE

Patterns of psychological development are assessed in a wide variety of situations, and different settings call for different forms of assessment. There are, however, general principles that should guide assessment regardless of setting.

The form of assessment will be influenced by the following factors:

- The physical resources available space, privacy, equipment (e.g. to test sight and hearing).
- The time available to the clinician.
- The expectations of the person or people who initiated the contact. In primary care this is usually one or both parents. In secondary care any one of a number of agencies may refer and each will have different expectations.

- The composition of the group that attends. In primary care usually only mother and child attend. In a psychiatric setting the whole family is likely to be involved.
- The motivation of those who attend. The group may vary in motivation—parents, for example, being highly motivated, a child negative towards attendance. Some families only come because they are sent by other agencies.
- The nature of the problem. Clearly some presenting problems will be more complex and require more intensive assessment than others.
- The skill and orientation of the clinician.
- The follow-up and treatment facilities available. If, for example, the type of treatment available is limited, for example, to brief counselling and/or medication, then assessment will need to be modified accordingly.

1.5.2 GENERAL PRINCIPLES OF ASSESSMENT

Physical setting

Ideally the room in which a child is seen should be big enough to take both parents, the referred child, and at least a couple of sibs. The clinician will achieve greater rapport if he does not sit behind a desk, but beside or away from it. Equipment should be available to carry out a physical examination, to test hearing and vision, etc. There should be a supply of drawing paper and coloured pencils available. Useful toys include three or four jigsaws of varying levels of difficulty, a post-box with different shapes, a set of small family dolls, and a set of farm animals. Toys available should be robust and carefully looked after. It is also useful to have three or four books of graded difficulty to check the child's reading level. It is an advantage if all these can be kept in a cupboard or drawer so that they can be brought out as required.

Preparing the referral

In primary care or a busy paediatric clinic, little or no preparation is likely to be possible. However, the staff of a child psychiatric team may achieve a more satisfactory assessment if careful preparation is undertaken. The letter to the family should make it clear that it is highly desirable for both parents to attend and that it is often helpful for sibs also to be present at the initial interview. Obtaining permission to request a school report prior to the assessment has the advantage that the clinician will then have most relevant information available by the end of the first interview. If the assessment is to take place under unusual conditions, for example with the use of a one-way screen or video equipment, or if it is intended that students should be present at the interview, then again the family should be warned beforehand.

Initial greeting

Whatever the setting, the clinician should first introduce himself if he has not met the family before. It is usually advisable to see together all family members who have attended in the first instance. This might be just the mother and child, or both parents and four or five children. A clinician may prefer to see a referred adolescent before other members of the family, especially if he has prior knowledge that the teenager is resentful about the referral. In general, however, at least a brief interview with the whole family or all those members who have attended is desirable. An initial step should involve asking the children how they would like to be addressed. The question 'What do you like to be called?', if the child's first name has a common abbreviation, often reduces initial tension and anxiety. The clinician should make sure he introduces anyone else in the room and explains what they are doing there. If, as is the case in some psychiatric facilities, a one-way screen is used, the family should be introduced to those behind it, and reassurance concerning confidentiality should be given.

1.5.3 APPROACHES TO ASSESSMENT

For an assessment in primary or specialist care, the mother and child may be the only informants who are easily accessible. A very considerable amount of information can be gathered from them, enabling the clinician to make a formulation of the problem and intervene usefully. However, for more complex and intractable problems seen in specialist child psychiatry clinics, information gathering will need to be much more extensive. In these circumstances, parents, children themselves and teachers will be the main sources of information (Achenbach and McConaughy 1997). In the following sections an approach suitable for use in specialist centres by psychiatrists and psychologists will be provided. The primary care clinician or paediatrician will need to extract from this comprehensive account the elements that are most relevant to his or her own setting, and some guidance is provided for this purpose in the text.

Interviews with parents

This can be divided into four parts: an exploration of the presenting problem, a developmental history, a biography of family members and an account of the structure and function of the family, and an account of the current functioning of the child in areas not covered in the exploration of the presenting problem.

- *Exploration of the presenting problem.* The following are likely to be relevant:
  — What is the reason for referral?
  — Whose idea was it to seek help?
  — What do the parents expect from professional help?
  — What is the nature and severity of the presenting problem?
  — What is the effect of the problem on the child's functioning at school, in the family, and on the child's relationship with other children?
  — How have others reacted to the child's problem?
  — What has been the course of the problem over time?
  — What do the parents think are likely causes of the problem, and what makes it better or worse?
  — What have the parents done already to improve the situation?
  — Have the child and family received professional help previously?

- *The developmental history.* In primary care, many clinicians will already be aware of many of the aspects covered here because of previous contacts with the family. In specialist care, this will not be the case, and the following will need to be enquired about:
  - Pregnancy/delivery. Pregnancy complications, the mother's physical and mental health, consumption of alcohol, drugs, prescribed medication. Delivery complications, birth weight, gestation, need for special care. Family stress at the time.
  - First months. Parent–child relationship, temperamental characteristics of the young child, family stress.
  - Motor development. Delay in walking, co-ordination problems with spoon and fork, doing up buttons, etc.
  - Language/speech development. Delay in first words, putting words together.
  - Attachment and relationships. Reactions following separations; relationships with parents, siblings, other adults and peers; substitute care.
  - Toilet training.
  - Schooling history. Educational achievement, behaviour problems in school; school refusal; changes of school.
  - Life events. Illnesses, injuries, hospitalizations of child or other family member. Death or divorce of care giver. Other changes in family composition.
- *Family structure and function*
  - Family structure and history. Parents: ages, occupations, current physical and emotional state, history of mental or physical disorder, former marriages or cohabitations and children of these relationships, whereabouts of grandparents. Sibs, full, step or half: ages, presence of problems. Home circumstances, sleeping arrangements.
  - Relationships. Parent–child relationship; level of criticism, hostility, rejection. What kinds of punishments? Safety and supervision provided by parents. Parental supervision. Parental relationship. Mutual affection. Capacity to communicate and resolve problems. Sharing of attitude over child's problems. Sharing of responsibilities.
  - Overall patterns of family relationships. Alliances, communication. Exclusions, scapegoating. Intergenerational confusion.
- *Current functioning of child*
  - Physical functioning. Headaches, stomach aches. Chronic conditions. Handicaps. Hearing, vision. Fits, faints, other type of attacks.
  - School. Type of school. Grade. Attainments. Learning/behaviour problems, including problems with concentration. Homework. Relationship with teacher.
  - Current level of development. Language/speech: comprehension, complexity, grammar, articulation, stammering or stuttering, speech idiosyncrasies, stereotypes or repetitive use of language. Motor functioning: motor co-ordination, clumsiness. Cognitive functioning: comprehension, memory.

- Attention/concentration. Attention span. Concentration. Distractibility. Perseverance.
- Eating, sleeping, elimination problems. Weight gain. (Self induced) weight loss. Appetite. Binge eating. Rumination. Sleeping problems. Nightmares/terrors. Sleepwalking. Daytime drowsiness. Enuresis. Encopresis.
- Activity level. Overactivity. Impulsivity. Fidgeting. Underactivity.
- Behaviour. Oppositional and antisocial behaviours: aggression, disobedience, stealing, fighting, firesetting, truancy, lying, vandalism, temper tantrums, cruelty.
- Habits: nail biting, thumb sucking, tics, head banging, hair pulling, autoerotic behaviours.
- Compulsions.
- Reaction to frustrations.
- Mood. Sadness. Depression. Suicidal feelings. Worries. Crying. Anxiety. Specific fears. Nervousness. Feeling worthless.
- Relationships. Relationship with parents: affection shown, mutual enjoyment, communication, reaction to separation, dependence/independence. Relationship with siblings. Relationship with peers: quality of relationships, how many friends, special friends, bullied by other children.
- Sexual interests and behaviour.

Obtaining factual information from parents and children
There are various approaches to obtaining factual information. Most practitioners use an informal style of questioning, aiming to cover a number of areas systematically, but concentrating on particular issues likely to be relevant to the child in question. Such semi-structured interviewing (Bird and Kestenbaum 1988) has the advantage that it is flexible and allows the clinician to adopt a conversational approach. However, psychiatrists and psychologists are increasingly using a variety of more standardized questionnaires for this purpose (Orvaschel 1988). Such questionnaires as the Diagnostic Interview Schedule for Children (Shaffer *et al.* 1993) provide generally reliable information, but suffer the disadvantage that they may be perceived by the family as more mechanical and less tailored to their own needs. Highly structured interviews are more suitable for research than for clinical purposes, and, at this stage, it seems sensible for most professionals to use a more informal assessment but ensure that all relevant areas are covered.

Some experienced psychiatrists and psychotherapists hardly structure assessment interviewing at all and rely almost entirely on the spontaneous expressions of the family members. They are concerned that, if the clinician structures the interview, family members will be inhibited from expressing feelings. There is, however, evidence that semi-structured interviewing need not place constraints on emotional expression and ensures more reliable gathering of factual information (Cox *et al.* 1981). Such an informal approach can begin by listening to the spontaneous complaints and other information provided by family members, and then by asking direct questions. Open-ended questions, for example 'In what ways have you tried to deal with his ...?' produce more information than closed questions answerable with a yes/no, for example. 'Have you tried rewarding him for good behaviour?' It is never a good idea to submit a parent or child to a barrage of questioning without leaving a significant amount of time for the spontaneous expression of anxiety. In obtaining information about particular symptoms or problems, it is important to obtain an idea of the frequency of their occurrence, the details of what actually happened, provoking events, and the behaviour of parents and others that seem to make it better or worse. It is wise to concentrate on recent examples of the behaviour in question. Problematic behaviour is often situation-specific, i.e. it occurs in some settings and not in others. This often gives clues to effective management, so it is important to obtain as full information as possible.

Eliciting feelings and attitudes from parents

Often parents' feelings and attitudes are the crucial variables in assessment. Positive feelings (such as warmth, tolerance, acceptance) and negative feelings (such as criticism, hostility, and rejection) may be elicited by appropriate questioning, by suggesting the presence of feeling states and observing parental reactions, and by reinforcing expressions of feeling when these occur. One can ask questions such as 'How does that make you feel? Do you feel that gets on your nerves?' Suggestions such as 'That must make you feel very angry?' or 'It sounds as though you quite enjoy it when he does that sort of thing?' sometimes elicit strong emotional responses. Showing interest and sympathy when emotion is spontaneously expressed may have a similar effect.

Building family confidence

Parents who bring a child to a family practitioner, paediatrician, or psychiatrist for a psychosocial or psychosomatic problem not infrequently suffer from a deep sense of failure at what they imagine to be their own incompetence in dealing with the problem themselves. It is therefore particularly important to avoid conveying a critical attitude, and to take every opportunity to comment on the positive coping behaviour the parents are showing. One should assume, and in the great majority of cases this assumption is correct, that parents are doing their very best for their children. *An assessment interview should be perceived by parents as a supportive, not an undermining experience.*

Interview with the child

Adolescents should always be seen separately at some point; so should children from about 6 or 7 years to puberty if time permits. It is usually not desirable to attempt to see children younger than this without their parents.

An entirely verbal approach can be used in an individual interview with older children and adolescents. After setting the child at ease, for example by talking about leisure activities and favourite television programmes, the interviewer can go on to broach the presenting problem and the child's view of its occurrence. Questioning can then go on to more general anxieties, depression of mood, suicidal thoughts and feelings, etc. 'I see a lot of children who get worried and anxious about things. What sort of things do you feel anxious about?' 'What sort of things make you angry at school?' 'What sort of things get you upset at home?' 'A lot of boys/girls I see worry something terrible is going to happen to their mum. Do you ever feel like that?' are all useful probes. Very unresponsive or mute children can be reassured—'I see a lot of children who have difficulty talking. I wonder why it is hard for you. It could be because you are feeling angry, or mixed up ... or just because you can't think of anything to say?' If the child has come because of some misdemeanour, the clinician should avoid either condemnation or approval, but try to find out about the circumstances in which the wrongdoing occurred and the child's feelings about it in a morally neutral way. The interviewer should conclude by asking the child what else he or she would like to talk about.

For younger children, the supply of toys described above, especially family figures and farm animals, may well be a more effective trigger to elicit informative fantasies or anxieties the child may be experiencing. Many children of 6–10 years can, however, communicate well verbally without the use of toys and drawings.

Interviews with adolescents may need to include a number of topics not covered with younger children. Sexual concepts and behaviour and the possible use of drugs are examples. Adolescents may also be expected to elaborate to a greater degree than younger children on their mood states, relationships with peers, and special interests.

Before concluding any interview with a child alone, if it is thought desirable to raise any of the matters the child has discussed with the parents, then the child's agreement should be sought beforehand. If the child refuses (a rare event), then this should be respected unless the child would be put in danger as a result. The clinician may, however, say to parents that the child has expressed some private anxieties he would prefer not to communicate to them, and stress the normality of children sometimes having private thoughts they do not want parents to know about.

The following areas should be covered in a full assessment:

- *School*. What school do you go to? What year? What do you like best/least in school? Can you get along with your teacher? Which teacher do you like best/least? What grades do you get? What about homework? Does anyone help you with your homework? Do you have trouble paying attention? Do you have difficulty finishing tasks? Any subjects you have trouble with? Any special help? Do you get in trouble in school? Do you skip classes? If you could change something about school, what would you want to change?
- *Activities*. What do you do in your spare time, such as hobbies, sports, clubs? What do you do when you are alone? What is your favourite TV programme, music?
- *Friends*. How many friends do you have (give me their names)? Do you think that is enough or would you like to have more friends? Do you know them from school or from elsewhere? How old are they? How long have you been friends? What do you do with your friends? Do they come to your house or

do you go to their house? Do you have a special friend? Is there someone you don't like? Do you have troubles getting along with other children? What kind of problems? Do you get into fights? With whom? What usually starts the fights? Do you get teased? By whom? Do you ever feel left out? (If child reports problems with peers, ask child what he/she has done about it). If you could change something about your friends, what would you want to change?

- *Family.* Who lives in your home? Do you have a separate room? What happens when you do something you are not allowed to? Do you think the rules in your home are fair or unfair? What kind of punishments are there in your home? Who punishes you? What do you like to do with your mum/dad? What do you like your mum/dad to do for you? When you are away from home (staying with a friend overnight), how do you feel? How do your parents get along? Do they have arguments? What about? How do you feel when they argue? Who do you like best/least in your family? If you could change something in your family, what would you want to change?

- *Feelings.* What makes you scared/sad/lonely/angry? How often do you feel scared/sad/lonely/angry? When are you scared/sad/lonely/angry? Sometimes children worry about things they have done or things that might happen; what do you worry about? How do you feel most of the time? What sort of things make you have these feelings?

  Children sometimes think life is hopeless. Do you ever think that ... or that life is not worth living ... or about harming yourself? Do you think about harming yourself? Or even killing yourself? Have you ever tried to harm/kill yourself? (These questions should be asked in this sequence, stopping when the child answers with a negative.)

- *Self perception.* Tell me a little about yourself. What do you like most/least about yourself? If I asked your best friend to describe you; how would she/he describe you? What makes you proud about yourself? What makes your parents feel proud about you? If you could change something about yourself, what would it be?

- *Strange thoughts/experiences.* Do you ever have thoughts that other people would think are strange? Have you had experiences or things happened that you did not understand? Do you ever hear sounds or voices/see things that other people think are not there? Do you ever do things other people think are strange?

- *Physical complaints.* Do you have trouble falling asleep/waking too early? Do you have trouble eating/losing weight/ maintaining weight? Binge eating? Aches (headache, stomach ache), nausea, vomiting, dizziness, heartpounding, numbness, tingling. Tired? Bedwetting? Daytime wetting? Soiling? Other physical problems?

- *Antisocial behaviour.* Do you break rules; do things other people think you should not do such as stealing, fighting, running away from home, skipping classes, firesetting? If yes, do you do these things alone, or with others? Have you been in trouble with the police or law?

- *Alcohol/drugs.* Do you drink beer, wine or spirits? If yes, how often? Have you been drunk? Or stoned/high on drugs? Have you had a strong urge for more drugs? Do you think drinking/taking drugs is a problem? Do other people think that your drinking/taking drugs is a problem?

- *Stress.* Did any event happen that was very upsetting for you? Tell me about it. What happened? When? How old were you? What happened to you afterwards?
- *Fantasies.* If you had three wishes, what would you wish? What would you like to be when you are older? If you could read the future, how would you like things to be when you are older?
- *Screening tasks.*
  — Gross motor screening: catch ball, hop on one foot, show hand (right and left).
  — Fine motor screening: writing sample, drawing, making jigsaw, building blocks, using scissors.
  — Mathematics/reading: if possible, use standardized reading/math tests.

General
A great deal may be learned from observing the child during the interview. The following is a scheme that can be used for classifying such observations.

- *General appearance.* Signs of dysmorphism. Nutritional state. Evidence of neglect/abuse.
- *Level of awareness.* Orientation. Vigilance. Evidence of minor epilepsy. Memory.
- *Somatic complaints.* Somatic complaints during interview such as dizziness, headaches. Conversion. Developmental functions.
- *Motor functioning.* Gross motor difficulties, clumsiness. Fine motor difficulties or other unusual movements (stereotypes, mannerisms). Tics. Tremors. Mouth movements.
- *Language.* Difficulties understanding language. Difficulty expressing self verbally, including stuttering. Unusual or bizarre language, including echolalia, neologisms, babbling, nonsense words.
- *Thought.* Problems remembering facts. Intelligence. Concrete thinking. Disorganized thinking. Perseveration. Slow of thought. Flight of ideas. Abnormal thought. Delusions. Obsessions. Preoccupations. Limited fantasy or imagination. Poor reality testing. Daydreaming.
- *Perception.* Hallucinations. Illusions. Derealization. Depersonalization.
- *Attention.* Problems with concentration, paying attention. Easily distracted. Lapses in attention.
- *Activity.* Overactive. Fidgeting. Moves around. Underactive.
- *Impulsivity.* Impulsive. Impatient. Acts without thinking.
- *Interaction.* Overly anxious to please. Seductive. Inappropriate behaviour. Testing the limits. Shy. Withdrawn. Reluctant to talk. Overly dependent. Manipulative. Overly dramatic. Disinhibited. Lack of social reciprocity. Avoids eye contact. Resistance to comply. Interaction with parents. Ease of separation. Affection shown.

- *Mood and feelings.* Unhappy, sad, or depressed. Worries. Cries. Apathetic. Angry. Nervous. Sudden changes in mood. Fears. Anxiety. Flat affect. Feels guilty.
- *General behaviour.* Acts too young for age. Unmotivated. Verbal aggression. Physical aggression. Irresponsible behaviour. Stubborn. Unpredicted behaviour. Behaves like opposite sex. Repetitive behaviours (e.g. compulsions, rocking, hand flapping). Habits (e.g. nail biting, hair pulling, nose picking).

Information from teachers

Teachers can provide information on the child's achievements, the behaviour in the classroom and playground, the relationship of the child with other children and with teachers. Information can be obtained by letter or telephone and/or by sending a questionnaire. An easy-to-complete behaviour questionnaire such as the Rutter B Scale (Rutter 1967) can be sent, with some additional questions concerning the child's educational achievement and any other matters the teacher thinks worthy of comment.

Standardized interviews and questionnaires

Standardized interviews and questionnaires have been used in research studies for many years, and are now increasingly employed in specialist clinical practice. They have the advantage of greater reliability than less structured methods, and they can be administered by less skilled staff. However, they do not allow rapport to develop between clinician and client, and their use may mean important information is missed because the child has an unusual problem outside the scope of the interview or questionnaire.

In contrast to standardized interviews, questionnaires are not designed to replace the diagnostic process but can serve a valuable purpose. For example, they can be sent to parents, teachers, or young people themselves before the first appointment. If returned in advance, the information can be processed and used during the initial contact. This can result in saving valuable time. Examples of useful questionnaires that have been well standardized on normal populations include the Child Behavior Checklist (CBCL) (Achenbach 1991*a*), the Teacher Report Form (TRF, Achenbach 1991*b*), the Youth Self-Report Form (YSR, Achenbach 1991*c*), the Rutter Parent Behaviour Checklist (Rutter *et al.* 1970*a*), the Rutter Teacher Behaviour Checklist (Rutter 1967), and the Richman Pre-School Behaviour Checklist (Richman 1977).

Physical examination and investigation

Children with physical symptoms will always require a physical examination to identify organic disease. General practitioners and paediatricians would naturally carry out such an examination themselves. Psychiatrists vary in whether they carry out physical examinations or refer to others for this purpose. Most psychiatrists would feel it desirable to examine the child themselves on at least some occasions, though not necessarily to check all bodily systems.

A screening neurological examination alone can, for example, both rule out significant neurological disorder and identify developmental delays in motor co-ordination, visual perception, etc. The assessment may reveal the need for physical tests including blood count, urinalysis, plasma chemistry, skull radiography, electroencephalography (EEG), brain scan, or magnetic resonance imaging (MRI).

1.5.4 DIAGNOSIS

With the information obtained during the assessment, the clinician may be, and in many cases will be in a position to organize the information to classify the behaviour and emotional problems the child is showing is to make a diagnosis.

To do this there are two main approaches: the *clinical–diagnostic* and the *empirical–quantitative* approach. Traditional clinical–diagnostic systems such as the DSM (American Psychiatric Association 1994) and the ICD (World Health Organization 1992) employ criteria for disorders that are the result of consensus through negotiations among panels of experts. This approach can be characterized as working from the 'top down', because it starts from decisions about which disorders should be included and about the criteria for defining such disorders (Verhulst and Achenbach 1995). In this way, disorders reflect current clinical practice and are defined by a rather arbitrary set of criteria. The assessment strategy that is typically followed to derive DSM or ICD diagnoses is the clinical interview, either unstandardized or in standardized forms.

In contrast, the empirical–quantitative approach, which is derived from psychometric concepts, uses quantitative procedures to determine empirically which characteristics tend to co-occur to form syndromes. The empirical approach works from the 'ground up', because it starts with large numbers of items that describe a broad range of behavioural/emotional problems that are scored for large samples of subjects. Multivariate statistical procedures are used to identify which problem items go together to form syndromes.

The assessment strategy that is typically followed to obtain quantitative scores for the empirically derived syndromes are standardized rating scales such as the CBCL and related instruments. Rating scales have the advantage that normative data can be readily made available, and that decisions on the number and severity of problems which should be regarded deviant, are based on actual distributions of scores in populations rather than an arbitrary number of criteria.

The mere fact that the two approaches as described above exist together shows that neither of them fully satisfies the numerous questions with regard to assessment and diagnosis of child and adolescent psychopathology. The combination of both diagnostic paradigms may be valuable if they compensate for the weaknesses and augment the strengths for each approach (Kasius *et al.* 1997). The clinician will probably find it most helpful to use the clinical diagnostic approach, whereas for research purposes a combination of the two approaches will often be desirable.

1.5.5 FORMULATION

Following an assessment along these lines, the clinician is in a position to formulate the problem. A formulation should consist of a statement of the main presenting features, a diagnosis, an indication of probable causes, an opinion concerning desirable management, and a view on outcome. An example of a formulation might be as follows.

John is a 9 year-old boy who has been refusing to go to school for reasons of anxiety for the past month. He is also enuretic. The underlying problem is an over-close relationship with his mother, with father often away at work. A viral infection may have acted as precipitant. The diagnosis is school refusal. Family counselling sessions with a rapid but planned return to school are indicated. The outlook for return to school is good, but he will probably remain an anxious boy.

Ideally such a formulation should be written down, but, in primary care, if time does not permit this, the clinician will nevertheless find it helpful at least to establish a formulation in his own mind before proceeding further.

1.6 Psychological assessment

By convention, the emotional and behavioural disorders of childhood and adolescence are referred to as psychiatric disorders. This does not mean that one has to be a psychiatrist to assess and treat them. Indeed, most psychiatric disorders are dealt with by mental health professionals who are not psychiatrists, such as psychologists, and by other professionals such as paediatricians, family doctors, child health nurses, teachers, and social workers. These professionals also deal with other types of problems or disorders, including learning difficulties and both general and specific intellectual or cognitive deficits. The terminology used to describe these is confusing. But for most professionals it is only necessary to grasp that there are three types of psychological or psychiatric problem with which they may be faced:

- emotional and behaviour problems
- specific learning difficulties, as well as specific deviations, delays or deficits in psychological development
- mental retardation or general learning difficulties.

Broadly speaking, psychiatric assessment relates to the first of these and psychological assessment to the second and third.

Most psychological assessment arises from a need to examine whether a child or adolescent has a learning or educational problem. If assessment reveals that such a problem exists, the next task is to establish its nature. This accomplished, there is a need to find out what is causing the problem. The cause may lie in the way the child is being brought up at home or taught at school. Alternatively, the cause may lie in a deficit in an underlying psychological function or functions.

Such deficits may be found, for example, in the fields of memory, attention, visuospatial awareness, visuomotor development or so-called executive function, in which the capacity to integrate and control activity is impaired. The somewhat different roles of educational and clinical psychologists are described in Chapter 10, but it is worth noting here that, very generally, the educational psychologist is likely to focus most on the child's performance in school, the reasons for any difficulties there and the identification of appropriate remedial measures. The clinical psychologist is more likely to attempt to identify strengths and deficits in specific psychological functions, both with problems picked up in school and with those occurring in other settings and associated with other psychiatric and medical disorders. There is, in fact, considerable overlap in the work of these two professional disciplines, and the greatest differences are not in what they do, but in the context in which they carry out their work.

Both types of psychologist will use a range of assessment and remedial or treatment techniques, including naturalistic observation and structured as well as semi-structured or unstructured interviews. Both may also use psychological tests, and, as these are specific to psychological investigation, they will be described in more detail.

It should be emphasized that the administration of standardized psychological tests, if carried out at all, is only part of the appraisal of the nature and severity of the problem. Usually, more time is spent, for example, by educational psychologists in working directly with teachers, in setting up individualized targets for children to achieve, in devising interventions to help them achieve these targets, and in monitoring the effect of the interventions on the individual child (Leach 1980). Nevertheless, tests continue to have a valuable place in the psychologist's repertoire. They are helpful in monitoring progress or deterioration in children with conditions that might affect mental function (e.g. a cerebral degenerative disorder or leukaemia) or when treatment might be expected to produce intellectual change. They also remain useful as research tools. Consequently it is important for non-psychologists working with children (e.g. clinical medical officers, paediatricians, social workers, and psychiatrists) to be aware of their uses and limitations.

1.6.1 TYPES OF TEST

Skill to be assessed

Standardized tests vary according to the functions they are intended to measure. Such functions include:

- general intelligence
- special skills, for example language, perceptual ability, motor ability
- educational attainment, for example in reading or mathematics.

Those involved in systematically assessing children's performance in school tend to use three main types of test (Assessment of Performance Unit 1978):

- Comparative tests to discover where an individual child's performance stands in relation to that of other children. Appropriate normative data on the general population of children must be available if a test is being used for this purpose.

- Diagnostic tests to identify strengths and weaknesses.
- Curriculum related procedures to determine whether something taught has been learned (Cameron 1990).

In general, comparative tests are likely to be most useful where groups of children are being assessed, for example, to see whether a modification in diet has produced an improvement in overall intelligence in children with phenylketonuria, or whether a local educational authority is putting its remedial resources into schools with the highest rates of children having educational problems.

In contrast, diagnostic tests and curriculum-related procedures are most helpful when devising an educational programme for an individual child. The 'curriculum' may involve teaching a very basic skill such as doing up buttons, or acquiring a much more advanced set of information for a public examination. The principles are the same. One valuable 'curriculum-related' check-list approach to pre-school children with serious learning difficulties is the Portage guide to early education in the first 6 years of life (Bluma *et al.* 1976).

In carrying out a diagnostic test on a child failing in school, the psychologist will not only note the level of the child's performance and the particular cognitive problems such as deficits in attention and concentration that the child may be experiencing, but will also observe whether performance is impaired by undue anxiety or other emotional states.

Learning is a process that proceeds by stages (Haring *et al.* 1978), and children with emotional problems may be impaired in the initial acquisition of a task or skill, in achieving fluency in its performance, in maintaining such fluency, in generalizing beyond the setting in which the skill has been learned, or in applying the skill appropriately.

Construction of tests

Those involved in constructing standardized, norm-referenced tests of intelligence and attainment first identify the skills they wish to assess and the age range over which they wish the tests to apply. They then identify tasks that can be given to children that measure these skills and have high powers of discrimination, i.e. there is a suitably wide range of variation of achievement among children of the same age when given the task. They then develop criteria for scoring children's performance on the task. The reliability of the testing is then assessed by ensuring that children given the task twice perform in very nearly the same way on the two occasions (test–retest reliability) and that two observers watching the child perform the task rate the child in the same way (inter-rater reliability). They then examine the validity of the test, by using external criteria to determine whether the test does actually measure the skills intended. This can be done in a variety of ways, for example by seeing whether children who score highly on the task later achieve better in examinations than those who score poorly (predictive validity), or whether there is a correlation between the new test and another well-tried test assessing similar functions (concurrent validity). Finally, the test is standardized on a large representative population of children spanning the ages for which the test is to be applied.

1.6.2 TESTS OF DEVELOPMENT IN INFANCY AND EARLY CHILDHOOD

Bayley Scales of Infant Development

The Bayley Scales (Bayley 1993) are an American test covering the age from 2 months to $2\frac{1}{2}$ years. A range of items is assessed so that the child can be scored on a Mental Developmental Index and a Psychomotor Developmental Index. The scale takes about 45 minutes to administer and, given a skilled and experienced psychologist, provides a reliable, comprehensive record of the child's level of functioning.

Griffiths Mental Development Scale

The Griffiths Scale (Griffiths 1954) is a British test designed for children aged up to 2 years. There is an extension available for use above this age, but this is less satisfactory. The test has five sections: locomotor, personal–social, hearing and speech, eye–hand, and performance. It takes about an hour to administer. The test can only be administered by professionals who have been specifically trained in the use of the scale. It is currently being revised.

Denver Developmental Screening Test (DDST)

The DDST (Frankenburg *et al.* 1975) is a screening instrument for identifying children aged from birth to 6 years at risk for developmental delays and anomalies, so that they can be selected for further assessment. Four areas of development are assessed: personal-social, fine motor, language, and gross motor. The test takes about 20 minutes to administer. It can be applied by relatively inexperienced personnel, but is less accurate than the Bayley or Griffiths test.

1.6.3 TESTS OF GENERAL INTELLIGENCE

Wechsler Pre-school and Primary School Intelligence Scale

The Wechsler Pre-school and Primary School Intelligence Scale (Wechsler 1989) is a test applicable to children aged 4–$6\frac{1}{2}$ years. In the full form there are six verbal and six non-verbal tests, taking about an hour to administer, but a short form is available. Verbal IQ, performance IQ, and full-scale IQ scores can be computed. The test is reliable and well validated and provides a useful profile of the young child's pattern of abilities. However, as with the WISC (see below) the reliability of individual subtests is not high, and too much weight should not be put on isolated subtest results.

Wechsler Intelligence Scale for Children revised form (WISC-R)

WISC-R is a test of general intelligence applicable to children aged 6–14 years, which has been standardized on a UK population (WISC III UK, Wechsler 1992). There are 13 subtests, measuring different aspects of the child's abilities. Six of these (information, similarities, arithmetic, vocabulary, comprehension, and digit span) are used to obtain a 'verbal' IQ, and the other seven (picture completion, picture arrangement, block design, object assembly, coding, visuo-spatial, and mazes) are used to obtain a 'non-verbal' score. A 'full-scale' score is obtained on the basis of the results of the 13 tests. The test takes about an hour to complete, but a standardized, reasonably reliable short form of the test can be carried out in about 20–25 minutes. The child's scores on this can be 'prorated' to achieve a rough equivalent to a score obtained on the full test.

Scoring on the test has been computed to ensure that the mean is 100 with a standard deviation of 15. About 15% of the population therefore score below 85 and 2.5% below 70. Results on tests such as the WISC-R are used in defining levels of mental retardation.

British Ability Scale

The British Ability Scale (Elliott *et al.* 1997) is a test of general intelligence suitable for use with children aged 2–17 years. Testing takes about an hour, but shorter forms of the test can be used. A total of 24 scales are employed, and these assess speed of working, reasoning, spatial imagery, perceptual matching, short-term memory, retrieval, and application of knowledge. An advantage of the test is that it covers a wide age range, so that, if longitudinal assessment is required, its use, at least to some degree, overcomes the problems of relating results on one test to those obtained on another. Norms are so far only available for British children.

Goodenough–Harris Drawing Test

Also known as the Draw-a-Man Test (D. B. Harris 1963), this is a brief test to assess non-verbal intelligence in children aged 3–10 years. The child is asked to draw the best picture of a man he can, and the drawing is scored against carefully defined criteria. The test is reasonably reliable, but provides only a modest indication of the child's general intelligence as assessed in other ways.

1.6.4 TESTS OF EDUCATIONAL ATTAINMENT

Word Reading Subtest of the British Ability Scale

In this test (Elliott *et al.* 1997), suitable for children aged 6 years and upwards, the child is asked to read a series of words of increasing difficulty until he has made a number of consecutive errors. A reading age, mainly reflecting accuracy of reading, is then obtained. The test takes about 10 minutes to administer.

Neale Analysis of Reading Ability

In the Neale Analysis children aged 6 years and upwards are asked to read aloud a small number of stories, and are then asked questions about them (revised British edition, Neale 1988). The child can be scored for accuracy, speed, and comprehension, and reading levels for each of these computed. The test takes about 20–30 minutes to administer, but provides a broad, useful assessment of the child's reading abilities.

Wechsler Objective Reading Dimensions (WORD) test

WORD (Wechsler 1993) assesses basic reading, spelling, and reading comprehension and has the advantage that it is directly comparable with the Wechsler tests of general intelligence.

Wide Range Achievement Test (WRAT)

WRAT (Jastak and Jastak 1978) is a test suitable for children aged 5 years and over. There are two forms, one suitable for children up to 12 years and the other for older children. Reading, spelling, and arithmetic skills are assessed. It takes 20–30 minutes to administer. The test is useful and reliable, but norms are only available for North American children, so that the test is of limited applicability elsewhere.

Wechsler Objective Numerical Dimensions test (WOND)

WOND (Wechsler 1996) assesses mathematical reasoning and numerical operations and has the same advantage as the WORD that results are directly comparable with those obtained on the Wechsler scales of general intelligence.

1.6.5 ADAPTIVE BEHAVIOUR

Vineland Adaptive Behaviour Scale

The Vineland Adaptive Behaviour Scale (Sparrow *et al.* 1984) is a useful measure of a child's level of independence and self-help. It can be used to assess children from birth to adolescence. A parent, usually the mother, is asked a series of questions about the child's social and self-help skills and the information scored accordingly. A social age and a 'social quotient' can be obtained to define the child's level of independent functioning.

1.6.6 SPECIFIC SKILLS

A variety of other tests, such as the Reynell Developmental Language Scales, the Lowe–Costello Symbolic Play Test, and the Bruininks–Oseretsky Test of Motor Proficiency, are used to assess specific skills and abilities. These are discussed in the sections dealing with the relevant aspects of development.

1.6.7 APPLICATION OF TESTS

Indications

Psychological testing can play a most valuable part in the assessment of a child's mental functioning. In particular, results of testing will be helpful when:

- a child is failing educationally in relation to his peers
- although not failing educationally, a child appears to be functioning well below his level of ability
- there is reason to believe that a child is suffering from a condition likely to affect intelligence or educational attainment, and it is desirable to obtain a record of progress or deterioration.

The results of tests can be used, in conjunction with observations of the child in the testing situation (e.g. by noting his approach to tasks, distractibility, etc.), in the classroom, discussion with parents and teachers, and an appraisal of the child's responsiveness to different remedial approaches, for a variety of purposes. A specific programme of remedial instruction geared to the child's educational needs may be instituted. This may or may not involve a change in the child's class or school. The results of psychological testing may be one factor pointing to the need for a change in a child's treatment (e.g. anticonvulsant medication in a child with epilepsy).

1.6.8 RISKS AND DANGERS OF TESTING

These can be classified as follows:

- *Inappropriate test used.* The test employed may be for older or younger children, not relevant to the purpose for which it was administered, or not standardized on the population from which the child was drawn. Thus it is inappropriate to test children from developing countries on unmodified tests standardized in western countries.
- *Unsatisfactory test conditions.* The child may be tested in noisy, distracting circumstances, the tester inexperienced, or the child unmotivated or over-anxious. The child may not speak fluently the language in which the test is administered, or may be hampered by hearing or visual impairment or other causes of incomprehension. A child with poor attention may be difficult to test unless the test conditions are good and the examiner extremely patient.
- *Overgeneralization of conclusions.* There is an inherent unreliability in all tests. Inevitably children given a test on one day will not score the same if given it even a few weeks later. The tester should be aware of the margin of error involved in the test he is using.

  The tester should not draw inappropriate conclusions concerning the child's future. Especially in children under the age of 4 or 5 years, results of IQ testing are poor guides to later functioning unless the child's level is particularly low, and even then caution should be exercised in providing a prognosis.

Sometimes variations in functioning lead to inappropriate conclusions. Thus a child who is reading somewhat below what one would expect from his level of intelligence is not necessarily underachieving. Variation in test score cannot be used to diagnose brain damage, though tests have sometimes been used for this purpose. Certainly, however, results of testing can indicate that further physical investigation is necessary to establish whether indeed brain function or structure is impaired.

- *Labelling*. The risks of children being labelled on the basis of psychological test results as dull and expected to achieve only poorly are real enough. It is the responsibility of everyone involved in administering tests and talking about the results with parents and teachers, to explain their limited predictive value, so as to ensure that expectations about the child are not inappropriately fixed at a low level.

2

Maltreatment in the family

Four main types of child maltreatment occur: physical abuse (of which Munchausen syndrome by proxy is a variant), neglect, emotional abuse, and sexual abuse. More than one type of abuse may occur at any one time, and a child who has been subject to one form of abuse is more likely to suffer another in the future.

2.1 Physical abuse

2.1.1 DEFINITION

Physical abuse occurs when an adult inflicts a physical injury on a child more severe than is culturally acceptable. It is sometimes more difficult than one might think to draw the line between acceptable and non-acceptable violence. For example, in the UK, over 90% of both mothers and fathers have hit or smacked their children at some time, and over 75% in the previous year (Nobes and Smith 1997), so it is not reasonable to consider the use of physical punishment in itself as a form of abuse. Corporal punishment was only abolished in British schools in 1986, and remains tolerated in many American states. There are important cultural differences in what constitutes physical abuse, with some ethnic minorities viewing quite severe physical punishment as within the range of normal disciplinary practice, and others regarding almost any physical restraint as undesirable (Giovannoni and Becerra 1979). The situation may change as other countries follow the example of Sweden, Finland, Denmark, Norway, and Austria in the introduction of legislation to forbid the use of physical punishment in the home as well as at school.

2.1.2 PREVALENCE

The incidence of physical abuse is difficult to estimate, and will depend on the criteria used. In the UK, social services departments maintain child protection registers to record children at serious risk. In 1993, 4.5 per 1000 children were registered, of whom about a quarter had been physically injured.

A study from north-east Wiltshire, England (Baldwin and Oliver 1975), suggested that the annual prevalence rate of severe physical abuse was 1 per 1000 in children under the age of 4 years. Severe physical abuse was defined as that which resulted in bone fractures, bleeding into or around the brain, other severe internal injuries, repeated mutilation requiring medical attention, or death. Mortality from non-accidental injury in this study was 1 per 10 000 children. The prevalence of less severe physical abuse is uncertain, as it often does not come to medical attention. A national study of 3–17 year olds in the US (Straus *et al.* 1980) found that 14% had been kicked, bitten, punched, hit with an object, beaten up, or assaulted with a weapon by one or both of their parents. Few of these children would have come to professional attention because of child abuse. Cohn (1983) has estimated that about one million children are physically abused in the US each year, with 2000–5000 abuse-related child deaths and 2% of all families involved in child abuse.

2.1.3 RISK FACTORS

Particular social, family, parental, and child factors are strongly linked to child abuse (Graham *et al.* 1985).

- *Cultural factors* include exposure of the population to violence through the mass media and acceptance of violence within the family and school as normal.
- *Neighbourhood factors* include the support and help people in the locality or housing estate give each other, the general level of affluence and employment, standard of housing, and availability of play space.
- *Family attributes* of relevance include family size, quality of the marital relationship, quality of parenting behaviour, and level of communication regarding family problems and feelings.
- *Parental factors* include parental age (very young parents are more likely to abuse), parental personality, and mental health. Only about 10% of abusing parents have clear-cut forms of mental illness such as schizophrenia or depressive psychosis, but a high proportion of the remainder have relevant personality characteristics, such as impulsiveness, proneness to anger and irritability, and difficulty in forming relationships. Parental childhood experiences of early neglect and severe physical punishment are often present in the background of abusing parents themselves. Parental cognitive factors may also be of importance. Some parents regard their children in an egotistical way, merely as extensions of themselves, whereas others are able to accept that even their very young children have complex feelings of their own that deserve respect. The former are much more likely to abuse (Newberger and White 1989).
- *Child factors* include premature birth and early separation, need for special care in the neonatal period, congenital malformations, chronic illness, adverse temperamental characteristics, and style of obtaining attention. Most children subject to abuse are living in poor socio-economic circumstances, reared by young, inexperienced parents with personality problems. A minority, however, are living in well-to-do or comfortable circumstances and the main reason for abuse here lies in parental psychopathology.

In addition to these background factors, there are often triggering events such as an acute illness in the child or sib, a financial crisis in the family, or a marital dispute. It is rare to identify simple cause–effect mechanisms in child abuse. Personal environmental and triggering factors interact with each other to produce a situation in which abuse may seem an inevitable outcome.

2.1.4 CLINICAL FEATURES

The cardinal feature of the clinical presentation of physical abuse is a physical injury for which the explanation provided is unsatisfactory. The most common forms of non-accidental injury result in multiple bruising, burns, abrasions, bites, torn upper lip, bone fractures, subdural haematoma, and retinal haemorrhage. Other less common forms of physical abuse result in death by drowning or poisoning. The sudden infant death syndrome (cot death see Section 8.2) is produced by a deliberate parental act such as smothering in about 10% of cases.

The child may present to a variety of agencies. Parents may bring the child to the general practitioner or Accident and Emergency department either with the injury or with some other physical or behaviour problem. The complaint may be that the child will not stop crying or just does not seem well, and the injury may only be revealed on examination. Alternatively, neighbours, a relative, day nursery worker, teacher, or other person in the community may become concerned and report the matter to the police, NSPCC, or social services department.

Admission to hospital may reveal other supportive evidence. Insensitive parental handling of the child may be observed, or a child may appear frightened of his parents or unduly 'watchful' of strangers. The physical appearance of the child, who may be neglected and poorly thriving, is also relevant.

2.1.5 MANAGEMENT

Where it is the family doctor or clinical medical officer who suspects abuse or severe neglect, he should refer the child to hospital, informing either the paediatrician or casualty officer as well as the social services department of his suspicion. Children who present first to casualty departments and in whom non-accidental injury is suspected should, in all cases, be admitted to hospital for investigation. Parents should be told this is a necessary step so that further investigations can be carried out. If parents refuse, an Emergency Protection Order should be applied for. The patient's general practitioner and local social services department should be contacted (if they are not already involved) and relevant information such as previous injury, placement of the child or sibs on the local child protection register, or periods of time spent 'in care' should be sought.

History and investigations

A thorough assessment and complete record of details is particularly important in suspected cases of non-accidental injury, as records may well have to be produced in court at a later stage. An account of the circumstances surrounding the injury should be taken from the parents, together with a full medical history and details of the social background. A record of the nature of the injuries should be made with diagrams and photographs (Polnay *et al.* 1996).

Physical investigations will be necessary both to document the full extent of the injuries and to exclude conditions that may mimic non-accidental injury.

A full radiological survey (looking for old injuries and to exclude bony abnormalities such as osteogenesis imperfecta) should be performed. In some cases CT scanning of the head and ultrasound examination of the abdomen may be appropriate. The child's coagulation factors should be checked. Observations made by nursing and play staff of the parents, of the child, and of parent–child interaction are often very helpful.

Once all the relevant information has been collected, the consultant paediatrician or other senior doctor should, if non-accidental injury seems the most likely explanation, talk with the parents. The extent and nature of the injuries should be described, and the parents given an opportunity to explain how these injuries have occurred.

The social services department should be notified that the child is thought to be the subject of non-accidental injury. The decision whether to inform the social services department is often difficult in cases where non-acidental injury is suspected but the evidence is not strong, and medical staff are reluctant to involve themselves in the prolonged and sometimes painful procedures that such a case may entail. However, if in doubt, it is better to inform the social services department, and thus share the responsibility for the child's future safety. Further, if the parents at this, or any previous stage, indicate they might remove the child from hospital, then a social worker should immediately make an application to a magistrate for an Emergency Protection Order.

Case conferences

Once informed, the social services department will organize a case conference about the problem. This will be attended by representatives of hospital and community medical, nursing, and social work staff, a local authority social worker, the general practitioner, and a member of the police (usually an officer designated to this area of work). Other professionals who have had contact with the family, such as playgroup leaders, child or adult psychiatrists, or NSPCC officers, should also be present. If the child is of school age, a representative of the education service (usually an education welfare officer) will be present. Parents are usually informed of the timing of the conference, but not invited to attend, though the conclusions should be discussed with them as soon as possible afterwards. The aim of a case conference is to consider and share all the information available about the child and family, to make an agreed plan to ensure the child's safety and well-being in the future, to identify a 'key worker' to co-ordinate implementation of the plan, and to arrange a date to review progress (Department of Health 1989).

Various decisions need to be made:

- Should the child's name be placed on the child protection register? If so, this will require a member of the social services department to visit and monitor the situation regularly.
- Should the child be formally removed from parental care on a temporary and perhaps later on a permanent basis? If so, an application for a Care Order under Section 8 of the Children Act 1989 must be made to a court.

- Is the medical evidence of the cause of injury strong enough to stand up in court?
- Is it safe for the child to go home? If so, what level of supervision needs to be provided and who is to have responsibility for this? Are resources adequate to provide this level of supervision?
- How is the person taking main responsibility going to keep in touch with other professionals with whom the family may be in touch?
- Do other professionals, for example a child or adult psychiatrist, now need to be involved in further assessment and care?
- How are parents to be informed of decisions that have been reached? Usually a 'key worker' is nominated by the conference to ensure that decisions made are carried out.

Removal from parental care

In assessing whether the child needs to be removed, or whether the risk of returning the child home under supervision can be taken, a number of considerations are relevant (Oates 1984). These include especially

- evidence of recurrent trauma to the child and sibs
- the child's present physical state
- the understandability of the act of violence (did it occur when the family was under unusual stress that is unlikely to be repeated?)
- the general level of parental care quite apart from the abusive episode
- the presence of parental mental illness or personality disorder
- the personal qualities of the parents, and their apparent willingness to work with professionals and others who might be involved in helping them
- the degree of responsibility the parents accept for what has happened
- the availability of social work resources to ensure adequate monitoring.

In the end, the responsibility for the decision has to be taken by the social services department, but in practice the decision is usually a consensus one.

In a minority of cases it will be apparent at an early stage that the best interests of the child will not be served by a return to the family, as the risk of repeated abuse and serious neglect is too great. In this case, court proceedings are likely to be necessary. The paediatrician will need to assist the court by describing the injuries and the reasons for believing they were not accidentally caused. The social workers and, on occasions, other professionals such as a general practitioner or psychiatrist will provide evidence on the social background, caring capacities, and mental state of the parents. If it is decided the child needs to be permanently removed from parental care, then arrangements will need to be made for long-term fostering or adoption.

Return to the family

Assuming a child is returned home to the care of parents, either from hospital or after a period of temporary foster care, a programme of management or treatment needs to be agreed. The child's name will need to be placed on the child protection register, so that the case automatically receives a certain level of attention and, if the family moves, the social services department in the new area is automatically informed.

The key element to subsequent care will be the monitoring role played by a social worker, who will not only maintain regular contact, but will also attempt to help the family cope with material and other stresses and be available if, at any time, the parents feel they cannot cope and are reaching a situation where violence may occur again. Periods of temporary foster care may need to be arranged.

In addition, if resources are available, other types of intervention, perhaps requiring referral to a child psychiatric department, may be helpful. The parents may be given the opportunity to express their ambivalent feelings towards their child, and to understand how their own childhood experiences have failed to meet their own needs for nurture, and so made it difficult for them to care for their child. They may be helped by behavioural methods to develop skills enabling them to cope with their children's demanding behaviour (Gambrill 1983). Attendance at a day nursery, child psychiatric day centre, or other pre-school facility may be arranged.

2.2 Munchausen syndrome by proxy

2.2.1 DEFINITION

Munchausen syndrome by proxy (also known as illness induction syndrome, factitious illness) is an unusual form of physical maltreatment in which symptoms or signs of illness in children are deliberately fabricated or induced, nearly always by the mother. There may be no underlying physical condition or, alternatively, a physical illness may be present but its manifestations grossly exaggerated (Meadow 1982). Minor exaggerations of illness by parents are common. This condition can only be regarded as present if parental behaviour is persistent over time and results in social and/or physical disability in the child.

2.2.2 CLINICAL FEATURES

Children involved are usually of pre-school age, though occasionally a little older. Various methods of fabrication have been described, including false reporting of symptoms, falsification of specimens or charts, poisoning, smothering, and withholding food or medicines (Bools 1996). The child may be reported to have symptoms that in fact never occur. Epileptic fits and recurrent drowsiness are common examples. Alternatively, signs of illness may be artificially induced. Blood may be put in the child's urine or faeces by the mother using her own blood obtained by finger-prick or from menstrual products. The child may be covertly administered hypnotics, tranquillizers, or other medication, and become periodically drowsy or comatose. Administration of salt or diuretic medication can produce bizarre biochemical syndromes. Artificially induced rashes and fevers have been reported. Some children are put on highly restrictive diets, sufficient to produce malnutrition, for imagined overactivity or other behaviour problems.

The conditions produced in this way naturally present considerable diagnostic difficulties. Extensive investigations on an in-patient basis usually take place, and rare diagnoses may be suggested. Eventually, it is realized that the symptoms occur only when the mother (or occasionally the father) is present. It will also be noted that the mother hardly ever appears to leave the child's side, and resents attempts to encourage her to do so. At this stage there is often great reluctance on the part of medical and nursing staff to accept the possibility that the illness is factitious. Considerable ingenuity may be required to confirm the diagnosis by observing the mother produce the symptoms, and indeed this may turn out to be impossible, in which case the diagnosis remains presumptive.

The following features are characteristic of the syndrome:

- The perpetrator is nearly always the mother, but a number of cases have been reported in which the father has been involved (Meadow 1998).
- A previous child may have suffered or even died from an undiagnosed or very unusual condition.
- The mother has often obtained medical information earlier in her life. Usually this involves a period of nursing training.
- Mothers do not usually have overt psychiatric illness, although a minority show personality disorders with widespread maladaptation in a number of areas of their lives. Usually, however, their abnormal behaviour towards the child appears to be an isolated psychopathological feature.

2.2.3 ASSESSMENT

Although assessment will largely depend on the manner of presentation, there are certain common features (Meadow 1985):

- A high level of suspicion is required whenever a condition presents which is unusual, only occurs when the mother is present, or for which the only evidence is based on maternal report.
- Once suspicion has been aroused, there should be no further physical investigations. These may in themselves have an element of danger.
- Initial emphasis should be placed on careful recording of symptoms and checking of signs in relation to the mother's presence, and thought should be given to possible mechanisms whereby the symptoms might be artificially produced. Efforts should be made to check the mother's account by obtaining independent evidence from father, other relatives, nursery school staff, general practitioner, or health visitor. This should be done tactfully, without raising the mother's suspicions. The mother may also be fabricating about other areas of her life.
- An attempt should be made to separate the mother from the child to assess the effect on the child's symptoms. This may be resolutely refused by the mother, but is sometimes possible.
- A psychiatric assessment will often be helpful. This can sometimes be introduced to the parents as necessary to investigate possible behaviour or emotional problems in the child that may indeed be present. Such assessment may

reveal the presence of parental psychopathology, and may also uncover the reasons for the mother's behaviour. One common pattern is that the mother has herself suffered chronic deprivation in childhood, and now seeks from caring nurses the sympathy and interest that having a sick child elicits. The parent responsible may have suffered a somatizing or eating disorder in the past, or show a borderline personality disorder or Munchausen syndrome currently.

In some circumstances, forensic pathological laboratory investigations or even police surveillance may be indicated. Open or covert video observation of the mother's behaviour may be required, and this will raise difficult ethical issues requiring team discussions beforehand.

2.2.4 TREATMENT

Confrontation

As soon as the diagnosis has been sufficiently established such that court proceedings to protect the safety of the child could be successfully contested, the mother or both parents should be confronted with the diagnosis and the evidence to support it. A sympathetic rather than accusatory attitude should be taken up by the doctor (preferably the senior paediatrician involved). At the time of confrontation, help should be offered to the family. The father should at this point be involved in the discussions if he has not been previously involved.

Immediate protection of the child

In all circumstances the local social services department should be informed that the child is at risk; the family may already be known to this department. If the parents attempt to remove the child from hospital, an Emergency Protection Order should be obtained. In any event (see above) a case conference attended by the various professionals involved will be needed in order to plan for the future safety and care of the child, and allocate responsibility for further supervision of the family.

2.3 Neglect

Neglect involves a failure to provide adequate physical care, such as warmth or food, and/or a failure to provide the requirements for adequate psychosocial development, such as language or other cognitive stimulation.

2.3.1 PREVALENCE

About one fifth of children on child protection registers in England are recorded as suffering neglect. This amounts to around 1 per 1000 of the population. However, neglect is usually only noted if there are physical effects, such as failure to thrive, and the prevalence would probably be much greater if those children suffering inadequate psychosocial stimulation were included.

2.3.2 RISK FACTORS

Children living in poor socio-economic circumstances are at much greater risk of neglect, so parental unemployment, inadequate housing and poverty are commonly found. Parents are likely to have weak parenting skills, and may show some degree of learning disability. Alcohol consumption in the home may be high, and there may be violence between the parents. Occasionally children present with neglect from well-to-do families, and here parental mental illness or personality disorder are especially likely to be present.

2.3.3 CLINICAL FEATURES

The child is likely to present to the family doctor or in the Accident and Emergency department for reasons other than neglect, but to be noted to be poorly clothed, dirty, and failing to thrive. A dietary history may reveal the child is receiving an inadequate calorie intake. There will be poor weight gain in relation to height. The child is likely to be developmentally retarded, especially in language. There may be signs of other forms of maltreatment.

A home visit will reveal low standards of cleanliness and often inadequate protection and safeguards against accidents. The home is likely to be poorly heated. There will be an absence of books, toys, and other play material.

Physical examination may confirm the abnormal pattern of growth, and there will be catch-up growth in hospital when an adequate nutritional intake is provided. The child may be anaemic and show signs of chronic infection, such as impetigo. There may be contact dermatitis in the perianal region. Psychological investigation will reveal developmental retardation, often global, but possibly confined to language.

2.3.4 MANAGEMENT

The management of children suffering neglect causing significant harm will follow very similar lines to that in children suffering physical abuse (see above). However, there will be greater emphasis on improving the social and material circumstances of the home as well as the diet and level of social stimulation, and on monitoring physical progress through regular growth charting and psychosocial development through developmental or psychological assessments.

2.4 Emotional abuse

2.4.1 DEFINITION

Emotional abuse is said to be present when there is evidence of non-physical, but actively damaging behaviour by an adult towards a child, and the child's behaviour and emotional development have been seriously affected. Unlike physical and sexual abuse, emotional abuse refers to the quality of the parent–child relationship, rather than to an event or a series of events. Usually the emotional abuse involves hostility and rejection, but there may be other forms of active, non-physical abuse. Many parents criticize the behaviour, appearance, or other attributes of their children from time to time. Abuse can only be said to occur when such parental behaviour is persistent and generalized.

2.4.2 PREVALENCE

There is no definite information on the prevalence of emotional abuse, and doubtless difficulties in achieving a clear, agreed definition are important here. However, of children on child protection registers in England in 1996, 15% were thought to have suffered emotional abuse.

2.4.3 RISK FACTORS

These are usually multiple, and are similar to those occurring in physical abuse and neglect. They include:

- *Social factors*. Although these forms of abuse occur at all levels of society, they are commoner in families in economically deprived circumstances. Poverty, chronic unemployment, and poor, cramped housing are frequent accompaniments.
- *Parental characteristics*. Parents may have been abused in their own childhood, and have often had other damaging experiences at that time. They may be suffering from personality disorders or various forms of mental illness, especially depression, but occasionally less common types of disorder. In fact, diagnosable mental illness is not often present, but the family atmosphere may be characterized by violence between the parents, one or both of whom may show high consumption of alcohol. Their parenting skills will usually be poor, and, in particular, they will have especial difficulty in rewarding their children for good behaviour.
- *Child characteristics*. Children with chronic physical disorders or mental retardation are at slighter higher risk of abuse and neglect. Temperamentally 'difficult' infants and toddlers are also at greater risk, as are those with conduct disorders, but, in these circumstances, the primary problem is more likely to be the abusive parental behaviour.

2.4.4 CLINICAL FEATURES

Emotional abuse is often accompanied by other types of abuse (physical or sexual), or by neglect or absence of care.

Such abuse may be shown in many different ways. There may be:

- *Hostility and rejection*. Usually, when parents criticize a child, the criticism is temporary, and relates to a particular shortcoming or bad behaviour. Hostility is present when anything the child does elicits criticism, and even when the child's behaviour is good, it produces a negative reaction. 'He did do the washing up, but that's only because he wanted to get into my good books after

I told him off.' There are often constant belittling, pejorative remarks of this type.

- *Gross overprotection.* The child may not be allowed anything like the normal amount of autonomy that would be expected at his age. For example, a child might be prevented from going to school because of fear of infections he might catch there.
- *Other non-physical, but actively damaging behaviour.* This might involve the child being used as an emotional crutch by one or both parents, for example, by being expected to act as an emotional support for a chronically depressed parent. The child may be used as a message-carrier or spy by two separated parents. He may be exposed to emotional blackmail, for example by repeated threats of abandonment by one or both parents.

2.4.5 ASSESSMENT

The assessment of emotional abuse that is accompanied by physical maltreatment or neglect has been described above. However, in many circumstances, emotional abuse will be an isolated form of maltreatment, and both assessment and management may need to follow a different course.

- *Family interviews.* Emotional abuse is likely to be most evident when family members are seen together as a unit. It will be noted that one or both parents is openly and persistently critical of the child, perhaps with constant sarcasm and hostile comments. The child may be scapegoated, with other children in the family having their misdemeanours ignored or made light of. He may appear more disturbed in the presence of his parents than when he is away from them. It is often painful for clinicians to sit and listen while children are being discussed in their presence in such a negative way, but it should be remembered that the process is going on at home the whole time, and seeing the problem enacted before one is a necessary part of assessment.
- *Parental interviews.* Parents should also be seen separately, partly to establish the reasons for such negative attitudes, and partly to determine whether they are suffering from any form of mental illness. Parents may disfavour a particular child for a variety of reasons. They may have strongly wished for a child of the opposite sex, the child may be intellectually dull, physically unattractive, or deformed, or may remind the parents of another member of the family by whom they themselves were seriously rejected. For example a boy may remind his mother of her own father who sexually abused her, of an uncle with a criminal record, or, in the case of parental divorce and remarriage, of the biological father whom she now detests. It is important in addition to take a comprehensive history and, in particular, to determine whether the child has a significant emotional or behavioural problem.
- *Child interviews.* Children over the age of 7 or 8 years should, with parental consent, also be seen alone. They can be reassured at the onset of the interview that what they say is confidential. After time spent in discussion of neutral topics, they can be asked about parental behaviour as they see it with such

questions as: 'I wonder if you feel your dad gets on at you more than he does the others? What sort of things is it that he does that upset you most? How does it make you feel when that happens?'

- *Other sources of information.* In children of school age, the teacher will be a valuable source of information. If the assessment is made in hospital, the views of the family doctor and health visitor should be obtained.

2.4.6 TREATMENT

Treatment will depend particularly on the presence and nature of any psychiatric disorder present in the child or parent, and on the motivation of the parents to receive help. Many severely rejecting parents are unwilling to receive treatment for themselves and other family members. If emotional abuse is present, i.e. the child can be seen to be suffering a serious impairment of development as a result of constant rejection or neglect, then the case should be referred to the local social services department. As in the case of non-accidental injury this will lead to a social evaluation, and a case conference involving the various professionals concerned, at the end of which the child is likely to be put on the child protection register for regular surveillance or, in extreme cases, taken into care following legal proceedings. Magistrates are, however, often reluctant to make Care Orders where no sign of physical abuse exists. The decision of a doctor to refer such a case to the social services department is rarely easy, as referral will almost inevitably result in loss of the goodwill of the parents. However, when the child has been clearly suffering over a prolonged period already, and treatment is refused, a firm decision to refer should be taken.

Whether formal treatment is accepted or not, the aim should be to promote the child's welfare, if at all possible, within the family unit. If treatment is accepted, parent management training will be a central feature. This will often involve parents keeping a chart of the positive aspects of their child's behaviour over a period of time, with a built-in reward system for the child. Specific problems in the child and failure to thrive may require specific therapies. It is particularly important to give attention to ways of improving the child's self-esteem both within the family and at school, as this may have been severely affected.

2.5 Sexual abuse

2.5.1 DEFINITION

Sexual abuse has been defined as sexual behaviour between a child and an adult, or between two children when one of them is significantly older or uses coercion (American Academy of Child and Adolescent Psychiatry 1997).

Such abuse can be classified according to the nature of the activity involved:

- The child may have been assaulted or mutilated in the genital area. This can be seen as a form of non-accidental injury and is dealt with elsewhere in this book.

- The child may have been subjected to sexual stimulation or intercourse, or been persuaded to stimulate an adult sexually. Such inappropriate sexual activity may take place:
  — accompanied by violence (rape); or
  — with the apparent consent of the child. In these circumstances, even though apparently consenting, the child may well comply because of fear.
- The child may be involved in other sexual activities, for example posing for pornographic photographs or films.

The occurrence of abuse must be seen against the background of normal erotic behaviour and attitudes to nudity and sexuality within families. Studies in both the US and the UK have revealed a very wide range of attitudes and behaviour (Smith 1991). It is important that definitions of abuse do not affect normal, warm physical feelings that parents may have for their children. Further, cultural factors need consideration in defining abuse. For example, ritual circumcision in females is the norm in some cultures and is regarded with abhorrence in others.

2.5.2 BACKGROUND INFORMATION

The prevalence of sexual abuse is unknown because it so frequently never comes to light. In the US it has been estimated that about 19% of girls and 9% of boys are subjected to stressful sexual experiences during their childhood and early adolescence (Finkelhor 1979). In the UK it has been estimated from a survey of late teenagers that about 9% of children have been sexually abused and about 1% have actually had an incestuous sexual experience (Baker and Duncan 1985).

2.5.3 RISK FACTORS

- *Age and gender*. The subjects of sexual abuse are mainly adolescent boys and girls in their early teens. However, when a case involving a family member comes to light in a child of this age, it is often apparent that the sexual activity has been going on for several years. A significant number of younger children are involved, and in a small minority of cases children of pre-school age are the victims. Abuse occurs within the family and with strangers in about equal proportions. The family perpetrator is likely to begin by engaging the child in a non-sexual special relationship which then gradually proceeds to secret sexual behaviour of an increasingly intimate nature. The perpetrator often explains what he is doing as normal, and requests the child's co-operation on the grounds of affection. As time goes on, blackmail is often used to ensure secrecy.
- *Social factors*. Abuse may occur in all socio-economic groups, but is more likely to appear in socially deprived families living in cramped circumstances. Depression in mothers and a history of antisocial behaviour or heavy drinking in fathers is commonly present.
- *Family structure*. In many cases, when such abuse has occurred, it is between father or stepfather and daughter. However, other family members are not

infrequently involved. A minority of cases of sexual abuse involve rape by people from outside the family. Where boys are the subject of sexual activity, this usually takes the form of homosexual assaults by father or stepfather. Boys are less commonly involved in heterosexual activity with their mothers. Older siblings may be involved in sexually abusing their younger brothers or sisters and in some families a child may, at the same time, be both suffering abuse and perpetrating abuse.

- *Family function.* It has been suggested (Bentovim 1988) that sexual abuse within the family can best be seen by viewing the family as a system in which each relationship has an impact on others. For example, sexual activity between father and daughter may begin after there has been considerable strain in the marriage, when the father turns away from his wife and looks to his daughter, not only for sexual gratification but also for emotional support. The wife colludes with the development of this alternative arrangement, and may choose to ignore evidence of the sexual activity as it emerges. She may be emotionally distant from her daughter, and communication in the family about feelings is likely to be generally poor. Such families are often rigid and moralistic with a strong taboo on the open discussion of sexual matters. Consequently, they are slow to change. However, the sexual attraction to young children that perpetrators experience may also be understood by considering intrapsychic mechanisms. A perpetrator's erotic or painful experiences of being abused as a child may create a dissociated mental component which may be reactivated in adulthood under particular circumstances. Male adolescent perpetrators have frequently been abused themselves and there is often serious domestic violence in their backgrounds.

2.5.4 CLINICAL FEATURES

Sexual abuse may come to light for several reasons:

- An allegation is made by the victim or someone who knows the victim. For example, the child may tell another child who informs a teacher. A family member, friend, or neighbour may become suspicious and contact the social services department.
- The child presents with a behaviour problem or learning difficulty which raises suspicion of sexual abuse by professionals who are consulted. Any type of stress reaction may be present: physical symptoms such as abdominal pain with no organic cause, emotional withdrawal, aggressive behaviour, or difficulties in concentration. These non-specific symptoms should raise suspicion of sexual abuse if no other obvious stress is present. Certain types of behaviour, such as over-sexualized talk or play, compulsive masturbatory activity, an unexplained suicidal attempt, or running away from home, should raise particular anxieties. Refusal to communicate (mutism) and anorexia nervosa can also occur as a response to abuse.
- Physical signs suggestive or pathognomonic of abuse are present. There may be unexplained scratches, bruising, or bleeding in the genital area, or a foreign

body in the vagina. Recurrent urinary infection may be a sign of sexual abuse. Sexually transmitted diseases such as chlamydia and gonorrhoea are virtually pathognomonic of abuse when occurring in the prepubertal child.

2.5.5 ASSESSMENT

The assessment of sexual abuse will depend on the way in which the case has come to light. In particular, a doctor, especially a general practitioner or paediatrician, may be the first person to suspect that abuse has occurred; or he might be requested by another agency to confirm or refute the suggestion. In either event it is useful to observe the following principles:

- A high index of suspicion should be maintained. It is probably unusual for children to lie or fantasize about being sexually abused. Professionals are understandably reluctant to take seriously suggestions that sexual abuse has occurred in an apparently normal family, but this attitude is unhelpful.
- The comprehensiveness of assessment for child sexual abuse should depend on the level of suspicion. For non-specific problems such as bed-wetting or sleep disturbance, it is not appropriate to undertake specific investigations. On the other hand, when serious suspicion is aroused because of specific concerns (see above), physical investigation together with an interview with the child and parents will be required.
- Concerns about child sexual abuse should always be shared with other professionals. Anything that is more than a fleeting suspicion should be communicated to a colleague so that responsibility for deciding on the next step can be shared. Moderate or serious suspicion needs to be communicated to the social services or social welfare department.
- Detailed investigations, whether physical or psychological, into child sexual abuse are usually unpleasant for the child and family and may be traumatic. In children who turn out not to have been abused, such investigations may come to be seen as a form of 'secondary abuse' and even in children who have been abused, investigation is a serious ordeal. Such investigations therefore need to be carried out by skilful professionals who are experienced in the techniques they are using, the child needs adequate preparation and continuing explanation, and the assessment needs to be carried out in the least stressful circumstances that are possible. It is important for those involved in the early stages of assessment to remember that the use of leading or suggestive questions may prejudice subsequent, more skilled interviewing, so that it later becomes much more difficult to know what has actually happened and provide appropriate care.
- Physical examination of the genitalia. A brief examination of the external genitalia for bruising, scratches, forms part of an ordinary general physical examination. A more thorough investigation to determine the patency of the vulva and anus, with collection of specimens for forensic purposes, needs to be carried out by trained paediatricians or police surgeons in a paediatric setting with the mother or someone else of the child's choice present.

It is important to remember that most sexual abuse, for example licking or fondling of the child's genitalia, or forcing the child to masturbate the perpetrator, will not produce any positive physical findings.

- Interviewing the child. All family doctors, paediatricians, and child psychiatrists should feel competent to make general enquiries concerning the possibility of child sexual abuse by encouraging the child to talk about events that worry them and suggesting there might be problems the child may find it difficult to discuss. However, if responses to such questioning are positive, or if there are other strong grounds for believing the child has been sexually abused, then someone specially skilled in interview techniques will need to be involved.

Skilled interviewing in this area requires probing of the numerous ways in which the child might have been abused without asking leading questions or putting ideas into the child's mind. Helpful guidelines have been provided by Jones (1992) and by the American Academy of Child and Adolescent Psychiatry (1997). The child will require reassurance that he or she is doing the right thing by talking about the experiences and will not get into trouble because of it. It is vital to ensure that a complete record is kept of the interview, either by video-recording or by taking down what the child says verbatim.

2.5.6 MANAGEMENT

Immediate management of a case in which a child has been sexually abused will follow along similar lines to that occurring in physical abuse. In some cases, where the suspected perpetrator is in the home, the child will be admitted to hospital, though this will usually not be necessary if the perpetrator is not living in the home. The social service department should be informed, and a case conference or a co-ordinating meeting called. For success in management, it is vital that a co-ordinated plan should be made between the health personnel (health visitor, general practitioner, paediatrician, clinical medical officer), the social services department, and the police. It is widespread current practice in the UK for offenders to be charged. Minor and first offences are usually dealt with by cautioning, but more serious offences usually result in custodial sentences.

Continuing management will involve an attempt, as far as possible, to support the child within the family (Furniss *et al.* 1984). In a minority of cases, where care has been and promises to be generally inadequate and neglectful, the child will need to be removed from the home to the care of the social services department. In any event the child should be given the opportunity to continue to communicate her feelings about the experience. Depression and guilt are commonly experienced by girls who have been the victims of rape or incest, and a number will show post-traumatic stress disorder.

If the perpetrator is the father or stepfather, family breakdown is common, but by no means an inevitable outcome. A treatment approach involving initially separate interviews with the family members, then family interviewing, first with father absent, and then with father present, appears to have a positive influence in a significant number of cases. Group therapy (Section 9.2.4) for girls who have shared this experience may provide valuable emotional support. Parents whose children have been the victims of sexual assault from someone outside the family also need the opportunity to express their feelings and to be helped to understand their child's subsequent behaviour. Family interviews may be particularly useful in this respect.

2.6 Outcome following child maltreatment

The outcome of the different types of abuse described above is remarkably similar (Mullen *et al.* 1996). Women who report any forms of abuse in their childhood are found to show high scores on interviews assessing psychiatric disturbance, high rates of depression, and eating disorders as well as high rates of sexual problems when compared with non-abused control women. The commonality of outcome may be a reflection of the overlap between different types of abuse.

Nevertheless there are some specific findings. Children who have been physically abused have a 10–30% risk of re-abuse, and, in some cases, this will prove fatal. They have a high rate of physical problems, including cerebral palsy and accidental injury. Many will be developmentally delayed and have learning difficulties (Hensey *et al.* 1983; Lynch and Roberts 1982). There is a high rate of subsequent behavioural and emotional problems in childhood. Many of these problems found on follow-up are likely to be the result of emotional deprivation and lack of appropriate stimulation present in the abusive family rather than of the injuries themselves.

The outcome of children who are victims of Munchausen syndrome by proxy is variable. A poor outcome is probable where there are insufficient grounds to remove the child from home, the mother continues to deny responsibility, and the pathological mother–child relationship remains unresolved. On the other hand, reasonably good results have been reported when there is an acceptance of help from a multidisciplinary team (Bentovim and Gray in press).

The consequences of neglect have been less well studied, possibly because this form of abuse so often overlaps with other types. However, it seems likely that neglected children will often fail to achieve their full potential for growth, and that they will show mild to moderate learning disabilities as a result of unsatisfactory early psychosocial stimulation.

The outcome of emotional abuse will depend largely on the nature of the psychiatric problems produced, the presence of intractable or treatable personality disorder or mental illness in the parents and the motivation of the family to receive help. Children showing conduct disorders in a strongly rejecting family are likely to do particularly poorly.

The medium- and long-term psychiatric outcome for children who have been sexually abused frequently involves persisting dysfunction. Tebbutt *et al.* (1997) found that nearly half of a sexually abused group showed significant depression and low self-esteem 5 years after disclosure. In general, boys do less well than girls. In late adolescence, a history of sexual abuse is correlated with the presence of conduct disorder, anxiety, and depression (Fergusson *et al.* 1997). A number of runaway adolescents who live on the streets, some of whom have become involved in prostitution, have suffered sexual or other forms of abuse at home. Adult women who report having been abused in their childhood are more likely to suffer social, interpersonal, and sexual difficulties in their adult lives (Mullen *et al.* 1994). A very strong association has been found between sexual abuse in which penetration occurred and later depression in women (Cheasty *et al.* 1998), with a much smaller effect of less severe abuse.

Two additional points need to be made about the outcome of abuse.

- First, the quality of parenting when abused children grow up and have children themselves is likely to be both generally and specifically affected by their earlier experiences. Thus, sexually abused children are at higher risk of abusing, and especially sexually abusing, other children especially if they have, in addition, witnessed intra-familial violence (Skuse *et al.* 1998).
- Secondly, many children do, as a result of protective factors and the coping mechanisms they use, survive abuse without psychiatric disorder and without impairment of their parenting ability. The probability of problems later on by no means indicates that these are inevitable.

3

Neurodevelopment and neuropsychiatric disorders

3.1 Motor development and disorders of movement

3.1.1 NORMAL MOTOR DEVELOPMENT

Motor development commences well before birth, as witnessed by frequent and vigorous limb movements in the womb. Kick charts can be used to monitor fetal activity and well-being. Motor skills are a prerequisite to effective control of the environment and result from a complex interaction between genetic potential, opportunity, and personal attributes such as motivation and organizational skills. Complicated manoeuvres such as drinking from a beaker without spilling require execution of a series of sophisticated and co-ordinated movements. Thus intellectual capacity and the ability to plan ahead, anticipate, and respond remedially to circumstances are as important as muscle power and co-ordination. In addition satisfactory visual acuity, intact visual pathways, and perceptual skills are needed.

Tables exist which list the average ages at which certain motor skills are obtained. However, the exact age of acquisition varies substantially because of genetic and environmental factors. It is important to distinguish between the average age when children are able to perform a particular motor skill and the age at which, if the skill has not materialized, there is a need for further investigation. Table 3.1 lists such information. The significance of gross motor delay rests on the possible presence of underlying pathology, or a developmental delay which may be of a specific or more general nature. Even in children not walking at 18 months, only a minority of children will have identifiable pathology (Chaplais and Macfarlane 1984). However, many very low birthweight children have impaired motor skills on tests of manual dexterity, ball skills, and balance which persist into adolescence despite some improvement in early childhood (Powls et al. 1995).

Influences on normal motor development

The sequence and timing of motor development is largely genetically pre-programmed. Thus children tend to follow the same motor developmental trajectories irrespective of social and cultural context. Head control precedes thoracic and lumbar motor co-ordination, which is necessary to sit up unaided. This is followed by the ability to pull to standing, to 'cruise' around holding on to objects, and finally to walk unaided with increasing agility. Skilled fine motor movements such as finger–thumb opposition ensue. Racial differences in the speed of motor development, with black children progressing more rapidly than

Table 3.1   Performance of motor skills

Movement	Average age of performance (months)	Need for concern if not performed by age (months)
Gross motor movements		
Sits with head steady	3	5
Sits without support	7	10
Stands holding on	10	15
Takes 2–3 steps unaided	14	18
Walks up steps holding rail	20	30
Jumps up and down on 2 feet	30	42
Hops on 1 foot	48	72
Hand skills (fine motor skills)		
Grasps a rattle	3	5
Transfers a cube from hand to hand	7	10
Uses 'pincer' (finger-thumb) grip for small objects	9	12
Drinks from beaker	14	20
Builds tower of 4 cubes	20	33
Copies circle	36	42
Threads beads	40	48
Copies + sign	48	54
Copies square	54	66

white, irrespective of socio-economic status, are reported. However, it seems that while black children as a group achieve motor milestones at a significantly earlier age, the magnitude of difference is small, being less than 1 month on average for milestones prior to walking (Capute *et al.* 1985). Socio-economic status has a far smaller influence on gross motor development than on other areas of development. In contrast, fine motor development is thought to be more sensitive to social influences and opportunities for exploration and play.

Assessment

Motor development can be rapidly assessed with a minimum of equipment including a rattle, play bricks, lace and beads, and crayons and paper. It is important to distinguish between failure of skill acquisition, retarded skill development, plateauing of development, and loss of motor skills. There are numerous fuller accounts of technique and interpretation (e.g. Bax *et al.* 1990).

3.1.2 CAUSES OF DELAY IN MOTOR DEVELOPMENT

General developmental delay

Seriously delayed motor development is usually associated with delay in other spheres including cognition, language, and social functioning. The most common cause for such a situation is generalized learning disability (mental retardation). However, many children with learning disability have normal early motor milestones. Gross motor development is therefore a poor predictor of learning disability.

Specific motor delay

Motor developmental delay without learning disability may be caused by:

- cerebral palsy
- other central nervous system abnormalities
- muscle abnormalities (especially hypotonic disorders) e.g. Duchenne muscular dystrophy
- specific motor dyspraxia (clumsiness).

Clumsiness (specific motor dyspraxia)

As many as 5% of the school population are thought to be clumsy at least to some degree, with boys affected more than girls (Illingworth 1991). Many of these children are also delayed in other areas of development. Others, despite otherwise normal development, have a tendency to fall over, to trip over themselves and other objects, and to bump into things. There is often a history of delayed gross and fine motor development. Such children can be awkward with their hands and are usually poor at writing, tying laces, and buttoning. This leads to poor performance at dancing, PE, and other physical activities with a consequent risk of teasing and low self-esteem. Thus clumsiness may present with school refusal, poor academic progress, or other manifestations of insecurity (Henderson and Hall 1982).

There is wide normal variation in agility and dexterity. Delayed maturation is thought to reflect genetic factors rather than lack of opportunities or encouragement. Neuromuscular disorders such as muscle tone problems, muscular dystrophy, and joint hyperextensibility may predispose to clumsiness as may certain drugs including anticonvulsants, tricyclic antidepressants, and benzodiazepines. Intrauterine growth retardation, birth complications, and pre- or postnatal malnutrition may be of significance in the individual case.

The ICD-10 category 'specific developmental disorder of motor function' describes a serious impairment in the development of motor co-ordination that is not solely explicable in terms of general intellectual retardation or of any specific congenital or acquired neurological disorder. The term *dyspraxia* is usually reserved for instances where there is thought to be impairment or immaturity of the organization of movement—not just of movement itself. Such children have difficulty in planning and executing complex movements and often have language, perception, and thought problems as well. Language may be impaired or delayed and articulation may be immature. Thus, it is not a question of whether a child can accomplish a movement, but whether it can be accomplished with integration and quality. A popular theory is that there are problems with 'sensory integration'—the ability to understand and synthesize the messages that the senses convey and difficulty in relating those messages to actions (Ayres 1979).

Assessment includes getting the child to try to walk along a thin beam, to roll a ball, whistle, skip, clap, throw and catch a ball, tie laces, thread beads, and screw on bottle caps. There may be obvious tremor or ataxia while building with 2.5 cm (1 inch) cubes. More formal psychological assessment may be required to confirm the diagnosis and to exclude generalized learning disability. This may include tests of motor proficiency such as the Bruininks–Oseretsky test (Bruininks 1978, Hattie and Edwards 1987). Formal neurological examination and EEG are usually non-contributory, except where clumsiness has developed in a child with previously normal dexterity.

Management depends on the nature and severity of the problem. Explanation to child, parents, and teachers about the presence of a specific developmental difficulty and the fact that it is not the result of laziness is often sufficient. Slow improvement can be expected although some disadvantage in this area is likely to persist. Confidence, self-esteem, coping strategies, and useful problem-solving techniques can be gained from interested physiotherapists, occupational therapists, and speech therapists.

3.1.3 STEREOTYPIES AND HABIT DISORDERS

Stereotypies are involuntary, co-ordinated, patterned, repetitive, rhythmic, non-reflex, non-goal directed motor activity that are carried out in exactly the same way during each repetition (Tan *et al.* 1997). *Mannerisms* are similar although, with these, in contrast to sterotypies, the content of the movements suggests they have some meaning for the child. Stereotypies can occur in isolation (monosymptomatic) or can be part of a wider and more serious disturbance such as autism. They include head banging, rocking, posturing, spinning round or running round in circles, hair pulling, thumb sucking, nose picking, and nail biting. More rarely they can take a particular pattern indicative of a specific clinical condition, for example the midline hand wringing and hyperventilation seen in Rett syndrome (Hagberg 1993) or the hand flapping in response to anxiety or excitement witnessed in fragile X syndrome (Turk and Graham 1997).

A genetic tendency to show stereotypic behaviour may be triggered by adverse social circumstances including residential care, understimulation, and abusive experiences (Tröster 1994). The age of the child and the context or situation are important in determining the type of behaviour shown. For example, nail or lip biting/chewing occurs predominantly in concentration/demand situations, while pulling faces and scratching oneself is associated more with arousal/frustration situations. Head banging is more frequent in boys than in girls.

Stereotypies are seen more often in young people with learning disabilities and those with sensory impairments. These may be aggravated by having unreasonable demands made, or by the child being in unfamiliar, loud, or hectic environments, or by lack of sensory stimulation.

Head banging is common, occurring in up to 7% of children. It usually develops towards the end of the first year of life. The behaviour is usually shown when the child is put to bed but may occur repeatedly during sleep. Insecurity, attention-seeking, or neglect should be considered but often the behaviour has a comfort-seeking function and is self-limiting, stopping between 2 and 3 years of age. Protective cot-padding, rearrangement of night-time routine, and efforts to avoid inadvertently reinforcing the behaviour by undue attention may be helpful.

Hair pulling (trichotillomania) is rarer. It may occur as an isolated habit or may be symptomatic of underlying psychological problems such as anxiety or depression. Usually hairs are plucked out of the head but eyebrows and eye-lashes may be affected as well. Swallowing the plucked hair can produce a hairball (trichobezoar) which may cause intestinal obstruction requiring surgical removal. Behavioural management including exposure to situations that trigger the hair pulling with concurrent response prevention exercises, differential reinforcement of incompatible behaviours (DRI), and rehearsal of control postures (e.g. sitting on hands or keeping hands clenched in pockets) are the treatments of choice if the problem fails to respond to basic reassurance and explanation. Associated severe anxiety or depression may require treatment in their own right and may involve individual or family psychotherapy.

3.1.4 TICS AND TOURETTE SYNDROME

Definition

A tic is a sudden, rapid, recurrent, non-rhythmic, stereotyped motor movement or vocalization. Tics can be transient or persistent and can have voluntary as well as involuntary components. Individuals are often aware of increasing pressure to perform the tic just prior to doing so ('premonitory urge').

Mild and transient tic behaviours are common in childhood and are of very little clinical significance. In contrast, severe multiple motor and vocal tics can be profoundly disabling.

Clinical features

Age of onset is usually around 7 years—only rarely before 2 or after 15 years. Characteristic initial features are eye and facial twitching which may be precipi-tated or aggravated by psychological stress, such as entering a classroom with a disliked or feared teacher in it, or worry about an ill parent or sibling. Such tics can be suppressed briefly. They are often better during sleep or when the child is involved in enjoyable activities. They can be worsened by anxiety, stress, boredom, excitement, and stimulants. Many tics last only a few weeks or months. Frequently no medical input is needed. Reassurance and discussion of concurrent stresses and pressures in the child's life may be all that is required.

More severe forms develop around the same age, but persist and spread to affect other body parts. Complicated motor movements (e.g. brushing hair back, spinning round, touching) and vocal utterances of words or phrases may occur. The type of tic seems to stay constant over time and phases of development (de Groot *et al.* 1994). The presence of persisting combined multiple motor and vocal tics causing marked distress or significant impairment in social or other important areas of functioning is known as Gilles de la Tourette syndrome (Tourette syndrome) (Robertson and Stern 1997).

Tourette syndrome

Tourette syndrome is characterized classically by convulsive muscular jerking and explosive utterances. *Coprolalia* (obscene utterances) and *copropraxia* (obscene gestures) do occur but not as frequently as used to be thought (Goldenberg *et al.* 1994). Associated psychiatric problems are common and include social and relationship difficulties, obsessive–compulsive behaviour, impulsiveness, distractibility, and inattentiveness.

Prevalence

Mild tics occur in approximately 10% of children with boys being affected more often than girls. There is no association with social class or racial group. The condition may be more common in urban than in rural settings. Tourette syndrome affects 3–5 in 10 000 individuals, being 3–4 times more common in boys than in girls.

Aetiology

- *Genetics.* A genetic basis to Tourette syndrome has been confirmed although the exact nature of inheritance remains unclear. Both single gene and polygenic effects have been suggested.
- *Neurological.* Recent brain imaging studies suggest a loss of the normal asymmetry of the basal ganglia (Singer *et al.* 1993) and a trend toward smaller left lateral ventricles. PET scanning has shown metabolic and perfusion abnormalities in the basal ganglia and frontotemporal area (Baxter and Guze 1993). In contrast, EEG studies show only non-specific abnormalities. There are few postmortem studies, but these show changes consistent with defective striatal projections.
- *Neurochemical.* Abnormal dopamine metabolism is suggested by the beneficial effects of dopamine antagonists such as the butyrophenones (haloperidol), dimethylbenzylpiperadines (pimozide) and substituted benzamides (sulpiride). In contrast, psychostimulants and other dopaminergic agents can aggravate symptoms.
- *Familial environment and other stresses.* Undue parental or school pressures may aggravate problems. The child's bizarre behaviour may itself be the cause of severe family disturbance and it is often impossible to disentangle the multiple causal factors. It is important to emphasize that the child's behaviour is neither malicious nor wilful and that understanding rather than a punitive approach is required.
- *Individual psychopathology.* There is no evidence that repressed aggressive or sexual urges underlie these disorders, although this was suggested in the past. In severe cases individual psychopathology occurs secondarily to the problem. The content of the utterances seems to be related to their social unacceptability and associated anxiety.

Assessment

A detailed account of the tics, their nature and development should be obtained from the child, parents and if possible the class teacher. Factors which trigger or ameliorate the problem should be noted as should the child's personal experiences, including any premonitory urges. It is particularly important to identify family reactions to the presence of the problems. Check for any other emotional or behavioural problems or developmental delays. Physical examination is usually negative. Interviewing the child may exaggerate the movements because of the anxiety engendered, and it is important to obtain an account of the usual frequency rather than rely on observations in the clinic. Observe parental reactions to tics. Consider whether tic severity fluctuates according to the topic or person being discussed.

Diagnosis should not usually present difficulties. Differential diagnoses include other dyskinesias including the athetoid and choreiform movements witnessed in cerebral palsy and Huntingdon's and Sydenham's choreae. In these conditions the movements are non-repetitive and multiple muscle groups are affected. Stereotypies associated with severe learning disability and autistic spectrum disorders should be considered as should repeated compulsive behaviours.

Amphetamine derivatives, including those used for treating hyperkinetic disorders, may aggravate or unmask tics. Movements in myoclonic epilepsy are repetitive but usually involve larger muscle groups. The ability to suppress symptoms during certain tasks does not exclude the diagnosis.

Treatment

Mild tics usually respond to explanation and reassurance. Possible stresses and ways to remove them should be considered with parents and child. Parents should be counselled to avoid giving the tics undue attention. Prognosis is good, with mild tics disappearing within weeks or months.

Severe tics including Tourette syndrome require more intensive, protracted, and combined approaches. The above aspects should still be covered and families should be made aware of relevant booklets and put in touch with self-help groups.

Behavioural modification approaches begin with a functional analysis of factors triggering tics, and those which encourage their persistence. Charting of baseline tic frequency should be followed by an incentive scheme such as stickers or stars for periods of tic-free time. *Habit reversal training* utilizes incompatible muscular or vocal responses that do not physically allow the tic to be manifested during rehearsal (Peterson *et al.* 1994).

Family/individual counselling

The family should be sympathetically encouraged to explore the impact of the tics on their lives and how these might be minimized. Beliefs in a malicious or wilful basis to the problem should be dispelled. Attention conditional on the tics should be minimized.

Medication

Medication has been shown to be helpful and sometimes very helpful for severe tics and Tourette syndrome. Dopamine antagonists such as haloperidol, pimozide, and sulpiride produce at least some improvement for most individuals but side-effects, especially dystonic reactions, are common, especially with haloperidol. Haloperidol may be given in two divided doses increasing from 0.02 to 0.05 mg/ kg per day. Transient drowsiness to which the child habituates is common. Pimozide is useful where haloperidol is ineffective or where it produces unacceptable side-effects. Dosage is 1 mg twice daily increasing by 2 mg increments weekly to a maximum of 8 mg daily. Risperidone, the first of a novel class of antipsychotics, the benzisoxales, antagonizes brain 5-HT$_2$ receptors with weaker effects on dopamine (D$_1$ and D$_2$) and histamine (H$_1$) receptors. Successful responses in children have been reported but results to date have been mixed (Lombroso *et al.* 1995).

Clonidine, a selective α_2 adrenergic agonist, is useful in severe cases with associated hyperactivity. However, sedation and postural hypotension can be problematic. Dosage should be low—in the range 0.025–0.5 mg daily in single or divided doses. There is increasing interest in nicotine via gum or transdermal patches as a means of reducing tics. Tricyclic antidepressants and selective serotonin reuptake inhibitors such as fluoxetine and sertraline may occasionally be useful, especially when there are features of depression or obsessive–compulsive behaviour.

Outcome

Outcome is affected by tic severity, presence of associated psychiatric problems, level of intellectual functioning, developmental delays, presence of brain dysfunction and family disturbance. Mild tics in young children generally disappear over a few months. Recurrences are usually short-lived. About 50% of individuals with more severe problems will improve markedly in their late teens or early twenties, but the disorder persists into adulthood in a substantial number.

3.2 Normal language and speech development

• *Language* comprises the sum of skills necessary for the process of communication. It consists of the ability to understand and utilize communications, verbal and non-verbal, and to make such communications to others with meaning.
• *Communication* comprises the processes of transmission (expression) and reception of information.
• *Speech* is the oral production of language.
• *Non-verbal communication* includes gesture, facial expression, nature and degree of eye contact, and other aspects such as posture.

Communication begins at birth. Indeed awareness of speech, especially the mother's voice, is apparent *in utero*. Even before birth, awareness and responsivity can be demonstrated by the unborn baby's ability to react differentially to sounds and other stimuli.

In the first few hours of life babies begin to distinguish their mother's voice. Different cries for pain and hunger ensue rapidly. From 2 months of age babies move their lips in response to their mothers talking to them. By 3–4 months early babbling usually occurs. At 4 months the child is able to discriminate between all speech sounds in all languages. This ability is gradually refined until the child can only discriminate between the sounds of his own language. As this occurs the child's vocalizations become increasingly imitative. Mother and baby can be observed to be involved in conversational 'turn-taking' in which the child will respond by babbling when the mother stops speaking to him. A normal phase of automatic 'echoing' of adult speech and appearing to 'play with sounds' is common. At about 12 months the first words with meaning, such as **car,** 'bicky' (biscuit), **Mama,** or **Dada** usually occur. These first words are often holophrastic, i.e. they function not only as labels but also as whole phrases, such as '**Dad, carry me**', or '**Dad gone now**'. By 18 months the child is usually generating combinations of words, and shortly after this symbolic (make-believe) play can be observed. There is therefore a characteristic development of communicative ability before the onset of speech.

The fact that a child has not acquired a particular skill by the suggested age does not mean that the child's development will necessarily be impaired subsequently. It does mean that the child has, at that time, a significant language delay, is at risk for subsequent impairment, and requires assessment.

3.2.1 THEORIES OF LANGUAGE DEVELOPMENT

Various theories have been developed to explain the process of language development. B.F. Skinner proposed a behavioural model, whereby children learn language largely by imitation and selective reinforcement for correct utterances. Noam Chomsky emphasized innate mechanisms such as a 'language acquisition device' to help explain why children produce rule-based grammatical utterances (e.g. 'he bringed the money') that they could not have learned by imitation. Piaget and Bruner have attempted to explain language development in terms of more general cognitive processes and symbolic thought. However, none of these theories is fully explanatory. Imitation can only be of minor significance because children's language is so different from that of the adults they hear. Conversely, innate mechanisms do not explain the wide variations in language between children brought up in different cultures. However, there is now a large body of information about factors associated with and sometimes causing language problems (Bishop 1992, Rapin 1996).

Psycholinguistic studies suggest that it is useful to consider different levels of language development. This includes

- the pronunciation of individual sounds (*articulation*)
- the sound system of a particular language (*phonology*)
- the grammatical structure of words (*morphology*) and sentences (*syntax*)
- the representation of literal meaning (*semantics*)
- variation in language use (*pragmatics*).

All these levels of language have receptive and expressive components. Thus, instead of the medical diagnosis in traditional use (autism, learning disability, etc.), speech and language therapists use terms such as articulation disorder, phonological impairment, oral/articulation dyspraxia, oral dysarthria, receptive/expressive language delay or disorder, pragmatic disorder, or complex communication disorder. (The latter involves problems in several areas of language including that of pragmatics.) The distinction between a delay and a disorder refers to the difference between a slow, but normal pattern of development, and a departure from the usual pattern.

Influences on normal language development

- *Genetic factors* are particularly important in establishing the sequence with which different stages are reached, and in determining the pace of development.
- *Physical factors*. Intrauterine growth retardation or a prolonged second stage of labour are risk factors for slower than average language development. Recurrent otitis media occurring before 2 years of age is a common cause of mild receptive and expressive language delay. It can also account for articulation problems.

Quality of social environment is the other significant factor (Fundudis *et al.* 1979, Beitchman *et al.* 1986). Pace and quality of language and speech acquisition are linked to:

- *Social class*. Middle-class children are more advanced, especially after about 3 years of age.
- *Family size*. Children in large families are on average slower to speak, probably because adults have less time to talk and listen to them.
- *Multiple births*. Twins speak a little later than singletons, perhaps because twins often communicate a good deal together, and do not need to communicate with adults so much.
- *Sex*. Girls' early language development is slightly more advanced than boys, perhaps because girls are more socially responsive and therefore may elicit more conversation and social interaction from their parents than boys do early in life.
- *Quality of stimulation*. Children reared in social isolation or in institutions where they are severely neglected often show marked, but frequently surprisingly reversible delay in language development. More generally, the quality of language interaction between parents and child seems more important than the quantity of language stimulation in family-reared children. Children with parents who listen, react, and draw out their offspring conversationally are likely to be more linguistically advanced and sophisticated than those whose parents fail to acknowledge their attempts to communicate or just talk at rather than with them.
- *Bilingual households*. Children reared in families where two languages are spoken from the outset show no disadvantage and usually acquire both

languages well. The need to speak two languages may, however, be a disadvantage for children language-delayed for other reasons.

3.2.2 ASSESSMENT OF LANGUAGE

It is usually possible to gauge the rough level of an infant or young child's speech and language reasonably accurately by asking the carer, usually the parent, questions in the presence of the child about this aspect of development, and by observing the way the child uses language during history-taking. It is usually better for a clinician not to talk to pre-school children directly to begin with as the intrusion of a stranger may only serve to aggravate shyness and social inhibition—a common cause for discrepancies between parentally reported skills and those shown by the child on clinical observation. Encouraging the carer to use appropriate toys and puzzles with the child will give some idea of the quality of language interaction. Precise requests may be needed to get parents to co-operate in assessing particular aspects of language, for example to pick out a colour or an object without pointing. Imaginative play and sharing a picture book are good ways of facilitating direct interaction with a pre-school child in order to assess language development. For older children, conversation about a recent experience, favoured sports team, pop star, or television programme will often elicit responses useful for language assessment. By these means it should be possible to develop a reasonable idea of the child's capacity for comprehension, expression, use of inner language (as shown in capacity for make-believe play), and response to gesture.

Hearing needs to be assessed. This can be estimated in children up to 1 year of age by observing the child's ability to localize sounds, and later by making simple requests either face-to-face, or with older children by hushed voicing from behind. Hearing is now usually routinely assessed in population screening programmes undertaken by general practitioners or community paediatricians. However, hearing loss can be episodic. It is therefore unwise to assume that a child's hearing is currently unimpaired because a normal hearing test was previously undertaken, especially if there is a history of recurrent secretory or suppurative otitis media.

Children in whom there is an apparently significant delay in language development or in hearing ability should be referred for a more expert speech and language therapy assessment. There are various excellent tests of the language ability of the preschool child including the Reynell Developmental Language Scales (1997), the Renfrew Language Test, the British Picture Vocabulary Scale, and the Clinical Evaluation of Language Fundamentals—Preschool Version. The Illinois Test of Psycholinguistic Abilities (Kirk *et al.* 1968), the Test for Reception of Grammar (Bishop 1983), the Clinical Evaluation of Language Fundamentals—Revised, and many others can be used with older children. No one test is suitable for all children or is sufficient to assess all aspects of speech and language. They should therefore be used only by professionals with specialist knowledge in this area, ideally speech and language therapists. For an assessment of inner language, a test of symbolic play (Lowe and Costello 1976) can be useful.

3.2.3 LANGUAGE DELAY IN YOUNG CHILDREN

A child who is not talking or who is unusually slow to speak may be suffering from any of the following, either alone or (commonly) in combination:

- learning disability (mental handicap)
- specific developmental language delay and dysphasia
- autism
- hearing impairment
- elective mutism.
- very severe sensory deprivation.

3.2.4 LANGUAGE DELAY AND LEARNING DISABILITY

Children with learning disability experience language delay to roughly the same degree as the delays in other aspects of their development. Learning disability is the most common cause of significant language delay and is discussed in more detail in Section 3.3.2.

Specific developmental language delay and dysphasia

Both the DSM-IV 'communication disorders'(American Psychiatric Association 1994) and the ICD-10 'specific developmental disorders of speech and language' (World Health Organization 1992) classifications, include disturbed development not directly attributable to neurological or speech mechanism abnormalities, sensory impairments, mental retardation, or environmental factors. Both classifications divide developmental speech and language problems into articulation, expressive language, and receptive language disorders. ICD-10 includes an additional category of acquired aphasia with epilepsy (Landau–Kleffner syndrome). DSM-IV replaces the older term 'developmental articulation disorder' with 'phonological disorder' and in addition has a separate diagnostic category for stuttering.

Many children with specific language delay show immaturities in articulation, comprehension, and expression. Many are also generally learning-disabled but with their level of language development significantly below their non-verbal abilities. A few are of average or above average general intellectual ability. For example, a child may be unable to understand simple requests at a level expected for his age, and may have difficulty in naming common objects, but may be normal in other respects. However, small discrepancies between verbal and non-verbal ability are common in the first 2–3 years of life, and are usually of little significance.

Severe forms of specific language delay with particularly marked discrepancy between non-verbal and verbal ability, are often classified as forms of dysphasia, especially if the child is of average or above average general ability. Such dysphasias may be mainly sensory or mainly expressive in nature. In sensory dysphasias the child will not understand spoken language despite the presence of normal hearing (as assessed by special investigations), and will show well developed ability in non-verbal skills. Spontaneous speech is usually very limited.

In expressive dysphasia the child's hearing and understanding of speech is normal or near normal, but expressive ability is severely deficient.

Background factors

Significant specific language delay with or without associated learning disability is present in about 6–8% of 3 year old children (Silva *et al.* 1987). Developmental expressive language delay not associated with learning disability occurs in about 5–6 per 1000 children. It is two to three times as common in boys as in girls. There is a strong association with family size, social class, and the presence of emotional and behavioural disorders (Stevenson and Richman 1976). There is often a family history of similar delay. Severe, pure receptive dysphasia occurs in a much smaller proportion (about 1 per 10 000 children). Other forms of dysphasia are also rare. There is no specific association between dysphasia and social class.

Aetiology

Specific developmental language delay is usually caused by a combination of polygenic inheritance and poor quality of language environment.

Dysphasias may be congenital (present from birth) or acquired. Congenital dysphasias are usually genetically determined, and often a family history can be obtained in these instances. They may be secondary to perinatal birth trauma or severe hearing loss. Acquired dysphasias arise from brain trauma (usually sustained in a road traffic accident), cerebral infection, or cerebrovascular accident. Chronic receptive dysphasia may also arise following, or in association with, a cluster of epileptic seizures—the Landau–Kleffner syndrome (Mouridsen 1995).

Management

Children with developmental language delay often show multiple signs of deprivation and behavioural disturbance. Action to improve the social circumstances of the family should be taken if possible. Improved housing conditions and establishment of the right to financial benefit may result in a better environment for language stimulation.

If a child appears to be relatively neglected at home, other measures to improve the quality of care should be taken. Basic advice to parents, for example on ways to open up conversation with their children, may be helpful. Responding to the child's comments in ways that open rather than close the way to further communication should be encouraged, as should labelling and talking about everyday activities. Special time should, if possible, be set aside for play. Parents should be encouraged to let the child help with domestic activities and to talk with the child while these are going on. Particular patience is required in trying to understand a child with language delay and in helping him cope with the frustration of not being understood. Sibs and peers may be less patient than parents and this may lead the child to develop behavioural problems arising out of his inability to communicate effectively. Placement in a playgroup or nursery school may be helpful if the child is ready to separate, and the facility should be selected to ensure the curriculum is directed towards promoting language development.

More severely language-delayed children will benefit from advice and sometimes treatment from a speech and language therapist. Individual or group sessions may be helpful. However, of at least equal value is specific instruction given by therapists to parents and teachers on how to develop a particular aspect of verbal comprehension, achieve more effective social use of language or how to practice a particular sound, etc.

A few severely language-disabled children may benefit from special schooling specifically designed to meet the educational needs of children with language and communication problems who are of average or above-average intelligence. Such specialized schooling may be needed from early on or may only be considered necessary once less specialized educational measures have proved inadequate. Specialist speech and language units now exist in most local education authorities and complement educational units for young children with extremely poor or abnormal communication skills. These often take a mixture of children with autistic spectrum disorders, learning disabilities, and specific language delays. Repeated evaluation of language skills and hearing is required to ensure continued appropriateness of intervention packages.

Prognosis

Mild specific language delay has a good outlook, with most children catching up. More severely delayed children, in particular those with only a few words by 3 years, are at high risk for later behavioural and educational difficulties (Richman *et al.* 1982). Many of these will require special education. Problems include continuing language delay, specific reading difficulties, anxiety disorders, social relationship problems, and attentional deficits. The prognosis is worse for those with a lower level of intellectual functioning and for those with receptive rather than purely expressive problems. The prognosis for children with dysphasia is variable. Many will be chronically disabled by their language delay with later reading and writing difficulties. Acquired dysphasias can have a better outcome, with marked improvement occurring through the first 2 years after brain insult.

Hearing impairment

Hearing impairment arising from chronic recurrent suppurative or secretory otitis media is a very common cause of mild language delay and speech immaturity.

Differential diagnosis

The differential diagnosis of language delay involves five conditions: learning disability, specific developmental language delay, hearing impairment, autism, and selective mutism. These can occur in combination. Assessment requires careful history-taking and observation with particular attention paid to non-verbal abilities, responses to sounds, use of gesture, and other non-verbal means

Table 3.2 Differential diagnosis of language delay

	Learning disability	Specific developmental language delay	Deafness	Austism	Elective mutism
Non-verbal ability	Poor—similar to verbal ability	Average or above average	Average or above average	Average or below average	Average
Response to sounds	Normal for developmental level	Normal	Absent or poor	Variable	Normal
Use of gesture	Present	Present	Markedly present	Absent or impaired	Present
Neologisms and echolalia	Absent or transient	Absent or transient	Absent	Present	Present
Variability in language use	Absent	Absent	Absent	Present	Present
Speech intonation	Normal or immature	Often immature	Abnormal	Abnormal	Variable

of communication, presence of neologisms and echolalia, variability in language use, and the child's speech intonation (see Table 3.2).

3.2.5 DISORDERS OF SPEECH PRODUCTION

Articulation and phonological impairment (dyslalia)

Problems of articulation and phonological impairment involve immaturity of speech production. They are also characteristic of children who have developmental language delay. Some consonants, such as **b**, **d**, and **m**, are characteristically clearly pronounced early. Others, such as **s** and **r**, are developed later. Blends such as **sk**, **fl**, and **br** are harder to produce than single consonants. A child might omit or substitute consonants and will consequently be difficult to understand. If this occurs with only one or maybe two particular consonants, the child is said to have an articulation disorder (such as a lisp where **th** is substituted for **s**). If this occurs in isolation from a specific language delay the condition has a good prognosis. Advice from a speech and language therapist should be sought if the child is conscious of and worried about his articulation.

When lack of intelligibility is caused by the omission or substitution of a variety of speech sounds, it is possible that one or more immature phonological processes are operating. These include 'fronting', 'backing', 'velarization', and 'syllable harmony'. The child is then said to have a phonological impairment—a condition which is often linked with specific language delay and which will require assessment and advice from a speech and language therapist.

Stammering (stuttering)

Stammering involves hesitation, repetition, and prolongation of sound with word-blocking. Loose repetition of sounds and words is relatively common in the pre-school period and almost invariably starts around the age of 3–4 years, when it is termed 'normal non-fluency'. Around 3% of children are affected. It is about twice as common in boys than in girls. Mild speech hesitancies remain common in to middle childhood.

Genetic factors may be of importance in causation. Stammering tends to run in families in a manner suggesting polygenic inheritance. No specific adverse child-rearing practices have been clearly identified as being associated. However, it is thought that a family history of stammering may predispose parents to react differentially to their young child's normal dysfluency which may, in turn, result in the establishment of a true stammer. Stammering has been said to be linked to poorly established cerebral dominance and to attempts to convert left-handed children to right-handedness. However, there is no good evidence for this. Also, in countries where all left-handed children are persuaded to use their right hands, there does not seem to be an increased rate. Stammering is not particularly associated with emotional disorder, and, when severe, may lead to great anxiety and distress.

Management

Parents with young children who have mild or moderate forms of stammering should be encouraged to ignore it, to respond to the content rather than the form of their child's communication, to allow the child extra time and space for communication, and most importantly to avoid telling the child not to do it or punishing the child. This may prove difficult for older siblings and other children who may tease the stammering child mercilessly. Self-consciousness about the stammer with associated anxiety is the main cause of its perpetuation. Stopping thinking about the problem, and reducing the associated anxiety, help it go away. Any associated emotional or behavioural problems should, of course, not be ignored. Dealing with these effectively while ignoring the stammering will be additionally helpful.

Stammering occasionally persists beyond 5 years of age and is associated with movements of the face and other body parts. If at least moderately severe, special techniques applied by psychologists and speech and language therapists may help, even if they do not eradicate the problem. These techniques include the use of relaxation, speech and breathing techniques, and counselling. Haloperidol and pimozide may produce some symptomatic improvements in adolescents who stammer, although side-effects such as sedation and parkinsonism may be a problem.

3.2.6 ELECTIVE MUTISM

Definition

Elective mutism is defined in ICD-10 (World Health Organization 1992) as being characterized by a marked, emotionally determined selectivity in speaking, such that the child demonstrates language competence in some situations but fails to speak in others. Diagnostic criteria for DSM-IV selective mutism (American Psychiatric Association 1994) are five-fold:

- persistent failure to speak in specific social situations despite speaking in others
- disturbance interferes with educational or occupational achievement or with social communication
- disturbance has lasted at least 1 month
- disturbance cannot be explained by lack of knowledge of, or comfort with, the spoken language required in social situations
- disturbance cannot be explained by embarrassment relating to a communication disorder or having a psychiatric disorder.

Clinical features

Children with elective mutism may communicate by gestures, nodding, head shaking, pulling and pushing, or occasionally by monosyllabic short utterances. There is often mild or moderate early language delay in the first 2 or 3 years. Concern is usually raised when the child starts playgroup, nursery, or school. Refusal or inability to talk becomes apparent and is usually attributed to shyness. Persistent refusal to talk suggests more serious disorder. Occasionally mutism may follow a traumatic life event (MacGregor *et al.* 1994). Children with selective mutism usually talk normally at home though there may be selectivity in whom they speak to even when there. Associated features may include:

- *Unusual personality traits.* Some children may have been persistently obstinate, self-willed, manipulative, controlling, and oppositional from early on. However, recent research suggests this is probably an uncommon pathway to mutism (Dummit *et al.* 1997). Others may be excessively shy with fear of social embarrassment. These children may also show social isolation with withdrawal, clinging, and obsessive–compulsive traits.
- *Adverse family factors.* Parents may have been overprotective in the early years. A history of parental mental ill-health can often be elicited.
- *Teasing and scapegoating* by peers
- Occasionally there is an associated *communication disorder* or general medical condition causing articulation abnormalities.
- *Anxiety disorders*, especially social phobia and avoidant disorders (Dummit *et al.* 1997).
- *Learning disability* (Klin and Volkmar 1993).

Aetiology

The child's temperament is probably of major importance. Children with selective mutism are often excessively shy and withdraw from strangers at an early age. Developmental immaturity is suggested by the early history of language delay. Increasing parental pressure on the child to speak may exacerbate obstinacy and refusal. Members of some families with a child who has selective mutism may themselves opt out of conflict by becoming silent.

Prevalence

Excessive shyness on school entry is relatively common. Almost 1% of children at school entry aged 5 years may not utter a single word after 8 weeks there (Brown and Lloyd 1975). However, nearly all are speaking normally by the end of the school year. The prevalence of clinically significant selective mutism is probably around 1 per 1000 (Kolvin and Fundudis 1981). It is found in fewer that 1% of individuals seen in mental health settings. Selective mutism is slightly more common in females than males. There is no link with social class. Intellectual ability is very variable but is usually average or low average.

Assessment

An account that a child speaks normally or nearly so at home, and has not done so at all at school for more than two terms, is pathognomonic of the condition. Milder levels of non-speaking usually reflect pathological shyness rather than selective mutism. The possibility of autism is excluded by the child showing affectionate social relationships at home and the use of gesture to express needs and to share interests at school. Deafness is usually ruled out by normal responses to sounds within the home.

Evaluation of the child's temperament and the quality of family relationships form a necessary component of assessment. Psychological and speech and language evaluation may also be useful. Assessment of the child's comprehension and expressive language and speech should be carried out. A baseline for the quantity and quality of the child's talking in different situations and with different people should be established and documented.

Treatment

A small number of initial family interviews are often helpful to clarify patterns of communication within the family and to identify the presence of special alliances (especially between mother and identified child). It may also be possible to elicit the often considerable anger experienced by both parents and child.

Behavioural methods stand the best chance of success but by no means produce consistent improvement. Positive reinforcement schedules based on rewards for increasing use of verbal exchanges should be established along with the imaginative use of tape- and video-recorders with which the child can experience rapid feedback of verbal efforts in an enjoyable fashion. Individual psychodynamic psychotherapy with mute children is not usually effective. A small body of literature supports the use of low dose selective serotonin reuptake inhibitors such as fluoxetine for serious cases which have failed to respond to the above measures (Dummit *et al.* 1996). Benefits obtained probably relate to the antianxiety and antidepressant properties of these medications. In general, a school-based multidisciplinary individualized treatment plan is required, involving the combined efforts of teachers, clinicians, and parents with home- and clinic-based interventions (Dow *et al.* 1995). Even with quite young children progress is unlikely to be sudden or dramatic but it is reasonable to aim for slow steady steps towards an increase in talking.

Outcome

Many children who do not speak in certain settings will start to do so after a few months. However, a 5–10 year follow-up of children with narrowly defined selective mutism suggested that slightly less than half improve (Kolvin and Fundudis 1981). Long-term follow-up into adulthood does not seem to have been undertaken.

3.2.7 READING AND READING RETARDATION

The process of reading involves understanding the meaning of written or printed symbols. Most children can read single, short words by the age of 6 or 7 years. By 10 or 12 years they have acquired sufficient reading ability to cope with everyday tasks such as reading a tabloid newspaper. The acquisition of reading ability is a necessary requirement for full participation in a literate society.

Development of reading ability

In order to achieve a reasonable level of reading ability, a child must be able to:

- Make perceptual discriminations, for example to discriminate between **m** and **n**, **p** and **q**, and many other similar shapes.
- Discriminate between sequences, for example to distinguish between **bad** and **dab**, and **dog** and **god**.
- Achieve transfer of information from one sensory modality to another—visual symbols must be transformed into auditory internal or spoken speech.
- Blend sounds satisfactorily: for example, articulating the word **cramps** involves five blending tasks.
- Comprehend language at the level of the written material.
- Integrate information acquired from the new reading material into an already existing knowledge store.

The acquisition of reading ability probably arises in two main ways, so that there are two routes to reading. The first, which follows the use of visual cues and benefits from their presence, is phonological. This involves the slow and painful deciphering of the single letters or common combination of letters (e.g. **th, ing**) in words along the lines described above ('letter–sound correspondence'). The second, or lexical route involves the establishment of the meaning of a passage by using a variety of other higher-order skills. In this route whole words rather than single letters are perceived. Some words less essential to understanding meaning are either very briefly scanned or not scanned at all. Most children begin by using the phonological route, but soon adopt the lexical route, only reverting to the phonological when they have difficulty in deciphering an essential word, phrase, or longer passage.

Types of reading difficulty

Standardized tests of reading ability such as the Neale (1988), the Schonell and Schonell (1950) and the Wide Range Achievement Test (WRAT) (Jastak and

Jastak 1978) allow the establishment of a child's reading age. They may be consistent with the chronological age, or above or below it. Reading skills usually correlate strongly with the child's general cognitive skills. They also depend on a number of other factors including motivation, task involvement, learning opportunities, socio-economic background, birth order, parental interest, and the school attended (Maughan and Yule 1994).

General reading backwardness

Reading difficulties are often part of a picture of a generalized delay affecting all aspects of development. Most children with such problems have mild learning disabilities and would score in the 50–70 point range on tests of intellectual ability with a fairly even profile of attainments on subtests. The correlation between reading ability and intelligence is reasonably high but not perfect, so quite a number of children with learning disabilities will be found to read somewhat above or below the level expected from their general ability. General reading backwardness shows an equal sex ratio and is associated with a wide range of developmental difficulties including motor and praxic abnormalities. It is more common in socially disadvantaged homes.

Specific reading retardation

Specific reading retardation (SRR) is defined in ICD-10 (World Health Organization 1992) as a specific and significant impairment in the development of reading skills that is not solely accounted for by mental age, sensory impairments, or inadequate schooling. Diagnostic criteria for DSM-IV reading disorder (American Psychiatric Association 1994) comprise:

- *reading achievement*, as measured by individually administered standardized tests of reading accuracy or comprehension, that is substantially *below* that expected given the person's chronological age, measured intelligence, and age-appropriate education
- *disturbance* significantly interfering with academic achievement or activities of daily living that require reading skills
- *reading difficulties* in excess of those usually associated with any sensory deficit present.

One can predict expected reading age from a child's non-verbal intelligence. Thus if a child has a non-verbal IQ of 100, then there is a high probability that he will be reading at an average level for his age. However, if a child of 10 with an IQ of 100 has a reading age of about 13–14 years, then this represents approximately two standard deviations higher than expected. Similarly a reading level of 6–7 years in the same child would be approximately two standard deviations lower than expected. Specific reading retardation is said to exist when the child's reading performance is greater than two standard deviations below the predicted reading level. These children tend to have very persistent disability (Maughan *et al.* 1985).

Attempts have been made to define a syndrome of *dyslexia* from among children with SRR. Dyslexia has been said to exist when genetic or other constitutional factors cause neuropsychological deficits leading to reading failure—the level of instruction and social background having been judged as adequate and thus insufficient to explain the reading difficulties. However, it has proved difficult, especially in younger children, to distinguish such a group from other children with specific reading retardation. One study found no support for the concept of dyslexia at age 6–7 years. However, among older participants there was support for the concept of dyslexia as a phonological deficit. Other children with SRR show their reading difficulties as a form of developmental lag (Badian 1996). A further reason for problems in delineating a group of children with SRR who have dyslexia is that the word is often used as an umbrella term for the various manifestations of reading difficulties, each of which has its own type of complex neuropsychological dysfunction (Njiokiktjien 1994). Nonetheless many clinicians still find the concept useful in individual cases as it draws attention to the child's problems and emphasizes the need for special input.

Prevalence

The rate of SRR was found to be 4% in 10 and 11 year old children in the Isle of Wight, and approximately 10% in inner London (Berger *et al.* 1975). A more recent study from Lancaster confirms the figure of approximately 4% (Lewis *et al.* 1994), and also confirms the high proportion of boys to girls (3 : 1). Large family size and overcrowding are commoner in both SRR and general reading backwardness (Rutter *et al.* 1970a).

Background features

It is especially difficult in this condition to distinguish between those background factors that are causative and those that are merely associated. It should not therefore be assumed that all the factors listed below have aetiological significance, though a number probably do.

- *Familial factors*. Reading problems are strongly familial probably because of a mixture of social and genetic factors. 35–45% of parents of an affected boy will have experienced similar difficulties compared to less than 20% of parents of an affected girl (Vogler *et al.* 1985) suggesting possible gene imprinting effects. Conversely, affected children tend to be more severely impaired when father rather than mother is the affected parent (Wolff and Melngailis 1994). Twin studies suggest that 69% of the phenotypic variation in reading ability is due to heritable influences and 13% of the variation is due to shared environmental effects (Reynolds *et al.* 1996). It may be that mild common disorders represent extremes of normal variation, while severe, but rare problems are aetiologically distinct (Plomin 1991).
- *Social factors*. The importance of large family size, overcrowding, and urban living has already been emphasized. Lack of books at home and low familial interest in reading are also important. Encouraging parents of infant

school-aged children to listen to their children reading regularly has a definite preventive effect on the development of reading problems (Hewison and Tizard 1980).

Neuropsychological deficits

- *Perceptual deficits*. Reading retarded children often have poorly developed visuospatial ability with left–right confusion. The capacity for fine auditory and visual discriminations may also be impaired. These problems create difficulties in distinguishing similar but not identical sounds and visual patterns— skills necessary for fluent reading. There is controversy as to whether being ambidextrous predisposes to SRR. Mixed eye-handedness and mixed hand-footedness are not particularly associated with reading problems and neither is left-handedness.
- *Language deficits*. Reading retarded children are often slow to speak and subsequent language development may continue to be delayed. Both comprehension and expression are likely to be affected.
- *Sensory deficits*. Episodic partial hearing loss, usually due to recurrent secretory or suppurative otitis media, may be associated with delay in reading development. However, the relevance of secretory otitis media ('glue ear') in early childhood to later language delay and reading problems is uncertain. Visual defects, such as uncorrected refractory errors, are also occasionally of significance.
- *Behavioural disorders*. Children with conduct disorders characterized by antisocial behaviour are particularly likely to show specific reading problems (Rutter *et al.* 1970a). Further, children with reading problems have a particularly high rate of conduct disorders. This vulnerability extends to emotional disorders as well (Richman *et al.* 1982). There seems to be an age effect in that younger children with backward reading tend to manifest inattentive and overactive behaviours whereas older ones show more signs of conduct disorder, and low self-esteem. Research (Smart *et al.* 1996) suggests that although behaviour problems may exacerbate reading delay, there is little evidence that reading problems lead to the development of behaviour problems. Where children had reading and behaviour problems (as opposed to behaviour problems alone), the behaviours tended to be of an attention deficit hyperactivity disorder type. Sex differences were also noted. Two-thirds of reading-disabled boys had behaviour problems whereas two-thirds of reading-disabled girls did not. However, there do seem to be a number of children who fail educationally, become discouraged, and may turn to antisocial behaviour in frustration. Further, underlying impulsiveness and inattentiveness may lead to the development of both antisocial behaviour and learning problems.
- *Educational opportunity*. Children exposed to many changes of teacher, or to teachers who find it hard to maintain discipline and a positive approach to learning in their pupils, are more likely to have reading difficulties. School absence, unless prolonged, is unlikely to affect academic progress adversely in the early years of schooling.

Clinical features

- *Early identification.* Language delays, poor concentration, clumsiness, and visuospatial problems (e.g. drawing, jigsaws) are risk factors for later difficulties with learning. However, many children catch up and it is difficult to predict which children will later develop reading failure.
- *Reading retardation.* Parents may consult health professionals because of their child's failure to learn to read or because of very slow progress. The main purpose of such a consultation should be to rule out underlying medical causes such as sensory impairment. Requests to confirm or exclude diagnostic categories such as dyslexia should be referred to a suitably qualified clinical or educational psychologist once the clinician has confirmed that there is some evidence for SRR.
- *Associated or secondary disorders.* Children with severe reading problems may present with somatic symptoms such as abdominal pain or headaches produced by tension or anxiety arising from their educational difficulties. Attentional deficits and overactivity may coexist with reading problems and should always be enquired after. Antisocial behaviour and associated substance abuse may mask underlying reading or other learning difficulties.

Management

The identification, assessment, and remediation of SRR is largely an educational matter. However, health professionals are appropriately involved in a number of ways:

- *Early identification.* Child health surveillance procedures should identify individuals with early language delays and reading difficulties. Such information must be transmitted to school teachers so that the child can receive extra attention as early as possible.
- *Later identification.* Children presenting with physical or emotional problems, or later speech and language difficulties, may have underlying serious educational failure. Again teachers need to be alerted to such problems and educational psychology referral made if appropriate.
- *Assessing medical and psychiatric causes of learning failure.* Children who are failing to learn satisfactorily deserve a full medical assessment including careful checks of vision and hearing. Handedness should be established. General and specific tests of attainment, including tests of motor clumsiness and visuospatial ability, may be better undertaken as part of a comprehensive evaluation by a clinical or educational psychologist. Stressful factors (acute or chronic) in the home, neighbourhood and school should be tactfully enquired after as these often exacerbate tendencies towards learning problems. Associated psychiatric disorder should lead to appropriate referral and treatment.
- *Remediation.* The treatment of specific reading retardation is an educational matter unless there are associated medical (including psychiatric) problems. Systematic specialist educational assessment followed by small-group tuition

with understanding of the child's linguistic strengths and needs is essential. The sense of repeated failure and despair may require hard work over a long time by the teacher in order to build up a positive relationship with the child and to nurture a belief that he can succeed. No one approach is suitable for all children with this problem. Intensive personalized teaching with access to one-to-one tuition is most likely to be important. A popular approach is that of Reading Recovery (Clay 1985). This consists of a concentrated daily programme in the early school years with emphasis on phonological training as much as on reading *per se*.

* *Advocacy*. Doctors and other health professionals may be approached because of a child's lack of educational progress or because available remedial facilities are perceived as lacking. Enquiries regarding locally available specialist educational help, and the extent to which the child's educational needs have been assessed and are appreciated, is an important aspect of the doctor's support to the family. Parents can either be reassured that all possible reasonable steps are being taken, or can be put in touch with relevant local educational personnel and services that may be able to offer more assistance.

Outcome

Children with serious specific reading retardation are unlikely to make very rapid progress, the rate depending on the condition's initial severity, the child's general intellectual skills, and the child's social background (Maughan and Yule 1994). Given appropriate educational and other input they will usually make slow but steady progress, although most will continue to find reading difficult into adulthood. The best outcomes are obtained by children who have received support and encouragement at home, specialized attention at school, and where, in adulthood, they have found work appropriate to their personal strengths and limitations (Maughan 1995). The prognosis is similar for girls and boys.

A major aim for parents and professionals is the prevention of secondary antisocial and other problems. Guidance and support to the child and family in constructive decision-making at crucial points in the child's development are important, as is encouragement in less literacy-dependent skills such as sports and carpentry. Loss of self-esteem with consequent delinquency is a definite risk among children who are failing educationally. However, disruptive behaviour in childhood need not inevitably lead on to high rates of antisocial difficulties in adulthood.

3.3 Intelligence and learning disorders

3.3.1 INTRODUCTION

Definition

The concept of intelligence is difficult to define. It can be considered as the sum of those aspects of mental life which relate to general cognitive abilities necessary for appraising and adapting to the environment. Intelligence is often perceived as a unitary entity. However, research is increasingly clarifying different components. In particular, attention is increasingly given to the dimension of social intelligence, the capacity to demonstrate social skills. Ability levels in the various components of intelligence correlate reasonably well, and intelligence does seem to be distributed normally throughout the population. The development of intelligence is under both genetic and environmental control. However, the relative contribution of each will depend on the type of intelligence and environmental circumstances. For example, non-verbal abilities seem to be highly genetically determined whereas language aspects are largely environmental (Reznick *et al.* 1997). The mental state of parents may also be important so that, for example, boys of depressed mothers attain lower scores intellectually than those of non-depressed mothers (Sharp *et al.* 1995). The inheritance of intelligence is assumed to be polygenic, consistent with the normal population distribution. Exceptions to this general rule are specific chromosomal or genetic disorders where the specific genetic defect produces a general lowering of abilities. In western developed countries, twin and adoption studies suggest that polygenic factors contribute between 30% and 60% to the variance of intelligence. In developing countries, where environmental variations are more extreme, the genetic contribution may be smaller.

Continuity of intellectual development through childhood and into adulthood is variable. Predictive validity of testing undertaken before 5 years of age is poor, except for those with very low intellectual abilities. Predictive strength increases from 5 years onwards. This is probably the result of continuity of test material as much as genetic and environmental factors. It is important to distinguish continuity of intelligence scores as a group phenomenon from the sometimes considerable variation in an individual child's IQ as tested at different times. The relationship between IQ, educational attainment, and later occupational achievement is positive but tenuous. Highly intelligent people may perform only modestly whereas others with very average abilities may do exceptionally well. This is because of the myriad of other factors which are of major importance in achievement. These include drive, persistence, attentional skills, social abilities, inherited wealth, and useful social contacts.

3.3.2 LEARNING DISABILITY

Definition

Abnormal intellectual development may be due to slowness in development (retardation) or distortions in development, or a combination of these. One major functional consequence of intellectual impairment is learning disability (or disabilities)—a term commonly used in the UK for the problems experienced by people who would previously have been labelled as having mental handicap or mental retardation (see Turk 1996a). It is rare for intellectual functioning to be impaired to the same degree for all skills. However, where such skills are almost all significantly impaired, it is reasonable to consider the child as having learning disability or mental retardation.

A variety of synonyms have been used over time in an effort to counteract the stigma associated with intellectual impairment. Redundant categories such as imbecile, idiot, and feeble-minded were initially replaced with concepts of mental subnormality. Mental retardation is still the preferred term in the ICD-10 and DSM-IV classifications, as well as in North American clinical practice where 'learning disabilities' or 'learning difficulties' refer more to specific developmental delays such as dyslexia and dyscalculia. Pre-school children are often referred to as having 'generalized developmental delay'. Special schools and other educational services exist for children with moderate and severe learning difficulties, equivalent to IQ ranges of approximately 50–70 and less than 50 (Tables 3.3 and 3.4).

For a diagnosis of mental retardation or learning disability the developmental impairment should be global and long-term. In addition, the child's IQ should be less than approximately 70 and the child should be functionally impaired in everyday life skills. ICD and DSM classifications differ to some degree, and, as educational terminology is also different and some older terms persist, it is not surprising that confusion commonly occurs (see Table 3.3). Mild learning disability differs from more severe forms in presentation, aetiology, associated features, prevalence, appropriate management, and outcome. The distinction between the two on the basis of severity is therefore vital.

Table 3.3 Classification of learning disability by IQ

	ICD-10	DSM-IV
Mild	50–70	50–55 to approximately 70
Moderate	35–49	35–40 to 50–55
Severe	20–34	20–25 to 35–40
Profound	Below 20	Below 20 or 25

NB: Concurrent impairments in adaptive behaviour must also be present. DSM-IV defines adaptive functioning as comprising the following domains: communication, self-care, home living, social/interpersonal skills, use of community resources, self-direction, functional academic skills, work, leisure, health and safety.

Table 3.4 Education categories and IQ

Education category	IQ
Moderate learning difficulties (MLD)	50–70
Severe learning difficulties (SLD)	Below 50

NB: IQ is only one of many considerations in determining educational categorization and placement.

Clinical features

Learning disability may first be identified or suspected antenatally if there is a known family history of a specific genetic disorder which predisposes to such problems. Identification may occur immediately or soon after delivery when a condition known to be strongly associated with learning disability, such as Down syndrome, is diagnosed. Antenatal diagnosis by amniocentesis, chorionic villus sampling, or fetal blood analysis is becoming increasingly common. Biochemical population screening shortly after birth identifies nearly all children with phenyl-ketonuria and congenital hypothyroidism, allowing for the early instigation of preventive treatments. Occasionally, diagnosis may be delayed, sometimes for many years, until the consequences of generalized developmental delay become obvious.

The severity of learning disability, and sometimes underlying aetiology, will influence mode of presentation. Delayed gross motor milestones in the first year of life often indicate the presence of moderate or more severe learning disabilities. However, these are often unreliable, being influenced by familial, racial, and cultural factors. Delay in social milestones, e.g. smiling, attachment behaviour, or fear of strangers may be more informative, provided possible sensory and psychosocial reasons for such delay have been excluded. Many children with mild or moderate learning disability show normal motor development, presenting instead with speech and language delay. Deafness may be suspected because of lack of response to sounds, or lack of appropriate words or phrases at a particular age. Mild learning disability may not be detected until school entry age when the developmental delay that has been present from birth first shows itself as failure to make adequate educational progress. Learning disability occasionally arises from postnatal events such as head injury, cerebral infection, or the consequences of an intracranial space-occupying lesion. Developmental delays may only become apparent months or even years after birth. This results in frequent misattribution regarding causation which may sometimes be mistakenly regarded as organic (e.g. vaccination-induced) or psychological (e.g. birth of a sibling, parental separation). There is, however, increasing evidence for neurodevelopmental pre-programming whereby the trajectory of intellectual development is determined long before birth even though the consequences may only be shown much later. Once diagnosed the clinical features of children with learning disability will depend more especially on:

- the severity of the intellectual impairment
- associated physical and psychiatric conditions
- quality of care and education received
- aetiology of the learning disability.

Prevalence

IQ tests are designed and standardized to ensure that 2–3% of the population score in the mild learning disability range (IQ 50–70). Moderate to profound learning disability (IQ less than 50) occurs in 3–4 per 1000 children

(Abramowicz and Richardson 1975). There are more boys than girls in special schools for children with learning difficulties. This is probably largely the consequence of boys having higher rates of associated disorders, especially behaviour problems. It may also be the result of many genetically-determined learning disability syndromes being linked to the X chromosome, with boys at a developmental disadvantage because of their lack of a 'back up' healthy X chromosome. In the UK and other developed western societies mild learning disability occurs most commonly in children from low socio-economic groups. Middle-class children are under-represented in schools for children with moderate learning difficulties. Countries with less socio-economic inequality, such as Sweden, show little link between mild learning disability and social class (Hagberg *et al.* 1981). Moderate to profound learning disability is not associated with social class.

Aetiology

Mild learning disability (IQ 50–70)
Polygenic influences and multiple deprivation   Many children with mild learning disability come from deprived family backgrounds with shortcomings in the quality of parental care. There is a strong link between mild learning disability and low socio-economic status, large family size, and overcrowded housing. Overstretching of parental emotional, intellectual, and financial resources means that parents may be unable to provide a sufficiently rich language and intellectual environment to promote the child's development adequately. Parental intelligence is often below average, though only a minority of parents of children with mild learning disability will have learning disability themselves. Family and twin studies confirm that polygenic influences are of importance in the aetiology of mild learning disability. A multifactorial model of causation operates with these genetic variations interacting with environmental disadvantage. All specific causes of moderate, severe, or profound learning disability may, on occasion, produce mild learning disability if the insult to the brain is less serious. Conversely, approximately 10% of individuals with moderate, severe, or profound learning disability have no recognizable underlying medical condition and it is believed that this group may constitute the extreme end of the normal continuum (see Simonoff *et al.* 1996 for review). There is evidence that an increasing proportion of mild learning disability is caused by specific aetiological factors, and a lower percentage arises from polygenic influences interacting with environmental deprivation. This also occurs in developed countries with improving social conditions (Lamont and Dennis 1988). The trend is of clinical relevance because of the increasing numbers of children with mild learning disability who have an identifiable specific medical (as opposed to polygenic or environmental) reason for their slow development. Chromosomal abnormalities, especially Down syndrome and fragile X syndrome, and perinatal abnormalities, are the most common causes.

Other physical causes of mild learning disability include:

- *Malnutrition.* Maternal nutritional state during pregnancy affects fetal development, including development of the fetal brain. After birth, malnutrition can also cause psychological deficits or abnormal behaviour even in developed countries. Children who fail to thrive because of inadequate energy intake, especially in the first year of life, frequently show marked learning difficulties when they enter school. In developing countries malnutrition usually co-exists with infection and severe environmental deprivation. Thus the effects on mental functioning are both direct and indirect. Malnourishment exacerbates lethargy and slowness to respond to stimulation. Proneness to infection increases with increased risk of cerebral damage.

- *Toxins.* Controversy has persisted as to whether exposure to low levels of lead in the atmosphere and in dust created by vehicle exhaust is a hazard to children's mental development. Epidemiological studies carried out in the UK suggested the effect was very small or non-existent (Smith *et al.* 1983, Thomson *et al.* 1989). However, recent sophisticated meta-analysis of studies suggests a clearly significant, though still small causal association between lead exposure and children's IQ (Schwartz 1994). Lead interferes with GABA-ergic and dopaminergic neurotransmission, and it inhibits long-term potentiation in the hippocampal region of the brain. Alcohol intake in pregnancy producing the fetal alcohol syndrome is another important example of a toxin causing learning disability (Steinhausen 1995).

- *Specific trauma.* Specific physical trauma to the brain, for example perinatally or through a road traffic accident, may impair brain function sufficiently to cause learning disability, but not to such a degree as to cause more serious problems. Postencephalitic states can also fall into this category.

- *Idiopathic.* There remain a small number of individuals with mild learning disability who come from apparently non-deprived backgrounds with no family history of learning disability and no obvious physical condition present. There remains the possibility of 'hidden' deprivation or an as yet unidentified physical cause. Sensitive history-taking is necessary in these situations as the distinction is important for future management. However, sometimes uncertainty remains even after careful evaluation.

Moderate to profound learning disability (IQ less than 50)

The great majority of children functioning at this level of intelligence (Fig. 3.1) have organic brain pathology accounting for their learning disability (Bregman and Hodapp 1991, Harris 1995). It is important to remember that organic lesions can co-exist with social neglect and that both must be checked for.

Chromosomal defects account for approximately 40% of moderate or more severe learning disability.

- *Down syndrome* (trisomy 21) accounts for about three-quarters of this 40%, i.e. nearly one-third of all cases of moderate to profound learning disability. Down syndrome also occurs in a mosaic form where the individual cells are a mixture of normal and trisomy 21 cells. In this instance there is a relationship between the proportion of cells demonstrating trisomy 21 and the degree of learning disability. There is reasonable evidence for a common personality and temperamental profile based on good sociability and communicativeness

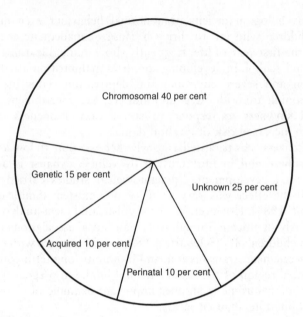

Fig. 3.1.   Causes of moderate, severe, and profound mental retardation in childhood.

with low levels of autism and hyperactivity (Gibbs and Thorpe 1983). However, autism can occasionally occur with Down syndrome and can be severe (Howlin *et al.* 1995).

- *Fragile X syndrome* accounts for approximately 10% of moderate or more severe learning disability; it is the most common inherited cause of learning disability and affects girls as well as boys despite its X-linked mode of inheritance. The degree of learning disability is very variable and there is an association with attentional deficits and with autistic-like features which often co-exist with a reasonably friendly and sociable personality (Turk *et al.* 1994).
- *Sex chromosome abnormalities. Turner syndrome* (XO) (El Abd *et al.* 1995), *Klinefelter syndrome* (XXY) (Mandoki *et al.* 1991), and other abnormalities of the sex chromosomes often manifest with levels of intelligence within the normal range. However, sometimes there are discrepancies between verbal and performance functioning, or other specific cognitive impairments. There is also evidence for an increased risk of emotional and behavioural problems (Robinson *et al.* 1983, Ratcliffe 1994).
- *Other autosomal abnormalities.* These include disorders in which there is a chromosomal deficit—e.g. *cri du chat syndrome* (Cornish and Pigram 1996), or excess—other trisomies, e.g. *Edward syndrome* (trisomy 18) and *Patau syndrome* (trisomy 13).

- *Genetic defects*. Single gene defects account for approximately 15% of moderate to profound learning disability. These are mainly metabolic disorders such as galactosaemia and phenylketonuria (Section 3.9). They exert their effects by altering the metabolism of amino acids, lipids, carbohydrates, and, rarely, other body constituents. Some endocrine disorders as well as a range of other rare genetic disorders are included in this category.
- Abnormalities of pregnancy and the perinatal period account for approximately 10% of cases:
  — infections of pregnancy such as rubella, toxoplasmosis, cytomegalovirus, herpes simplex virus, acquired immune deficiency syndrome (AIDS)
  — alcohol or drug abuse in pregnancy
  — maternal phenylketonuria
  — perinatal abnormalities, including birth trauma and postnatal hypoxia
  — neonatal disorders, including infective and metabolic conditions such as hypoglycaemia.
- *Postnatal causes* include head injury (accidental or non-accidental), cerebral or meningeal infections, severe and protracted epileptic seizures often with associated serious hypoxia, and exposure to toxins such as large quantities of ingested lead. Hypoxia causing learning disability also very occasionally follows cardiac arrest or respiratory tract obstruction, as in near-miss drowning or sudden infant death syndrome. Some endocrine and metabolic disorders (e.g. congenital hypothyroidism) may only become apparent well after birth. Medications such as anticonvulsants, sedatives, and tranquillizers can blunt cognitive functioning and concentration skills to a degree where the child may appear learning-disabled and will suffer from impaired ability to learn new material.
- *Other causes*. Approximately 25% of children with moderate to profound learning disability have no identifiable cause for their problem. In some of these children there are other signs of developmental abnormality such as deformities or organ malformations, making it likely that the learning disability has arisen from a single gene or chromosomal disorder, or as a failure of early fetal development. In others the presence of epilepsy confirms underlying cerebral abnormality. There remain some children who do not show such stigmata and indeed look perfectly normal. In the absence of a history of growth deprivation or non-accidental injury, however, it seems reasonable to assume that such children are suffering from an as yet unidentifiable organic disorder. Any unjustified assumption that such cases might be caused by covert parental neglect is likely to increase the already serious emotional burden on the family. Indeed, parents should be counselled that failure to uncover the cause for their child's problems does not imply that there is no organic cause—more, that we are not clever enough yet to work out what it is!

Table 3.5 provides information on the medical features of some different causes of learning disability.

Table 3.5 Causes and clinical features of learning disability

Syndrome	Aetiology	Clinical features	Comments
Chromosome abnormalities[a]			
Triple X	Trisomy X	No characteristic feature	Mild diminution in intellectual functioning. More severe learning disabilities with greater numbers of X chromosomes
Cri du chat	Deletion of short arm of chromosome 5	Low birth weight, slow growth, cat like cry, microcephaly, hypertelorism, epicanthic folds, abnormal palmar creases	
Inborn errors of metabolism			
Phenylketonuria	Autosomal recessive causing lack of liver phenylalaine hydroxylase. Commonest inborn error of metabolism	Lack of pigment (fair hair, blue eyes). Retarded growth. Associated epilepsy, microcephaly, eczema and hyperactivity	Detectable by postnatal screening of blood or urine. Treated by restriction of phenylalanine from the diet during early years of life. Important for expectant mothers with phenylketonuria to recommence low phenylalanine diet in order to prevent damage to foetus. Low phenylalanine diet may ameliorate behavioural problems even in those who have suffered adverse central nervous system effects.
Homocystinuria	Autosomal recessive causing lack of cystathione synthetases	Downward lens subluxation, tendency to fine sparse dry and fair hair, skeletal abnormalities similar to Marfan syndrome. Association with thromboembolic episodes	Learning disability variable. Forms responsive and non-responsive to vitamin B_6 exist. Low methionine, high cystine diet can prevent learning disability in individuals non-responsive to B_6 if begun neonatally

Galactosaemia	Autosomal recessive causing lack of galactose 1-phosphate uridyl transferase	Presents following introduction of milk into diet. Failure to thrive, hepatosplenomegaly, cataracts	Detectable by postnatal screening for the enzymic defect. Treatable by galactose-free diet. Toluidine blue test on urine
Tay-Sachs disease	Autosomal recessive resulting in increased lipid storage (the earliest form of the cerebromacular degenerations)	Progressive loss of vision and hearing. Spastic paralysis. Cherry-red spot at macula of retina. Epilepsy	Death at 2–4 years
Mucopolysaccharidoses (Bax and Colville 1995)			
Hurler:	Autosomal recessive, absence of lysosomal α-L-iduronidase	Physical features may be grotesque as in Hurler syndrome with protuberant abdomen, hepatosplenomegaly, associated cardiac abnormalities and hirsutism. Hearing problem, language difficulties and general delay are common presenting features in Hunter syndrome. Behaviour problems frequent in the Sanfilippo syndrome	Life expectancy highly variable. Death before adolescence is the rule in Hurler syndrome. Other conditions are compatible with more normal life spans
Hunter:	X-linked, deficiency of iduronate sulfatase		
Morquio:	Autosomal recessive, deficiency of N-acetylgalactosamine-6-sulfatase (type A) or β-galactosidase (type B)		
Sanfilippo:	Enzyme deficiencies resulting in urinary heparan sulfate excretion		

Table 3.5 (continued)

Syndrome	Aetiology	Clinical features	Comments
Lesch–Nyhan syndrome	X-linked recessive leading to enzyme defect affecting purine metabolism. Excessive uric acid production and excretion often manifesting as 'sand crystals' in urine	Often normal at birth. Development of choreoathetoid movements, scissoring position of legs and severe self-mutilation including knuckle gnawing and lip-biting	Antenatal diagnosis possible by amniotic fluid culture and enzyme level estimation. Postnatal diagnosis possible by blood or single hair root analysis. Death in second or third decade frequent from infection or renal failure. Self-mutilation extremely resistant to psychological or medical treatments
Williams syndrome (infantile hypercalcaemia)	Autosomal recessive	Learning disability and social impairments often with a superficial veneer of good social function and highly developed and articulate language (cocktail party chatter)	
Other inherited disorders Neurofibromatosis (von Recklinghausen syndrome)	Autosomal dominant inheritance	Neurofibromata, café au lait spots, vitiligo. Associated with symptoms determined by site of neurofibromata. Astrocytomas, meningioma	Learning disability in a minority. Some may have attentional deficits
Tuberous sclerosis (epiloia)	Autosomal dominant (very variable penetrance). Familial and sporadic forms	Epilepsy, facial angiofibromata, hypopigmented skin patches, shagreen skin, retinal phakomata, subungual fibromata. Associated multiple tumours in kidney, spleen and lungs. Frequent autistic features, hyperactivity and sleep disturbance	Learning disability in about 60%

Lawrence–Moon–Biedl syndrome	Autosomal recessive	Retinitis pigmentosa, polydactyly, sometimes with obesity and impaired genital function	Learning disability usually not severe
Prader–Willi syndrome	Microdeletion on long arm of paternally inherited chromosome 15	Neo-natal hypotonia and failure to thrive followed by developmental delay, hyperphagia and gross obesity with impulsive tantrums and skin-picking. Predisposition to diabetes mellitus	Over-eating and other challenging behaviours are best treated by strict behaviour modification programmes and occasionally appetite suppressants. May also arise from 'uniparental disomy' (inheritance of both chromosome 15s from mother)
Angelman syndrome	Microdeletion on long arm of maternally inherited chromosome 15	Learning disability, severe speech and language delay with autistic features, jerky ataxic gait, frequent paroxysmal laughter. Eyes often bulge, large mouth with tongue protrusion. Epilepsy common	May also arise from 'uniparental disomy' (inheritance of both chromosome 15s from father)
Infection			
Rubella embryopathy	Viral infection of mother in first trimester	Cataract, microphthalmia, deafness, microcephaly, congenital heart disease. Autistic disorders common	If mother infected in first trimester 10–15% infants are affected (infection may be subclinical)
Toxoplasmosis	Protozoal infection of mother	Hydrocephaly, microcephaly, intra-cerebral calcification, retinal damage, hepato-splenomegaly, jaundice, epilepsy	Wide variation in severity
Cytomegalovirus	Virus infection of mother	Brain damage. Only severe cases are apparent at birth	
Congenital syphilis	Syphilitic infection of mother	Many die at birth. Variable neurological signs. 'Stigmata' (Hutchinson teeth and rhagades) often absent	Uncommon since routine testing of pregnant women. Infant's Wasserman positive at first but may become negative

Table 3.5 (continued)

Syndrome	Aetiology	Clinical features	Comments
Cranial malformations			
Hydrocephalus	Sex-limited recessive inherited developmental abnormality, e.g. atresia of aqueduct, Arnold–Chiari malformation. Meningitis. Spina-bifida	Rapid enlargement of head. In early infancy, symptoms of raised CSF pressure. Other features depend on aetiology	Mild cases may arrest spontaneously. May be symptomatically treated by CSF shunt. Intelligence can be normal
Microcephaly	Recessive inheritance, irradiation in pregnancy, maternal infections	Features depend upon aetiology	Evident in up to a fifth of institutionalized individuals with learning disability
Miscellaneous			
Spina bifida	Aetiology multiple and complex	Failure of vertebral fusion Spina-bifida cystica is associated with meningocele or, in 15–20%, myelomeningocele. Latter causes spinal cord damage, with lower limb paralysis, incontinence, etc.	Hydrocephalus and learning disability in four-fifths of those with myelomeningocele. Proconceptual and antenatal folic acid preventive
Cerebral palsy	Perinatal brain damage. Strong association with permaturity	Spastic (commonest), athetoid and ataxic types. Variable in severity	Majority are below average intelligence. Athetoid are more likely to be of normal IQ. Increased prevalence of emotional and behavioural disturbances
Hypothyroidism (cretinism)	Iodine deficiency or (rarely) atrophic thyroid	Appearance normal at birth. Abnormalities appear at 6 months. Growth failure, puffy skin, lethargy	Now rare in UK. Responds to early replacement treatment
Hyperbilirubinaemia	Haemolysis, rhesus incompatibility and prematurity	Kernicterus (choreoatheotosis), opisthotonus, spasticity, convulsions	Prevention by anti-Rhesus globulin. Neonatal treatment by exchange transfusion

[a] For Down syndrome and X-linked learning disability see text.

Assessment

There are four components to assessment of the child with learning disability:

• investigation of the cause of learning disability
• identification of associated physical and psychiatric problems
• determination of level and profile of cognitive functioning
• assessment of family functioning, care, expectations, and coping capacity.

Establishing a cause

Identifying a cause for a child's learning disability may not be possible. However, it is most important to make a diagnosis wherever possible because:

• the individual and family have a basic right to know what the cause of the child's learning disability is, if this is identifiable
• awareness of a cause provides relief from uncertainty
• a physical diagnosis may give relief from guilt feelings arising from beliefs that the family and/or social factors were the cause of learning disabilities or developmental or behavioural disturbance
• the existence of a diagnostic label facilitates the bereavement process relating to having a child with learning disability, and assists in grief resolution
• it assists the family in focusing towards the future
• genetic implications become clearer and genetic counselling can be provided where appropriate
• very occasionally a treatable cause may be found, and more often knowing a cause allows for more effective multidisciplinary interventions relevant to the individual's profile of strengths and needs
• family members can, if they wish, join an appropriate support group.

In moderate to profound learning disability, the level of intellectual functioning provides important clues to aetiology. Mild learning disability rarely has an identifiable cause, although some studies have suggested that as many as 10% of children with mild learning disability of unknown aetiology could have a specific cause identified if sufficient investigations were undertaken (Thake *et al.* 1987). Moderate to profound learning disability more often has an identifiable physical cause. Some aetiologies, for example phenylketonuria, may be suspected before a birth because of a previously affected sibling. Alternatively they may be diagnosed soon after birth through population screening programmes. Antenatal amniocentesis may have diagnosed a condition sometimes linked to learning disability such as spina bifida. Physical examination at birth may reveal stigmata consistent with an obvious chromosomal abnormality such as Down syndrome. Traumatic birth, peri- or postnatal hypoxia, or hypoglycaemia may alert the clinician to the possibility of later developmental delay. Routine biochemical investigations soon after birth will reveal disturbances of amino acid metabolism such as phenylketonuria, and readily treatable endocrine disorders such as congenital hypothyroidism. Hypotonic postural abnormalities or asymmetrical movements shortly after birth should alert the clinician to possible cerebral palsy which may be associated with learning disability, as well as a greater likelihood of emotional and behavioural problems and peer relationship difficulties (Yude *et al.* 1998). Many causes of moderate to profound learning disability should therefore be established by the time the baby is a few weeks old on the basis of routine history-taking, thorough physical examination, and biochemical, genetic, and other laboratory investigations.

The remaining instances of moderate to profound learning disability will be identified as a result of increasingly evident, unusually slow development. Motor milestones, although widely documented and assessed, are relatively poor indicators of general developmental functioning. Social and language development are more sensitive markers. Affected babies are often passive and are frequently described by the parents as having been unusually 'good' babies in that they rarely cried for attention or were demanding in other ways. They lack the normal spontaneity and inquisitiveness which most babies and toddlers have, and this may raise initial suspicions of hearing or visual impairments. These need to be evaluated and may be present in association with learning disability.

All children with learning disability should be investigated in order to exclude identifiable causes. Chromosomal analysis and specific DNA testing for fragile X syndrome are the most likely investigations to produce positive findings. Plasma and urinary amino acids, skull radiograph, computed tomography or magnetic resonance imaging (if available) and viral antibody screen will rule out the most common causes. The decision whether to investigate further will depend on results of history-taking and clinical examination as well as on the availability of resources. However, if the above investigations are negative, then even the most thorough and expensive subsequent testing will uncover aetiology in only a tiny minority of cases. It must also be remembered that unnecessarily heroic efforts to identify a cause may raise unrealistic hopes and expectations in parents that an aetiology will ultimately be discovered that will lead to treatment or cure. It may also distract families and professionals from the more important issues of establishing appropriate medical, psychological, educational, and social support and interventions at an early stage.

Mild learning disability is usually suspected and subsequently investigated much later, often when children commence school and are noted to be falling behind their peers educationally. Occasionally the history and physical examination provides some clues to a specific physical cause, and further investigations can be requested as appropriate. Where no physical cause is suspected, investigation should be limited. The presence of obvious social factors such as disadvantage, neglect, or abuse may suggest non-organic aetiology. However, it must be remembered that psychosocial disadvantage can often co-exist with biological determinants so these should still be checked for. Carrying out chromosomal investigation, DNA testing for fragile X syndrome, and plasma and urinary amino acid evaluation will at the very least be reassuring to parents. Further physical investigation as described above may be justified if the major cause of the child's difficulties remains obscure, especially if the child is at the lower end of the mild learning disability range.

Identification of associated physical and psychiatric problems

Sensory disorders, especially hearing and visual defects, are very common in children with learning disability. Sight and hearing should therefore be checked carefully whenever learning disability is suspected. These checks should be repeated regularly because sensory defects may arise during the child's development, or may become more evident or more detectable. General physical and neurological examination is also necessary to identify abnormalities, deformities, or other stigmata which might give a clue to aetiology. These often require treatment in their own right. Cerebral palsy occurs in approximately 25% of children with moderate or more severe learning disability. Epilepsy is common. Episodes of altered consciousness, strange behaviour, and other attack phenomena should therefore be enquired about and investigated appropriately (Corbett 1981).

Emotional and behavioural problems are particularly common in children with learning disabilities, especially in the more seriously disabled (Bregman 1991; Kaminer *et al.* 1984). Systematic and detailed questioning to elicit the presence of such problems is therefore essential in this group so that difficulties can be determined and appropriate multidisciplinary interventions instituted at an early stage.

Certain genetic aetiologies predispose to particular psychological and psychiatric problems (O'Brien and Yule 1995; Turk and Sales 1996). Knowing the aetiology of the child's learning disability is therefore important in raising suspicions of possible psychiatric problems which should be checked for. The hyperkinetic syndrome (attention deficit hyperactivity disorder) and autistic disorders are much more common in children with learning disabilities than in the general population (Wing and Gould 1979). About 10% of moderately or more severely learning-disabled children show the hyperkinetic syndrome, and roughly the same proportion demonstrate autistic spectrum disorders (about 300 times the rate of the general population). About the same proportion (10–15%) of severely learning-disabled children show self-injurious behaviour. This tendency is aggravated by unstimulating institutional lifestyles, but it is also definitely more common in certain genetic conditions such as Lesch–Nyhan syndrome, de Lange syndrome, Smith–Magenis syndrome, Prader–Willi syndrome and fragile X syndrome (see Table 3.6).

The family's psychological functioning, and the presence of social problems should also be established. Parents and siblings are often profoundly affected psychologically and have substantial extra care and support requirements as a result of having a family member with learning disabilities, perhaps associated with challenging behaviour (Turk 1996a; Tunali and Power 1993; Gath and Gumley 1987). The clinician must try to determine whether the child with learning disability is being neglected or inadequately stimulated, either deliberately or by default, because of familial distress, depression, exhaustion, or 'burnout'. Advice from a social worker can be invaluable here.

Determination of level and profile of functioning

Multiple aspects of the child's functioning require detailed evaluation: general intelligence, speech and language, gross and fine motor development, attentional

Table 3.6 Genetic conditions with associated self-injurious tendencies

Syndrome	Nature of self injury
Lesch–Nyhan syndrome (Nyhan 1972)	Knuckle gnawing, hand-biting, lip-biting
de Lange syndrome (Johnson *et al.* 1976)	Lip-biting, head-banging
Fragile X syndrome (Turk *et al.* 1994)	Hand-biting, especially at the base of thumb ('anatomical snuff box') usually in response to anxiety or excitement
Prader–Willi syndrome (Dykens and Cassidy 1995)	Skin-picking and scratching
Smith–Magenis syndrome (Colley *et al.* 1990)	Head-banging, nail pulling, object insertion into orifices

skills, and social and personal development. The child with generalized learning disability will need assessment in all these different areas.

An experienced clinician with a small amount of available equipment will be able to make a reasonably accurate assessment of a child's developmental level in each of these areas. More precise estimates can be obtained by the application of standardized developmental or psychological tests, or an instrument more specifically designed for this purpose.

The decision whether or not to refer a child to a psychologist will depend largely on local practice and availability of psychological time. In theory, any child who might benefit from specialist advice on education or the promotion of development should be referred. In practice, it is desirable to refer all children in need of, or likely to need, special schooling. As a rough guide this would include all 2 year olds functioning at less than a 15 month level, all 3 year olds functioning at less than a 2 year level, all 4 year olds functioning at less than a $2\frac{1}{2}$ year level, and all 5 year olds functioning at less than a $3\frac{1}{2}$ year level. Some of these will not, in fact, require special schooling, but there is a high enough risk to justify referral.

The child's level of functioning in daily life skills is at least as important as an assessment of ability on standardized tests. Some children who appear very slow on testing are capable of a much higher level of functioning and vice versa. Parents should be asked about what their child can and cannot do, using a standardized developmental assessment sheet such as the Denver Developmental Screening Test (Frankenburg *et al.* 1975).

Assessment is not a once-for-all exercise. Children with developmental delay require regular monitoring of progress. The aetiology of the condition may give clues to the pattern of development that may be expected. For example, children with fragile X syndrome, despite having learning disabilities, tend to develop cognitively at a rate parallel to their non-learning-disabled peers until adolescence when the discrepancy widens (Dykens *et al.* 1989). This is attributable to specific problems with the processing of *sequences* of information (in contrast to simultaneous information processing) being increasingly required as development progresses.

Family care, expectations, and coping capacity

Useful information about the quality of parental care provided will be given by the way in which parents speak of the child, dress, and undress him, and answer questions about the way the child responds to being talked to and played with. Parental expectations regarding the child's future development should also be assessed by asking questions about how they think the child is doing compared to other children of similar age and backgrounds, and how they think the child will develop over time. A major source of familial difficulty is a mismatch between the child's abilities and potential, and parental perceptions of what the child is and will be capable of.

The parent's coping capacities are of major importance in relation to future management. At initial assessment these will often be quite uncertain. One should never underestimate the enormous and life-long burden of raising a child with severe developmental delay. Parents can rightly feel affronted by professionals who seem to believe they have an infinite capacity for coping and psychological stability in the face of overwhelming care needs and challenging behaviour. Nevertheless, with time, it is possible to work collaboratively with parents to consider the extent to which they can cope with the multiple and intense demands of their child's developmental difficulties. The nurturing of a strong and supportive relationship between professional and family is essential for discussion of such sensitive issues as to whether parents feel they can ultimately cope with such demands or whether the child would receive more appropriate support and care elsewhere. The most vulnerable families are likely to be those experiencing multiple stresses, or where there have been relationship difficulties prior to the birth of the affected child (Byrne and Cunningham 1985). Much which has been written on the psychosocial aspects of chronic physical disorder is relevant to families of children with learning disability (see Chapter 7).

Management

Important components of management include:

- breaking the news
- counselling on promotion of development
- dealing with associated disabilities and behaviour problems
- advising on appropriate education
- genetic counselling
- providing social and emotional support.

Breaking the news

Imparting information to parents about the nature, likely causes, and likely further developments of their child who has learning disability is one of the most difficult tasks for the clinician. Even allowing for faulty memory, parental reports obtained after the event suggest that it is still often badly done, but that a thoughtful and systematic approach can markedly reduce the rate of dissatisfaction (Cunningham *et al.* 1984). Where the condition is diagnosed immediately or shortly after birth, it is important for the news to be broken as soon as possible to both parents with the affected baby present in the room. This is a critical time which the parents will remember. It is therefore important that it should be undertaken by the most senior professional, usually the consultant paediatrician, accompanied by other relevant staff who will be involved in follow-up, such as junior doctors and the health visitor. The interview should be planned in advance and conducted in privacy without fear of interruption, and sufficient time should be set aside for it. Written information should be provided at the end of the interview. Its content should be considered carefully. Many syndrome support groups now provide excellent pamphlets outlining the nature and implications of the condition. Giving a recent scientific paper will usually be less satisfactory, as this may be jargon-ridden or almost impossible to understand, and may instil fear because of stark descriptions of the most serious problems likely to occur. A subsequent meeting between family and paediatrician should be arranged for a day or so after initial disclosure in order to repeat the information imparted and to provide the family with an opportunity to ask questions. Towards this end the family should be encouraged to make written notes of any questions which come to mind in order to combat the risk of their mind going blank upon meeting with the professionals. Close liaison between hospital specialists, community midwife, health visitor, and general practitioner should continue over the ensuing months to ensure further support, advice, and counselling.

Counselling for parents who have a child with a recently identified learning disability covers a number of aspects, psychoeducational and psychotherapeutic. Psychoeducational aspects include genetic counselling during which information on the child's condition (if present) and likely implications for the child in the future, and for future parental pregnancies, can be imparted. A difficulty here is that parents often go into genetic counselling expecting a clear statement about the consequences of their child's genetic disorder and clear advice regarding further pregnancies. In reality, knowledge about these aspects is often severely limited, leading to further uncertainty. However, there is an increasing number of conditions where much is known about likely developmental progress and likely behavioural and other challenges to be faced. In these instances it does seem that the early imparting of information is useful in preparing parents to deal with these later challenges. It does not appear to lead to the development of 'self-fulfilling prophecies', and can be helpful in the prevention of avoidable secondary developmental and psychiatric handicaps in children with long-term incurable developmental disabilities (Turk 1996b). Psychotherapeutic aspects of counselling can be further subdivided into directive and non-directive approaches. Non-directive counselling consists of sympathetic and supportive listening, with clarification of feelings and problems in a warm, genuine, empathic, and non-judgemental fashion. The aim should be to facilitate the family's task in reflecting on their predicament and in developing their own perspective of their situation and how best to cope with it. The clinician should make efforts to try to understand exactly how the family must be feeling rather than merely expressing concern. Giving the family time to express their feelings, and even tolerating moments of quiet in a consultation ('meaningful silences') are important. However, discussion and psychotherapeutic counselling must be directive as well—moving the family towards practical solutions to their problems by means of methodical problem-solving approaches whereby pathways to potential solutions to the difficulties they will face can be clarified and tested out (Turk 1996a).

There are a number of specific aspects to breaking bad news and counselling of families which require particular consideration.

- Parents quite understandably often request information on the 'cause' of their child's problems. They may be requesting information on the underlying aetiology (e.g. Down syndrome or fragile X syndrome). Alternatively, they may be searching for insight about the cause of the particular problem, e.g. challenging behaviour which has triggered the current consultation. The doctor will often be mainly interested in identifying aetiology. Failure to diagnose an organic condition may lead to erroneous suggestions that there is 'nothing wrong with the child' or that 'we cannot find any problem' or 'all the tests are negative'. It may be true that even where a cause is discovered it frequently does not significantly influence management. Even so, parents are usually aware of this and are searching for something else—the basic human need to gain further understanding of why things are the way they are. The possession of bad news is usually better than the uncertainty of no news at all. Indeed, the saddest families are often those where no cause is ever discovered for their child's disability. The clinician must therefore be careful to emphasize that failure to identify an underlying cause is very different from suggesting that there is no cause or even that there is no serious problem.
- Parents usually have some idea what is wrong with their child before they are seen. It is always helpful to discover 'where they are at' in their understanding and expectations of their child's condition. It is, for example, useful to ask them what sort of age they think their child has reached as far as his functioning is concerned. They may have known a similar child, read a relevant book, seen a relevant video or film, etc.
- Information is poorly absorbed and only partially retained when parents are anxious and upset. They need repeated opportunities to ask questions and to check out their own level of understanding.
- Communication that 'nothing can be done' for a child with learning disability is untrue and misleading. There may indeed be no medical cure, but parents should be encouraged to believe that there is a great deal that can be done. It is useful to have some clear ideas of the positive steps that parents, often with the help of teachers, doctors, psychologists, and other professionals can take to promote development and minimize associated physical, behavioural, and social problems.
- Many people may be involved in imparting information about a child with developmental delay. They may include the health visitor, midwife, paediatrician, general practitioner, social worker, clinical medical officer, and teacher. Whoever is involved must check out with parents what they have previously been told and by whom before imparting their own views. If a

professional provides different information from that previously given, it is important to indicate that it is not unusual for professionals to hold varying views and, in the end, the parents, who are the only real experts in their own child's development, have to work out for themselves what the real nature of the problem is. Efforts to maximize free and frequent communication between professionals will do much to prevent different information being provided unintentionally. Many parents are confused by the complexity of the organizations providing services, and there are considerable advantages if the professionals involved can agree on a 'link-person' who can take responsibility for imparting and sharing information with the family, co-ordinating services, and explaining their delivery to the family.

• Parents will want to share the information provided with relatives and friends. They may lack the skills to do this, and it is helpful to ask if they feel confident about it, and, if not, whether they would like to rehearse it. This also provides an opportunity to check the accuracy of their understanding. An offer to meet with family and friends at least once is often welcomed enthusiastically by parents. They then feel confident that they are not conveying misinformation.

• Parents faced with painful knowledge react in a variety of ways. Most are able to absorb the knowledge, cope with the loss of the normal child they had hoped to bring up, and get on with rearing the child they do have as best they can. A minority are persistently angry, depressed, unrealistic, inappropriately guilty, or show other, more complex reactions. The management of such reactions is discussed in more detail in connection with parents of the physically handicapped in Chapter 7. There is good evidence that parents of a newly diagnosed child with learning disability go through a similar set of emotional reactions to individuals suffering bereavement reactions. In this instance it is the parental grief for the anticipated normal child which never materialized, and the need to adjust to the less than perfect child they now have. Many parents labelled 'difficult', 'demanding', or 'neurotic' are probably experiencing pronounced grief reactions which can be helped by acknowledgement of what they are going through, with reassurance that their reactions are not abnormal—more that they are reacting normally and understandably to an abnormal situation. Grief recurs at times in the child's and family's development when events occur which remind parents of their differences from others, for example when their child has to receive a statement of special educational need or go to a special school, or a younger sibling overtakes the learning-disabled child developmentally. These episodes of chronic sorrow are common and often missed. A fluctuating course of familial adjustment with negligible improvement is often the rule. Professionals tend to underestimate these later stressful experiences while overestimating the initial stress at the time of diagnosis (Wikler *et al.* 1981).

• All parents want to know what is ultimately going to happen to their learning-disabled child. As the child gets older, the future becomes more certain, but, in the pre-school period, unless the child is profoundly disabled, it is often quite uncertain how well a child will develop later. In general, and there will be exceptions, parents should be encouraged to look no more than 3 or 4 years ahead at a time until the child reaches teenage, when planning for a longer span of post-school life becomes appropriate.

• In considering outcome, parents often want to know whether a child will 'catch up'. Figure 3.2a, although very simple, may be found helpful in explaining why it is that children appear to fall further and further behind normal children, even though they acquire new skills each year. If a learning-disabled child has a sibling, say a couple of years younger, the modification shown in Fig. 3.2b may be helpful.

If the diagram in Fig. 3.2b is drawn, it is important to point out that the line drawn for the retarded child will be affected to some degree by his particular pattern of development, and by the quality of home care and education he gets. The lines drawn are only a rough guide to development. Further, it is important to say that development can be expected to continue, albeit at a slow rate, into the late teenage period and early adulthood. Indeed development may continue well into adult life, and this is reflected by the statutory provision of school education until 19 rather than 16 years for children with special educational needs, and by the presence of adult training centres and colleges of further education thereafter. However, overoptimistic predictions can be as damaging as overnegative views, if not more so (Carr 1985). The clinician must make it clear, as sympathetically as possible,

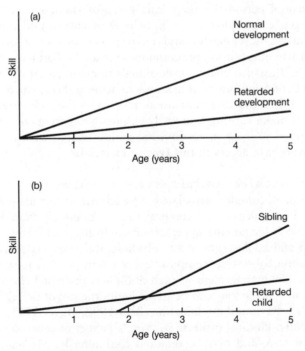

Fig. 3.2. Simple graphs of normal and retarded development.

that although the child will indeed make progress, the rate is likely to be very slow and the final level of intellectual functioning will fall well short of that of the general population. This message is important in order to avoid unrealistic parental hopes and expectations.

• If the learning-disabled child is present, it should not be forgotten that he may be capable of understanding much that is being discussed and will almost certainly have taken in the 'emotional atmosphere'. In these circumstances the child should be included in the consultation, though at a level the child can comprehend. Many young people with learning disabilities are able to understand information about their condition which can be invaluable in helping their own emotional and practical adjustment.

Counselling on the promotion of development
Children with learning disabilities take longer to learn new material and, once they have learned something new, they usually forget more easily than do ordinary children. Consequently they need more help, and more systematic help from parents, teachers, and others in the acquisition of skills. In particular, they often fail to learn by observation, and therefore need more structured teaching.

This help needs to be provided at an appropriate level for the child. It is worse than useless to try and teach skills too far ahead of the child's existing level, so parents should, for example, be discouraged from trying to teach their children to read when they cannot discriminate simple shapes or label common objects correctly.

In the pre-school period the main role for professionals such as teachers, speech and language therapists, etc. is in helping parents to find ways to stimulate their children's development and interest in constructive activities. The availability of early intervention programmes such as the Portage scheme (Revill and Blunden 1979), which enable professionals to guide parents in setting realistic targets and choosing practical methods to achieve them, has done much to help parents feel they can carry out useful tasks with their children. Clinicians should therefore make sure that, as early as possible, parents of children with learning disabilities are put in touch with professionals such as teachers and psychologists who have access to this type of material.

Dealing with associated deficits and behavioural problems
As already indicated, common associated physical deficits include impairment of vision and hearing, epilepsy, and cerebral palsy. Commonly linked psychiatric deficits (Turk 1997) include the hyperkinetic syndrome, and infantile autism. In later childhood and adolescence, other psychological and psychiatric problems such as aggression, obsessive–compulsive behaviour, and depression become more prevalent. The management of each of these is discussed elsewhere in this book. Self-injurious behaviour can be treated with the use of protective devices, medication, and behavioural modification (Blair 1992, Oliver 1995), though not always successfully. Physical protection, using a helmet or other device, is often a necessary first step, and may be required continuously. Medication, though widely used, is often ineffective and commonly produces undesirable side-effects,

especially oversedation. However, neuroleptic medication does sometimes have a useful role to play in this condition as do selective serotonin reuptake inhibitors (Garber *et al.* 1992) and opiate antagonists such as naltrexone (Winchel and Stanley 1991). Medication needs careful monitoring if it is not to have prolonged and possibly irreversible side-effects. Particularly in institutionalized children, but also in those living at home, whatever may have been the original reason for prescribing drugs, there are risks of children remaining on medication for years, sometimes with multiple drug combinations, long after there is evidence for their effectiveness. Behavioural therapies (Section 9.2.1), especially differential reinforcement of other more positive behaviour and extinction, have probably had greater success, but put more demands on staff. Gains are often difficult to generalize to different settings, and the programmes often have to be continued indefinitely.

Children with learning disabilities are not only prone to the development of psychiatric syndromes such as autism, the hyperkinetic disorder, and self-injurious behaviour but also show an excess of the commoner behavioural and emotional problems seen in children and young people. Assessment and treatment in these cases should follow similar lines to that in children with more normal intelligence. Having learning disabilities is no longer seen as a contraindication for psychotherapeutic procedures. They can be helpfully applied at least in the mildly and moderately learning-disabled group. Psychotherapeutic techniques similar to those used with younger children of the same mental age can be readily applied to children with learning disabilities.

Advising on appropriate education
Decisions on appropriate education should be taken by teachers, educational psychologists, and other educational professionals in active collaboration with parents. Clinicians will very often need to provide advice to enable sensible decisions to be made. In the UK such advice is formally sought when a full assessment is made for a child with special education needs. However, it is desirable to provide information before this stage is reached. The clinician will be expected to provide information on medical matters such as the need for medication, physiotherapy, hearing aids, spectacles, etc. In addition, the clinician's observation of the child's attention span, persistence, level of activity, capacity to form relationships, language and communication skills, etc. will enable useful suggestions to be made about whether the child has a particular need for individual attention, or for a more or less structured setting.

The clinician must make clear to parents that he does not have responsibility for final decisions on education, but only for advising the education authority. It is usually unwise to say that a particular named school would be best for a child, but if a clinician has a view about this, then mention can be made of the school in the report to the authority as a possible placement. Medical reports to education authorities are made available for parents to see either in full or abstract form, so it is sensible to tell parents what it is intended to put in a report before it is written, or to give them a copy.

Once the child is placed in a particular school, any change in the child's medical and psychiatric management needs to be made known to the school either directly to the head teacher or via the school doctor.

Genetic counselling

All parents should receive information about the risks involved if they have further children, even if it is improbable that they will. Further, if the learning-disabled child has siblings, parents should be encouraged to discuss the genetic implications with their normal children for their own progeny once they reach their mid-teens. The extended family will also need to be contacted and possibly screened for asymptomatic carrier status for various disorders. In most cases such information can be reassuring. If it is not provided, there is a likelihood that unnecessary anxiety will be experienced, and that it will be more difficult for parents to make valid and informed choices whether to have children or to undergo specific antenatal tests.

The risks involved in some common conditions for further full siblings of the learning-disabled child and for the children of full siblings are shown in Table 3.7. The figures in Table 3.7 may need to be modified if there are special features present (e.g. if there is a further learning-disabled person in the family, the child has an atypical form of the condition, etc.). In these cases, in particular, specialist genetic advice is highly desirable.

Risks involved in less common conditions and principles of genetic counselling including specialized techniques for antenatal diagnosis are described in detail elsewhere (Gardner and Sutherland 1996).

Providing social and emotional support

Parents with learning-disabled children will usually obtain emotional support from a variety of sources, but especially from relations, friends, neighbours,

Table 3.7 Genetic risk for conditions associated with learning disability (was d)

Condition	Risk (%)	
	Further full siblings of the child with learning disabilities	Children of full siblings of the child with learning disabilities
Down syndrome (trisomy 21)	1% (NB: risk increases with increasing maternal age)	As in general population
Down syndrome (translocation type)	2–10% if parent a carrier	As in general population (if not a carrier)
Phenylketonuria	25%	As in general population
Fragile X syndrome	50% (boys more likely to be affected, girls more likely to be unaffected carriers, but both can have learning disabilities)	50% if mother a carrier
Unidentified cause	4%	As in general population

health visitors, social workers, and, as the child gets older, teachers. Health professionals and those working with them such as hospital social workers can provide valuable support and, in some cases, the help they give in this respect can be crucial to maintaining family unity and facilitating familial adaptation to their new circumstances.

Parents often feel a special relationship with the clinician who made the original diagnosis and wish to return to him for help when subsequent crises arise. Some paediatricians, clinical medical officers, and psychiatrists make a practice of offering parents of children with moderate to profound learning disabilities regular annual appointments to review the child's progress. They can offer encouragement despite the fact that often any progress has been painfully slow. Such a review, which may form part of a monitoring of the special education that the child is receiving, also provides an opportunity to check the possibility that further assessment and treatment of associated deficits (e.g. hearing, vision), are required. The child may have developed new problems (e.g. behavioural difficulties) or be entering a new phase of life (e.g. puberty) which raises fresh anxieties in the parents and new challenges to be confronted and overcome. Problems may arise not only in the handicapped child but also in other members of the family, such as the child's siblings (Gath 1989). Again review appointments offer an opportunity for counselling and, where necessary, appropriate referral.

Many of the principles mentioned in relation to the counselling of parents of children with chronic physical handicap are also relevant in connection with parents of the mentally handicapped.

3.3.3 GIFTED CHILDREN

Definition

Children with unusual intellectual gifts fall into three main categories:

- Those with high measured intelligence. It is generally accepted that an IQ of over 140 on one of the standardized tests such as the Wechsler Intelligence Scale for Children marks a child out as having unusual all-round ability.
- Children of any level of general intellectual ability with an unusually well-developed isolated gift, for example in mathematics or music. Children with unusual athletic ability, who undergo prolonged periods of intensive training, share many features with this group.
- Children with learning disabilities who have one or two exceptional, isolated capacities, for example for complicated computation, drawing, or musical skills. These are referred to as 'idiots savants' and some, but not all, are autistic. However, most people with autism do not show such unusually highly developed islets of ability.

Psychiatric aspects

Contrary to popular belief, highly intelligent children have either the same or somewhat lower rates of behavioural and emotional problems than do children in the general population (Freeman 1983). There is no good evidence for the view that is sometimes stated that gifted children have particularly low needs for sleep and are prone to overactivity. They are likely to be active, inquisitive children with bright, intellectual parents, but not all fit this stereotype. When they do have problems, these may be related or unrelated to their giftedness. Related problems include boredom at school (sometimes leading to behavioural problems there), due to an inappropriate curriculum or teachers failing to recognize a child's special capacities, or frustration at the lack of intellectual stimulation. Parents who are told that their children are gifted may develop unrealistic expectations about their performance. Although a minority do become very high achievers academically, most gifted children do not become gifted adolescents or adults and this often leads to disappointment and bitterness towards education services which are seen as having let the child down. Social isolation, arising because of the child being set apart from others less talented, may also be a problem.

Emotional problems unrelated to the giftedness are more common in this group. Parental marital disharmony and maternal depression are among the most common features.

The management of problems related to giftedness is largely educational. Most young gifted children can be well educated in ordinary schools, provided special attention is given to their curriculum and social needs. A variety of enrichment and accelerating educational strategies can be used for exceptionally able pupils (Cohn 1988). A minority thrive better in schools (e.g. music schools) in which their special capacities can be nurtured. Problems arising from factors other than the giftedness can be dealt with as in the non-gifted group with family or individual assessment and treatment.

3.4 Attention and attention deficit hyperactivity (hyperkinetic) disorder

3.4.1 DEVELOPMENT OF NORMAL ATTENTION

The development of attention follows a characteristic pattern throughout childhood. Newborn babies are equipped to pay attention to certain kinds of stimuli rather than others. Thus they will selectively attend to moving objects more than stationary ones, to intermittent rather than monotonous tones, and, within the first few weeks, to a picture of a human face rather than a picture of a jumble of facial features. The development of attention is characterized by change along a number of dimensions.

- *Exploration.* The attention of infants and toddlers is dominated by features of the environment. The young child is highly exploratory and, above all, his attention is captured by novel stimuli he has not met before. As he gets older, the nature of the child's environment and what is happening in it becomes less important, and the child's attention becomes more related to a preconceived internal plan or intention. Relatively undirected exploration is replaced by more systematic searching. The child's scanning of the environment becomes increasingly logical, systematic, active, exhaustive, and organized.

- *Search.* A child's tendency to search for certain features in his environment is affected by his needs and motivation. These aspects therefore become increasingly important to his attention span. Success in searching will often be rewarded, so that his capacity to attend will be reinforced and thus lengthened.
- *Distraction.* A feature of the young child's attention to novelty is that he remains open to distracting stimuli. As children get older and work more to a preconceived plan in their searching, distracting stimuli have to be excluded. The capacity to inhibit irrelevant stimuli comprises the ability to attend selectively to certain stimuli. It involves central attentional processes which are developmentally determined.
- *Span of attention.* An increasing span of attention is a characteristic feature of development. Older children sustain attention for longer periods of time.
- *Links with other cognitive skills.* Attention allows absorption of information and ensures better adaptation to the environment. An older child attends to a book because he enjoys reading it and wants to know how the story develops. If his short-term memory or his visuospatial ability (e.g. capacity to discriminate letter shapes) are poor, or if he has some degree of language delay or other learning difficulty, then attending to the book will be unrewarding for him, and his attention will not be sustained. The development of the capacity to attend is therefore dependent to a large degree on the development of other abilities.

3.4.2 ATTENTION DEFICIT HYPERACTIVITY DISORDER (ADHD, HYPERKINETIC SYNDROME)

Definition

Hyperkinetic disorder is characterized by an early onset (before 7 years of age), and the combination of overactive, poorly modulated behaviour with marked inattention, lack of persistent task involvement, restlessness, impulsive tendencies and a high degree of distractibility. These characteristics are pervasive across situations and persistent over time (World Health Organization 1992). The DSM-IV classification criteria for attention deficit hyperactivity disorder (American Psychiatric Association 1994) are similar, but the presence over a 6-month period or more of at least 8 out of 14 types of behaviour, including especially fidgetiness, difficulty in remaining seated, high distractibility, and impulsivity, are required. The presence of either overactivity/impulsiveness or inattentiveness is sufficient, unlike the ICD-10 criteria which require both. This is one reason why more children in North America than in Europe are diagnosed as having these disorders.

The term 'minimal brain dysfunction syndrome' was once used (Clements 1966) to explain on physiological grounds (unspecified brain dysfunction) a behavioural syndrome very similar to or identical with the attention deficit disorder/hyperkinetic syndrome described below. Most clinicians now believe that it is undesirable to use the term minimal brain dysfunction to describe this behavioural syndrome because it says little if anything about aetiology, and evidence of central nervous system dysfunction is usually lacking (Taylor 1985).

Clinical features

Onset

Children usually present to health services between the ages of 3 and 7 years. Identification often coincides with starting school because of the greater pressures to sit still, concentrate, and behave there. However, sometimes in children who present with other problems later in life, it will be clear from the story that the child was overactive and lacking in concentration earlier on.

Complaints about the child's behaviour may come either from the parents or from playgroup organizers or teachers. This is partly because people vary in their capacity to tolerate difficult behaviour and partly because the child may show considerable variability from situation to situation in his activity level and attention span.

Behavioural characteristics

Characteristically the child will, from babyhood, have been a restless and difficult feeder, sometimes sleeping poorly and irregularly. Some mothers even report antenatal overactivity, with high levels of intrauterine kicking and restlessness. As walking begins and the child becomes more mobile, he is noted to be unusually active and into everything in an unfocused fashion. He may only be able to sit for a moment or two at a mealtime. This high level of activity, often in association with clumsiness, means that the child is particularly prone to accidents. As the child is expected to spend more time on pursuits involving concentration, it is seen that he is highly distractible and cannot settle to any activity for more than a brief period. Puzzles, construction toys, and picture books do not engage his attention. Though he may be able to sit in front of the television for an indefinite period, it is notable that he is restless and fidgety and seems to take little in.

Entry to a pre-school facility may bring to light a problem that has been present for some time, because the child is suddenly expected to conform and to cope with more structured expectations. Many severely overactive children are unusually uninhibited in their response to strange people, failing to show normal stranger anxiety. They may show associated developmental problems, especially language delay and other behaviour problems, particularly a tendency to aggressive behaviour.

As the child gets older, overactivity usually becomes less of a problem, but defects of attention and concentration may persist and may lead to continuing learning problems. Impulsiveness and lack of inhibition may result in antisocial behaviour, relationship difficulties, a tendency towards substance abuse and a poor work record.

Differential diagnosis includes the possibility that the child is showing normally active behaviour that is perceived to be abnormal by parents or, less commonly teachers. Both hyperkinetic disorder and ADHD (see below) are at one end of a continuum rather than clearly defined entities, so that inevitably the distinction between normal and abnormal will be arbitrary in borderline cases. Distinction between ADHD and oppositional defiant disorder and conduct disorder may present problems, but often there is co-morbidity with both disorders present.

Background information

Prevalence has been found to vary widely, especially between North America and the UK, with prevalence rates for children with hyperkinetic disorder in the UK being 0.5–1.0% while rates for ADHD in the US are approximately 3–5% (Cameron and Hill 1996). Reasons for this discrepancy include differences in parent and teacher perceptions of behaviour, differences in clinic referral rates, and differences in diagnostic practice. Systematic differences in diagnostic practice due both to the classification systems used and to the training of clinicians have indeed been demonstrated (Prendergast *et al.* 1988). When applied to a total population of around 250 000, the above prevalence figures mean that approximately 200 children will have hyperkinetic disorder and about 2000 will have the milder and broader diagnostic category of ADHD (Taylor and Hemsley 1995). Prevalence rates for these two conditions are converging as the diagnostic systems become increasingly similar.

Boys show hyperkinetic problems about three or four times as commonly as girls. There is no strong link between social class and the condition. Children showing the hyperkinetic syndrome who also show aggressive behaviour have high rates of family disharmony, parental mental illness, and other indices of family and social disruption in their background, than those without antisocial features (Taylor 1986).

Aetiology

Causative variables thought to be of importance include:

- *Genetic factors.* There is now reasonably good evidence that attention deficit hyperactivity disorder is associated with a D4 receptor gene polymorphism (Gill *et al.* 1997). Adoptive studies (e.g. Alberts-Corush *et al.* 1986) as well as family studies (Biederman *et al.* 1986) and twin studies (Goodman and Stevenson 1989, Levy *et al.* 1997) also suggest that there is a strong genetic contribution, especially in boys. Monozygotic twins show greater concordance than dizygotic in activity levels, and the biological parents of affected children have a strong history of hyperkinesis in their own childhood. Genetic factors may operate by their effect on temperament and on neurochemical processes (see below). Also, certain genetic syndromes have been found to have a particular association with hyperactivity and attentional deficits. These include fragile X syndrome, tuberous sclerosis, Turner syndrome, and Smith–Magenis syndrome (Turk and Hill 1995).
- *Brain dysfunction.* Children with evidence of brain damage, for example those with epilepsy and cerebral palsy, show high rates of the hyperkinetic syndrome. Rates are even higher in children with associated learning disability (especially

if this is severe), with around 10% so affected (Corbett 1981). It is important, however, to stress that most children with the hyperkinetic syndrome do not show overt evidence of brain dysfunction.

• *Neurochemical processes.* Brain dysfunction is also suggested by the presence in some studies, but not all, of a high rate of non-epileptic EEG anomalies. In addition, abnormalities of dopamine metabolism have been described in ex- perimentally induced hyperactivity in rats, although this mechanism has not been confirmed in affected children. Dopamine is a neurotransmitter sub- stance, found in considerable concentration in the activating system of the brain, and is therefore important in the control of the level of arousal. There have also been less well confirmed reports of abnormalities of serotonin and noradrenaline metabolism. Focal cerebral hypoperfusion has been reported in children with hyperkinesis, especially in fronto-striatal regions (Lou *et al.* 1984, 1989). SPECT imaging has demonstrated diminished activity in left frontal and parietal areas in individuals with ADHD (Sieg *et al.* 1995).

• *Diet.* Hyperactivity has been related by the US allergist, Feingold (1975), to the presence of various additives and naturally occurring substances in the diet. Tartrazine and salicylates are said to be particularly noxious. Attempts to prove this theory by removing these substances from the diet and then re- introducing them in controlled clinical trials using double-blind techniques have been unsuccessful. However, more systematic attempts to identify the specific substances affecting a particular child and then remove them from the diet suggest that behavioural effects may be significant and substantial for a minority of individuals (Egger *et al.* 1985; Carter *et al.* 1993; Schmidt *et al.* 1997). Additive-free diets remain widely used. It is likely that some of their effectiveness relates more to the fact that their use requires parents to be firm and more consistent, at least over their children's food, than to any direct action arising from withdrawal of noxious substances.

• *Lead.* Lead ingested or inhaled in high concentrations can produce severe brain damage. It has been claimed that lead in much lower concentrations, previously considered to be within the normal range, can produce hyper- activity (Needleman *et al.* 1979). The evidence for this claim has been called into question, and it is uncertain whether removal of lead from the environ- ment would produce any lowering at all in the rates of hyperactivity (Smith *et al.* 1983).

• *Temperament.* Children who have been active from the first few months of life are likely to remain so at least during their childhood years (Thomas and Chess 1977). This tendency does seem to have a genetic basis, as shown by twin studies (Torgerson and Kringlen 1978). Continuity of behaviour that sometimes seems relatively impervious to outside influences has been taken as evidence that the child's temperament or personality plays an important part in the development of the syndrome.

• *Psychological factors.* Psychological mechanisms implicated include inclin- ation to seek immediate reinforcement, arousal modulation problems (children sometimes showing unduly low and sometimes unduly high arousal), poor inhibitory control, an aversion to delay (Sonuga-Barke *et al.* 1996), abnormally severe distractibility (Leung and Connolly 1996), basic impairments of attention, and possibly deficient somatosensory processing (Parush *et al.* 1997).

- *Social factors.* Young children are more likely to show behaviour disorders, including disorders characterized by high levels of activity, if they are living in poor social conditions, with inadequate housing and in families with stretched financial resources (Richman *et al.* 1982). It is likely that these factors operate by their influences on parental health and parental behaviour.

- *Parental behaviour.* It has been observed clinically that mothers of children showing the condition are sometimes relatively unresponsive to their children's demands. It may, therefore, be that some of the child's overactive behaviour is undertaken in order to elicit a response in the caring adult, or in severe cases may even reflect attachment problems between mother and child. Parents of hyperkinetic children also sometimes show inability to provide consistent control for their children, and are occasionally passive and unusually accepting of difficult behaviour. However, the role the parents play in producing hyperactivity should be considered cautiously. It has been shown that parental behaviour becomes more appropriate when children are successfully treated with stimulants (Barkley 1989), suggesting that inappropriate parental behaviour may be secondary to the child's behaviour problems.

- *Early childhood experiences.* Children separated from their parents in early life, then reared in institutions for 2 or 3 years, and finally settled in good adoptive families may continue to show behavioural problems that are sometimes of hyperkinetic type (Tizard and Hodges 1978). Further, some parents date the development of hyperkinetic problems from stressful events such as a hospitalization occurring in the first year of life. There is no systematically gathered evidence of the later effects of traumata of this type, but it is certainly possible that they occur.

Interactional effects

The above contributors to hyperactive behaviour usually operate in combination with the child suffering from a multiplicity of adverse influences. It is very common, for example, to see overactive children in whom adverse temperamental characteristics interact with parental stress or personality problems making it harder for them to provide consistent control and affectionate care. The pattern of interaction may be even more complex with, for example, adverse experience producing neurophysiological dysfunction and problems in modulating and monitoring experience. The child may then develop learning difficulties that have a secondary disturbing effect on his behaviour. Hyperkinetic behaviour often coexists with more general behavioural difficulties and defiant tendencies. However, when these co-occur the genetic evidence is similar to that for 'pure' hyperkinetic disorder (Silberg *et al.* 1996). It is easy to envisage how adverse experiences and repeated senses of failure with accompanying low self-esteem might lead to the development of conduct disorder in a child with hyperkinetic disorder. Family studies also suggest that as many as one-third of first degree relatives of children with ADHD have (or have had) the condition themselves. Thus a substantial proportion of these children's parents have at least some

ADHD-related disabilities which will impinge on their own parenting abilities and behavioural and social functioning. Adult ADHD is now being increasingly recognized (Toone and van der Linden 1997).

Assessment

As precise as possible an account of the level of activity, degree of inattention, and related problems should be obtained. Because of the situation-specific nature of much hyperactivity, it is particularly important to obtain separate accounts of behaviour from both parents and teachers, or, for example, playgroup leaders. It should be noted whether the child's behaviour varies within situations:

• At home, is the child better when his father is around?
• At school, is he more difficult in the structured classroom than in the play-ground, or in less structured classroom activity?
• Has any response to dietary constituents been noted?

A parental complaint that a child is overactive does not necessarily mean that the child's level of activity is unusually high. One or both parents may perceive quite ordinary levels of activity to be pathological.

An account of the child's past level of activity should be taken with particular reference to the possibility of brain damage—perhaps from a very difficult birth or a prolonged epileptic fit. However, sustained and pervasive hyperactivity is rarely attributable to such physical traumas. Definite developmental delay, either general or specific (e.g. language delay or clumsiness), would support a bio-logical component to the problem. The child's developmental level and learning ability also require assessment.

The family background, quality of family relationships, and way in which the parents respond to the problem are all relevant. Observation of the interaction between parents and child when the child is being difficult is also likely to be revealing. It is important to remember that child–parent interaction in a consult-ing room may not be representative of what goes on at home. The parents should be asked about this.

Finally, it is often helpful to ask the parents to keep a chart over a week or fortnight of a particularly troublesome type of behaviour that they have described. Brief rating scales such as those developed by Conners (1973), although not diagnostic, can be useful in gauging severity of behavioural prob-lems and in monitoring progress.

Treatment

Specific therapies (medication and behaviour modification) are usually given most attention in discussions of management of this syndrome. However, it is equally important to help parents to see the problem in perspective, and to facilitate environmental manipulations of one sort or another.

Counselling of parents should focus first on an acknowledgement of the extent of the problem, the probable importance of biological factors, and the way these interact with the reactions of those around the child. The fact that the child is not going to change rapidly, but that the long-term outcome may well be good providing one can avoid the child becoming discouraged and low in self-esteem, should also be emphasized.

Environmental manipulations that may be helpful if they are feasible include (in school) providing more opportunity to engage in free play, and ensuring that, in structured settings, the opportunities for the child to be disruptive are reduced. This can sometimes be achieved by careful attention to classroom seating arrangements, and by not expecting prolonged periods of sustained attention too soon. Praise should be given if the child's level of attention improves even slightly. There should be a minimum of distractions and the availability of small-group tuition with clear incentives and reward for even short spells of attentiveness and on-task behaviour. At home the parents should be encouraged not to overstimulate a hyperkinetic child. Having only one or two toys out at a time, and limiting the visits of friends to small numbers, may be useful. Any foodstuffs which seem to have an obvious and predictable detrimental effect on behaviour should be excluded from the diet as far as possible.

Formal behaviour modification programmes can take place either at home or at school. Whether these are feasible or not will largely depend on whether the parents are sufficiently motivated and organized and whether skilled psychologist support is available. An operant approach can be embarked upon which follows the principles described in Section 9.2. The child's behaviour in one or two especially troublesome respects, for example sitting at table or concentrating on a puzzle, should be charted by parents and teachers. Rewards agreed with the child should be instituted for appropriate behaviour, and inappropriate behaviour should be ignored. Even though inappropriate behaviour may demand attention, care should be taken to ensure that the child receives more attention at times when his behaviour is more appropriate.

Medication should be limited to cases where the child's behaviour is seriously affected both at home and school and where it has failed to respond to psychological, educational, and social interventions. The child should have been personally observed by the clinician to have high levels of inattention and overactivity and, although there may be adverse circumstances in the family, there should be a lack of evidence that these are the prime causes of this type of behaviour.

Stimulant medication was reported many years ago to have a beneficial effect on hyperkinetic children. It remains a well-evaluated form of treatment for the severely affected child. Methylphenidate (Ritalin) should be prescribed morning and lunchtime in doses increasing by small amounts every 3 or 4 days. It is sensible to begin with methylphenidate 5 mg in the morning and increase by 5 mg at these intervals while parents and teachers monitor the child's behaviour—preferably with the help of rating scales. Benefits are less clear for children under 5 years of age but may occur. There is substantial variation in the dosage required for optimal response, and hence maintenance doses may range from 5 to 20 mg twice daily. Side-effects are common and include tearfulness and depression, irritability, twitchiness, reduction of appetite, growth retardation, insomnia, headaches, dizziness, and sometimes a worsening of symptoms. This worsening may occur over 2 or 3 days and is then followed by definite improvement, so it can be worth persisting with medication even if it seems ineffective to begin with. Some of the side-effects may be mitigated by 'drug holidays' at weekends, or for more prolonged periods. Where the child's growth is temporarily affected, there appears to be catch-up growth once the drug is stopped (Roche *et al.* 1979).

With all these side-effects, it is often a matter of careful negotiation with parents to determine whether the drug should be prescribed or persisted with. Parental feelings on the matter are obviously of great importance. Nevertheless, a number of children receive clear benefit from the use of stimulant medication. In most children, a period of medication lasting several months or a year or two is necessary. It is often the child or the parents rather than the clinician who decides when the drug has outlived its usefulness. Parents can be reassured that addiction will not occur, but they should keep tablets out of the way of teenage sibs. Where methylphenidate proves ineffective or produces unacceptable side-effects it is worth considering dexamphetamine. This has a slightly longer half-life and can be better tolerated although the same range of adverse effects is possible. Tricyclic antidepressants, such as imipramine, have also been shown to be of benefit. They have the advantage of facilitating rather than hindering sleep and do not suppress appetite. However, potential cardiac side-effects mean careful monitoring is required. Clonidine in night-time doses of 25–50 µg can be beneficial behaviourally but probably has less impact on concentration skills and freedom from distractibility.

Medication is more likely to produce adverse effects in children with learning disabilities, autism or other evidence of central nervous system dysfunction. However, such children can benefit from very carefully balanced and monitored medication regimes and their chances of being helped by such means should not be overlooked (Payton *et al.* 1989a).

Parents commonly try to remove food additives, colourings, and flavourings from their children's diet if they suspect hyperactivity. It is unhelpful for professionals to be dismissive about this form of treatment and more appropriate for them to help parents to apply and evaluate such approaches systematically. Some guidelines are provided in this section.

The following foods are most likely to contain additives, the commonest substances to which children react:

- processed ham, bacon, salami, sausages, ready-cooked and frozen meat, frozen fish
- ice-cream, ice-lollies, and all forms of confectionery, flavoured crisps, sauces, etc.
- fizzy drinks and fruit squash (except those specially labelled as free of additives and artificial colourings)
- most types of wrapped bread and breakfast cereals
- shop-bought cakes, biscuits, desserts, jellies
- margarine, processed or coloured cheese.

If the application of a diet free of additives and artificial colouring, or the avoidance of one or two specific foods, such as orange squash, chocolate, sweets, lollies, or ice cream, appears to be helpful in improving a child's behaviour, it would not be sensible to discourage its use. Such a diet will result in a child's life being somewhat socially restricted, but will have no other ill-effects.

In considering initiating more systematic and drastic dietary treatment, the severity of the problem as well as the presence or absence of features suggestive of dietary aetiology should be taken into account. Other measures should be used in managing mild levels of hyperactivity.

Positive indications for more systematic dietary treatment include:

- episodic changes of behaviour, especially if these are associated with intake of specific foods, rather than the child being frustrated
- changes of behaviour that result in the child being in an episodic, excited, explosive, or tense state
- the absence of obviously stressful factors in the background
- a consistent and predictable adverse behavioural response to the ingestion of a specific foodstuff
- negative parental attitudes to medication, and a positive attitude to a dietary approach.

A systematic approach to dietary restriction involving a systematic identification of foods or additives has been shown to be effective in some children (Carter *et al.* 1993; Schmidt *et al.* 1997). This treatment, which has also been used in the management of severe migraine, requires the services of a dietitian. The child is put on a small number of foods (perhaps one or two vegetables, one or two types of meat, and a source of carbohydrate such as rice) with added vitamins and calcium gluconate. The child is maintained on this restrictive diet for about 3 weeks, and, if improvement occurs, foods are reintroduced one by one at about weekly intervals, in order to identify positively activating items of diet. Foods most commonly identified as harmful using this approach are wheat, milk, and eggs. Chocolate is also often implicated by parents but its total exclusion from a child's diet will be difficult.

This restriction/reintroduction dietary approach does, however, have dangers. Unless properly supervised, growth failure may occur as a result of malnutrition. Some parents have appeared to restrict diet quite unnecessarily on the grounds of imaginary hyperactivity—a form of Munchausen syndrome by proxy (Section 2.2). Dietary approaches may distract attention away from important social or familial factors affecting the child. Finally, reintroduction of foods after a long period of abstinence may, very occasionally, produce anaphylactic shock.

Outcome

A number of follow-up studies have been carried out and the prognosis is variable. Overactivity in the pre-school years tends to predict conduct disorder in middle childhood (Richman *et al.* 1982). Mild, pure forms of the condition have a reasonably good outcome, though there may be persisting restlessness. Followed up to adolescence, children who have been diagnosed as severely hyperkinetic show impaired cognitive test performance and poor scholastic achievement. Later, in adult life, a high proportion develop antisocial behaviour disorders, increased risk of substance abuse, poor work records, and relationship difficulties (Barkley *et al.* 1991; Klein and Mannuzza 1991). Sadly, the evidence that early institution of medication and other treatments alters the prognosis is limited. However, the importance of at least giving the child the opportunity to experience more normal social and educational opportunities at critical times of development should not be trivialized. The prolongation of ADHD into adulthood has now been well described (Toone and van der Linden 1997).

3.5 Pervasive developmental disorders

3.5.1 CHILDHOOD AUTISM

Definition

Childhood autism is characterized by the early onset (before 3 years of age) of delay and deviation in three critical areas of development: the ability to form social relationships and to share interests and emotions, the use of language and communication (both verbal and non-verbal), and the presence of often severely incapacitating ritualistic tendencies including a highly restrictive, stereotyped, repetitive behavioural repertoire. Children with autism are likely to show mannerisms such as hand flapping, rocking, spinning, and toe walking, resistance to change in daily routines such as sitting on a different chair at table or taking a different route to school, attachment to unusual objects, and acute emotional reactions of excitement or anxiety in situations which do not usually provoke such responses. There is a dislike for novelty and surprises—for children with autism, variety is not the spice of life! Repetitive unimaginative play is common—for example stacking up dolls or placing them in lines rather than nurturing them, or twirling the wheels on toy vehicles and looking at them closely from many different angles rather than pushing them along the ground uttering 'vroom vroom' car-like noises.

Autism is now classified (World Health Organization 1992; American Psychiatric Association 1994) as a 'pervasive developmental disorder'. The DSM-IV diagnosis of autistic disorder requires a qualitative impairment in reciprocal, social interaction, qualitative impairment in verbal and non-verbal communication and in imaginative activity, and a markedly restricted repertoire of activities and interests, with onset during infancy or childhood. The ICD-10 diagnosis of autism is based on similar criteria but abnormal or impaired development must be present before the age of 3 years. The term 'pervasive developmental disorder' is somewhat misleading, as the deficits shown are, in fact, not usually fully pervasive. For this reason many clinicians prefer the umbrella term 'autistic spectrum disorder'.

The condition may first become apparent in the first few months of life with an assumption that it has been present from birth. In other cases there is a period of normal development usually lasting no longer than 3 years, followed by the gradual appearance, usually over a few weeks or months, of the classical features. The most severe forms of the disorder have a prevalence of only approximately

5 per 10 000 individuals (Fombonne *et al.* 1997). However, when one acknowledges that there is a spectrum of severity which merges imperceptibly with 'normality' at its mild end, then prevalence figures increase to 20 per 10 000 (Wing 1993).

Behavioural features

Social relationships

Some babies are 'different' from birth, are slow to smile, appear generally unresponsive and passive, and do not seem to enjoy being picked up. They do not put their arms up to be cuddled, and may wriggle and squirm when taken into their mother's arms. Eye contact is often abnormal, with features of indifference which may take the form of looking away or a blank unfocused stare. There may be active avoidance of eye-to-eye contact with others. The usual selective attachment to mother with accompanying development of fear of strangers around 8 months of age often fails to materialize. By 2–3 years of age the child shows a preference for his own company and, if he hurts himself, may not come to his parents for comfort. He will be slow to distinguish his parents from other people. Pointing is used to get needs met but not in order to share something interesting.

These social abnormalities change with age. As the child gets older he may, much later than normal children, become very attached to his parents and be distressed by their absence. He is still, however, likely to show little interest in playing with other children or developing friendships with them, though he may play alongside them. There is often a preference for older or younger children rather than those of the same age. As he moves into puberty, the child's social relationships are likely to remain unusual. There will be no imitation of other people's activities. He will probably still prefer his own company and, even if he has reasonable language, it is likely that his social relationships will be marked by lack of awareness of the feelings of other people, and by an incapacity to take on another person's point of view. He will make no real friendships with others his age.

Speech and language development

Impairment occurs in both verbal and non-verbal communication. Both comprehension and expression are usually markedly delayed, especially when considered in relation to other aspects of the child's development. About half the children diagnosed as autistic are not speaking single words by the age of 5 years and, of these, only a minority later develop any useful speech. When speech does occur, it shows various abnormalities including persistent echolalia (mechanical repetition of sounds or words) and neologisms (use of words the child has made up). Echolalia may be immediate, or of the delayed type—the child repeating a word that has been said to him some time previously over and over again. The echolalia may be partly responsible for pronominal reversal, the child saying, for example, 'you want' when he means 'I want'. There is often an associated abnormality of voice production. A source of particular distress to parents is the fact that the child's language usage is often highly sporadic. The child may, for example, utter one or two well-formed phrases, and then not speak again for several weeks or months. The child may make requests by taking an adult's hand and leading in the required direction to a cupboard or door. There is usually no use of gesture. Where speech is more developed there is often a disregard for the content of conversation, with a lack of appreciation of the conversational partner's perspectives and needs. Such difficulties constitute major problems with the social use of language (pragmatics). This may lead to the individual appearing rude, insensitive, and unable to participate in conversations because of failure to appreciate the conversational partner's point of view including the need for turn-taking. Individuals with reasonable expressive language still often show a failure to appreciate metaphor—for example interpreting proverbs in a concrete fashion. The child shows no or very little make-believe play, and there is usually an absence of imaginative activity, probably because of deficient symbolic thought processes.

As the child gets older, expression and comprehension continue to improve, but usually at a disappointingly slow rate. Further, the child's intonation may remain mechanical, monotonous, stereotyped, and repetitive. Speech often has a highly pedantic quality (Ghaziuddin and Gerstein 1996). It is impossible for the child to sustain a meaningful conversation for more than a sentence or so.

Mannerisms
In this condition mannerisms take a variety of forms, but particularly characteristic are rapid flapping movements of the arms and hands, occurring especially when the child is excited or upset. Twirling of the body and walking on tiptoe are also characteristic, as are repetitive rocking and jumping. There may be a whole range of other mannerisms involving, for example, speech and gait. The child may examine objects by sniffing them or may show abnormal fascination with the texture of objects or materials such as peoples' hair, smooth plastic, or nylon tights. There can be preoccupations with sounds (e.g. water hissing in pipes) or sights (e.g. clothes tumbling in a washing machine). Aversions to such sights, sounds, and other sensations also occur. Sometimes one set of mannerisms follows another in time.

Resistance to change
The child often develops a stereotyped pattern to his life and becomes very distressed if there is any deviation from it. Food has to be prepared in a particular way, the table must be laid just so, the child insists on being dressed in a particular order, a walk to the shops or a journey to school must follow a particular route. Sometimes these rituals threaten to constrict family life to a serious degree and they result, of course, in considerable restriction in the child's range of activities. There is also often marked resistance to changes in the child's environment, so that rearrangements of furniture or toys at home can cause catastrophic reactions.

Attachment to particular objects
Normal toddlers show attachments to cuddly objects they like to have around them at bedtime or when they are upset. Autistic children sometimes become

attached to unusual non-cuddly objects, for example bits of wire, tin cans, twigs and leaves, or bunches of keys, from which they hate to be separated at any time.

Acute emotional reactions
Frequent outbursts of excitement, anxiety, misery, or anger may be precipitated by alterations in the environment that would not be expected to cause more than a slight ripple in the emotional life of an ordinary child.

Other behavioural symptoms
There may be a wide range of other symptoms including sleep problems, over-activity, distractibility, impersistence, soiling, and wetting.

Intellectual development

General intellectual development
As language is specifically delayed in autism, this is best gauged by considering non-verbal development. Non-verbal development may be within the average range, but is much more likely to be delayed. About 70% of autistic children have non-verbal IQs below 70, about 50% below 50. Only about 5% have IQs over 100 (Wing and Gould 1979).

Specific deficits other than language
The child is likely to be particularly poor in tasks involving symbolic thought, and in those that require him to perceive how other people are thinking or feeling (Baron-Cohen 1991). There are also problems in organizing information, planning ahead and being able to shift with ease from one topic or idea to another without being distracted ('executive function deficits') (Bishop 1993).

Special abilities
Islets of ability have been described in autistic children. These usually involve mechanical tasks such as rote memory—learning things off by heart. In general these abilities only take the child into the normal range and are not exceptional, except in relation to the generally low level of ability. Very occasionally, however, some abilities are developed to a most unusual degree. These may be mathematical (e.g. the capacity to multiply two four-figure numbers together in the head, or to calculate the day of the week of a date several years ago) or they may just involve rote memory. Not all children with these unusual abilities (idiots savants) are autistic, but a proportion are (O'Connor and Hermelin 1984).

Physical conditions
Usually children with autism have no identifiable physical abnormalities. However, they may show an underlying cerebral disorder (see below). About 15% of children with autism develop epilepsy in infancy or early childhood. A quarter to a third of children with autism who have not had seizures in early life develop them during adolescence or adulthood. Seizures usually take the form of complex

partial (psychomotor) epilepsy. They can occur in individuals with any level of intellectual functioning but are more common in those with learning disabilities. Fits are usually not severe and respond to standard anticonvulsant medication (Gillberg and Schaumann 1989).

Background factors

Autism occurs in about 3–5 per 10 000 children and is about four times commoner in boys than in girls (Steffenburg and Gillberg 1986). However, the rate of autistic disorders in children with learning disability, but with a triad of similar social, language, and relationship impairments is much higher, increasing to as many as 21 per 10 000 (Gillberg *et al.* 1986). Autism occurs in all countries throughout the world where it has been looked for. It was thought to be commoner in middle-class families, but this was almost certainly the result of ascertainment bias—middle-class children with autism being more likely to be identified. At present, it seems most likely that the basic deficits in autism are cognitive ones, in particular involving the ability to appreciate the point of view of others, and that this will differ from one's own (Baron-Cohen 1989). Affected children also have particular difficulty in accurately identifying the emotional expressions of other people—an inability to read emotions ('alexithymia') (Hobson 1986). Other cognitive deficits are also being identified and researched, including difficulties in organizing information, planning ahead, and shifting from one theme to another ('executive functions') (Happé and Frith 1996). Such evidence implies that the problems in social relationships, mannerisms, language, acute emotional reactions, etc. are secondary to the child's difficulties in making sense of his environment as a place filled with other human beings with whom he should be interacting. However, the unusual nature of the deficits in autism makes it unlikely that there is a simple or straightforward link between one or more cognitive deficits and the developmental disabilities observed.

Although the basic psychological defect is uncertain, there is now agreement that a degree of brain dysfunction, however subtle, underlies the condition rather than it being a reaction to adverse environmental influences. The evidence for this view arises from knowledge of:

- *Genetic factors.* The condition runs in families with 2–3% of siblings affected. Siblings of autistic children also have a higher than expected rate of language delay (Bailey *et al.* 1996). Parents of children with autism have been found to differ from matched comparison group parents on a number of psychological criteria including executive function skills, reading measures, speech and pragmatic language deficits, friendship difficulties, and being more rigid, aloof, hypersensitive to criticism, and anxious (Piven and Palmer 1997; Piven *et al.* 1997). Concordance for autism is much higher in monozygotic than in dizygotic twins (Le Couteur *et al.* 1996; Steffenburg *et al.* 1989). Studies of extended families also support a strong genetic component to aetiology (Jorde *et al.* 1990). A small number of cases have been described with chromosomal defects, especially the fragile X syndrome (Turk *et al.* 1994), but probably this does not account for more than about 5% of cases of autism

(Wahlstrom *et al.* 1989). However, there is some evidence that certain profiles of autistic-like features may be associated with particular underlying medical conditions which should be checked for (Gillberg 1992).

- *Underlying physical conditions.* Autistic children have been found to suffer from an excess of complications of pregnancy and delivery. However, these complications are usually mild and their role in causing autism is questionable (Bolton *et al.* 1997). In a minority of cases, the condition arises on the basis of a well-identified physical condition. This may be infective (congenital rubella), metabolic (phenylketonuria), genetic/developmental (tuberous sclerosis, fragile X syndrome, Rett syndrome), toxic (fetal alcohol syndrome), or of unknown aetiology (e.g. infantile spasms). Numerous, so far unsuccessful, attempts have been made to identify a specific neuroanatomical, neurophysiological, or neurochemical cause for the condition. Various anatomical abnormalities including hypoplasia of specific cerebellar lobules and widening of the fourth ventricle have been described. When autism occurs in children with tuberous sclerosis, tubers are particularly likely to be located in the temporal lobes, and this may give a further clue to anatomical localization of autistic dysfunction (Bolton and Griffiths 1997). Abnormalities of catecholamine and endorphin metabolism have also been inconsistently reported (see Ciaranello and Ciaranello 1995 for review).
- *Parent and family factors.* There is no evidence that abnormal parental attitudes or behaviour are responsible for the development of autism, though this has been alleged in the past (Koegel *et al.* 1983). Clinical impressions that fathers of autistic children tend to be schizoid in personality have been confirmed by systematic study (Wolff *et al.* 1988), but the link is likely to be genetically determined. On the other hand, the impact of having an autistic child on family life and parental health is often substantial. Children with autism can be extremely unrewarding to bring up because of their lack of affection and slow progress in social relationships and language development. Parents can react by distancing themselves emotionally from their child and this can be mistaken as the cause of the child's autism rather than a consequence of it.
- *Link with schizophrenia.* A small number of autistic children develop schizophrenia (and indeed other psychotic conditions) in later life (Petty *et al.* 1984). However, the distinctive clinical characteristics and family studies make it clear that autism and adult schizophrenia are genetically distinct syndromes with very different treatment implications (Kolvin 1971).

Assessment

Most children with autistic disorders come to attention in the second or third year of life because of developmental delay—usually noticed initially in language development. Tell-tale features can be picked up in infancy by trained individuals. These include failures to develop a desire to share interesting things, to demonstrate make-believe and imaginative play, and to use pointing to share something interesting the child has seen, not just to get needs met (Baron-Cohen *et al.* 1996). The diagnosis is made on clinical grounds using the criteria described above. Atypical cases are common, but it is unwise to make a diagnosis of autism unless both significant language delay and the characteristic disturbances of social relationships are present.

The condition needs to be differentiated from a number of other possible diagnoses:

- *Learning disability.* Social and communicatory difficulties may be part of a generalized developmental delay. Autism is a likely diagnosis where social and language problems are greater than would be predicted for the general level of intellectual functioning.
- *Asperger syndrome* (Attwood 1998). Individuals with this diagnosis are usually of higher intellectual ability with more advanced language skills than those shown by children with autism. However, they do show empathy difficulties and eccentricities with impaired understanding of social convention, severe impairment in reciprocal social interaction, and circumscribed interests of a non-social nature. Superficially excellent language skills usually co-exist with stilted or pedantic speech, poor understanding of metaphor and emotion, and non-verbal communication difficulties. Clumsiness is common. The term is often used to describe the milder end of the autistic spectrum.
- *Disintegrative disorder/disintegrative psychosis.* This rare condition, previously known as Heller syndrome, usually has an onset at 3–8 years of age following a phase of normal development. There is progressive loss of language and play skills with the development of social aloofness and self-preoccupation. Some social relationship skills (e.g. good eye contact) may be preserved. The cause is unknown. The condition appears to have a prognosis similar to, or rather worse than, autistic disorders of later onset. It is uncertain whether the condition can be meaningfully distinguished from autism (Volkmar and Cohen 1989).
- *Rett syndrome.* This condition occurs only in girls. Normal developmental progress for the first 1–2 years is followed by skill loss with the development of autistic features, associated with jerking or writhing, involuntary movements, abnormalities of muscular tone, midline stereotypies including persistent hand wringing, and hyperventilation (Olsson and Rett 1987). A similar picture of regression after a normal period of development in the first 1–2 years, followed by very slow subsequent mental development, may also occur in children of both sexes in the absence of autistic features.
- *Developmental dysphasia/developmental language disorder/selective language impairment.* These various labels for developmentally determined speech and language problems describe conditions which may be congenital or acquired. The language difficulties may lead to abnormal socialization and solitariness.
- *Semantic–pragmatic disorder.* This term is controversial. It should really be reserved for children who show the characteristic language and communication abnormalities without the accompanying social impairments and ritualistic tendencies. In practice the label is often applied to socially and emotionally odd children. There is increasing evidence that semantic–pragmatic disorder lies on the autistic spectrum (Shields *et al.* 1996).

- *Childhood schizophrenia.* Schizophrenia before puberty is rare. It presents similarly to adult schizophrenia with formal thought disorder, delusional perceptions, passivity phenomena, and hallucinations (See Section 5.6.2). There is usually a family history of schizophrenia. The characteristic cognitive, social, and language impairments of autism are absent.

Management

Management should begin with an explanation to the parents of the nature of the diagnosis, its probable cause, the ways in which the child can be helped, and the likely outcome. It is important to reassure parents that their behaviour and style of parenting have not produced the condition, though this does not mean that, in the future, there is not much they can do to help the child. In the pre-school years it will not be possible to predict outcome with any degree of certainty, but it is important that parents should be prepared for a chronic and often seriously disabling course to the condition. Positive aspects of the child's development, and the fact that he will continue to make progress, albeit slowly, need to be stressed. It is important to put aside sufficient time to discuss parents' questions about the condition and to be prepared for follow-up appointments for the same purpose.

Neither medical treatment (medication) nor interpretive forms of psychotherapy directed towards the child have a significant place in management. However, brief courses of medication may sometimes be useful to reduce the impact of associated behavioural problems (Gilman and Tuchman 1995). For example, major tranquillizers such as haloperidol and risperidone may sometimes be beneficial in reducing severely aggressive behaviour. Opiate antagonists such as naltrexone may help associated self-injurious tendencies. Selective serotonin reuptake inhibitors such as fluoxetine, sertraline, and paroxetine may ameliorate obsessional tendencies particularly when associated with depressive symptoms. Psychostimulants such as methylphenidate and dexamphetamine may reduce associated hyperactivity but often worsen autistic features. In contrast, behavioural and educational methods have been demonstrated to be helpful. Rutter (1985) suggests four goals of such treatment:

- fostering of normal development
- reduction of the rigidity and stereotypy that often dominate the life of the child and family
- removal of maladaptive behaviours
- alleviation of family distress.

These goals are most likely to be met by a combination of counselling, behaviour modification, and special schooling (Howlin and Rutter 1987).

Normal development is fostered by encouraging parents to provide intensive, stimulating experiences more consciously geared to the child's developmental level than would be necessary with an ordinary child. For example, if parents take obvious pleasure in early vocalization, label objects verbally when they use them, communicate with their child in every possible way (with gesture and signs as well as words), the child's language will be given its best chance to develop. Special schooling with a favourable teacher–pupil ratio, and teachers experienced in teaching children with social and communication difficulties in a highly structured and predictable setting and routine, play a most important part in the encouragement of normal development (Rutter and Bartak 1973; Jordan and Powell 1995; Quill 1995).

Both at home and at school the reduction of stereotypies and other maladaptive types of behaviour can best be approached by behavioural methods. Operant methods involving consistent and systematic rewards for appropriate behaviour or responses are effective in enhancing communication skills and in improving eating and sleeping patterns. The technique of 'graded change', introducing alterations in the child's environment in very small but firm and maintained steps, may be effective in reducing the rigidity which some autistic children insist on in their environment. Differential reinforcement of other behaviours (DRO), with simultaneous ignoring of undesired behavioural tendencies wherever possible, is a particularly powerful treatment for maladaptive behavioural tendencies. Methods of this type need to be applied by parents at home, teachers at school, and other supporting and caring individuals wherever they meet the child, as generalization of change from clinic or hospital to other settings is always difficult.

Parental counselling to alleviate distress and promote coping skills is particularly necessary in the first few months after the diagnosis is made, but remains important subsequently. Parents take a very variable time to overcome their grief at 'losing' the normal child they expected to rear. They react in a variety of ways to their distress—especially with anger and depression and often disbelief regarding the diagnosis. Anxiety about the future, often largely based on realistic concerns, sometimes becomes preoccupying and gets in the way of potentially useful interventions. Health professionals, with their capacity to understand and accept parental reactions, can support and advise about ways of fostering normal development and tackling behavioural problems. With knowledge of the likely outcome they can often play a helpful part in supporting parents of such children (Howlin and Rutter 1987; Turk 1996*a*). Family therapy can play an important role regarding grief work, the need to adapt to life-long support of a disabled family member, and the need to address the often substantial effects on siblings (Howlin 1988).

Social interventions are of importance in alleviating the family's burden and facilitating more normal development. These include ensuring that all allowances the family is entitled to are being claimed, respite care has been offered, and the family has been supplied with appropriate information and the potential to link with supportive organizations such as national autistic societies.

Outcome

Autism is almost always a life-long condition. Approximately two-thirds of children so diagnosed remain dependent as adults throughout their lives and require continuing care at home or in hostel accommodation. Only about 10% achieve a really significant degree of independence, and a somewhat smaller number are able to obtain a job on the open market (Lotter 1978); 50% remain without spoken language and those that do develop speech show continuity over time in their styles of language deviance. Personality problems involving impairment of social relationships are usually prominent. Progress in social functioning does occur, but most develop a pattern of being 'aloof', 'passive', or 'active but odd' (Gillberg 1991). About 1 in 6 children develop occasional attacks of epilepsy, and 50% of individuals experience aggravation of their behavioural problems as they enter adolescence. Less than half this number show signs of stagnation or deterioration in daily life and language skills. A minority of children develop more serious aggressive problems or marked mood swings, sometimes amounting to manic–depressive or schizophreniform psychoses during adolescence, and these will require treatment in their own right. The best predictors of outcome for independent living are the measured intelligence of the child (those with a non-verbal IQ over 70 do best later on), the presence of socially useful language by 5 years of age, the early development of constructive play, and harmonious and supportive family relationships.

Three provisos need to be made to this bleak account of prognosis:

- First, some instances of apparently classical but mild autism diagnosed in the pre-school period and associated with normal or high intelligence, do seem to abate in middle childhood.
- Second, although progress is very slow, in nearly all cases there is continuing improvement throughout childhood and adolescence, so that each year the child gains some new skills.
- Third, the quality of parental care and education is important in outcome. Autistic children who are neglected or who do not receive the correct educational input will not make the gains of which they are capable. This applies as much to those with more severe learning disabilities as to those with higher intellectual functioning (Rutter and Bartak 1973).

3.5.2 ASPERGER SYNDROME

Definition

Asperger syndrome is an increasingly diagnosed condition which is characterized by a lack of empathy and capacity for social relationships, pedantic speech (Ghaziuddin and Gerstein 1996), and preoccupation with special interests about which the child may accumulate extensive information in a mechanical fashion (Wing 1981; Tantam 1988), The condition has sometimes been described as schizoid personality or autistic psychopathy (Wolff 1991*a,b*).

Clinical features

After what is usually a relatively normal early development, the child is usually noted to lack warmth and interest in social relationships round about the third year of life. Intellectual functioning is often normal, language is not usually delayed, but the quality of speech is often impaired with lack of variety in intonation. The combination of a monotonous delivery of speech, and often laborious emphasis on exactitude in the use of language gives a pedantic quality to the child's verbal output. As the child gets older he is likely to be isolated socially both by the fact that other children find him odd, and by the fact that he appears to have little interest in making friends. Lack of social sensitivity is prominent, and this sometimes leads to the child giving offence when none is intended. The child is likely to spend more and more time reading about a special interest, such as railway timetables or characters in space-fiction epics. These children are often clumsy in motor movement. They may show mannerisms, though these are usually not prominent. Physical health is generally good, and there are usually no specific learning disabilities. Frequently the most striking features, which influence style of treatment, are the resistance of the core deficit to change, the often highly developed personality and the partial, but often anguished, insight into the difficulties (Green 1990).

Prevalence

The condition occurs in about 3–4 per 1000 children (Ehlers and Gillberg 1993). It is about four times more common in boys than in girls. There may be a slight tendency for the condition to be more common in middle-class families but, as for autism, this is probably the consequence of more middle-class children with the condition being diagnosed. Intelligence is usually within the normal range. Parents may show some social and language difficulties themselves.

Aetiology

There is controversy as to whether the condition differs significantly from high-functioning autism. Indeed, in careful studies comparing children with the syndrome and autistic children, it has not been possible to identify consistent clear-cut differentiating features (Szatmari *et al.* 1995). However, detailed neuropsychological assessments have revealed multiple significant differences between individuals with Asperger syndrome and those with higher-functioning autism, particularly in the area of non-verbal learning difficulties (Klin *et al.* 1995). As with autism, the aetiology is unknown, but it is suspected that genetic factors are of major importance. Occasionally Asperger syndrome and autism occur in the same family, suggesting a common aetiology.

Assessment

Assessment of the condition involves taking a full family and developmental history as well as an account of the presenting social, communicatory, behavioural, and emotional problems. Physical examination is usually unremarkable, though clumsiness can often be detected. Physical investigations are not usually indicated.

There is often difficulty in distinguishing the condition from autism, in which language delay is prominent and learning disability is often present. It has been suggested that the term 'Asperger syndrome' should be reserved for those children who would otherwise be diagnosed as autistic, but who use language more freely yet fail to make language adjustments to fit the social context, and who wish to be sociable but fail to make deep and enduring relationships with peers. In addition they are usually clumsy, develop idiosyncratic but engrossing interests, and have marked impairments of non-verbal expressiveness affecting their facial expression and gesture.

Most clinicians continue to find it useful to make a distinction between Asperger syndrome and autism. In children with a mild variant of Asperger syndrome, it may be in their interests not to make a daunting sounding diagnosis, but to consider them merely as showing a personality variation. The point at which one can make a distinction between a normal and abnormal personality is arbitrary.

Treatment

There is no medical treatment for this pattern of personality. Parents and teachers can, however, protect children with such unusual personalities in a variety of ways. Acknowledging that the child's personality is unlikely to change very much over time and accepting the child for who and what he is are important first steps. Such children respond badly, with fearful reactions or aggression, to unpredictable events, so establishing a routine and minimizing surprises is helpful. Any unavoidable changes in routine such as moving from primary to secondary education or moving home should be anticipated, planned, and worked on well in advance. Tactful explanation to other children in the neighbourhood or classroom about the child's vulnerability, with firm handling of any bullying, reduces the stress to which the child is exposed. Most such children will cope in an ordinary school, but special educational arrangements are occasionally necessary.

As children get older they may be helped by supportive counselling about the nature of their condition, and ways in which they can improve their relationships with others. Depressive symptoms are common as the individual becomes increasingly aware of his difficulties, his differences from other people and the problems in adapting socially. However, most people with Asperger syndrome can develop a suitable niche for themselves, often based on their particular skills and interests and minimizing the need for unnecessary socialization.

Outcome

The outcome in these cases depends on whether the child's personality is widely deviant or whether he merely shows some mild personality characteristics of the type described. Most individuals will be able to obtain employment in a fairly routine job which fits in with their skills and interests, though they may not be able to cope with complex or changeable work situations. Successful relationships with the opposite sex leading to marriage are uncommon. For more severely affected individuals, sheltered employment and residence in hostel accommodation may be necessary.

There is an increased tendency towards various forms of mental illness, including anxiety and depressive reactions and obsessional disorders. A group of children with 'schizoid personality' (a closely related condition), followed up into adult life, showed a similar persistence of their personality problems with some increased tendency to antisocial behaviour (Wolff *et al.* 1991).

3.6 Sensory development

3.6.1 DEVELOPMENT OF NORMAL HEARING

The development of hearing enables a child to understand better and to respond to the world around him, and is especially vital in the development of language. Even antenatally, babies respond to loud sounds such as music or traffic (Bax *et al.* 1990). The newborn baby responds to sounds throughout the whole range that the human ear can detect. At birth, hearing babies show a startle response to a loud sound, and by 1 week they can discriminate the voice of their mother from other people. By about 6 weeks they will quieten or 'still' to the sound of the mother's voice. At 4–7 months, the infant will attend to weak auditory stimuli in his near environment. Between 10 and 15 months, the baby will be able to locate sounds above and below ear level without the aid of visual cues. The young child's ability to discriminate new speech sounds is partly determined by what is heard at home, indicating the importance of a wide range of early language experience.

Screening for deafness

Auditory responsiveness of newborns can be tested, using an auditory response cradle. This measures movements and changes in respiratory rate in response to 85 dB sound and can detect hearing impairment reliably. High-risk cases (e.g. with a family history of deafness) should be screened in this way. Turning in response to sound develops slowly in the newborn and early detection of deafness in the UK still mainly depends on screening procedures using a distraction test between 7 and 9 months (Hall 1989). The baby's capacity to localize sound by head turning to quiet sounds made just outside his visual field is assessed. Parental doubts about their child's hearing expressed before this age should, however, always be taken seriously. There is some controversy concerning whether screening for hearing impairment should continue between 1 and 5 years, but it is agreed that parents should always be asked if they suspect their child's hearing may be affected when the child is screened for other purposes during this time. Parental concern about hearing loss, the presence of language delay, and recurrent otitis media are indications for repeated testing. Children thought possibly to be suffering from hearing impairment require audiometric procedures, a description of which is beyond the scope of this book, but it should be noted that the sooner detection occurs and remedial measures instigated, the better the prognosis.

Auditory perception continues to mature throughout childhood. For example, the child's capacity to discriminate between consonants and different musical sounds increases up to the age of puberty.

3.6.2 HEARING IMPAIRMENT

Deafness can be classified according to its cause (conduction or sensorineural) or according to its severity (mild, 15–30 dB loss; moderate, 30–45 dB loss;

severe, 65–95 dB loss; profound, greater than 95 dB loss), or according to the frequency-range loss. Severity may vary depending on the pitch and tone of the sound. A particular pattern of loss, for example loss of high or low frequency, may make generalization from average loss misleading.

Mild conductive hearing loss is relatively common, and is usually caused by secretary otitis media ('glue ear'). Conductive loss may also occur in association with certain syndromes, such as Down syndrome, fragile X syndrome, and cleft palate in which the middle ear is often affected.

More severe degrees of deafness commonly have a sensorineural cause. Sensorineural deafness occurs in about 1 per 2000 children (I. G. Taylor 1984). Genetically determined conditions and fetal infection (especially rubella and cytomegalovirus) are responsible for a high proportion. It is important to remember that congenital rubella infection may be reactivated after birth causing progressive hearing impairment in a child whose hearing has previously been normal or less severely affected.

Psychological development

In deaf children who do not have associated disabilities such as cerebral malformations, cerebral palsy, and visual impairment, non-verbal intelligence does not differ early on from that found in the general population, but may begin to decline even in the pre-school years (Sonksen 1985). Early conceptual development of hearing-impaired children usually proceeds normally. Deaf children show normal make-believe play, confirming that language development is not a necessary requirement for the development of some forms of symbolic thought. Language development is, however, likely to be impaired even in the mildly hearing-impaired child, and will be seriously affected in more severe forms of deafness.

The causes of language delay in the mildly deaf child are often complex. Recurrent ear infections are more likely to occur in understimulated children living in deprived and overcrowded circumstances. A child with mild hearing loss living in a chaotic household with the television or radio on loud all the time is much more likely to have difficulty in making sense of verbal messages and making himself understood than a child with a similar level of hearing loss living in more fortunate circumstances. The former child is not only more likely to show early language delay, but also difficulties in reading later on.

It has been frequently suggested that chronic secretory otitis media (CSOM) is a common cause of reading failure. However, rigorously controlled studies (e.g. Webster *et al.* 1989) suggest that this is probably not the case, although there may be small effects on language and reading development (Haggard and Hughes 1991). It is more likely that the adverse social conditions linked to CSOM are more likely to be responsible for educational problems. Nevertheless, CSOM is an unpleasant condition that impairs communication while it is present, and it certainly deserves early identification and treatment.

Severe deafness affects both comprehension and expression. The child's inability to hear diminishes his capacity to monitor his own vocalizations. His capacity to understand what is going on around him and to communicate with others, especially members of his own family, is thus potentially seriously threatened.

Early management of the severely deaf child

Parental suspicion of deafness can precede diagnosis by several months. The intervening period is one of uncertainty for the family, although the diagnosis is less often accompanied by hopelessness and despair than is the case with visual impairment. Help from competent professionals (such as audiologists, speech therapists, and psychologists) will reduce secondary problems.

Assessment of the intellectual development of deaf children requires special skills. Psychologists will use intelligence tests, such as the Merrill Palmer, Hiskey–Nebraska, or Leiter, which require little or no language ability.

Mild or moderate degrees of deafness can usually be compensated for to some degree by hearing aids, so that communication with the family need not necessarily be seriously affected. With more severe degrees of deafness, especially in the pre-school years, parents may need to be helped to understand and cope with behaviour problems associated with impaired communication and lack of coping skills. There is controversy as to whether parents should be encouraged themselves to learn one of the various sign languages, but most now agree that all forms of facilitating communication, both in the family and in the school setting, should be promoted. Unusual degrees of dependence may arise because the child cannot use auditory cues to locate his mother and so needs to be physically close to her or at least within eyesight. Temper tantrums arising from frustration because of inability to make needs known are more common in young deaf children. Special care needs to be taken to encourage the deaf child to mix with other children who, in the early years, are likely to ignore a child who does not respond readily to requests and social overtures. Efforts should be made to encourage communication and to minimize forms of behaviour that may be off-putting to others. Hospitalization of the seriously deaf child also requires special preparation because of the child's impaired level of verbal understanding.

With modern aids, the education of all but the most severely deaf or multiply disabled children can take place in normal school or in a special unit attached to a normal school. For a small minority of children, more specialized day or residential education will be required. Wherever the child is educated the staff need to have a comprehensive appreciation of the hearing-impaired child's strengths and weaknesses as they interact with the academic, psychological, and social demands of the school setting and routine.

Psychiatric disorders

The rate of emotional and behavioural difficulties in the hearing-impaired child is higher than that in the general population. Children with fluctuating hearing impairments are at greater risk of behavioural problems and language and reading delay; children with permanent hearing impairment experience similar mental health problems to hearing children although presentation, treatment, and outcome differ because of differences in communication and language use (Hindley 1997). Hindley *et al.* (1994) found that approximately 50% of hearing-impaired or deaf 11–16 year old young people had psychiatric disorder—rates being greater in those attending hearing-impaired units than in those attending a deaf school. The use of verbal speech as well as sign language, which may indicate increased hearing ability, has a protective effect in adolescence (Vostanis *et al.* 1997). Freeman (1977) found deaf children were particularly likely to be described as restless, possessive, and destructive. Causes consisted mainly of disturbances in family relationships and inappropriate child-rearing practices and attitudes. Such problems are, however, heightened by difficulties in communicating with the deaf child. For example, studies which use teacher or parent questionnaires find a preponderance of conduct disorder while direct interviews with hearing-impaired children show a preponderance of anxiety disorders (Hindley and Brown 1994). Significant differences have also been identified in the patterns of fears experienced by hearing-impaired young people (King *et al.* 1989). Whereas hearing children are more fearful of failure and criticism, hearing-impaired children are more afraid of the unknown, injury, and small animals. Divorce is not more common in parents of deaf children, but when family conflict occurs it often focuses around problems of communication with the child in question.

Assessment and treatment of disturbance in deaf children pose unusual problems for the professional. It has been suggested (Freeman 1977) that mental health professionals who are involved should either be able to sign or to have a competent interpreter, that they should be sure to collect information from more than one source, and that they should be wary of wrongly interpreting deviant verbal expression as a sign either of thought disorder or intellectual impairment. Not surprisingly, it has been found that the interviewer's linguistic competence has a significant effect on the range of symptoms elicited at interview—poor competence leading to the masking of the child's emotional difficulties (Hindley *et al.* 1993). In general, once communication problems with the deaf child or adolescent have been at least partly overcome, the principles of assessment and treatment need not vary greatly from those employed with hearing children. In serious instances the services of a highly specialized team for young deaf people with psychiatric disorder may be required.

3.6.3 DEVELOPMENT OF NORMAL VISION

The development of visual skills allows children to explore and learn about their environment, and to integrate information obtained from the other senses in a way that enormously increases their capacity to adapt to the world around them. It is not surprising that blindness is one of the handicaps most feared by parents for their children.

The pupillary reflex is present from about week 28 of gestation. At birth, newborns can see objects best at 23 cm (9 inches) away, conveniently enabling them to observe their mother's face while feeding. They will also turn their head to a diffuse light source such as a window at this time. The newborn is also capable of visual fixation, and by 4 weeks can be seen to watch his mother carefully when she speaks to him. Visual input during the first 3 months of life leads to the development of integrated circuits at cortical level which are revealed by behaviour such as reaching for an object in the field of vision, and turning to a sound source at 4 months, blinking to a threat at 5 months, and searching for a recently lost object at 8 months. Smooth convergence of both eyes and binocular vision develop by 4–6 months.

Visual perception also shows rapid maturation in the first year of life. At 2 months an infant will look more at a picture of a face than at a shape with 'scrambled' facial features on it. By 6–7 months, and often earlier, a baby can tell familiar from unfamiliar faces. Perceptual maturation continues at least during the first 10 years of life. As children get older they become more capable of distinguishing shapes such as letters that are similar but somewhat different from each other (Walk 1980).

Screening for visual defects, for example congenital cataract, should take place through careful inspection of the eyes after birth. Parents should be asked at all subsequent screening examinations (recommended in the UK at 6 weeks, 8 months, 21 months, and 39 months) whether they have any concern about the child's sight. Any parental anxieties about the child's vision should be taken seriously and would normally indicate referral to an ophthalmologist. Squints can often be detected at the 8 month examination. Visual acuity should be checked periodically by the school nurse throughout the school years in case the child has need of spectacles (Hall 1989).

3.6.4 VISUAL IMPAIRMENT

Visual defects to a degree requiring special education occur in about 4 per 10 000 children. They are caused by a wide variety of physical conditions. Optic atrophy, cataract, and diseases of the macula, retina, and choroid account for over 50% of cases of registered blindness (Fine 1979). Most causes of blindness or partial sight are present at birth, and about half are genetically determined (Jay 1979). Visual difficulties may be caused by cortical visual impairment, a condition in which the ocular structures are normal, but the occipital lobes are damaged (Jan *et al.* 1987). The condition is difficult to diagnose because many such children have some residual vision and visual impairment may vary considerably depending on the task in question, being better in familiar environments and when the child understands what to look for and where to look for it.

Additional handicaps are common among children with visual defects. Rates of associated handicap depend on the severity of the visual defects involved, but in some series as many as 70% of visually handicapped children have been found to be suffering from some degree of learning disability. It is, however, often uncertain how far such retardation is organically determined (see below). Cerebral palsy, hearing loss, language delay, and related congenital abnormalities are also relatively common.

Psychological development

Children with visual defects present from birth are often not identified immediately. Their parents only gradually realize that there is something wrong, perhaps because of delay in the smiling response, or the fact that the baby seems surprised when a bottle touches his mouth. In fact, in the first 6 or 8 weeks of life, the baby may indeed show perioral movements that resemble a smile but do not depend on visual stimulation and have no social function. It is only at around 2 months that the 'reflex' smile to visual stimuli and, later, the smile of recognition, become established. Professionals are often slow to accept that parental anxieties are soundly based.

Even in the absence of organic causes for slow development, children with visual deficits are often slow in their motor, language, and social development. This may be due to the fact that, ordinarily, vision-assisted learning takes place in achieving skills such as the location of sound and touch which do not obviously require an intact visual pathway for their performance (Sonksen 1985). It may also, at least in some cases, be related to the fact that visually impaired children receive inappropriate stimulation or too little stimulation from their parents. The infant's apparent lack of responsiveness may lead the mother and others around to avoid attempts at social interaction. The depression experienced by mothers after the diagnosis has been confirmed may also contribute to such stimulus deprivation. Mothers should be strongly encouraged to respond actively to their child's vocalizations, using touch as well as verbal stimulation. Initial expectations after diagnosis may be too low, and the lack of visual cues may lead to delay in the development of attachment (Fraiberg 1977). Toys should be carefully selected for their tactile and auditory qualities. The development of object constancy (the capacity to retain an image in the mind when the stimulus is no longer present) is slow to develop in the visually impaired child, so that, once attachment has occurred, even brief separations from the mother can be more upsetting than they would be to a sighted child of a similar level of maturity (Hunt and Wills 1983). Hospitalizations therefore need especially careful planning to ensure that the child is not left unaccompanied by a familiar figure who can interpret what is happening to him. Assessment of intellectual level in blind or partially sighted children can be carried out using specially designed tests (e.g. Reynell and Zinkin 1975).

Psychiatric disorders

The rate of behavioural and emotional disorders in visually impaired children is higher than in the general population (Jan *et al.* 1977) with 45% showing a moderate or severe disorder, but there is no reason to think that these are inevitable consequences. Factors relating to disturbance include the severity of the visual loss, the presence of multiple disabilities, the frequency and duration of early hospitalization, parental anxiety, and depression, as well as the quality of family relationships (Freeman 1989).

Psychiatric problems characteristic of this group include feeding and sleeping difficulties as well as social isolation. Mannerisms, not necessarily related to other behaviour or emotional problems, are common. The most common are stereotypies, especially rocking, eye pressing, repetitive noises, and hand flapping. The term 'blindisms' has been used for these mannerisms, but, in fact, with the exception of eye pressing they also occur in other conditions such as autism. They are much more characteristic of blind than of partially sighted children. They appear related to the level of stimulation the child receives, and may represent a form of self-stimulation when understimulated or a response to overstimulation or tension.

Management of psychological and psychiatric problems in children with visual defects requires more than ordinary skills and experience of, for example, the ways in which the visually impaired child responds to frustration. Mannerisms may, however, respond well to operant behaviour modification programmes.

The special educational needs of a child with a visual defect require careful planning to reflect individual needs and especially the stage of development. This should be achievable with the child living at home but an older child or adolescent may benefit from the special facilities available in a residential placement.

Follow-up studies of blind children into adolescence and early adulthood suggest that a significant proportion are able to obtain employment and make rewarding social relationships, but this is less likely to occur in the multiply handicapped. It is certainly more difficult for the blind teenager to make and sustain friendships, but this may be made easier if the young person has the opportunity, at least part of the time, to mix with others with similar disabilities. The causes of occupational success or failure in adolescents with visual impairments are multiple and complex, including distance visual acuity, the individual's attitude to visual impairment, and interaction with the normally sighted (Wolffe and Wild 1984). The acquisition of sexual knowledge and appropriate sexual behaviour is problematic and requires special attention. Indeed a high proportion (nearly a quarter) of blind teenagers report having been sexually molested (Freeman 1989).

3.7 Chromosomal abnormalities

The most common defects involving chromosomes are:

- *numerical*: there are one or more additional chromosomes, or a chromosome is absent
- *mosaic*: in a single individual, some cells have normal chromosome patterns, others abnormal
- *deletions*: part of a chromosome is missing
- *translocations*: part of a chromosome has transferred to another one
- *DNA expansions*: there is abnormal amplification of a DNA sequence on a chromosome.

Abnormalities may affect either one of the two sex chromosomes or one or more of the 22 pairs of autosomes.

The relevance of these conditions for a child psychiatric perspective has been substantially increased by growing awareness that many syndromes have an associated 'behavioural phenotype' a characteristic profile of behavioural features and other developmental tendencies attributable to the underlying genetic anomaly (Turk and Sales 1996). Any one individual with a genetic syndrome may or may not show the characteristic behaviour, but is more likely to show the behaviour than individuals without the syndrome (Dykens 1995).

3.7.1 AUTOSOMAL ABNORMALITIES

Down syndrome (trisomy 21)

Down syndrome is the most common chromosomal abnormality which is compatible with life. It accounts for about one-third of all cases of learning disability with IQ less than 50. In 95% of instances the syndrome is caused by an additional chromosome 21 arising from an abnormality of germ cell division. About 1% of cases are due to mosaicism where there are two cell lines, one with two copies of chromosome 21 and the other with three. In this situation there is a relationship between the proportion of cells showing trisomy 21 and the severity of learning disability. In the remaining 4% (translocation type) there is an exchange of genetic material between two adjacent chromosomes. The trisomy (but not the translocation type) is associated with increased maternal age, with the condition occurring in about 1% of babies born to mothers aged over 40 years, but only about 0.1% in births overall. However, most babies with Down syndrome are born to younger mothers. The translocation type can be inherited, emphasizing the need for chromosomal confirmation of diagnosis even when it may seem obvious from physical and developmental features.

Physical features

The condition is usually evident at birth. Children have up-slanting eyes with epicanthic folds, a short nose with flat nasal bridge, brachycephaly (short head), white (Brushfield) spots in the iris of the eye, and a large tongue. The fingers are short and stubbed with an incurved little finger and the hands display a single palmar crease rather than the double crease normally found. The children are of short stature and show muscular hypotonia. There is a high rate of associated abnormalities, especially malformations of the heart (septal defects) and gut (e.g. duodenal atresia), some of which are incompatible with life. Upper respiratory tract and ear infections may produce chronic hearing difficulties. The risk for hypothyroidism rises with increasing age. Atlanto-axial instability has also been reported but is not usually of clinical significance (Morton *et al.* 1995).

Intellectual development

The very early development of children with this syndrome is often rather little below average (Carr 1970). However, by the age of 5 years the level of development is nearly always definitely retarded with a mean IQ of about 45 and a range from 25 to 70. Higher IQ levels have been recorded and a small number of children with Down syndrome can be educated in mainstream schools. Early stimulation programmes such as Portage help to promote development, and home-reared children achieve higher educational attainment in reading and arithmetic (though not higher IQ) than do non-home-reared children (Carr 1988), but there is no evidence that achievement of intelligence within the normal range is other than a most unusual outcome. The number of children with Down syndrome who are educated in mainstream schools has increased, partly as a result of more intensive early stimulation programmes, and partly because of new policies integrating children with learning disabilities into the mainstream of education. There are usually no specific cognitive deficits, although visuo-motor skills and tactile discrimination may be particularly impaired. The IQ level tends to remain stable during middle childhood, though it is influenced, within limits, by the quality of care provided. Institutionalized children generally do worse, and those given extra stimulation programmes do rather better than average.

In adulthood, individuals with Down syndrome are particularly prone to develop presenile dementia of Alzheimer type (Oliver and Holland 1986). In the early stages this condition may be mistaken for depression (also more common in people with Down syndrome than in other individuals with similar degrees of learning disability), 'challenging behaviour', or a psychological reaction to life circumstances.

Impact on family life

The presence of a child growing into adulthood but achieving only partial independence will alter the lives of parents and siblings in a most significant way. Depression in mothers of affected children is more common than it is in the general population, and this is often related to the experience of loss of the normal child the mother expected to have. Guilty feelings are not usually a prominent feature, though they may be present. Rates of divorce are not higher in parents (Gath and Gumley 1984; Carr 1988), though evidently the quality of family life is often profoundly altered, and sometimes diminished. Nevertheless, a significant number of parents speak very positively of the experience of bring-ing up a child with this condition. Behaviour problems in siblings, whose life is often markedly affected, are more often found if the child with Down syndrome has disturbed behaviour (Gath and Gumley 1987). There is a higher rate of psychiatric problems in the older sisters in these families, possibly due to their carrying an undue burden of care. Academically and socially, siblings do as well as their peers (Gath and Gumley 1987).

Behavioural development

Many children with Down syndrome are unusually good-natured, contented, and warm in their personalities, characteristics that have been confirmed in systematic comparisons with siblings and with other children who have similar degrees of intellectual impairment (Gibbs and Thorpe 1983). A minority are aggressive and difficult, and these are more likely to have the translocation abnormality. The rate of significant behavioural disturbances is, if anything, slightly higher than that in the general population, but lower than that found with other children with learning disabilities (Gath and Gumley 1984). This remains true for adults with Down syndrome when compared with their learning-disabled peers (Collacott *et al.* 1998). However, serious conditions such as autism (Howlin *et al.* 1995) and hyperkinetic disorder (Green *et al.* 1989) do occur in children with Down syndrome, can often be neglected because of problem behaviours being attributed to the associated learning disability, and can be very difficult to manage.

Management
The general assessment and management of these children should follow the lines described under the heading of general learning disability. Identification of the specific chromosome abnormality is important because the translocation type is more likely to recur in subsequent children than is the more common trisomy form.

Other trisomies

Trisomies at other chromosomal sites also cause multiple congenital abnormalities and intellectual impairment, but occur much less frequently. Trisomy 18 (*Edwards' syndrome*) is the most common. It is not usually compatible with life, although some babies with this condition do survive for several months.

Other autosomal abnormalities

Deletions and absences of chromosomes usually result in early spontaneous abortions, but there are occasional survivors. New genetic technologies such as fluorescent *in situ* hybridization (FISH) and DNA probe analysis by Southern blots are revealing increasing numbers of microdeletion and DNA expansion abnormalities associated with genetic syndromes, many of which show characteristic developmental and behavioural profiles (McGuffin 1987).

Cri du chat syndrome
The rare cri du chat syndrome occurs in approximately 1 in 50 000 live births. It is associated with a partial deletion of the short arm of chromosome 5. Affected individuals have severe developmental delay and a number of physical features including microcephaly, hypertelorism, epicanthic folds, oblique palpebral fissures, posteriorly rotated low-set ears, and a small jaw. There is infantile hypotonia as well as the characteristic cry which has been attributed to abnormal laryngeal development. Individuals who develop speech often display a characteristic relatively high-pitched, monochromatic voice timbre. Neonatal poor sucking and vomiting with failure to thrive are common, with continuing growth retardation. Cardiovascular and gastrointestinal abnormalities occur. Cognitive assessments frequently show marked discrepancies between verbal and non-verbal abilities with language development being particularly delayed (Carlin 1990). However, recent research (Cornish and Pigram 1996) has shown that over three-quarters of individuals can use basic sign or gestural language to communicate their needs. Also, receptive language skills are often more advanced than expressive ones (Cornish and Munir 1998). Other commonly witnessed behaviours include self-injury, overactivity, distractibility, repetitive movements, and hyperacusis (Dykens and Clarke 1997).

Prader–Willi syndrome

Prader–Willi syndrome demonstrates the phenomenon of imprinting, in which parental origin of the affected chromosome is critical in terms of the consequences caused by the genetic abnormality. It is produced by a deletion on the long arm of *paternal* chromosome 15. A proportion of individuals do not show this microdeletion but have inherited both copies of chromosome 15 from their mother—so-called *uniparental disomy*. Physical features include short stature, hypogonadism, infantile hypotonia, and a tendency to develop diabetes mellitus. Intellectual activities are uneven. Visuospatial skills seem good, yet numeracy and short-term memory present difficulties. Early language and articulation problems and poor feeding in early life are rapidly replaced by a voracious, insatiable appetite leading to extreme obesity. Increased food intake is aggravated by reduced total energy expenditure attributable to reduced activity levels (Schoeller *et al.* 1988). Self-injurious skin picking is common and there is some evidence that this and the overeating may respond to selective serotonin reuptake inhibitors such as fluoxetine (Hellings and Warnock 1994) or to fenfluramine (Selikowitz *et al.* 1990). The special psychological feature of this condition is the management problem posed by the severe obesity. The main intervention for this problem is strict, consistent, long-term behavioural modification programmes. Results are improved if strict food restriction is undertaken from an early age. As with other forms of obesity, it may be possible to obtain weight reduction, though difficult to sustain it. Management is complicated further by individuals' proclivity for sweet foods (far more so than the general population) and their tendency to frequent, unpredictable, violent outbursts (Dykens *et al.* 1992). Parents need a great deal of support long-term, and in many developed countries including the USA and UK there are parent support associations specifically for this condition.

Angelman syndrome

Angelman syndrome is usually caused by a similar chromosome 15 microdeletion to that found in Prader–Willi syndrome but inherited *maternally*. The condition can also be caused by uniparental disomy for *paternal* chromosome 15. There is severe learning disability, typical facial features, an abnormal jerky 'puppet-like' gait, a tendency towards an open mouth with tongue protrusion and specific EEG changes (Clayton-Smith 1993). Repetitive paroxysmal laughter with no obvious precipitant is common. Speech and language development is extremely delayed with children developing very few words and having difficulty in using gestural or sign systems (Joleff and Ryan 1993). Abnormal social interactions with autistic features have been reported (Sales and Turk 1991). The typical lack of speech may not only be due to severe intellectual impairment, but also to oral-motor dyspraxia and deficits in social interaction and attention (Penner *et al.* 1993).

Smith–Magenis syndrome

Despite its rarity, with a prevalence of about 1 in 50 000, Smith–Magenis syndrome is receiving increased attention. It is caused by a microdeletion on the short arm of chromosome 17. Physical features can be very subtle and degree of intellectual impairment highly variable, making diagnosis difficult. Individuals are prone to severe sleep disorders with problems settling and repeated waking throughout the night. They often demonstrate self-injury in the form of head banging and nail pulling (Colley *et al.* 1990). Overactivity and attentional deficits are marked and autistic features are common (Vostanis *et al.* 1994).

Tuberous sclerosis

Tuberous sclerosis is an autosomal dominant condition caused by deletions on either chromosome 9 or chromosome 16. As well as being associated with learning disability and infantile spasms which may prove very difficult to control (Riikonen and Simell 1990), it is strongly associated with autism and hyperactivity (Harrison and Bolton 1997). However, a substantial minority of people with tuberous sclerosis function intellectually within the normal range with few if any obvious behavioural problems and no more than one or two of the characteristic skin stigmata such as facial angiofibromata or shagreen patches.

3.7.2 SEX CHROMOSOME ABNORMALITIES

The effects of sex chromosome abnormalities are usually less obvious and more readily compatible with life than the above chromosomal abnormalities. As with autosomal abnormalities, diagnosis is confirmed by microscopic examination of the chromosomes using special techniques and sometimes by specific DNA tests. Screening for sex chromosome abnormalities may be achieved by examining cells obtained from a buccal smear. Where more than one X chromosome is present, so-called *Barr bodies*, or clumps of chromatin, can be seen at the periphery of the nucleus. This technique is therefore often helpful when a male is suspected of having an extra X or a female an absent or extra X chromosome.

Turner syndrome

Turner syndrome is one of the commonest chromosomal anomalies, with an incidence of at least one in 1850 live female births. Approximately 50% of these girls have 45 chromosomes, one X chromosome being absent. Most of the remainder show a mosaic chromosomal pattern with some cells containing XO and others XX sex chromosomal material (Chu and Connor 1995). Occasionally one of the X chromosomes suffers loss of its extremities, the remaining material forming a 'ring'. In this condition the developmental and behavioural features are very different from that of XO Turner syndrome (El Abd *et al.* 1997).

Clinical features

The child is likely to be short and stocky. The neck may be webbed and the carrying angle at the elbow increased. External genitalia remain infantile, and the internal reproductive organs do not develop. Other congenital abnormalities (especially coarctation of the aorta) are common. Menstruation does not occur at puberty and the girls are infertile. The condition usually presents with growth delay, but, surprisingly, bearing in mind the short stature, the diagnosis is not infrequently delayed until puberty when individuals present with amenorrhoea. Recent work indicates the importance of parental inheritance of the single X chromosome. The 70–80% of girls who have a maternally derived X have more cardiovascular abnormalities and neck webbing and their height correlates very strongly with maternal but not paternal height (Chu *et al*. 1994).

Psychological aspects

General intelligence is not usually affected, but there is often a specific defect of visuospatial ability, and mathematical skills are also frequently impaired (Ratcliffe *et al*. 1991). Moderate and severe learning disability does not, however, appear in excess (Silbert *et al*. 1977).

Opportunities are needed to express concern about appearance and stature. This is all the more necessary as the diagnosis is so often delayed, and the girl is unprepared for the future in store for her. There may be anatomical problems with sexual intercourse, and infertility is certain. Menstruation can be induced with cyclical oestrogen therapy, and this may be desirable to help the girl feel more normal. Recent treatment with oestrogens, androgens, and growth hormones holds promise for improving growth and sexual development.

Social relationships are often impaired, and there may be other problems including language difficulties and attentional deficits (Skuse *et al*. 1994). These do not appear to be due to the short stature itself, as comparisons with children with other types of short stature suggest that girls with Turner syndrome are specifically at risk for these difficulties (McCauley *et al*. 1986). Girls with the syndrome are said to show a stronger feminine sex-role identity than do girls with constitutional short stature (Downey *et al*. 1987). Chromosomal imprinting is of importance psychologically as well as physically. Paternal derivation of the X chromosome is associated with better psychological adjustment and superior verbal and higher-order executive function skills which mediate social interactions (Skuse *et al*. 1997). Conversely, maternal X chromosome derivation is said to be associated with rates of autistic spectrum disorders approaching that seen in males generally. The ring Turner anomaly is probably more often associated with more severe intellectual impairment and autistic-like social, communicatory, and ritualistic problems as well as structural brain abnormalities such as agenesis of the corpus callosum (El Abd *et al*. 1997).

Noonan syndrome

Noonan syndrome is caused by an abnormality on the long arm of chromosome 12. It is inherited in an autosomal dominant fashion, 50% of cases being new mutations (Jamieson *et al*. 1994). Although the condition is clearly not attributable to a sex chromosome abnormality, individuals have most of the features of Turner syndrome. About one-third of pregnancies with a Noonan syndrome fetus are complicated by polyhydramnios. Cardiac lesions are common, especially pulmonary stenosis and hypertrophic cardiomyopathy. Individuals frequently show motor inco-ordination and three-quarters have significant feeding difficulties in infancy (Sharland *et al.* 1992). Short stature, motor milestone delay, and vision and hearing problems are common. There is a wide range of intellectual functioning with a slight general shift downwards so that approximately 10% require special educational input. Performance IQ exceeds verbal IQ. There are high levels of parentally reported emotional problems which may be attributable to the common early feeding difficulties. Questionnaire surveys suggest that children with Noonan syndrome tend to be clumsy, stubborn, and irritable with communication difficulties and food fads (Wood *et al.* 1995).

Klinefelter syndrome

Klinefelter syndrome occurs in boys who have an XXY chromosomal structure. It is the most common single cause of hypogonadism and infertility, affecting about 1 in 500 males. The appearance in childhood is not particularly abnormal, although individuals tend to be rather tall. At puberty the testes remain small, other secondary sexual characteristics may only partially develop, and breast development occurs in about half the affected individuals. Diagnosis usually occurs in adulthood when individuals present with infertility.

Psychological aspects

Retrospective and total population information suggests that children with Klinefelter syndrome are more likely to be anxious, dependent, socially withdrawn and introverted, and to have increased rates of emotional disorder (Mandoki *et al.* 1991). They tend to have speech and language impairments but relatively intact non-verbal intellectual skills (Ratcliffe *et al.* 1991). Claims that adults with Klinefelter syndrome do not show such deficits suggest that pubertal maturation may eliminate them (Stewart *et al.* 1991). Less than 20% have an IQ below 90 so intelligence is usually within the normal range (Ratcliffe *et al.* 1991). Boys with Klinefelter syndrome tend to be apprehensive and insecure with more peer group relationship problems and low sexual interest in girls.

XYY syndrome

Children with XYY karyotype are often unusually tall, but show no other clearly characteristic physical features. The condition was once thought to be associated with criminal behaviour, but the evidence for this is weak. In fact children in the general population with the karyotype are definitely more likely to have early language delay and later reading (but not arithmetical) difficulties (Ratcliffe *et al.* 1991). In childhood they do show high rates of temper outbursts and social relationship problems, and psychiatric referral occurs more frequently than in the general population, often because of oppositional and conduct disorders. Intelligence is mildly depressed in comparison with close relatives but almost always remains within the normal range. Psychological intervention should not be influenced by the presence of the karyotype which will, in any case, usually be unsuspected (Ratcliffe and Field 1982). However, presence of an XYY karyotype may explain deviant development and behaviour which might otherwise be attributed to poor parenting or social adversity.

Study of psychosocial adaptation of adolescents with sex chromosome abnormalities shows persisting lower mean IQ scores, lower overall psychosocial adaptation scores and increased incidence of psychiatric disturbance, usually depression. However, some individuals, whatever their karyotype, demonstrate relatively strong psychosocial adaptation—usually associated with a stable and supportive family environment (Bender *et al.* 1995).

Fragile X syndrome

The fragile X syndrome owes its name to the appearance of a pale, ragged, and partially detached-looking site just before the tip of the X chromosome's long arm at position Xq27.3 when cells are cultured in a folate-deficient medium. Laboratory diagnosis based on this cytogenetic test was frequently problematic because even in fragile-site-positive individuals, only a relatively small proportion of cells show the defect. Diagnosis is even less certain in female carriers and for antenatal testing. Highly sensitive and specific diagnosis is now possible using DNA Southern blot and polymerase chain reaction (PCR) technology (Oostra *et al.* 1993). The test is based on identification of an abnormal expansion of CGG base triplet repeats which exceeds 55 in so-called *premutation carriers* and 200 in so-called *full mutation* individuals who manifest the characteristic physical, developmental, and behavioural features. The abnormal DNA expansion is associated with hypermethylation of an adjacent gene site and suppression of its gene product—a protein which has important neurodevelopmental functions in terms of transfer of material from nucleus to cytoplasm and binding of messenger RNA to ribosomes (Brown 1996). This test identifies almost all individuals with fragile X syndrome but does not show up any other genetic disorders. The test is only undertaken if specifically requested, hence chromosomal analysis is still important and the need for DNA evaluation for fragile X must be explicitly requested.

Although the condition is sex-linked, the pattern of inheritance is not that of a simple sex-linked Mendelian disorder. Only four-fifths of affected males show cognitive defects, and about one-third of 'carrier' females are themselves learning-disabled (Hagerman and Cronister 1996). Fragile X has been shown to account for almost 10% of all boys with moderate to profound learning disabilities and for about 6–10% of otherwise unexplained mild learning disability (Thake *et al.* 1987). However, recent estimates put its prevalence at between 1 in 3000 and 1 in 6000 boys and approximately 1 in 8000 girls (Turner *et al.* 1996). It is therefore the most common inherited cause of intellectual impairment and the second most common cause of learning disability after Down syndrome (trisomy 21).

Affected children show a number of characteristic physical features including a large head with a long face and nasal bridge, 'simple' protruding ears, a large jaw, high-arched palate, hypermobile joints with ligamentous laxity, soft velvety skin, and postpubertal macro-orchidism (testicular enlargement) (Simko *et al.* 1989). Hearing and visual impairments have been reported as being common

(Hagerman 1996). Recurrent secretory otitis media ('glue ear') has been said to be a substantial problem for 60%. Common eye problems reported include squint, short- and long-sightedness, nystagmus, and ptosis (Maino *et al*. 1991). There may be an increased risk of mitral valve prolapse and aortic root dilatation (Puzzo *et al*. 1990). Epilepsy is said to affect approximately 20% of males. Seizures usually present in early childhood as staring spells, akinetic episodes, complex partial seizures, or generalized tonic–clonic episodes. They are usually infrequent and usually respond well to anticonvulsants, particularly carbamazepine. However, it is rarely possible to make a diagnosis on the basis of physical features (Thake *et al*. 1985) and early gross motor milestones are often unremarkable.

General level of intellectual functioning is very variable but is usually in the mild to moderate learning disability range corresponding to an IQ of 35–70. There is a verbal/performance discrepancy with relatively well-developed skills in language areas but poor numeracy and visuospatial functioning. The rate of intellectual development remains parallel to that of non-learning-disabled peers up until puberty when the discrepancy widens because of specific difficulties in the sequential processing of information which become more marked over time (Hodapp *et al*. 1991). All these intellectual anomalies are seen in female carriers, most of whom have average intellectual functioning. There is an association with autism. Fragile X syndrome accounts for 2–3% of cases of autism (Bailey *et al*. 1993) and a substantial minority of children with fragile X syndrome can be diagnosed as having autism (Turk 1992). There is a stronger association with a characteristic profile of autistic-like features including delayed symbolic and imaginative play, delayed echolalia, repetitive speech, hand flapping, hand biting, gaze aversion, and social anxiety in the presence of a usually friendly and sociable personality (Turk and Graham 1997).

Speech is frequently 'cluttered' (rapid and disrhythmic) with frequent dysfluent, rapid, tangential remarks and poor topic maintenance (Ferrier *et al*. 1991). Perhaps 50% or so of individuals display 'jocular litanic phraseology', so-called because of the humorous quality to the perseverative and repetitive speech which shows up-and-down swings of pitch and palilalia (multiple repetitions of phrases with increasing speed and diminishing volume). Speech disturbance is complicated further by central information processing difficulties, macrognathia, and temporomandibular joint laxity, emphasizing the need for early specialist speech and language evaluation and intervention (Abbeduto and Hagerman 1997). Care must be taken with any plans to eliminate 'deviant' speech and language patterns. It has been argued that some of the language impairments such as echolalia and repetitiveness may be serving important functions in maintaining other peoples' attention while giving the fragile X individual sufficient time to compensate for the information processing difficulties (Ferrier *et al*. 1991).

Children with fragile X syndrome often show unexpectedly extreme levels of inattentiveness, restlessness, fidgetiness, impulsive tendencies, and distractibility even when their level of general development is taken into account (Turk 1998). Some are also overwhelmingly overactive. Many of the remainder are very active as well but probably no more so than other children with similar degrees of intellectual impairment who do not have fragile X syndrome. There is some evidence that these features do not necessarily improve with age (in contrast to most children with these traits), emphasizing the need for early diagnosis and multidisciplinary intervention.

A positive result from an experienced laboratory requires explanation to the parents, who should be advised that further male children have about a 1 in 2 chance of learning disability and female children a roughly 1 in 6 chance of being affected. (These figures are based on knowledge that about 10% of males and 70% of females with a fragile site are of normal ability.) Multidisciplinary intervention will be determined largely by the degree of learning disability and the presence or absence of autistic features. However, teachers should be aware of the implications of the often strikingly uneven cognitive profile, the characteristic trajectory of intellectual development with sequential information processing difficulties, the gaze aversion, and the frequent attentional deficits (Gibb 1992).

Other sex chromosome abnormalities

There is a large number of sex chromosome abnormalities, all of which are extremely rare. Most of them are incompatible with survival of the fetus to term.

3.7.3 SYNDROMES WITH LIKELY BUT UNPROVEN GENETIC AETIOLOGY

There are some conditions where evidence for a genetic basis seems overwhelming yet identification of the gene(s) responsible remains elusive.

Rett syndrome

Rett syndrome (Hagberg 1993) affects only girls, occurring in approximately 1 in 15 000 live births. Normal development for 6–12 months is followed by gross motor and cognitive deterioration with language loss, seizures, and the emergence of stereotypic hand movements, overbreathing, and autistic features. Life expectancy is limited by physical decline including kyphoscoliosis which compromises respiratory function, often severely. The most plausible hypothesis is of an X-linked dominant abnormality which is always incompatible with life in the hemizygous male state.

Sotos syndrome

Sotos syndrome (cerebral giganticism) consists of excessively rapid growth including large head circumference which commences antenatally, non-progressive cerebral disorder, and learning disabilities (Rutter and Cole 1991). Overactivity and attentional deficits, inco-ordination, and poorly articulated speech have been reported as well as social solitariness, peer relationship difficulties, tantrums, and sleep problems.

3.8 Disorders of the central nervous system and muscle

3.8.1 CEREBRAL PALSY

Definition

In this group of conditions there is a permanent, non-progressive disability of movement arising from damage or dysfunction of the immature brain. Motor impairment affects muscular power and tone as well as posture, and there are often involuntary movements. The brain damage present is often responsible for associated sensory, language, and visuospatial disabilities, and sometimes epilepsy. If the damage is widespread, there may be global mental retardation. Paralysis may involve all four limbs (*quadriplegia*), one side of the body (*hemiplegia*), or the lower limbs (*diplegia*). The main disability may be postural involving balance (*ataxic cerebral palsy*), or there may be involuntary athetoid or choreoathetoid movements (*dyskinesia*).

Aetiology

The likely cause of the condition varies with the type of cerebral palsy (Hagberg and Hagberg 1984). Most cases of hemiplegia have a prenatal, third trimester cause. Spastic diplegia and quadriplegia are frequently related to prematurity, often extreme prematurity. Dyskinesias are likely to be due to severe birth asphyxia. Simple ataxia, especially if linked to mental retardation, is often inherited.

Prevalence

The overall rate is between 1.5 and 3 per 1000. Boys are slightly more affected than girls, and there is no particular association with social class.

Clinical features

These vary considerably, depending on the nature of the condition and its severity. A child with cerebral palsy may be handicapped by no more than slight weakness and inco-ordination in an upper limb. Alternatively, the child may be quadriplegic, blind, and grossly mentally retarded. Commonly there is a stormy birth, but the child appears to have made a good recovery after receiving intensive care. There may be serious feeding difficulties. Subsequently, later in the first year of life, the child is noted either to be unusually stiff or floppy. Motor milestones are delayed, but the child may appear alert and responsive. Disorders of articulation are common. A diagnosis is made on the basis of the history and clinical examination. It is often difficult to predict outcome in terms of disability in the first 3 or 4 years of life, but by about 5 years, the degree of likely future disability is usually reasonably clear.

Psychological development

The cognitive development of the child with cerebral palsy is often hampered for two main reasons. First, the brain damage or dysfunction may have affected parts of the brain necessary for adequate intellectual function to occur. Such damage may have an effect on both general and specific cognitive functions. Second, the fact that the child has cerebral palsy may seriously limit his experiences and thus his opportunities for learning. A child who, because of his disability, is confined to one room in his home may well have difficulty learning about spatial relationships.

General intelligence

Survey evidence suggests that about 50% of children with cerebral palsy have IQs below 70 (the proportion is about 2.5% in the general population). Some children with cerebral palsy, however, have normal or even superior intelligence. The type of cerebral palsy is relevant. Children with hemiplegia are less likely and children with diplegia and quadriplegia more likely to be mentally retarded. As a group, children with choreoathetosis have the best-preserved intelligence. Verbal intelligence is likely to be at a higher level than non-verbal intelligence.

The degree of physical disability is related to IQ level, so that the more physically handicapped the child, the more likely he is to be retarded. However, physical disability can be a very misleading guide to intelligence. Some mildly physically handicapped and apparently alert children may, on testing, turn out to be profoundly retarded. Many cases also occur in which gross physical disability, especially of dyskinesic type, is accompanied by high ability. This means that systematic assessment of cognitive skills is necessary.

Specific abilities

It is very common for the child with cerebral palsy to have a wide scatter of skills. In general, verbal skills are more highly developed than non-verbal, but there is wide variation.

Language disability

Articulation problems may be severe because the orolaryngeal musculature is affected by spasticity. Such articulation problems may be accompanied by difficulties in the comprehension or expression of language at a higher level. Aphasia is not common, but does occur.

Perceptual abnormalities

Even in the absence of damage to the eye, ear, or other related structures, the child may have a problem in perceptual discrimination. Children with auditory perceptual deficits may be unable to distinguish like-sounding consonants such as **p** and **b**, **t** and **d**. Even if able to perceive differences, they may be unable to perceive the meaning of different sounds. Thus a child may be able to perceive that a doorbell makes a different noise from a running tap, but in the absence of visual cues, be unable to recognize that the one sound means someone at the door and the other that someone in the kitchen is washing up or getting a drink.

Perceptual problems may be visual, auditory, or tactile. Visual perceptual problems can be divided into those that are visuospatial, and those that are visuomotor. Visuospatial difficulties may show themselves, with inability to distinguish right from left or below from above. Distortion of body image may also result from a visuospatial deficit. Visuomotor difficulties occur when the child fails to perceive the changing visual stimuli produced by his own movements (for example, in drawing and writing) to help him co-ordinate further motor activity

Abnormalities of motor co-ordination
Disability in the execution and co-ordination of movement (clumsiness or motor dyspraxia) may be present to a degree unexplained by muscular weakness or abnormality of muscle tone. This may give rise to particular difficulties in using a spoon and fork, drawing, writing, and dressing. Oral motor dysfunction, present in the majority of children with cerebral palsy, causes serious problems in sucking and swallowing, so that a high proportion of these children show feeding difficulties especially in the first years of life (Reilly *et al.* 1996).

These motor and perceptual abnormalities may result in the child showing educational retardation in relation to his measured intelligence. Specific reading retardation is, for example, common in children with cerebral palsy.

Psychiatric aspects

Prevalence
Children with cerebral palsy have a higher than expected rate of psychiatric disorders. In the Isle of Wight Survey, about 40% of children with cerebral palsy showed significant emotional or behavioural problems, the rate being slightly lower in children without associated epilepsy and higher if epilepsy was also present (Rutter *et al.* 1970*b*). Hemiplegia is very strongly associated with the presence of psychiatric disorder, with about 60% affected (Goodman and Graham 1996), compared with 15% in the general population.

Cerebral-palsied children with associated mental retardation are likely to show high rates of the hyperkinetic syndrome and autistic syndromes. Those with hemiplegia show especially irritability, anxiety and hyperactivity/attention problems (Goodman 1997*b*).

Reasons for the high rates of psychiatric disorder in the cerebral-palsied group include:

- *Direct effect of brain damage and dysfunction.* Children with physical disabilities not involving the brain do not show such high rates of psychiatric disorder even when their disabilities are severe, so some direct effect of brain damage on behaviour in the cerebral-palsied child seems probable. There is no difference in the rates of behaviour disturbance between children with lesions in the dominant and non-dominant hemisphere, but dominant lesions are more often associated with 'externalizing' behaviour (e.g. aggression, disobedience) and non-dominant lesions with 'internalizing' problems (e.g. anxiety, fearfulness) (Sollee and Kindlon 1987). In children with hemiplegia, the likelihood of psychiatric disorder increases with the degree of mental retardation, itself an index of the amount of brain damage (Goodman and Graham 1996).

- *Rejection by peers and siblings.* Children with physical disabilities are less frequently chosen as friends by other children. It is not clear whether cerebral-palsied children are particular likely to be rejected (Richardson and Royce 1968), but certainly they often have serious social problems. When young, they are likely to be subjected to teasing and ridicule, and as they reach adolescence, although teasing decreases, they are less able to participate in the increasingly mobile social lives of their contemporaries.
- *Poor self-concept and low self-esteem.* From the age of 4 years onwards (Teplin *et al.* 1981), cerebral-palsied children see themselves as different from others, and, as time goes on, they are increasingly likely to perceive themselves to be less valuable than others.
- *Parental attitude.* Disturbed cerebral-palsied children may have parents who have unrealistic ideas about their disability, either denying or exaggerating its extent (Minde 1978). Some parents also withdraw warmth and emotional commitment from their physically handicapped children as they get older.
- *Family relationships.* The rate of divorce and separation is not raised in parents of cerebral-palsied children. However, when arguments and tension do occur they often focus over problems in the management of the handicapped child, and this predisposes the child to become disturbed.
- *Educational failure.* Children who, in addition to their physical disability, are failing at school in relation to their apparent ability, are more likely to show disturbance.

Implications for management
Various measures taken by health professionals are likely to reduce the rates of psychiatric disorders in cerebral-palsied children (Freeman 1970).

- Early identification with involvement of both parents in the assessment process is likely to help parents to value their handicapped children appropriately. If parents are given practical advice how to help their children gain mobility and communicate, this also will be helpful.
- Comprehensive assessment, especially by a physiotherapist, speech therapist, and psychologist, will ensure that associated handicaps are identified. Systematic assessment for the presence of perceptual and perceptuomotor skills and disabilities will assist teachers and parents in promoting development. Continuing emphasis on what the child *is* able to do, rather than on what the child cannot do, and on developmental progress rather than on deficits, is also supportive.
- Promotion of social development can be achieved by ensuring that the child is given every opportunity to improve his communication skills. The use of an alternative communication system involving signing, such as Makaton, may be helpful here. The child needs opportunities for non-rejecting interaction with others of his own age that will result in avoidance of social isolation. Whether the child is placed in an ordinary or a special school may be less important than whether parents and teachers are aware of the child's social needs and go out of their way to encourage friendship. In the UK, PHAB (physically

handicapped/able-bodied) clubs for mixed groups of handicapped and non-handicapped adolescents have established themselves as useful in this respect. Again in the UK, there is a self-help group (Hemi-Help) specifically for children with hemiplegia and their parents.

• Providing opportunities for the physically handicapped child to express anxieties and worries should ensure that communication about the disability is adequate. Health professionals can provide older cerebral-palsied children and adolescents with such opportunities, listen to their concerns, and, with the agreement of the child or teenager, feed back information to those who might be able to help. Sexual counselling is particularly important for adolescents who, because of reduced contact with other youngsters, may experience guilt concerning sexual feelings and masturbation.

• The management of established psychiatric disorders is no different from that required in the non-handicapped population, and is likely to be at least as rewarding. Family approaches, as well as individual and behavioural psychotherapy, may be indicated. It is important to establish how the disturbed child and parent perceive the disability, and to what degree misperceptions and poor communication about the handicap are responsible for emotional disturbance. Children with such physical disorders are often disturbed for reasons that have little or nothing to do with their disability.

3.8.2 EPILEPSY

Definition

Epilepsy is present when there is a repeated paroxysmal discharge in the brain producing sudden episodic involuntary alterations of movement or sensory experience. Epilepsy is the most common but not the only cause of seizures (sudden episodes of loss of muscle power). Seizures may be produced by other organic as well as non-organic conditions, such as hysterical or 'sick role' disorders. Non-organic seizures are, by convention, known as 'pseudo-seizures'.

Classification

Epileptic attacks can be classified in a number of different ways according to their clinical and EEG features, their duration, their origin in the brain, their cause, and their association with fever (Table 3.8). Seizures may be generalized or affect the patient only partially.

• Major generalized seizures (*tonic–clonic*) usually involve a brief warning sensation (the *aura*) followed by loss of consciousness with spasmodic twitching of the limbs, clenching and unclenching of the jaws, and sometimes incontinence of urine. Afterwards there is usually a period of disorientation and sleep, often followed by headache.

• In generalized *absence attacks* there is usually a brief (10–15 seconds) episode of impaired consciousness with staring of the eyes, blinking, and rarely facial twitching. Such attacks often occur in clusters.

Table 3.8 Classification of epilepsy

Modified international classification	Clinical and EEG features of the attack
I	Generalized seizures
	Tonic, clonic, and tonic–clonic
	Absence
	Myoclonic
	Infantile spasms
II	Partial seizures
	Simple (motor, sensory)
	Complex
III	Unclassified

- In *myoclonic* seizures, there are sudden jerky movements and loss of muscle power often producing a brief fall to the ground or a fall back in the cot or bed.
- *Infantile spasms*, which nearly always occur in the first year of life, involve attacks of sudden flexion of the head, knees, and arms, associated with gross EEG abnormality of characteristic type.

Partial seizures may be simple or complex.

- A *simple partial seizure* may consist of an isolated disturbance of sensation or movement, for example twitching of a limb.
- A *complex partial seizure* involves some impairment of consciousness; for example, the child may be able to stand, but not to respond to questions. Such partial loss of consciousness may be followed or accompanied by a variety of movements and sensation including, for example, brief flicking of the eyelids, sucking movements, spasmodic jerking of one limb and/or one side of the face. In seizures arising from epileptic activity in the temporal lobes, the child may experience a variety of symptoms including a constriction or feeling of fear in the lower chest, strange sensations of taste or smell, other hallucinations, giddiness, mood changes, and automatic behaviour.

Duration of the attack

Most epileptic attacks last a few seconds to a few minutes. Prolonged seizures, referred to as *status epilepticus* for generalized seizures, or, for partial epilepsy, *epilepsia partialis continua*, call for immediate medical treatment.

Site of the epileptic activity in the brain

The paroxysmal electrical activity may arise from the deeper central brain structures (*centrencephalon*) and spread in a generalized fashion over the whole substance of the brain. This will produce a generalized seizure described above. Alternatively, the epileptic attack may arise from a circumscribed part of the brain such as the frontal or temporal lobe (see above).

Cause of the attack

Most epilepsy is not symptomatic of an underlying condition. It probably occurs because of an inherited disposition to attacks. All individuals have a disposition to epilepsy and, under certain conditions (e.g. if given an injection of insulin and made hypoglycaemic), would suffer an attack. The reason why some people with non-symptomatic epilepsy have an unusually strong disposition is usually unknown, and it is often unclear why attacks occur at particular times, though sometimes triggering factors, including psychological stress and exposure to flickering light, can be identified.

Some epilepsy, however, arises from an identifiable cause, for example from infection, intoxication, neoplasm, trauma, or vascular disorder. One common cause is the presence of a scar that acts as a focus or trigger for electrical activity. Such a scar may occur if a part of the brain dies as a result of anoxia occurring in an earlier prolonged seizure. Temporal lobe epilepsy is believed sometimes to occur in this manner following prolonged febrile convulsions (see below).

Association with fever

Febrile convulsions are attacks that commonly occur in infants and young children aged from about 6 months to 4 years that are accompanied by fever. Non-febrile convulsions may occur at any age. About 3% of children with febrile convulsions go on to develop epilepsy—the remainder are subsequently asymptomatic.

Background factors: psychosocial aspects

Epilepsy is one of the most common physical disorders occurring in childhood. Apart from febrile convulsions (3% of children) the rate is about 7–8 per 1000 in school-aged children (Rutter *et al.* 1970b). Both sexes are equally affected, and there is a slight tendency for working-class children to be more at risk.

There are various important ways in which psychological and social factors interact with the presence of epilepsy.

Behavioural changes

- For a day or two preceding a seizure, a child may become more excitable, moody, and irritable. This change in mood may be terminated by the seizure. Observation of the benign effect of an epileptic seizure on difficult behaviour in mentally ill adults led to the development of electroconvulsive therapy as a treatment for depressive psychosis.
- Epileptic seizure (ictal) activity in the brain may be reflected in an alteration of mood and behaviour that can be mistaken for a non-epileptic psychiatric disorder. Children who are experiencing absence attacks with brief lapses of concentration may be mistakenly thought to be inattentive for other reasons. Surprisingly, this most commonly occurs in children who are known to have epilepsy because they are also having major attacks, but it does also occur in children not suspected to be suffering from epilepsy. In psychomotor attacks, usually arising from the temporal lobes or other parts of the limbic system, the

child may experience a sudden acute sensation of constriction and fear in the lower chest and retrosternal area, and may run or cling to the nearest person. This may be mistaken for a non-organic anxiety attack. Hallucinatory experiences may be thought to arise from a psychotic disorder. Automatic behaviour may be thought to reflect a dissociative or hysterical state. In frontal lobe seizures there may be trance-like states and screaming attacks, especially occurring in sleep (Stores *et al.* 1991). In each of these cases, diagnosis will be assisted by the presence of the acute onset, by the apparently inexplicable nature of the symptoms, and by corroborating EEG changes. The increasing availability of telemetric and ambulatory EEG apparatus allowing EEG recording to be obtained during an attack is a significant advance in investigative technique.

• Seizures may be followed by behavioural change. In the period of neuronal quiescence after an epileptic attack, the child may wander around in an apparently purposeless manner, still mildly disorientated. This behaviour may also be mistaken for a psychiatric disorder of hysterical type, especially as the seizure disturbance itself may not have involved a major attack.

Precipitation of seizures by psychological stress

Probably about a quarter of children suffering from epileptic seizures have attacks brought on by stressful changes in the environment. There is no specific type of stress likely to be involved, though in schoolchildren, examinations are often an important factor. Family arguments are also occasional triggers. It has been suggested that epilepsy is more likely to persist when parental attitudes to the child are both intrusive and rejecting. The significance of stress and the precipitation of attacks is often difficult to confirm because of the possibility that stress is coincidental. However, experimental EEG controlled studies have made clear that neurophysiological changes of an epileptic type can indeed be stress-induced, even though strong clinical evidence for the importance of stress in an individual child may be hard to come by (Stevens 1959).

Children are sometimes able to control the frequency of their attacks to some degree. Some children can inhibit attacks by controlling their thoughts in a particular way. It is always worth asking children if they can stop an attack if they want to, and useful to find out why they will sometimes do this and sometimes not. Others are able to induce fits. The most common method of fit induction is by finger or hand flicking while looking at the sun or other bright light. This behaviour occurs most commonly in mentally retarded children, but is not unknown in children of normal ability. Clearly, in these cases the occurrence of a fit is a rewarding experience for the child. Further evidence in favour of the possibility of at least a small self-control element in epilepsy comes from studies demonstrating that, in selected cases, behavioural intervention can reduce seizure frequency (Dahl *et al.* 1988).

Associated behavioural and emotional disorders

The rate of psychological problems in children with epilepsy has been found to be over four times that in the general population (Rutter *et al.* 1970*b*). If the epilepsy is associated with evidence of an anatomical brain lesion (e.g. if the child also has cerebral palsy), then the rate of psychological disorders is even higher. These rates of psychological problems are much higher than those occurring in children with other physical disorders not involving the brain, such as diabetes mellitus and asthma. Psychological problems in children with epilepsy therefore probably arise partly because of the specific effects of brain dysfunction, rather than merely as a reaction to the presence of physical disability. Further evidence to support this view is provided by the fact that children with epilepsy have more psychological problems than children with other physical conditions at the time of onset of the fits (Hoare 1984a), and that subclinical epileptiform discharges do seem to affect psychological function (Siebelink *et al.* 1988).

There is no specific type of psychological problem linked to epilepsy. Such children are just as likely, if not more likely to show emotional problems with withdrawal and anxiety as aggressive behaviour disorders (Hoare and Kerley 1991). At the same time, children showing some relatively uncommon psychiatric disorders, such as autism, do have a high risk of the development of epilepsy.

Children with epilepsy are more likely to show psychological problems if their attacks are of psychomotor type, especially if they are of low intelligence (Harbord and Manson 1987). There are a number of possible reasons for this. Children who suffer such seizures often have experiences, such as unexplained anxiety and other mood changes, and strange sensations that are near enough to reality to be confused with it. It may be easier for children with generalized attacks which do not involve such strange but near-normal experiences to see their disorder in an objective, detached manner. Second, most psychomotor attacks arise from the limbic system of the brain, deep to the temporal lobes. The main nuclei of this system are the hippocampal formation, the amygdala, the hypothalamus, and the septal area. The brain neurotransmitters, especially dopamine, noradrenaline, and serotonin, that have been shown to have specific effects on mood and behaviour, exist in considerable concentration in these nuclei. This may explain why dysfunction in these areas of the brain may be especially likely to produce psychological problems. A proportion of teenagers with psychomotor epilepsy develop confusional psychotic states, sometimes following a run of seizures. Further, children with chronic temporal lobe seizures are at an increased risk for the development of paranoid schizophrenic disorders in later life. Such psychotic states occur, on average, 7–8 years after the onset of seizures (Slater *et al.* 1963). Finally, a very high proportion of children with infantile spasms (see above) later show developmental retardation with associated autistic features and/or hyperkinesis (Riikonen and Amnell 1981).

Most children with epilepsy have normal intelligence, and the mean IQ of children with this condition is only a little below average, provided that children with evidence of associated brain damage (e.g. cerebral palsy), are excluded from consideration (Rutter *et al.* 1970b). However, children with epilepsy have a high rate of specific reading disability and those with focal spike discharges (especially those with left temporal spikes) are particularly likely to show such a deficit (Stores 1978). The rate of learning and behavioural problems of schoolchildren who have previously suffered a febrile convulsion is slightly higher than that in the general population (Wallace 1984). The presence of neurodevelopmental abnormalities before the convulsions and the occurrence of frequent febrile fits increases the risk of such later problems.

Other background factors that make children with epilepsy more prone to psychological problems include low socio-economic status and depression or anxiety in the parents. This suggests that children with epilepsy have heightened vulnerability to the same sort of factors that produce psychological problems in children without epilepsy.

Anticonvulsant drugs, behaviour, and learning

Anticonvulsants are given with the intention of altering brain function in a specific manner—by raising the threshold for the development of epileptic attacks. It is not surprising that their effects, when administered, are less specific than this, and spread over into other areas of brain functioning, affecting behaviour and learning.

Phenobarbitone, sometimes used in the prophylaxis of febrile convulsions (see above), often produces irritability and overactivity, especially in the young child, though long-term effects on cognitive development and behaviour do not persist when the drug is discontinued (Wallace 1984). Phenytoin overdosage is occasionally accompanied by a confusional state, and long-term administration of phenytoin may produce chronic intellectual deterioration, which is not necessarily reversible. These effects may be produced by their influence on folate metabolism. Other anticonvulsants, including those others most commonly used—carbamazepine, ethosuximide, primidone, sulthiame, and sodium valproate—have all been described as having adverse effects on behaviour and learning in a minority of children to whom they are administered (Corbett *et al.* 1985). Inattention, lack of concentration, and minor disorientation and irritability are the most common effects observed. There is no anticonvulsant drug of which one can say with confidence that mental side-effects do not occur, but side-effects affecting intelligence and behaviour are most common with phenobarbitone and phenytoin, and least common with carbamazepine (Trimble 1987). Of the newer antiepileptic drugs, vigabatrin, gabapentin and lamotrigine, the first two have been reported as having behavioural side-effects, especially agitation and hyperactivity (Appleton 1996).

Surgery for epilepsy

In children with a clear-cut, unilateral temporal or frontal focus who do not also suffer from generalized seizures, temporal or frontal lobe surgery may be indicated. Results are variable but sometimes, especially in temporal lobe surgery, they are excellent (Fish *et al.* 1993). Such children often show serious psychiatric disorders before operation, but, given careful rehabilitation, if the operation reduces seizure frequency, the majority can be expected to be free of psychiatric symptomatology subsequently. Hemispherectomy can similarly be helpful in those unusual cases of hemiplegic epilepsy when unilateral paralysis is severe and fits are poorly controlled. Again, surgery that is successful in fit control will also relieve severe psychiatric disorders. It is likely that, with the use of advanced imaging techniques, the frequency with which successful surgery for epilepsy is carried out will increase.

Impact on the child and family

Epileptic seizures are frightening to witness, and even doctors who are not frequently involved in coping with them would agree they feel anxious when they see one. The affected individual appears in the grip of an unseen force, and the onlooker, especially in the presence of a grand mal fit, feels helpless. In many developing countries now, and in western industrialized societies not so long ago, epilepsy indicated possession by an evil influence, causing children with fits to be kept from going to school and mixing with other children. In 1949 a representative survey of American adults revealed that 43% of them would object to their child playing with an epileptic child, though by 1974 this proportion had dropped to 14% (Caveness *et al.* 1974). In 1949, 55% believed that people with epilepsy should not be employed (19% in 1974). Community prejudice against epilepsy is therefore widespread, although decreasing.

The impact of seizures on the child cannot readily be gauged by examining rates of emotional and behavioural disorder, as some children are probably disturbed not as a psychological reaction to the fits but as a more direct result of brain dysfunction. Nevertheless, there is ample clinical evidence to suggest that the impact is considerable (Ferrari *et al.* 1983). Children with generalized seizures are frequently made anxious by the fact that they do not know what goes on when they have a fit. They may fear that they will lose control, betray secrets, or make fools of themselves. Adolescent girls may be frightened that they will be sexually assaulted. It is common for youngsters to be worried that they will not be able to obtain a job or get married. Sometimes there are realistic fears of being teased or bullied at school if the fits are witnessed.

School performance may be affected. Although the mean IQ of children is well within the average range, underachievement at school is common, and is related to visuomotor impairment and the presence of psychiatric disorder (Sturniolo and Galletti 1994).

Other members of the family are sometimes profoundly affected. Many parents of infants and young children having their first febrile convulsion think that their child will die in the fit and some never forget the experience (Baumer *et al.* 1981). Parents often become depressed, especially if the fits prove difficult to control or affect the child's capacity to lead a normal life. There is an increased rate of psychological problems in both the parents and sibs of children with epilepsy (Hoare 1984*b*).

This account should not obscure the fact that most children with epilepsy do not show psychological problems, and that the majority of parents develop realistic ideas about the nature of their children's disorder and cope remarkably well with the problems it produces.

Management

Assessment of the child with seizures begins with an appraisal of the nature of the attack, a physical examination, and laboratory investigations including an EEG (Stores 1985). The possibility that the epilepsy is a manifestation of an underlying disease should always be considered, as should the possible role of psychological factors as precipitants.

In counselling parents and children in cases of so-called 'idiopathic' epilepsy, or epilepsy of unknown cause, various specific points need to be considered (Voeller and Rothenburg 1973).

The nature of the condition and its usually benign prognosis should be repeatedly explained to parents and children in appropriate language. The family should be encouraged to use a term like 'fits', 'attacks', or 'convulsions' when describing the seizures to friends, relatives, and teachers. Some explanation along the lines of a temporary excess of electricity in a particular part of the brain is often helpful. Parents should be encouraged to express their own views of the nature and causes of the fits, and this may reveal inappropriate fantasies concerning brain damage and the hereditary nature of the condition that require further discussion. The purpose and limited value of an EEG, and what happens when the child has an EEG, need explanation. Some children think the EEG puts electricity into the brain rather than recording it. Parents and teachers will be helped by being given precise instructions about what to do if a fit occurs, and should be reassured that they are coping appropriately if this is indeed the case. Limitations of exercise, for example swimming, need to be regularly reviewed, and it is useful to check on each attendance what the child is allowed to do. Parents and teachers may be overrestrictive or, much less frequently, may fail to take sensible precautions to safeguard a child who is having frequent attacks. Monitoring of anticonvulsants should include parents or the doctor checking with teachers whether the child is unduly drowsy or inattentive. As indicated earlier, any anticonvulsant may cause side-effects in particular children.

Children with epilepsy whose primary care has been well handled will be at reduced risk for the development of psychological disorders, but inevitably a significant number will show signs of disturbance, mainly emotional and behavioural disorders. In general, the management of such problems will follow similar lines as in cases without epilepsy. Indeed, the psychiatric problems of many children with epilepsy will be unrelated to their epilepsy and more closely linked to factors such as disturbances of family relationships. However, particular attention will need to be given to the possibility that behavioural disturbance is a manifestation of epileptic activity, that the child is being overprotected or rejected because of his attacks, that medication is producing adverse behavioural or learning side-effects, or that either the child or other family members are being made anxious by inaccurate fantasies about the nature of the condition.

The differential diagnosis of seizures and hysterical 'pseudoseizures' sometimes presents problems, in particular because pseudoseizures not infrequently occur in children with epileptic attacks. Children with pseudoseizures have high rates of physical and sexual abuse in their background and often both affective and dissociative features in other respects (Bowman 1993). The seizures are likely to be atypical in form and the child will probably show obviously purposeful movements. There may be inconsistent reactions to stimuli during an attack. EEG recording is likely to be helpful only if the child actually has an attack during the procedure, but this will only rarely occur unless telemetric ambulatory EEG is available. Plasma prolactin, raised following an epileptic attack, may be helpful in differentiating between generalized seizures and pseudoseizures (Singh and Jana 1994). Assessment and management of pseudoseizures should follow the same lines as that described under the heading of conversion or sick-role disorders (Section 5.5.2).

3.8.3 CEREBRAL TUMOURS

Brain tumours are a relatively common form of malignancy in childhood, second only in frequency to cancers of the blood-forming tissues. Even so, they are rare, with an annual incidence of 26 per million children under the age of 15 years (Stevens *et al.* 1991). Types of cerebral tumour seen are quite different from those found in adults. About two-thirds occur in the subtentorial part of the brain, and of these, most are medulloblastomas and cerebellar astrocytomas. The remainder consist of supratentorial tumours and tumours of the brainstem and adjacent structures (Till 1975). Only 3% of childhood tumours are metastic from other parts of the body.

Clinical features

The clinical features depend on the site of the tumour and the rapidity of its growth. Most subtentorial tumours present with headache, vomiting, and unsteadiness of gait. Psychological symptoms such as irritability and aggressiveness may be present, but almost always the physical symptoms are so prominent that there is little possibility of diagnostic confusion.

The presentation of supratentorial tumour will largely depend on the site where it occurs. Again psychological symptoms are not prominent, and epileptic fits or unilateral weakness of the limbs are much more common presenting features.

By contrast, children with brainstem tumours, in which cranial nerve involvement is usually an early sign, may show more marked behavioural symptomatology with lethargy, irritability, inability to concentrate, enuresis, and sleep disturbance sometimes present (Panitch and Berg 1970). Pontine gliomata may show even more striking behavioural changes and these may precede physical symptoms and lead to misdiagnosis. There is characteristically a period of withdrawal, apathy, and lethargy, followed by aggression, overactivity, and temper tantrums (Lassman and Arjona 1967).

Treatment

Surgical removal may be possible, depending on the site and nature of the tumour. Radiotherapy is used both as an adjuvant to surgery and, where surgery is impracticable, as in most tumours of the brainstem, as the main mode of treatment. The prognosis varies according to the type of tumour, the age of the patient, and treatment employed. The 5 year survival rate for all cerebral tumours in children is 51% (Stevens *et al.* 1991). The survival rate for children with medulloblastomas, the most common form of tumour, is 40–75% at 2 years and 30–50% at 10 years after diagnosis.

Psychosocial aspects of outcome

Among survivors, some degree of physical disability is common and, in addition, the rate of behavioural and emotional problems is high, with nearly half the children showing such difficulties. These vary in type and include both aggressive and emotional disorders, with occasional occurrence of psychosis (Kun *et al.* 1983).

Intellectual function is highly likely to be impaired, with a variety of specific learning disabilities (Johnson *et al.* 1994). About a third of the survivors require education in special schools. The intelligence of younger children is most seriously at risk, and this may be because intellectual function is most affected not by the tumour or surgical treatment, but by the subsequent irradiation to the immature brain. There is strong evidence from follow-up studies of children with leukaemia that young children are particularly susceptible to postirradiation effects on intelligence. The longer-term outcome of survivors of paediatric brain tumours is also often problematic (Lannering *et al.* 1990), with moderate or severe disability occurring in about one-third, when studied 5–16 years after diagnosis.

The postoperative course and psychosocial outcome of the rare craniopharyngiomata are somewhat different from other tumours. Postoperative hormone replacement therapy is always required in these cases. Intellectual deterioration is less common, but non-specific psychiatric problems (neurotic as well as aggressive in type) are more severe (Galatzer *et al.* 1981).

3.8.4 HEADACHE

Classification

Pains and aches in the head occur commonly in childhood, and are of three main types: organic, migrainous, and non-organic.

- *Organic* headaches are those with a recognizable organic cause and disappear when this cause is removed.
- *Migraine* headaches have certain characteristic features—their aetiology is usually multicausal, partly organic and partly non-organic.
- *Non-organic* headaches, which may be only poorly distinguishable from migraine, can be divided into those where the cause is psychological and those where it is unknown. Non-organic headaches are more frequently termed *tension headaches*, but this implies that the cause is known, and this is by no means always the case.

Clinical features

Headache of organic origin may arise for a large variety of reasons:

- infection of the teeth and sinuses
- cerebral causes such as tumours and abcesses; refraction errors, especially short sightedness
- vascular causes such as cerebral haemangiomata and hypertension.

In general, pain due to such causes is reasonably well localized and, because few of the causes are benign, increases in intensity day by day. It is usually worse in the evenings and frequently wakes the child at night. There is often no family history of recurrent headache. Children under the age of 5 years rarely suffer from non-organic headaches or migraine, so headache in this age group is particularly likely to be organic. Any change in behaviour with this type of headache is usually fairly obvious, and secondary to the pain rather than just associated with it.

Migrainous headaches do not usually start until 8 or 9 years of age, but may occur earlier. In childhood auras are infrequent, but occasionally headaches are preceded by a scotoma (blind spot), blurring of vision, or simple hallucinatory phenomena. The headache itself usually lasts less than half an hour, but occasionally goes on for hours or even days on end. It is pulsatile in quality, unilateral or bilateral, and may be accompanied by nausea and occasionally vomiting. Photophobia is often present. There is often a family history of migraine and, in many cases, a parent or sib has typical attacks.

Such migrainous headaches may be precipitated by a variety of factors including psychological stresses as well as the ingestion of certain foods, especially chocolate, cheese, nuts, and food containing glutamates. Fatigue and strenuous physical exercise may also be triggers. Occasionally, migrainous headaches occurring over a period of some months may be precipitated by trauma to the head.

Non-organic headaches are usually of daily occurrence and do not vary much in intensity throughout the day. They are usually experienced as tightness or pressure around the head, and may be accompanied by mild throbbing. They do not wake the child up at night. A family history is common. When the cause is psychogenic, there is likely to be a relationship between circumstances and the occurrence of the headache. For example, the headache may be a presenting sign of school refusal, occurring only on school days and not at weekends or in the holidays. Psychogenic non-organic headaches are usually accompanied by other behavioural and emotional changes, especially anxiety, depression, and other psychosomatic symptoms such as abdominal pain. Such headaches may also form part of a conversion (hysterical) reaction. In these circumstances, the child will be seen to benefit from the 'sick role' he has adopted. The complaints of pain will seem greater than the appearance of discomfort.

Differentiation between migraine and non-organic headaches is not always easy. Often, for example, children have only one or two of the features of migraine and there are associated symptoms suggesting a psychogenic cause.

It is also likely that the pathophysiological basis of some 'non-organic' headaches is similar to that of migraine.

Prevalence

Headaches of non-organic or migrainous origin are very common in children. The exact prevalence is unknown, but Sillanpaa (1983) found that over one-third of 7 year olds and over two-thirds of 14 year olds had suffered from headaches. There is some evidence that the prevalence of headaches among schoolchildren is increasing, and is greatest in areas of social instability (Sillanpaa and Anttila 1996).

Mechanisms

Organic headaches are produced by a variety of mechanisms depending on the cause. Migraine headaches are thought to arise as a result of vasoconstriction and then vasodilatation of the branches of the external carotid, internal carotid, and, rarely, basilar arteries. The reason why these arterioles undergo such changes is uncertain. Histochemical alterations occurring as a result of immunological reactions, themselves triggered by stress, ingestion of certain foods, etc., seem one likely explanation. Non-organic headaches may occur as a result of muscular tension, or undue sensitivity to normal pain receptor stimulation. The physiological processes involved in the development of such commonly experienced discomfort are poorly understood.

Assessment

In obtaining an account of the symptoms, focus should be on the frequency and nature of the headache, the presence of associated physical symptoms, especially nausea, vomiting, and abdominal pain, the relationship of the pain to psychological stress and ingestion of certain foods, and the presence of emotional or behavioural problems. The presence of headache in other family members should be noted.

In all cases of headache, physical examination should involve screening for neurological abnormality, including refractive errors, and observation of the fundi. Local causes of pain should also be excluded. An EEG is usually non-contributory, but skull radiography and CT scan may be indicated by any suggestion of possible cerebral pathology.

In the great majority of cases, physical examination will be negative and either migraine or non-organic headache diagnosed.

Treatment of migraine and non-organic headaches

As already indicated, these two types of headache are poorly distinguished from each other, and can be considered together in relation to treatment. Attention to possible stress factors at home, at school, or in the neighbourhood is always worthwhile. The child is sometimes perfectionist in nature, and parents are occasionally unnecessarily pressurizing. Counselling both parents and child to find less-than-perfect performance acceptable is sometimes helpful.

Attention should be drawn to the possibility that certain foods (e.g. chocolate, cheese, nuts, etc.) precipitate the headache. Avoidance of these can be useful.

With disabling migraine, a severely restrictive diet with gradual reintroduction of possibly offending foods may produce useful results.

Symptomatic relief may also be obtained by analgesic medication. Paracetamol often alleviates the pain, especially if taken early in the attack. If this is ineffective, ergotamine tartrate may be indicated if classical migraine symptoms are present. Pizotifen, a serotonin antagonist, may also be helpful (Gillies *et al.* 1986).

When headaches are but one manifestation of an anxiety or depressive state, the treatment should be directed towards the underlying condition. If the headache is the presenting feature of school refusal or a conversion reaction, the treatment should follow the lines described elsewhere. If, despite these measures, disabling symptoms either of migrainous or of non-organic type, persist, then hypnosis, progressive muscle relaxation, or cognitive behaviour therapy are frequently effective (McGrath and Goodman 1998). Cognitive behavioural approaches are probably most useful. They involve prospective recording of pain and coping strategies before commencing treatment, identification of negative thoughts with a conscious attempt to replace these with positive ones, examining unrealistic beliefs, distraction strategies, use of relaxing imagery, and problem solving. Richter *et al.* (1986) have shown this approach to be of value.

3.8.5 SPINA BIFIDA

Definition

Spina bifida is a condition present at birth, arising from a failure of fusion of the arches of the vertebral column. In most cases (*spina bifida occulta*), the failure of fusion is minor and of no pathological significance. In a minority, between 0.5 and 4 per 1000 births, there is herniation of the meninges and spinal cord as well. A *meningocele* or *myelomeningocele*, depending on the contents of the herniated tissue, is thus formed. Primary neurological defects comprise motor and sensory deficits (depending on the level of the lesion), partial or complete paralysis of the bladder and bowel, and sexual dysfunction. Hydrocephalus is usually associated with spina bifida, and there may be secondary neurological problems relating to this.

Surgical treatment at birth of newborns who, from the extent of the malformation, can be predicted to have a poor quality of life ahead of them, is controversial (Surana *et al.* 1991). Assessment of the child born with spina bifida to determine its likely prognosis is a skilled technique that is carried out in specialized centres. Children thought suitable for surgery generally have a reasonable quality of life subsequently, although many do have significant physical, behavioural and learning problems. The great majority (nearly 80%) of children thought unsuitable for surgery die within the first 3 months of life, but the management of survivors is highly problematic.

Psychosocial aspects

The early management of children born with spina bifida requires sensitive handling with involvement of both parents in any decisions that are taken.

Most parents will want to leave the responsibility for decision-making with the paediatrician and surgeon, but discussion with parents of the reasons for recommendations is likely to improve the chances of later psychosocial adjustment.

The terminal nursing of infants rejected for surgery usually takes place in hospital, but a few parents prefer to take their children home. In either event, emotional support for parents from the paediatrician and primary health care team should be provided. The situation is also distressing for nurses caring for the rejected child in hospital, and they too will need emotional support. A minority (see above) of such children survive, and are subjected to surgery later. These have a poorer intellectual outcome than those operated on earlier. The uncertainty associated with these children's future is particularly distressing for parents.

Developmental progress and intelligence

About two-thirds of children with surgically operated spina bifida show retarded development at 3 years of age (Spain 1974). However, only a small minority of surgically operated cases develop severe mental retardation, and the majority are within the low average, mildly, or moderately retarded range, with a mean IQ around 75–80 (Minchom *et al.* 1995). A smaller proportion are of average or above-average ability. Spina bifida is not associated with any specific cognitive deficits, but older children with the condition have been reported to show 'hyperverbalism' or the 'cocktail party syndrome' (Swisher and Pinsker 1971). These sometimes falsely convey greater verbal facility than they possess.

Poor intellectual development is associated with the presence of central nervous system infection and with the level of the lesion. The lower the lesion, the better is the intellectual outlook (Hunt and Holmes 1976). There is a reasonably high correlation between early development in the first 2 years of life and later IQ (Fishman and Palkes 1974).

Psychiatric disorder

Although not all investigators have found children with spina bifida to show high rates of psychiatric disorder (Spaulding and Morgan 1986), most have obtained positive findings. Thus, Connell and McConnel (1981) found prepubertal children with hydrocephalus to have high rates of behaviour and emotional problems, probably partly related to the organic brain dysfunction and partly to environmental, especially family, influences. Adolescents with spina bifida have high rates of depressive disorder. Dorner (1976) found 85% of 13–19 year olds with this condition reported feeling miserable and unhappy to the point of being tearful and wanting to 'get away from it all', and a quarter of the girls had suicidal ideas. Depression in adolescents is related to problems of mobility and feelings of isolation. Children with spina bifida tend to have low levels of self-esteem and, surprisingly, those with the least physical disability show the lowest feelings of self-worth, and the most disabled show higher levels of self-esteem (Minchom *et al.* 1995). Children with bowel problems frequently report social embarrassment and feelings of shame. Concerns about sexual function and fertility are common in this age group, and these are not made easier to manage by the fact that medical and surgical opinion as to what the future holds for the individual in these respects is often unclear. Many teenagers with spina bifida are ignorant of the sexual facts of life (Anderson *et al.* 1982).

Education

Most children with spina bifida are able to attend normal school, but a minority require special schooling, either because of general or specific learning difficulties, or because it has not proved possible to modify school buildings, for example to take wheelchairs. As integration of handicapped children into normal schools continues, a smaller proportion will be excluded for this reason. However, attendance at both mainstream and special schools is problematic if resourcing is inadequate (Wasson *et al.* 1992).

Implications

In the early years, parents need emotional support as well as a good deal of practical advice to deal with problems of mobility and incontinence. The genetic implications of the condition require careful explanation. The risk of recurrence, together with the possibility of detection of spina bifida *in utero* with subsequent abortion if the child is affected, should be explained before further pregnancies occur. The possible preventive role of vitamin supplementation in the periconceptual period also needs to be understood and appropriate dietary advice given.

In middle childhood and adolescence, many of the issues discussed in Chapter 7 concerning the psychosocial problems of handicapped children in general will be relevant to this group. Specific problems, especially concerning children and adolescents with spina bifida (Thomas *et al.* 1985), include concerns for the social embarrassment arising from continuing incontinence. Practical advice over menstruation and contraception will be necessary, especially if there are sensory deficits in the pelvic area. Sexual information and counselling is currently lacking, but national voluntary organizations often produce helpful booklets on these subjects for affected individuals, their parents, and professionals. Health professionals should check that advice concerning further education and employment is available to the teenager. As the child gets older, it will often be helpful to arrange that he or she has the opportunity to talk about feelings concerning the disability and the future with someone outside the family. Mental health professionals who may be providing this service need to have a good knowledge of the practical difficulties experienced by those suffering from the condition.

3.8.6 MUSCULAR DYSTROPHY (DUCHENNE TYPE)

Definition

Duchenne type muscular dystrophy is the most common type of progressive muscle disease in childhood, occurring in about 1 per 3500 boys. It is often inherited as a sex-linked recessive, so that if one boy in a family is affected, the chances of another boy having the condition may be as high as 1 in 2. However, the gene has now been cloned, and accurate antenatal diagnosis is possible. It usually presents with muscle weakness, especially of the legs, between 1 and 5 years. By 12 years, the majority of boys are wheelchair-bound, and death usually occurs by the age of 20. Other forms of muscular dystrophy, usually with a more benign prognosis, may occur in children of both sexes.

Psychosocial aspects and intellectual development

There is a tendency for boys with this condition to be of less than average intelligence, and there is a higher than expected rate of severe mental retardation. Many, however, are of normal ability. If cognitive impairment does occur, it is particularly likely to affect verbal ability with defective auditory processing (Dorman *et al.* 1988; Billard *et al.* 1992). Indeed, the condition may present with language delay. Most boys can be educated in ordinary school until their physical condition prevents it. Subsequently they should as far as possible be educated in special schools rather than have home tuition and lose contact with other children.

Boredom, apathy, depression, and angry reactions are common psychological problems shown (Fitzpatrick *et al.* 1986). These are less likely to occur if a positive attitude to learning, education, hobbies, and contact with friends is maintained by the child's parents and teachers; much ingenuity is required to retain a positive approach when the child becomes very weak.

Diagnosis

Because the condition is rare (and there are many other causes of boys tending to be slow to walk or to fall frequently once having learnt to walk) the diagnosis is often delayed. Inevitably this leads to parental distress. When parents are told that their son is suffering from this devastating condition, they need to be told together; unfortunately this does not often occur (Firth *et al.* 1983).

Communication

Parents often complain they are not given enough information about the condition. In fact they need repeated opportunities to express their own ideas and fears as well as to receive factual information. The genetic implications are not easy to grasp, and again many parents will need more than one explanatory session.

Principles of communicating with parents and children where the child has a fatal condition are discussed elsewhere. Parents will wish to communicate between themselves and with their child and his siblings about the muscular dystrophy in their own way, but it may be helpful for professionals to suggest early on that the more open the communication about the illness and its implications, the easier the family atmosphere is likely to be. Psychological disorders in sufferers and their sibs are more common where there is lack of open communication.

3.9 Metabolic disorders

There is a very large number of metabolic disorders occurring in infancy and childhood. Most are very rare and occur as a result of inborn errors affecting amino acids, carbohydrates, protein, lipid, purine, and other aspects of metabolism. Psychosocial aspects of a small number of the less rare disorders with particular psychiatric or developmental significance, are described here.

3.9.1 PHENYLKETONURIA

Definition

Phenylketonuria is a disorder of amino acid metabolism in which there is a deficiency in phenylalanine hydroxylase, the enzyme responsible for converting dietary phenylalanine to tyrosine.

Aetiology

Phenylketonuria occurs in about 1 in 15 000 births, and is an autosomal recessive disorder. The enzymatic defect results in excessive production of phenylpyruvic acid, phenylacetic acid, and phenylacetylamine. There is consequent interference with maturation of grey matter, defective myelination, and cystic degeneration of white matter in the central nervous system.

Clinical features and treatment

If untreated, affected children are usually markedly developmentally delayed and become severely or moderately mentally retarded. Normal intelligence has, however, occasionally been reported in untreated cases. Epileptic fits, eczema, and behavioural disturbances (especially hyperkinesis and autism) are common accompaniments.

The condition is treatable if diagnosed within the first few days of life. Universal screening at day 5–8 of life now ensures that virtually all children born with the condition are identified. Treatment involves a low-phenylalanine diet, with close monitoring of blood phenylalanine levels throughout the first 7 or 8 years of life. Subsequently, a relaxed diet with some restriction of phenylalanine intake is usually advised until mid-adolescence (but see below).

Dietary treatment should be instituted in a specialized centre. Specially manufactured low-phenylalanine milk substitutes provide the main source of nutrition in the early years, and other foods have to be severely restricted. This means that the child is unable to lead a normal social life. In the pre-school years this is not usually problematic, but in older children conflict over the diet may occur, especially if family relationships are tense for other reasons, or if the child is temperamentally difficult (Kazak *et al.* 1988). Counselling can be helpful in both preventing and managing these kinds of difficulties.

Treated children are virtually always within the normal range of ability, though their mean IQ is slightly lower than that of their siblings, and they have an increased likelihood of minor neuropsychological anomalies. Relaxation of diet in mid-childhood results in a small but definite decrement in intelligence (Holtzman *et al.* 1986). Rates of behavioural deviance are raised in treated children with phenylketonuria (Smith *et al.* 1988) when compared with class-room controls. Affected children show more mannerisms, fidgetiness, restlessness, and poor attention, as well as being more anxious, solitary, and miserable. Behavioural deviance is inversely related both to IQ and to the quality of bio-chemical control in the early years. Residual abnormality of phenylalanine metabolism, or the effect of having to take a rather unpalatable diet, may be responsible for high rates of behavioural deviance. Genetic counselling is an important component of family management.

Outcome

The outcome of early treated cases is usually good and, in adulthood, a normally independent life is to be expected. Affected women are, however, likely to give birth to children with congenital abnormalities and mental retardation as a result of the exposure of the fetus to high levels of maternal phenylalanine, unless they return to a diet before conception (Lenke and Levy 1980). Phenylketonuric women planning to have a baby should therefore go on a carefully monitored low-phenylalanine diet, which should be monitored from before conception to delivery.

3.9.2 GALACTOSAEMIA

Galactosaemia is a rare disorder of carbohydrate metabolism in which there is a deficiency of the enzyme galactose 1-phosphate uridyl transferase. Insulin production is stimulated so that the brain is exposed to persistent hypoglycaemia and other metabolic abnormalities, producing brain damage and dysfunction. Damage to the liver, spleen, and eye (with cataract formation) also occurs. It is transmitted as an autosomal recessive condition. Brain damage can be largely prevented by the administration of a galactose-free or low-galactose diet, but this is highly restrictive and is necessary for the whole of the individual's life.

Intellectual development in treated cases is satisfactory, although compared with their normal sibs, affected children have a slight decrement in IQ with specific visuospatial deficits (Komrower and Lee 1970).

Studies of emotional and behavioural development have found that treated children have high rates of problems (Fishler *et al.* 1966). Younger children tend to be fearful and anxious, and older children are more aggressive and anti-authority in their attitudes. It is likely that these difficulties arise partly as a result of residual brain dysfunction, and partly as a reaction to social problems arising both in the family and outside from the need to persist with an unusual diet.

3.9.3 MUCOPOLYSACCHARIDOSES

The mucopolysaccharidoses are a group of disorders affecting storage of carbo-hydrate. They are classified according to the precise type of enzyme deficiency that is present. The terms *Hunter syndrome* and *Hurler syndrome* and, more descriptively, *gargoylism* were used to describe varieties of the condition before the metabolic defects were identified.

The conditions are often identifiable by the characteristic facial appearance at or shortly after birth. In all the mucopolysaccharidoses there is a normal early development for about 6–12 months, followed in some types by a failure to develop further and subsequent mental deterioration. There are associated skeletal and other organ defects. Severe behaviour problems are common (Bax and Colville 1995) They include destructiveness, restlessness, sleep problems, and aggressiveness. Children aged 5–9 years are particularly likely to be affected. Sufferers may die in childhood or survive into early adulthood. A precise metabolic diagnosis is desirable, as different variants have different genetic implications—the conditions may be inherited in an autosomal or sex-linked recessive form.

3.9.4 LESCH–NYHAN SYNDROME

The Lesch–Nyhan syndrome is a very rare disorder of purine metabolism, in which there is a defect of the enzyme hypoxanthine-guanine phosphoribosyl transferase. It is of particular psychiatric significance because of the association with mental retardation and severe self-injurious behaviour. It is a sex-linked condition, and all reported cases have been boys.

Affected children show choreoathetosis and moderately severe mental retardation as well as self-destructive behaviour. Self-mutilation is of a different order from that occurring in other forms of mental retardation and autism. Biting of the child's own lips and cheeks produces loss of tissue with sinus formation. Severe head-banging can produce further brain damage.

Treatment of the self-mutilation can be extremely difficult. External restraint is nearly always necessary. Behavioural modification with removal of attention from the undesirable behaviour has produced short-term improvement (McGreevy and Arthur 1987). The use of carbidopa and tryptophan has also produced short-term beneficial change (Nyhan 1976).

4

Development and developmental psychopathology

4.1 Fetal and infant development

4.1.1 PSYCHOLOGICAL ASPECTS OF PREGNANCY AND THE PERINATAL PERIOD

During pregnancy, parents, and particularly the mother, experience complex psychological changes. Adaptation to parenthood can be seen as a transitional experience in which men and women come to see themselves taking on new responsibilities, as well as developing love and attachment to their new baby. Changes in the marital relationship commonly occur, with couples sometimes coming closer emotionally, but women sometimes becoming preoccupied with their baby-to-be and withdrawing from their husbands. A high proportion of pregnancies are unwanted in the early months, but most mothers are looking forward to their baby by the time of birth, though even at this time ambivalent feelings are not at all uncommon.

Psychosocial factors with effects on fetal development

Emotional state of the pregnant mother-to-be
Persistent negative attitudes to the pregnancy are associated with high rates of certain physical complications of pregnancy. For example, essential *hypertension* occurring during pregnancy has been linked to the occurrence of depression and ambivalent feelings in the pregnant woman (Wolkind 1981). By contrast, hypertension occurring in later pregnancy is not associated with these emotional problems and is more likely to be physiologically determined. *Vomiting* in early pregnancy is not associated with neurotic difficulties, whereas persistent vomiting throughout pregnancy appears to occur more frequently in women living in deprived social circumstances with inadequate social support. The causation of nausea and vomiting in pregnancy is often uncertain, but an ambivalent attitude to the pregnancy may be the most common causative factor (Macy 1986).

Minor psychological and psychosomatic symptoms are common in pregnant women and their partners. Although some women experience an improvement in their sense of well-being in pregnancy, the reverse is more common. Condon (1987) found only 15% of women felt better than usual during pregnancy, whereas 50% felt worse. Prospective fathers also commonly experience psychological change during their partner's pregnancy; in the same study 10% reported an improvement in well-being compared to 20% who sensed a deterioration.

Psychiatric disorders in pregnancy consist mainly of anxiety and depressive states. Between 5% (Cox *et al.* 1982) and 25% (Kumar and Robson 1978) of pregnant women have been found to show such conditions. Palpitations, free-floating anxiety, chronic feelings of tension, and emotional lability at a level not amounting to psychiatric disorder are even more common. Mothers who are anxious during their pregnancies may be likely to have babies who, in the first few weeks of life, are irritable and cry easily: the mechanism is uncertain (Ottinger and Simmons 1964). Depression in pregnancy may occur as an isolated episode, or merely reflect predisposition to mood disorder before the pregnancy that is likely to persist after it.

Pregnant women who are depressed are likely to neglect their physical condition, eating irregularly and perhaps becoming overweight. They are less likely to attend antenatal check-ups regularly. Consequently their babies are more likely to be at risk for perinatal hazards that may themselves produce psychological sequelae in the children later on.

Smoking, alcohol consumption, and drug addiction in pregnancy
Substance abuse is a serious hazard to pregnancy, especially if usage is heavy. *Smokers* have a higher rate of miscarriage during pregnancy, and low birth weight is more common. After birth, there are much higher rates of respiratory infection in the child (Stevens *et al.* 1988). Working-class women are more likely to smoke, as are women with psychiatric disorders. However, smoking has a clear, independent effect on birthweight even after socio-economic factors and psychosocial stress have been taken into account (Brooke *et al.* 1985). There are effects of smoking on later development, with babies of mothers who smoke having lower developmental quotients, and later, lower scores in tests of educational attainment. This is probably mediated by effects on fetal blood supply affecting nutrition and brain development.

Heavy *alcohol* consumption in early pregnancy results in babies born with the so-called *fetal alcohol syndrome*, a condition in which there is prenatal and/or postnatal growth retardation, central nervous system involvement as shown by developmental delay and characteristic facial dysmorphology, especially microcephaly, microphthalmia, or short, palpebral fissures, a poorly developed philtrum (median groove between the upper lip and nose), and a thin upper lip (Chasnoff 1988). Average reported IQ is around 68, but there are no specific cognitive deficits. Short attention span and learning difficulties are prominent in the school situation. It is likely that the mental retardation and attentional difficulties are at least partly organically determined, although the fact that many of these children live in deprived circumstances often makes it difficult to disentangle causative influences.

The effect on the fetus of lesser amounts of alcohol consumption is uncertain, but may be a good deal more widespread than is generally recognized (Weinberg 1997). In one study, maternal binge drinking early in pregnancy was associated with learning difficulties and behaviour difficulties in adolescent children (Olson *et al.* 1997). At this stage of knowledge, it seems improbable that consumption involving a glass of wine a day or less is harmful (Smithells and Smith 1984), but women planning a pregnancy are probably best advised to abstain from alcohol for about 2 weeks before the planned conception, and then to drink no more than a glass of wine or its unit equivalent a day throughout pregnancy (Royal College of Physicians 1995).

A variety of *drugs* administered to the mother during pregnancy may affect the fetus (Johnstone and Forfar 1984). In particular, lithium and valproate can produce congenital abnormalities. It is, however, sensible to avoid the use of all inessential psychotropic medication in the first 3 months of pregnancy. Although sporadic reports of fetal malformations occurring with use in early pregnancy of a variety of psychotropic agents are of only anecdotal value, it does not seem reasonable to take risks by using drugs with uncertain therapeutic benefit. For a woman planning a pregnancy, it also seems sensible to avoid the use of medication in the preconceptual period as soon as she ceases to use birth control.

Drug withdrawal effects in the newborn baby may occur up to 14 days after birth if the mother is addicted to amphetamines, barbiturates, heroin, cocaine, methadone, or morphine. Withdrawal effects from *alcohol* are less common. A high pitched cry, sweating, tremulousness, and gastrointestinal upsets are the most prominent symptoms in the neonate born to an addicted mother. The management of withdrawal effects in the addicted neonate requires the skills available in a specialist neonatal unit.

Direct effects of physiological responses to maternal stress on the fetus

Fetal heart rate increases if pregnant women experience fear, but there is no good evidence that stress in itself affects fetal development. Indirect effects through an influence on smoking and alcohol intake are much more likely (Newton 1988). There is also no evidence that mothers experiencing stresses in pregnancy are more likely to produce babies with malformations, nor that major life events can, except indirectly, trigger premature births. There may, however, be an effect on the later development of behavioural problems in the children. Maternal anxiety has also been linked to the later occurrence of *pyloric stenosis* (Dodge 1972). The evidence linking stress in pregnancy to later problems in children does not suggest that major delayed effects are at all common.

Effects of low birthweight on later psychological development

There have been many follow-up studies of low birthweight babies to assess whether later impaired psychological development is linked to the low birthweight itself, or is produced by premature birth or intrauterine growth retardation. The results are difficult to interpret for a variety of reasons:

- Low birthweight babies come from low social class groups more often than one would expect by chance. Consequently lowering of intelligence may be due to social rather than physical factors.
- The low birthweight may itself have been caused by an abnormality in the baby, and this abnormality may be responsible for poorer intellectual performance later on.
- The quality of care for babies born too small is improving year by year. Consequently, results obtained a decade or more ago may not be accurate reflections of the present situation.

Despite these problems, some reasonably firm conclusions can be drawn:

- If the birth is otherwise uncomplicated, and treatment for respiratory problems or convulsions has not been required in the neonatal period, then the outcome of low birthweight babies weighing over 1.5 kg is as good as normal birth-weight babies from similar social class backgrounds. The presence of respiratory distress (often associated with haemorrhage into the periventricular region) indicates a poor outcome in those babies who survive.
- The outcome of very low birthweight babies weighing less than 1.0 kg at birth, although also often good, is definitely more problematic. They are more likely to show minor neurological signs, lower intelligence quotients, and more behavioural difficulties than matched controls when examined shortly after school entry (Marlow *et al.* 1988). However, the mean IQ even of these children is within the average range. Although it is possible to predict the development of later neurological abnormalities from ultrasound investigation using technology available in the early 1980s, it is not possible to predict cognitive abnormalities (Costello *et al.* 1989).
- Babies suffering intrauterine growth retardation and born at a weight significantly lower than that predicted for their gestation (i.e. those babies who are 'light for dates') have a somewhat poorer outcome in terms of later behaviour and learning problems than those who are born early but at a weight appropriate for their gestation (Neligan *et al.* 1976). However, the evidence for this is not clear-cut (McBurney and Eaves 1986).
- If they receive the advanced technology available in most obstetric centres in the western world, about a third of babies born even at very low birthweight do well from a psychological point of view, providing they do not show evidence of cerebral palsy, blindness, or other gross physical defect. About a third show minor cognitive and behavioural problems and about a third more serious difficulties requiring special educational approaches.

Effects of perinatal complications other than low birthweight on
later psychological development
The impact of other complications of pregnancy and delivery on the psychological development of the child is often difficult to evaluate. In general, a history of a single adverse event, whether it be haemorrhage in early pregnancy, toxaemia of pregnancy, a breech delivery, or a caesarean section, is usually of little significance in the appraisal of a child with a learning or behavioural problem (Davie *et al.* 1972). If, however, multiple complications have occurred, or a single complication (such as traumatic birth) followed by a major neonatal problem (convulsions, respiratory distress, etc.), then this may well be of significance as an indicator of underlying brain dysfunction. Single pregnancy complications (such as early haemorrhage) may, however, be of considerable significance if associated with intrauterine growth retardation and a baby born small-for-dates.

Babies with multiple perinatal complications born into families of low socio-economic status are more likely to show psychological deficits later on than babies with similar obstetric problems born into more socially advantaged families. Thus there is an interaction between the effects of birth complications and social factors (Werner *et al.* 1967).

Psychosocial aspects of the neonatal period

Psychologically, the first month of life is often a period of great emotional intensity for the parents, especially for the mother. The establishment of a satisfactory feeding pattern, the development of a mutually rewarding relationship with the new baby, and adjustment to a changed sleeping pattern are all tasks that must be mastered over a relatively short period of time.

Problems in the neonatal period may occur as a result of factors affecting the baby or the mother. Unsatisfactory and insensitive professional care may also produce problems. These factors may interact so that, for example, depression in the mother may elicit unsympathetic or negative attitudes from professional staff who would otherwise have been more positive in their behaviour. Cumulative disadvantage may thus occur.

Factors affecting the baby

- *Physical illness.* The baby may suffer from a variety of physical conditions, including apnoeic attacks, respiratory disorders, vomiting, jaundice, bleeding conditions, convulsions, and metabolic disorders. Any of these will require specialist assessment and treatment. The management even of those conditions with a benign outlook will inevitably interfere at least to some degree with the development of the mother–child relationship. Babies requiring admission to hospital in the postnatal period may suffer from a variety of physical and psychological trauma. Minor adverse effects have been detected at 3 years of age in children undergoing neonatal surgery (Ludman *et al.* 1990).
- *Neurobehavioural factors.* Hyperexcitability and irritability, as well as apathy and somnolence in the newborn baby, are common after a traumatic birth, or a birth in which the mother has been heavily sedated during labour. They may also occur for other reasons, presumably physiological, which prove impossible to identify. In any event, such behavioural patterns may make the establishment of the early mother–child relationship more difficult.

Factors affecting the mother

- *Physical illness* in the mother in the immediate postpartum period is not common, but may occur. Breast abscess, gynaecological complications of the birth, and exacerbations of problems associated with pre-existing physical illnesses such as hypertension and diabetes mellitus are those most commonly experienced. If the mother needs specialist treatment in hospital, this will threaten the early development of her relationship with her baby.
- *Emotional problems.* Transitory mood disturbances (postnatal 'blues') affect about 50% of women in the immediate postpartum period. Crying, emotional lability, and feelings of ambivalence towards the baby lasting 2–3 days may

occur. Puerperal depressive states occur in about 1 in 8 mothers. These are likely to occur in the first month or so after the birth (Cox *et al.* 1982), especially in mothers who are under stress for other reasons. There is, in fact, no evidence of a rise in non-psychotic psychiatric disorder in women in the year after childbirth (Cooper *et al.* 1988), but when such disorders do occur, symptomatology often focuses around the baby. Excessive anxiety about the baby, self-blame, irritability, sleep problems, suicidal thoughts, and fear of harming the baby are prominent features. Such conditions usually respond fairly quickly to counselling and antidepressant medication and, if reasonable social support is available from husband, neighbours, and friends, separation from the baby is not usually necessary. Untreated, these disorders are likely to last several months.

- *Puerperal psychoses* of schizophrenic, schizoaffective, and affective type, in which there are delusions, often involving the baby as well as paranoid and other bizarre ideas, are often associated with inappropriate mood. They occur in about 1 in 500 women in the postpartum period, when there is a rise in the rate, though not a change in the type of psychotic disorders (Kendell *et al.* 1981). Separation is often necessary for the safety of the baby, but this may be avoided if strict supervision is available in a specialist unit for mentally ill mothers and their babies. Successful intensive community nursing care at home has also been described, and found to be suitable for all but actively suicidal or infanticidal women, provided they are not living alone and are within easy reach of hospital (Oates 1988). Prognosis for the acute phase of puerperal psychotic disorders is good, but about 1 in 7 mothers relapses following a further pregnancy. Psychotropic medication for mothers who are breast-feeding needs careful monitoring for its effects on the baby. Chloral, chlorpromazine, diazepam, and lithium prescribed to nursing mothers have all been detected in breast milk. If the baby appears drowsy, then the mother's medication should, in any case, be reviewed.

Factors in obstetric and neonatal units
The policies of obstetric units vary widely in the degree to which they foster or hamper positive development of the early mother–child relationship. Encouragement of early mother–infant contact, facilitation of breast-feeding, awareness of and sympathy for maternal anxiety, and a willingness to appreciate that normal babies vary widely in their early behaviour are all factors likely to promote good early relationships.

The development of attachment is discussed in more detail when early social relationships are considered (Section 4.1.2). The first few days of the child's life have sometimes been suggested to be a vital period in the process of early 'bonding' between mother and child, upon which the success of later attachment depends (Klaus and Kennell 1976). In fact, attachment is a continuous process, and there is no good evidence that babies who, for one reason or another, are deprived of satisfactory early opportunities to develop relationships with their mothers in their first few weeks, cannot develop good relationships later on both with their mothers and with other adults and children (Sluckin *et al.* 1983).

Nevertheless, there seems every reason why policies in obstetric and neonatal units should be carefully considered to encourage mutually rewarding mother–infant contacts in the first few days of life (see below).

Psychosocial aspects of health care in pregnancy and the neonatal period

Care in pregnancy

Pregnancy represents the start of life for one individual and a transitional phase in the life of others, especially the prospective parents and sibs. A problematic pregnancy can set the scene for later psychosocial difficulties. However, there is much scope for preventive activity by professionals (Newton 1988).

Women are more likely to produce healthy babies if, during their pregnancy, they receive regular and sympathetic antenatal care. Continuity of care is a considerable advantage. Mothers who see different doctors and midwives at each visit to a clinic are unlikely to receive very personalized attention. Virtually all mothers have anxieties about whether they will produce a normal baby. Sympathetic handling of anxiety, with regular, prompt feedback of information concerning the progress of the pregnancy, especially after a complication or an investigation such as a scan, will reduce unnecessary worrying.

Advice concerning smoking and alcohol intake will alert mothers-to-be of the dangers of heavy smoking and alcohol consumption. Such advice should, however, be linked to practical help, especially to reduce smoking. Early identification of heavy illicit drug use (often difficult because of poor antenatal attendance) will allow preparation for treatment of withdrawal effects in the newborn baby.

Identification of depressive states in pregnant women is of importance so that appropriate treatment can be provided to reduce distress. Women who have suffered such states before the pregnancy began are more likely to show continuing problems after the baby is born, so these should receive special attention. The Edinburgh Postnatal Depression Scale (Murray and Cox 1990) is a brief, reliable questionnaire, useful for screening depressive states both in pregnancy and in the postnatal period. Practitioners should be aware that the presence of a depressive state is one reason for non-attendance at antenatal clinics. Careful follow-up of non-attenders, if necessary by domiciliary visits by the primary health care team, is therefore indicated.

Women may be vulnerable for reasons other than poor mental health. They may be socially isolated, in conflict over continuing their careers, in marital conflict, or fragile following a previous perinatal loss. Women who have previously suffered a loss of this type are understandably unusually anxious about their present pregnancy, though not generally anxious or depressed (Theut *et al.* 1988). The provision of extra social support for vulnerable women in pregnancy may well improve the psychosocial outlook and there is some evidence that it may improve birthweight (Oakley 1988). Such social support has effects on the rate of accidents and the mood of the child, as well as on the helpfulness of the father when the child is 7 years of age (Oakley *et al.* 1996).

Identification of mothers-to-be who are unlikely to be able to care for their babies after birth, because of severe mental illness or personality problems, should also be undertaken. If this is a real possibility, early contact with the social services department needs to be made, so that discussion with the parents can, when this is necessary, helpfully lead to family support and, if this is clearly going to be unsuccessful, rapid permanent foster or adoptive placement of the baby shortly after birth.

Postnatal care

The policies of neonatal units caring for mothers and babies in the immediate postnatal period should encourage early mother–child contact, while taking account of the mother's need to rest and recuperate after a physically and emotionally exhausting experience. Arrangements for caring for babies of low birthweight or with other physical complications should not involve more separation than is absolutely necessary. Mothers of sick neonates interact less with their babies than mothers of normal children, unless special measures are taken to stimulate interaction (Minde *et al.* 1983). If the baby has to stay in a special care unit, then mothers should be encouraged to room-in and visit regularly, and to feel they have a valuable part to play in the care of the baby. Wolke (1987) has suggested a series of measures that can be taken to improve the environment for the sick infant in a special care baby unit. These include careful observation of the individual infant to detect reactions to noise, light, handling, and attempts at social interaction. There should be an individual care plan with readiness to change the pattern of care as the baby matures. In general, parents are able to cope with the uncertainties about their fragile baby if they are kept well informed of changes in the baby's state and expectations for the baby's future as they occur. Other measures that can help parents include encouraging them to use soothing techniques to calm their baby when agitated, to keep records of their baby's progress, and to have access to a picture gallery of previous graduates of the unit with 'before and after' photographs.

Many mothers, especially those with first babies, feel isolated and incompetent in the first few months of their baby's life. Regular visiting from health visitors, with emotional support and practical help, can reduce distress. In addition, mothers often feel benefit from attendance at groups run by voluntary organizations or at general practitioner health centres.

Although the occurrence of transitory mood states is of only trivial significance, there is a real need for early identification of puerperal depressive disorders, so that appropriate treatment can be provided (see above). Identification of the early signs of puerperal psychosis should lead to immediate psychiatric referral.

Babies at risk for later abnormality by virtue of their perinatal history should be carefully followed up. In the absence of overt signs of brain damage, most such babies will develop normally, but follow-up will result in early identification of those with a less satisfactory outcome. Parents are, in any case, likely to be anxious about the development of such babies over the first couple of years, and regular monitoring is likely to reduce rather than increase their anxiety.

Finally, those involved in perinatal care should identify babies at serious risk for later abuse. In the perinatal period, it is possible to predict with some accuracy the occurrence of later maltreatment (Leventhal 1988). However, the modest sensitivity and specificity of such prediction means that the impact of professional intervention to 'high risk' babies on the frequency of later abuse is rather slight. Nevertheless, it is clear that young, inexperienced parents who have premature babies or babies with other early problems in development are at particular risk, especially if they have a history of psychiatric disorder or anti-social behaviour. In these circumstances, assuming the parents are agreeable, involvement of the social services department is indicated. If the baby is thought to be at definite risk, the social services department should, in any case, be informed and a conference arranged.

4.1.2 ATTACHMENT

The development of relationships can best be understood using attachment theory (Section 1.2.9). In this section the processes whereby attachment occurs are described.

Attachment of family members

Parents, older sibs, and grandparents, especially if they are living with the family, will develop fantasies about the sex, appearance, and personality of the unborn child during the pregnancy. The appearance of the child and his early behaviour will dispel many of these fantasies, which will be replaced by perceptions based on reality. Intensity of feelings will, however, be heightened. In general, most family members—especially the mother who has had so much more close and physical contact with the child than the rest of the family, and who has under-gone the usually intensely painful experience of giving birth—will rapidly develop strong unconditional positive warm feelings towards the child. These are some-times mixed with ambivalence or even negative feelings, though normally positive feelings predominate.

Linked to these positive feelings are a number of other phenomena, all of which are likely to be most strongly experienced by the mother, especially in the first few months of life. Family members are likely to show:

- Strong *protective feelings* towards the child, especially if the child has been in danger during pregnancy, has been born after a long period of infertility, or prematurely, or has suffered physical illness.
- A need for *proximity* to the child. This is especially likely to show itself at night, when, in the early months, the parents may wish to have the child sleeping in the same room.
- *Exclusion* of other relationships. Not only may the mother pay less attention to the father and to other children, but older sibs may themselves wish to play less with their friends while the new baby is very young.
- *Empathic feelings* with the child. A tense, anxious child is, for example, likely to make other family members feel the same way. This is not just a reaction to the child but a sharing of the child's feelings.

These feelings, linked to the attachment process, and experienced by family members, will be present in varying degrees of intensity throughout the child's early years. As the child gets older and takes his place in the family, they are likely to remain present but to a diminished degree.

Attachment of the child

The process of attachment of the child to other family members is governed by the child's level of perceptual and other abilities, and the way in which these develop. The child's contribution to the development of social interaction is of great significance. These abilities develop at a much faster rate than has previously been realized. For example, in the first few days of life the child will distinguish his mother from other people by smell and by the sound of her voice.

Evidence that the child is becoming attached to other family members is shown by:

- *Recognition* of other family members as special people. Recognition of family members as different from each other and different from outsiders is accompanied by differences in the child's behaviour towards the various people concerned. In particular, in the first 6 months of life, the child may smile differentially and may cry when some people, but not others, pick him up. Subsequently, from about 7 or 8 months to 3 years, the child usually goes through a phase of acute anxiety over separation from familiar figures. This anxiety will gradually diminish in intensity, but most children continue to experience unpleasant effects when they are separated from their families and, of course, separation from loved figures remains difficult for most people throughout their adult lives.
- Expression of especially *intense feelings* towards family members. This is likely to be shown by demands for kisses and cuddling, but also by the fact that when the child is frustrated by family members, protest is likely to be more intense than with other people.
- *Expectation* that the family members will meet all needs. The child will, in the first few months of life, turn automatically to his mother for food, warmth, and comfort in distress. In the second and third year of life, the child will often 'test out' the capacity of members of his family to be all-providing by showing difficult behaviour. Thus the child learns that parents will continue to provide for him even when under testing circumstances.
- *Empathy* with the feelings of other family members. Especially in the first few months of life, just as the parents, especially the mother, are likely to be directly responsive to the mood of the child, so the child is likely to be directly responsive to the mood of parents. Children can be observed, for example, to become tense when their mothers are tense.

Attachment interaction between child and family members

Attachment is shown less by the individual behaviour of the child and other family members than by the development of interactions between them.

Characteristically these are likely to occur especially between mother and child in the first few months of the child's life. These interactions can be summarized as the establishment of:

- Mutually satisfactory *biological rhythms*. In the early days and weeks of the baby's life, its sleep needs will probably differ from those of the mother. Normally babies of a week old sleep about 17 hours a day, but waking occurs at intervals of 3–4-hours. By 3 months, most babies are sleeping for 6 continuous hours at night. Mother and baby (if the child is breast-fed) and parents and baby (for the bottle-fed) will by this time usually have adjusted their sleep patterns to each other's needs, though dissonance of sleep rhythms may mean that this continues to be an exhausting time for parents. If the baby is breast-fed, again a rhythm is set up which meets the needs of both mother and baby for frequency and quantity of feeds.
- *Bodily interplay*. Family members and the baby will gradually establish mutually satisfactory patterns of behaviour, involving holding and cuddling, to which even the young baby, by moulding his body and later by putting his arms up for holding, will contribute. Both parents and baby engage in mutual *en face* gazing and smiling at each other, again from the early days of life.
- *Communicative interplay* (Brazelton *et al.* 1974). Observational studies using split-screen video techniques have established the way in which, from the first few weeks of life, vocalizations of mothers and babies complement each other. Although formed expressive single-word utterances do not normally occur much before the age of 1 year, parents and babies will normally have established a system of preverbal communication long before this time. The baby will be communicating its needs for being held, for food, warmth, and dryness, and the parents their own needs for body contact, talking, and indeed gossiping with the baby.

Factors affecting the development of attachment

Factors within the child

- *Developmental maturity* of the child. In the absence of specific defects such as autism (Section 3.5.1), the child's level of social maturity is likely to be roughly similar to his development in other respects, so that mentally retarded children will be socially immature.
- *Temperament*. A number of specific temperamental characteristics are of relevance. A temperamentally anxious child will maintain close proximity to the parent. This may result in the parent becoming irritated and rejecting. A child with strongly positive emotional responses—a ready smile and a sunny disposition—may elicit strongly positive emotional responses in return. Twin studies reveal evidence of genetic factors in the infant's capacity to attune to its mother's affect (Szajnberg *et al.* 1989).
- The presence of *sensory defects* (such as impairment of hearing or vision) or other physical problems affecting the child's capacity to respond to signals put out by the parents.

Factors within family members, especially parents

- The *wish for the child* in the first place. The birth of many children is unplanned, and the discovery of pregnancy greeted with dismay. In most cases, as the pregnancy proceeds, much more positive feelings are experienced. In a minority this does not happen. It has been shown that when mothers are refused abortion and such pregnancies are carried to term, a high proportion of the children develop behaviour and learning problems (Forssman and Thuwe 1966).
- *Parental personality, physical and mental health.* The presence of a warm, outgoing personality, good physical health, and the absence of parental mental health problems such as depression and anxiety, will facilitate attachment. Infants are acutely sensitive to the affective behaviour of their mothers (Cohn and Tronick 1989).
- *Behaviour of older brothers and sisters.* This can facilitate or impair attachment in a variety of ways. An unduly jealous older child may, for example, distract parents from their younger developing baby. The behaviour of older sibs at the birth of a baby is dependent on a variety of factors (Section 1.3.2).
- *Quality of family relationships.* Parents who find each other's company mutually rewarding will find it easier to relate to their children.
- *Living conditions.* Attachment is more likely to occur when parents are not pressed by overcrowded living conditions and financial stress. However, very satisfactory attachment can occur in families living in materially deprived circumstances, providing that there are good quality family relationships.

Characteristic patterns of secure, insecure, resistant and disorganized/disoriented attachment shown by infants and young children are outlined in Section 1.2.9, where attachment theory is described. In general, the presence of a secure attachment will occur when positive infant characteristics interact with favourable environmental conditions. The other forms of attachment displayed in the 'strange situation procedure' (see page 11) are inconsistently linked to less favourable environmental circumstances. Abused children usually show one of the more worrying types of attachment.

4.1.3 ATTACHMENT DISORDERS

Attachment disorders can be classified as:

- primary attachment disorder:
  — reactive attachment disorder
  — disinhibited attachment disorder
- other disorders in which disturbances of attachment play a major role:
  — oppositional defiant disorder (Section 4.5.2)
  — conduct disorders (Section 4.5.3)
  — pre-school anxiety and depressive disorders (Section 4.4)

— elective mutism (Section 3.2.6)
— school refusal (Section 4.4.3).

Disturbed social relationships are prominent in many other psychiatric disorders, but are of central relevance in those listed above.

Reactive and disinhibited attachment disorders

Definition
In reactive or disinhibited attachment disorders the child, despite adequate intelligence, has failed to make specific attachments to a small number of care-givers, and instead shows either a complete lack of interest in initiating or responding to other children and adults, or indiscriminate but superficial attachment to any adults with whom he comes in contact.

Classification
In the ICD-10 classification (World Health Organization 1992), these two types of attachment disorder are classified separately as two forms of disorder of social functioning with onset specific to childhood and adolescence. In the DSM-IV classification (American Psychiatric Association 1994), both types are termed 'reactive attachment disorder of infancy or early childhood' and form part of a group of miscellaneous conditions. In this scheme, the presence of grossly pathogenic care is a necessary condition for diagnosis.

Clinical features
- In the *reactive* type, the child looks miserable, frightened and may be hypervigilant. Self-injury is common, and the child may refuse to eat, resulting in failure to thrive. The child shows no interest in making age-appropriate attachments to adults or other children.
- In the *disinhibited* form of attachment disorder, the child is unconcerned who is looking after him and approaches other adults and children in an unduly friendly way. The relationships so formed are superficial, and the child does not become sad or worried if his care-givers change. Such children are often very popular on hospital wards, where they make friends with nurses, and appear to cope with brief admissions extremely well. Overactivity, short attention span, emotional lability, poor tolerance of frustration, and aggressive behaviour are common accompaniments. A sharp distinction between the hyperkinetic syndrome (attention deficit disorder), conduct disorder, and this condition is often not possible. Learning difficulties often arise which are usually at least partly secondary to poor concentration.

In both types of attachment disorder, the child has usually been reared in his or her early years in a series of institutions and/or foster families, or has been seriously neglected in his own home. There may be a history of recent abuse, and this is more likely if the child is hypervigilant and watchful. Very occasionally, the clinical features occur in children reared in normal families who have sustained brain damage usually as a result of head trauma or cerebral infection.

Assessment

Direct observation of the child's behaviour towards the clinician is often sufficient to suggest, if not to confirm, the diagnosis. Assessment should include a consideration of the quality of care provided by the present care-givers, and an account of the child's behaviour in a pre-school facility as well as when he is with his family at home.

Attachment disorders must be distinguished from pervasive developmental disorders in which the child has little capacity for social reciprocity, fails to improve significantly when placed in a normal social environment, and shows associated characteristic language disorder, as well as stereotypies or mannerisms.

Management

Attachment disorders will usually be identified in the context of seriously inadequate parental care. The child may already have been removed from parental care, or still be living in unsatisfactory circumstances.

The primary aim of treatment should be, through family support, to provide the child's care-givers, whether these be the parents, foster or adoptive parents or staff in a children's home with help to improve their capacity to promote healthy development when this has been impaired. The focus will often be on the provision of consistent warmth and limit-setting, as well as on the improvement of peer relationships and communication with others. The provision of emotional support to parents or substitute care-givers, linked to a behavioural approach will usually be appropriate.

If the quality of the child's care at home remains poor and the child's development remains at risk of significant harm, then child protection procedures will need to be invoked (Section 2.1.5). However, even if the child with an attachment disorder is removed from a 'pathological' environment, his new care-givers are likely to continue to need help with his management.

Outcome

There is a lack of specific information on the outcome of children with attachment disorders, but the findings from studies of maltreated children are relevant (Section 2.6). Children placed with adopted families can do well even after a period of institutionalization lasting up to the age of 4 years. Their lack of generalized behavioural disturbance is likely to be reduced after placement (see Tizard 1977), but the capacity of the children to develop appropriate social inhibitions and to make and sustain relationships often remains impaired. Long-term follow-up of children placed out of institutions into permanent homes suggests that such improvement may be maintained at least into mid-adolescence (Hodges and Tizard 1989), but some degree of impairment, shown especially by deficiencies in attention and concentration, will remain.

4.2 Feeding and eating control disorders

4.2.1 ESTABLISHMENT OF FEEDING

The establishment of a satisfactory feeding relationship between a baby and its mother in the first few days of life depends largely on instinctively determined behaviour, based on physiological mechanisms. It is gradually shaped, however, by the experience of the feeding couple, whether this be mutually satisfying or unsatisfying, enjoyable or unenjoyable. Interaction in the feeding situation between mother and baby, and later between mother and toddler, is a reflection of their relationship more generally. It is also a situation in which the development of autonomy and independence is negotiated smoothly or with difficulty (Hammer 1992).

In breast-feeding, the secretion of milk into the breast is under hormonal control, and ejection is stimulated by the baby's sucking, which triggers the milk-flow reflex. Generally, after a few days, a rhythm is established between mother and baby so that there is a balance between the baby's requirements and the mother's flow and ejection of milk. Similarly, in artificially fed babies, a pattern of feeding times is established with gradual lengthening of the period between the late night and early morning feeds over the first few weeks or months. There are a number of good descriptions of the physiology of infant nutrition, the composition of breast and artificial milks, with discussion of early feeding patterns and problems (e.g. Wood and Walker-Smith 1981).

Satisfactory establishment of early feeding depends on:

- *Factors in the child.* An intact and well-functioning feeding apparatus and gastrointestinal tract, as well as good general health are required. Intact neurophysiological mechanisms are also necessary, and babies who have suffered perinatal trauma to the brain may show temporary or more permanent feeding problems. The use of intrapartum medication may impair the baby's capacity to suck after birth. Finally, feeding provides an early opportunity for the baby to demonstrate individual temperamental characteristics. Some babies are placid and relaxed; others fussy and irritable.
- *Factors in the mother.* The mother's capacity to supply sufficient breast milk or appropriate artificial feeds is obviously relevant. This may be impaired by local problems affecting the nipple or breast, or by impairment of physical health. More commonly, feeding will be adversely affected by the mother's emotional state, especially by undue depression or anxiety (see p. 176). The mother may be generally anxious and have a specific anxiety about feeding. Such emotional changes may be hormonally or psychologically induced.

Breast- or bottle-feeding: psychosocial considerations

There are advantages and disadvantages to both breast- and bottle-feeding. In developed countries, breast-fed babies are less likely to develop obesity, have a slightly lower incidence of asthma, eczema, and cot deaths, and, if they develop gastroenteritis, have a lower mortality rate. (In developing countries breast-fed babies have considerable added advantages in relation to infection and growth.) Psychological satisfaction also appears greater in mothers who breast-feed, though it is possible that this is because relaxed, contented women find it easier to breast-feed in the first place.

By contrast, bottle-feeding allows the feeding to be shared by other family members, and this makes it more feasible for a mother to return to work earlier. This will be a major consideration if there is economic pressure on the mother and, as is regrettably sometimes the case, breast-feeding at work is not feasible. Many mothers also find breast-feeding embarrassing.

There is no evidence that breast- or bottle-feeding influences the rate of subsequent behavioural or emotional problems in the child, though small later intellectual advantages have been detected in children who have been given breast milk as pre-term babies (Lucas *et al.* 1992). As there are small but clear physical advantages to breast-feeding, professionals should obviously encourage this practice. It is, however, neither kind nor rational to induce guilt in mothers who, for economic or social reasons, decide to feed their babies artificially. An increasing number of working mothers do, however, find it possible, once breast-feeding is well established, to breast-feed their babies morning and evening, while the baby receives artificial feeds during the day.

4.2.2 FEEDING PROBLEMS IN EARLY INFANCY (0–3 MONTHS)

Minor, transient problems and setbacks in early feeding are very common. Persistent, more severe difficulties are less normal and require careful assessment. Physical disorders may be present and, even if they are not, an unsatisfactory early feeding relationship may be a prelude to serious behavioural difficulties later on.

- *Rejection of the bottle or breast*. If a baby is active and otherwise well, this is usually only a transient problem occurring in the first few days of life. It is most likely to be due to faulty technique, and to be amenable to practical advice from an experienced health visitor or family doctor. A faulty feeding position, too large or too small a hole in the teat, may be responsible.
- *Failure to suck*. A baby showing general apathy and lack of interest in sucking may be suffering from neurological dysfunction following a traumatic birth, the late effects of intrapartum medication, a neurodevelopmental disorder, or a generalized physical disorder such as an infection. It may be associated with nausea related to other chronic disease. Very occasionally, failure to suck appears unassociated with any identifiable physical condition. This problem is difficult to explain. It is improbable, but not impossible, that even at this early age, the baby has developed unpleasant fantasies about the breast or bottle that deter sucking. More probably, the baby has had an adverse early experience in sucking, and sucking avoidance has become a conditioned response.
- *Crying*. Normally babies only cry for relatively brief periods before and occasionally after feeds. Longer periods of crying may be due to hunger, discomfort from the cold or a wet nappy, or lack of sufficient attention. Crying due to

pain is discussed below. Although prolonged crying in the first 3 months of life is often attributed to poor parenting, this is not true of most infants with this problem, in whom the difficulty is physiologically determined (St James Roberts 1991)

- *Diarrhoea*. Persistent passage of loose stools in infants may be due to *over-feeding*, *infections* (especially gastrointestinal or systemic infections), *cow's milk allergy*, *drugs*, or the *malabsorption syndrome*. Older children sometimes go through a phase of passing some undigested food (toddlers' diarrhoea). Psychosocial factors may be of significance in this form of disorder (Dutton *et al.* 1985).
- *Constipation*. Most commonly this is due to underfeeding, and especially inadequate fluid in the diet. Unusual physical causes include *cystic fibrosis* (although this more commonly presents with diarrhoea) and *Hirschsprung disease*. Occasionally babies withhold faeces if potting is attempted in the early months, though most babies do not appear to object to this futile practice.
- *Vomiting*. Slight regurgitation, often of no significance or due to overfeeding, needs to be distinguished from actual vomiting of whole feeds. The latter may be due to *infectious conditions*, *pyloric stenosis*, *cow's milk allergy*, or *hiatus hernia*.
- *Abdominal pain*. If unaccompanied by vomiting or failure to thrive, this may be a distressing symptom, but one of no organic pathological significance. The characteristic pattern of '3 month colic' is that the baby cries with pain and is unsettled in the early evening over the first few months of life, but then gradually improves. Usually, no physical cause is identifiable, and it must be assumed that physiological factors, probably affecting the motility of the gastrointestinal tract, are producing the prolonged pain-induced crying. Psychosocial factors may, however, be relevant (see below) in causation and, even if they are not, parents can become very distressed by the constant crying and require support through a difficult time.

Management of feeding problems in early infancy

Management of these early difficulties first involves an assessment of the likely cause, together with treatment of any underlying physical condition. Necessary procedures in the assessment and management of physically determined problems are well described elsewhere (Wood and Walker-Smith 1981). In many cases, however, such physical factors are absent or insufficient to account for the problem. In these circumstances, psychosocial factors may well be of relevance. These include:

- *Adverse living conditions*. Mothers living in crowded, insanitary conditions will inevitably have greater difficulty in feeding their babies adequately and safely, especially if they are bottle-feeding.
- *Problems in social relationships*. Among the most common of these are unsupportive husbands or boyfriends, and intrusive, critical grandparents.

The inexperienced mother needs all the sympathy and support she can obtain in the first few weeks of her new baby's life, and this may be lacking.

- *Generalized maternal anxiety or depression.* Postpuerperal affective states are relatively common. Irritability, apathy, and agitation are frequent features and will be shown in behaviour outside the feeding situation.
- *Anxiety focused on the baby.* Exaggeration of normal, maternal preoccupation with the baby may result in concern being expressed about quite ordinary aspects of the baby's feeding behaviour.

A common outcome of any of these psychosocial problems is that the mother is so anxious in her handling of the baby at feeding times that the baby becomes unsettled, cries excessively, refuses to suck, and eventually develops behaviour that reinforces the mother's anxiety so that a vicious cycle is established.

Psychosocial aspects
This will obviously depend on the circumstances, and, in particular, on the mother's social and material conditions and emotional state. It is necessary to exclude physical factors in the mother as well as the baby, but, even if these are present, psychosocial factors may be relevant. It should be emphasized that most such problems will be dealt with by primary care professionals, especially health visitors and family doctors. Only occasionally, where difficulties are serious and persistent, will advice from a paediatrician be sought, and psychiatric advice will be taken even more rarely.

- *Practical help.* Observation of the feed may immediately reveal the nature of the problem. An inappropriate feeding position is relatively common. Alternatively, the feeding position may be satisfactory, but the mother so tense and anxious that the baby is unsettled. Practical advice on the way the nipple is presented or on the size of the hole in the teat may be invaluable. An anxious mother may rapidly become more relaxed when, as a result of a simple tip, she becomes successful in her feeding. More subtle problems which direct observation may reveal include a lack of sensitivity to the baby's feeding behaviour—for example, an insistence that the baby continues to suck, when obviously he wants to take a break. Mothers can be helped by suggestions about altering the timing of feeds, so that the baby is not too hungry at the time the feed commences.
- *Mobilizing social support.* It may be useful to discuss a mother's feelings of isolation and insecurity with, if possible, the husband or boyfriend present. A health visitor may be able to encourage visiting from neighbours to provide company for an isolated mother. A self-help group of mothers at the local clinic or health centre can perform a similar function. Especially for a young and inexperienced mother, a health visitor may provide the nurturance the mother herself may need while trying to give it to her baby.
- *Counselling.* Some mothers, especially if seriously depressed and anxious, may benefit from the opportunity to express their ambivalent feelings towards their difficult baby to a sympathetic listener. Wider issues, such as concerns over

loss of femininity and attractiveness, can be discussed. The mother may have previously expressed regrets at giving up her work or worries about what is happening at her place of employment while she is on maternity leave. Such counselling also allows identification of circumstances which might lead to the possibility of non-accidental injury.

- *Psychiatric referral*. Mothers who show persistent disturbances of mood that fail to respond to counselling should be referred for psychiatric assessment and management. It is important, however, that the primary health care team should remain in touch with the family as well as the psychiatrist involved, as the type of help provided for the individual needs of the mother may need to be supplemented by continuing monitoring of the feeding relationship.

4.2.3 FAILURE TO THRIVE IN LATER INFANCY AND EARLY CHILDHOOD (3 MONTHS–3 YEARS)

Definition

Minor feeding problems in young children are common, occurring in around 20% of the population. They include finicky eating habits, overeating, mouthing non-food substances, spitting up and vomiting, and colic. They usually respond to management approaches such as regularly presenting the child with new foods, praising appropriate behaviour, and providing the child with opportunities to observe other children behaving more appropriately (Budd and Chugh 1998).

However, more serious problems may ensue, of which failure to thrive is the most frequently encountered. This involves a failure to grow and gain weight either from birth or after a period of normal physical development. Standardized centile charts are available (Child Growth Foundation 1994) by which an individual child's growth can be compared with others of his age. Those who are consistently below the second centile in weight, who have documented weight loss over time, or who have a reduction in growth velocity (as shown, for example, by the crossing of two or more major centiles on a growth chart), should be regarded as requiring serious concern and investigation. Some who are of low birthweight, but continue to grow, albeit at a slow rate, may be regarded as 'small normal' children. These have constitutional or genetic reasons for their size, and suffer neither from disease nor from environmental deprivation—the two major reasons for inadequate nutrition and failure to thrive.

Clinical features

If organic disease is present, the presenting features will depend on its nature. The failing-to-thrive child, appearing for a routine appointment at a follow-up clinic for low birthweight babies, may present with breathlessness due to a cardiac or other physical condition, or with symptoms referable to the gastrointestinal tract such as chronic diarrhoea and vomiting.

In the majority of children failing to thrive, who do not have organic causes, the presentation usually occurs from 2–3 months of age up to the third year of life. Feeding problems are common, and there may be regurgitation of food, vomiting, or chronic non-specific diarrhoea. Alternatively there may be no complaint at all from the mother, but the child may be found on a routine check to be falling below the second centile or faltering in growth velocity. The dietary intake of the child may be described as adequate, although careful investigation may reveal the child is, in fact, not getting enough to eat, and this is the commonest cause of failure to thrive. Nutritional inadequacy is often caused by a combination of failure of adequate provision of food and inadequate intake. The child is likely to be mildly or moderately delayed in cognitive development, especially in language comprehension and expression.

On examination, if physical disease is present, the child may show characteristic abnormalities. Failure to thrive for other reasons is not associated with particular behavioural characteristics, although developmental immaturity may well be present.

Prevalence

The prevalence of failure to thrive will depend on the criteria used. In theory there will be exactly 2% of children at or below the second centile, together with a number of other children who, although taller and heavier than this, are failing to achieve their expected growth. In practice, there are some children (small normals) a little below the second centile, whose parents are of short stature and whose birthweight suggests that they are just born to be small. These will not be a cause for concern. Mitchell *et al.* (1980), using multiple criteria, found that nearly 10% of children under the age of 5 years attending a primary health care centre in the US, showed failure to thrive. About 5% of paediatric admissions in the UK are for failure to thrive, and the problem also frequently presents to general practitioners.

Aetiology

Traditionally, causes of failure to thrive have been classified as organic and non-organic. This terminology is misleading (Frank and Zeisel 1988). All failure to thrive is produced by inadequate food intake or malnutrition, and is therefore organically determined. However, in a minority of cases observed in primary and secondary care (perhaps 5–10%), the malnutrition is related to physical disease such as infection, heart failure, cystic fibrosis, food allergies, or the malabsorption syndrome. In the remainder, physical disease is absent and the causes of malnutrition lie in the behavioural or developmental characteristics of the child, in the environment, or perhaps most commonly in the interaction between the child and the mother, an interaction that may be specifically maladaptive to the feeding situation (Skuse 1989). Community studies have shown that, compared to controls, infants and toddlers in the general population who fail to thrive, are often unusually 'good' babies, who sleep long hours and may, in addition, show subtle abnormalities of chewing and swallowing mechanisms. They are not more socially deprived, and their parents are often not especially deficient in parenting skills, though they may not stimulate their children sufficiently (Wilensky *et al.* 1996). Physiological anomalies may play a large part in the development of the poor growth rates of these children. However, those infants who present to clinics do tend to come from families with multiple social problems, and to be in touch with social agencies.

- The social background of young children who present with non-organic failure to thrive is often, though by no means always, socially deprived. The families are living in unsatisfactory accommodation, perhaps on housing estates with a bad local reputation. They may be in financial difficulties made worse by the burden of another child. In some cases, the social circumstances of the families may provide a large part of the explanation of the problem.

- In other families, living in more fortunate social circumstances, the main causes may lie in the mother's mental state or in the quality of parenting—the feelings of the mother and the way in which these are shown in her behaviour when feeding the child. A mother's difficulties in being warm and sensitive to her child's needs while it is feeding may be part of a general problem she has in making relationships, part of a specific difficulty in child-rearing, or only relate to the child in question. Some mothers become depressed because, although living in materially privileged circumstances, they are socially isolated—alone all day at home while the father is away at work. General personality problems are most likely to be explained by deprivation in the mother's own early background, often compounded by a lack of good current support from her husband or her own family. Specific problems with the child may be related to the fact that the baby was and perhaps is unwanted. More generally, relationships within the family may be disturbed by tension, and there may be an overt family conflict or a more covert, mutually unsupportive relationship between the parents.

- The child's characteristics may be of greatest importance. The exclusion of physical disease does not mean that the primary pathology lies in the family or wider environment: non-disease factors in the child may be of great significance. These include adverse temperamental characteristics: the child may be constitutionally lethargic, or unusually active or restless. Minor degrees of oro-motor dysfunction leading to difficulties in chewing and swallowing may be of major importance.

- Often the circumstances in which feeding takes place provide the best clues as to the real nature of the problem. The mother may sit the child in an inappropriate position (semi-supine rather than sitting upright). The child may be constantly distracted during feeding, for example, by television, pets, or other children. Feeding may be an event the mother regards as something to be concluded as quickly as possible, so that an attempt is made to press the child to eat at a quite inappropriate pace. Conversely, the child may require more encouragement to feed than the mother is prepared to provide.

It is most common for social circumstances, parental factors, and child difficulties to be present in combination rather than in isolation.

Assessment

The assessment of the problem will begin with an attempt to construct a growth line for the child from birth to the present time so that a judgement can be made concerning whether there has been a fall-off from expected growth. The birth-weight and child health clinic records will be invaluable for this purpose. A significant minority of children who fail to thrive have been born prematurely or show intrauterine growth retardation. Where this is present, consideration should be given to these factors in assessing the child's growth pattern.

Although the findings are likely to be negative, a physical examination of the child is essential. Particular attention should be given to the presence of dysmorphic features, signs of infection, and dyspnoea, all of which may indicate an organic explanation. Physical investigations should be limited unless there are positive indications. Normally, a routine blood count and urine examination will be adequate, though in areas where lead poisoning is endemic, lead levels should be estimated.

Enquiries should be made into the circumstances in which the family are living. Overcrowding, severe financial constraints, and lack of social support may all be relevant. Enquiries should be made about the mother's own mental state. Questioning about the mother's mood can most tactfully be achieved by asking whether the child's problem (or anything else) is making the mother feel low, unhappy, or anxious. Maternal mood may indeed be secondary rather than primary in these circumstances.

A dietary history should be obtained, if possible with the help of a dietitian. In some children a dietary history will make it clear that the child is not obtaining sufficient to eat. In some cases this will simply be due to ignorance, but in others enquiries concerning the mother's feelings about the child and the feeding situation will clarify the reasons. Useful information may be obtained by requesting the mother, with the help of a dietitian, to keep a record of the child's dietary intake over a week or fortnight. In mild cases of non-organic failure to thrive a sympathetic explanation with advice on diet given in the consulting room or out-patient department will, on follow-up, turn out to have been sufficient intervention.

Observation of feeding, ideally in the home, but if not in the consulting room or clinic, is often the most illuminating part of the assessment. The child may be seated inappropriately, subjected to major distractions, fed too rapidly or too slowly. The food may be unattractively prepared or presented. The child may be observed to have difficulties chewing or swallowing, even though the food is appropriately prepared and presented, and this may be an indication of the presence of oromotor dysfunction. The involvement of a speech and language therapist, skilled in the assessment of chewing and swallowing, will be helpful.

Where a child is more severely affected or there is a suspicion of undiagnosed organic disease, despite primary care and out-patient investigation, either because of the symptomatology or because of the absence of evidence of a psychosocial explanation, then the child should be admitted to hospital with the mother. Intensive physical investigations should, however, be avoided until it has been established that the child will not gain weight even though getting enough to eat.

Assessment of weight gain in hospital

Most children admitted to hospital will gain weight on a normal diet. Children who fail to gain weight despite normal intake have an organic cause for their poor growth. Children who do not receive an adequate intake may have an organic explanation, such as a neurological disorder, affecting their sucking or chewing capacity, or a chronic infection impairing appetite, but they are more likely to be showing food refusal for psychological reasons. The single most important investigation in the assessment of 'failure to thrive' is a trial of feeding, and other investigations should be held in abeyance until it is established whether the child is able to gain weight on an adequate intake.

Assessment of feeding behaviour of mother and child

Where a physical explanation remains the most likely cause, a range of further physical investigations will need to be carried out in hospital. Even in these, however, positive organic findings may not emerge. Berwick *et al.* (1982) noted an average of 40 laboratory tests carried out in infants admitted to hospital for failure to thrive. In only 0.8% was relevant diagnostic information obtained. A hospital assessment of physical state and response to adequate diet should therefore be accompanied by a further evaluation of the mother–child relationship, the feeding behaviour of the mother, and the behaviour of the child during feeding. In some cases the child will not feed with the mother but will feed with nursing staff. The mother may be noted to be stiff, uncomfortable, and perhaps uninterested or even disgusted by feeding her baby. Alternatively, she may be overconcerned, anxious, and intrusive.

Management

Most cases of failure to thrive can be managed in the primary care setting, and indeed the opportunity for home visits will often make primary care management more rewarding than treatment delivered from hospital.

Assuming physical disease has been excluded, management will centre on those features of the family circumstances, parental relationships, attitudes and behaviour, or—most commonly—the feeding situation, which assessment has revealed to be most relevant.

Where growth has fallen seriously behind, in order to achieve catch-up growth, the child will require 1.5–2 times the expected calorie intake for age (Frank and Zeisel 1988), and this will often not be easy to achieve.

Parents may need more accurate information about the amount of food their child needs to grow properly and, in some cases, this will in itself be sufficient intervention. More commonly, more active intervention is required, and this may call for the combined professional input of the health visitor, family doctor, and, where available, dietitian, speech and language therapist, social worker, psychologist, and psychiatrist.

The most rewarding form of intervention is likely to involve direct impact on the feeding situation. Simple behavioural measures including establishing a good feeding position, as far as possible excluding distraction when the child is feeding, ensuring the food is appropriately prepared and presented, making allowances for any difficulties the child has in chewing or swallowing, may all lead to improvement. A useful behavioural approach to the treatment of feeding problems in children who are failing to thrive has been provided by Iwaniec *et al.* (1985).

In children admitted to hospital, a plan of management will also require the combined skills of those with medical, social work, nursing, psychological, and dietetic expertise (Fig. 4.1). The mother is likely to get especially valuable help from supportive nursing staff. If the baby will not feed for her, but will feed for the nursing staff, the situation should be dealt with sympathetically and not critically. It should be explained that it is natural for babies to be more difficult with their mothers, because they are more emotionally involved with them. A mother who is deprived herself and consequently finds it difficult to care for her child will need a nurturant and not a critical relationship with nursing staff and social worker so that her self-esteem can grow and she can feel she has more to contribute to her baby's care than she thought. Practical advice from nursing staff in the feeding situation, if offered tactfully, can often be positively taken up by the mother. The establishment of feeding programmes with very gradual introduction of solids in small, frequent feeds, can be useful. Help may also need

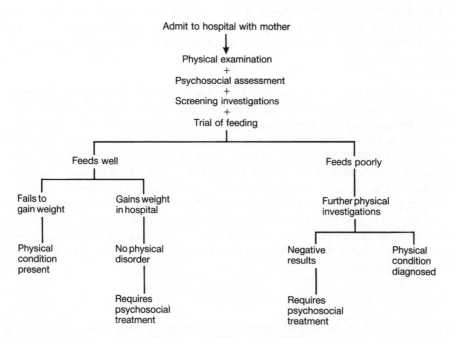

Fig. 4.1. Failure to thrive, failure to respond to out-patient care—plan of management (adapted from Campbell 1984).

to be given to ensure that the young child is adequately stimulated between feeds. Many children with failure to thrive show mild to moderate developmental delay, probably partly because of inadequate stimulation. It has been shown that malnourished children gain weight faster if active play and language stimulation programmes are instituted, and if the mother can be helped to undertake this type of activity, she may be able to continue once the child leaves hospital.

Whether management is conducted by the primary care or hospital team, depression in the mother is an indication for an evaluation of the family and other circumstances that may be involved in lowering mood and energy. Counselling from social worker or psychiatrist and possibly antidepressant medication may need to be arranged. The social worker may also be able to arrange for the alleviation of some of the social stresses acting on the mother by recruiting support from other family members, advising on financial benefits, etc. In cases where it is thought that the child is in serious danger of severe chronic neglect, the procedures described earlier for dealing with non-accidental injury need to be invoked (Section 2.1.5).

In brief, the treatment of severe failure to thrive occurring for psychosocial reasons requires the combined skills of a multidisciplinary team. Follow-up should ensure the child is indeed now thriving physically and is receiving adequate nutrition. The frequent occurrence of developmental delay and behaviour problems in children who fail to thrive means that attention in management should not be solely focused on the child's physical growth. Cognitive development should also be monitored and, where necessary, additional stimulation provided either at home or in a pre-school facility. Counselling should also be provided for any behaviour problems that may be present, and referral to a psychiatrist or psychologist for more intensive treatment arranged if this is not effective.

Outcome

Non-organic failure to thrive is likely to improve slowly with appropriate treatment, but most children will remain small for their age. This is particularly likely to be the case where growth faltering has occurred early in the child's life, especially in the 3–6 months period, perhaps because of the rate of brain growth at this time and/or because maladaptive feeding patterns, once established, are particularly difficult to alter. A high proportion of children with short stature in middle childhood will have first presented with failure to thrive in infancy. Further, perhaps due to subnutrition or family adversity, there is a high rate of developmental delay with subsequent behavioural and learning problems in children who have, in infancy, failed to thrive. There is surprisingly high continuity between early feeding problems and eating control difficulties in adolescence (Marchi and Cohen 1990).

4.2.4 PICA

The mouthing and chewing of inappropriate objects is an uncommon presenting problem, although toddlers and young children often put small toys, buttons, pencils, and anything else available into their mouths. Persistent mouthing of earth and scavenging occurs in young, deprived children. Older children who continue to put objects in their mouth are usually, but not always, mentally retarded. The dangers of pica include acute and chronic accidental poisoning. Children with pica are more likely to ingest tablets, bleaches, etc. if they are left lying around. They are also more likely to show high levels of body lead concentrations, although pica is now a very rare cause of lead poisoning, at least in the UK (Smith *et al.* 1983).

The management of children presenting with pica depends on the nature of the problem. The removal of dangerous substances from the child's whereabouts is an important precaution. If the pica is a sign of chronic deprivation, then attention should be given to improving the social conditions in which the child is living. Behavioural methods are sometimes effective in treatment of pica in older mentally handicapped children.

4.2.5 OBESITY

Definition

Both objective and subjective criteria are important in the definition of overweight. Using standardized weight and height charts (Child Growth Foundation 1994) it can readily be ascertained whether a child is over the 97th centile for weight (or 20% over expected weight for given height and sex). A body mass index over the 90th centile is sometimes taken as an objective criterion for serious concern. Similarly, a child's degree of adiposity can be assessed using skinfold callipers (Tanner and Whitehouse 1975) and compared with standardized tables. There is a reasonably good correlation between an observer's subjective comparison of a child's degree of obesity and these standard measures. The subjective judgement of the child and family may, however, be very different. Older girls may regard adiposity well within the 'normal' range as objectionable, and many parents of children with worrying objective evidence of obesity do not perceive their child as having a problem.

Clinical features

There are four main modes of presentation of obesity in children, each of which has somewhat different implications for management. The child may be noted to be overweight during a routine procedure such as immunization, or when presenting with an acute physical disorder such as a respiratory infection. Second, the child may be noted to be overweight by teachers or others outside the family. Third, the parents may become concerned about the rate at which the child is gaining weight. Finally, in older children, and especially in adolescent girls, the child herself may express concern. A presentation in which the family or child have themselves been motivated to seek help is more likely to respond to attempts at treatment than where only others have been worried.

The degree of overweight is rather poorly correlated with the amount of concern expressed by family members. Some grossly overweight children are never brought to attention by their parents, while other parents express considerable anxiety over rather minor degrees of overweight. Motivation to attend is often enhanced by a child's unhappiness at school because of teasing.

Prevalence

Obesity is the most common nutritional disorder in developed countries. Because of varying standards, precise prevalence figures cannot be stated, but estimates vary between 2 and 15% (Lloyd and Wolff 1976). In fact, probably the lower figure is more realistic if considering those children whose health is definitely at risk because of obesity. On the other hand, the higher figure is an underestimate if one considers all those teenage girls who consider themselves overweight.

Objectively defined obesity is more common in girls than in boys and, probably because of their greater intake of cheap starchy foods, the condition is more common in working-class than in middle-class children (Wilkinson 1975).

Aetiology

Clear-cut single-factor organic causation is rare, though obesity does occur as part of the Prader–Willi and Laurence–Moon–Biedl syndromes, both associated with mental retardation. Hypothalamic syndromes affecting the appetite mechanism may also result in obesity, but again these occur very rarely, and other signs of hypothalamic and pituitary malfunction are obvious.

Most obesity is multifactorially determined (Woolston 1987). Obesity certainly runs in families. Genetic, as well as environmental factors, are important. Although the evidence from twin studies is conflicting, a large investigation of Danish adoptees (Stunkard *et al.* 1986) clearly pointed to the importance of genetic factors. Obesity was related to the weight of biological parents (especially the mother), but not to the weight of adoptive parents. Nevertheless it is likely that environmental factors play a part in determining which genetically vulnerable children become obese.

Obesity occurs when there is an excess of calorie intake over energy output. By the time obese children are professionally assessed, their dietary intake is often not unusually high, though it is sufficient to maintain the degree of overweight. In this case, either the intake at some previous point in time must have been excessive, or the child is predisposed from an early age to put on excessive weight with a normal intake. Artificially fed babies are more likely to be overweight, both currently and in mid-childhood than breast-fed babies. In many children, the dietary intake is excessive at the time of presentation.

Obese children exercise less than the non-obese, but the differences do not appear great enough to suggest that low energy output is largely responsible for obesity and, in any case, obesity is quite as likely to be a cause of taking little exercise as the other way round. It is, nevertheless, interesting that the prevalence of obesity increases according to the number of hours of television viewed by the child. It has been claimed (Gortmaker *et al.* 1996) that over 60% of overweight incidence in 10–15 year olds in the US can be attributed to television watching.

Inappropriate patterns of eating in the family are probably of significance. The artificial feeding of babies and excessive intake of cheap, starchy foods in an unbalanced diet occur more commonly in working-class families. More specifically, the intake of bread, potatoes, and between-meal snacks of crisps, biscuits, and sweets is encouraged in some families, and restricted in others. Family patterns of overeating are probably the single most important cause of obesity.

Family and individual psychopathology is thought important by many clinicians, but good evidence is lacking. It has been suggested that mothers who feel guilty about some aspect of their own behaviour may overprotect their children and fail to allow them autonomy. The child is never allowed to feel hungry, and so loses the capacity to determine its own need for food. There is no evidence that obese children are unusually aggressive, as one might expect if their autonomy was severely restricted. Certainly some obese children, like some obese adults, do overeat when they are miserable, and prepubertal obese children are indeed more depressed than age-matched controls.

Many very overweight children have good cause to be miserable. They are often derided by other children, teased, bullied, and called names to a degree that leads to a serious degree of social isolation (Tobias and Gordon 1980). Sociometric studies have shown that obese children are less likely to be wanted as friends than children with other physical disabilities, even those with conspicuous deformities. Obese adults have been shown to be self-denigrating, anxious, and sensitive to social criticism, and the same is probably true of overweight children. However, much psychopathology in obese children may be caused by factors such as maternal depression and poor social circumstances that are also responsible for the obesity (Epstein *et al.* 1996).

Assessment

An adequate history should attempt to clarify the onset of obesity. If the onset is recent, was it associated with any particular event? Details of the child's intake at mealtimes and between meals should be obtained. The dietary history is likely to be inaccurate unless the focus is on the last couple of days. The intake of other family members, and their own degree of overweight, will be relevant. The presence of any behavioural or emotional problems should be established and, in particular, it is helpful to know whether the child's relationships with other children have been affected by his or her appearance. Finally, it is useful to know what dietary measures, if any, have been tried to date, and how motivated the child and family are to achieve loss of weight.

Physical examination should establish accurately the height and weight of the child for baseline purposes. The presence of any endocrine disorder can usually be excluded purely on physical examination.

Management

Management depends particularly on the degree of obesity and on the motivation of the child and family. In all children over the 97th centile, it is reasonable to point out the health hazards of remaining overweight, but in many cases this, in itself, will not be a sufficient motivating factor. In those who are motivated, usually either because of teasing at school or because the degree of obesity has reached even more alarming proportions, a positive treatment approach is indicated.

- *Dietary restrictions.* Under the supervision, or with the help of a dietician, a 3.3–4.2 MJ (800–1000 kcal) per day diet taking into account the child's food preferences should be recommended. This is most unlikely to be a sufficient treatment measure in itself, and even for short-term success a variety of other measures will need to be implemented.
- *Behavioural measures* involving cognitive self-management have proved modestly effective in the short-term (Duffy and Spence 1993). This approach involves obtaining a clear account of the stimuli that normally precede eating, so that alternative responses can be achieved. When, for example, the child feels miserable or has reached a time when he would normally take a snack, he is given some alternative activity to eating, which is then reinforced. In adults, behavioural methods have been shown to have more long-lasting effects than appetite-suppressant drugs (Stunkard *et al.* 1980). Focused treatment programmes involving behavioural control of eating patterns, education of the child and family concerning calorie intake, and encouragement of exercise do appear to have at least a short-term effect, and there are encouraging suggestions of long-lasting effectiveness (Epstein *et al.* 1994).
- *Family and group approaches.* An attempt should also be made to change family patterns of eating behaviour, for a child is unlikely to reduce his intake if the behaviour of the rest of the family is unchanged. The family should eat the same meals as the child. Family sessions, in which behaviour at mealtimes is discussed, may be helpful in this respect, particularly by stimulating involvement if one of the parents appears unconcerned and indifferent to the problem. Some older children and adolescents will also benefit from attendance at groups run on 'weight-watcher' lines, and this is probably the most useful approach overall.
- *Hospitalization.* In-patient treatment is indicated for a variety of reasons:
  - First, when there is scepticism among family members that excess intake is responsible, an admission may demonstrate that weight loss is indeed possible without any more complicated procedures.
  - Second, it may be necessary for life-saving purposes when the very seriously obese child is showing hypoventilation (Pickwick syndrome), and useful results can be obtained by admitting the child.
  - Third, if family patterns of eating are inappropriate, a period away from home may allow an older child to develop autonomy in the realm of eating behaviour so that, when he returns home, he has the capacity to refuse food when it is pressed upon him.

More drastic forms of treatment applied in adults to the very severely obese include jaw-wiring and the ileal bypass operation. These have also been used in older adolescents with reasonably successful results. Clearly, however, these can only be contemplated when the obesity has become life-threatening.

Outcome

Obese children have a high risk of remaining obese in adulthood. Thus Stark *et al.* (1981) found that 4 out of 10 obese children became obese adults. Long-term obesity is associated with hypertension, cardiac disease, diabetes, emphysema, varicose veins, and poor operative risk. These adverse outcomes are, however, only common in the severely obese. Most forms of treatment produce immediate short-term improvement, and treatment effects can be demonstrated from a combination of self-monitoring and family approaches (Epstein *et al.* 1994).

4.3 Sleep and its disorders

4.3.1 NORMAL SLEEP PATTERNS

The newborn baby sleeps on average 16–17 hours a day, though there is rather wide variation. Cycles of sleep and waking are relatively brief. Over the first 3 months of life the total amount of sleep declines little, but the cycles are longer, so that, by the age of 3 months, 70% of babies are sleeping right through the night. By 6 months 85% of babies sleep through the night, but 10% are still waking every night by the age of 1 year. By this age the great majority of babies have established a stable pattern of sleep and wakefulness, with a long sleep at night and a nap in the morning and afternoon. Social class and the parity or experience of the mother are not related to wakefulness, but breast-fed babies are more likely to wake at night than bottle-fed ones (Eaton-Evans and Dugdale 1988).

Developmental neurophysiology of sleep

The neonate has a characteristic EEG sleep pattern that gradually approaches but does not attain the adult pattern by the age of 1 year. Adults show two types of neurophysiological activity during sleep—*quiet sleep* and *rapid eye movement* (*REM*) sleep.

- So-called *quiet sleep* has four stages, proceeding from stage 1 with low-amplitude, fast-frequency waves, to stage 4 with high-amplitude, low-frequency waves.
- For about 20% of sleep time adults show REM sleep in which the EEG shows low-amplitude fast-frequency waves, associated with decrease of muscle tone, variations in pulse rate, respiration rate, and blood pressure, as well as bursts of rapid eye movements. A sleep cycle from the beginning of one phase of REM sleep to the beginning of the next lasts about $1\frac{1}{2}$ hours. By contrast, neonates show nearly 50% REM sleep and a good deal of sleep that is poorly differentiated in EEG terms. Cycles are of short duration, lasting about 45 minutes. The adult, when falling asleep, goes through a prolonged phase of quiet sleep before a REM phase, while the neonate goes straight from wakefulness to a REM phase. By 3 months, however, the infant, on going to sleep, does pass through a phase of non-REM sleep. From 3 months to 1 year the

infant's sleep EEG pattern also becomes much more clearly differentiated with increasingly prolonged periods of slow-wave quiet sleep.

Infant sleep in the first year of life gradually comes to be increasingly modified by environmental influences. By 6–8 months, a change in sleeping arrangements, anxiety or depression in the mother, or an alteration in the bedtime ritual may result in an increase in wakefulness. Disrupted quiet sleep is commoner in babies who have suffered pregnancy and birth complications (Blurton-Jones *et al.* 1978) and in babies born to diabetic mothers.

At about the age of 18 months, and perhaps earlier, infants show signs of dreaming. Dreams occur largely in REM sleep. When woken from REM sleep, adults will report a dream on about 80% of occasions, whereas in non-REM sleep they report dreams on only about 10% of occasions.

Influences on sleep in early childhood

In the second and third year of life, normal children often show difficulties in getting off to sleep. During the night, wakeful periods occur and a high proportion of children do not go back to sleep without calling for their parents. In one population study (Crowell *et al.* 1987) more than a third of children aged 18–36 months woke their parents during the night at least once or twice a week. Unwillingness to go to sleep in this phase of life may be related to a variety of developmental factors. In order to go to sleep the child must stop paying attention to the world outside him, withdraw into himself, and think his own thoughts in his internal world. Many children go through a phase when they are unwilling or frightened to give up the external world. As they go to sleep they may wish to carry an image of their mother or some other familiar person with them. But their capacity to retain an image in their minds (their capacity for *object constancy*) is limited, so they may need to recall their mother for a brief reminder. The presence of a doll or bit of blanket—a *transitional object* (Winnicott 1953)—may ease the journey over the bridge from wakefulness to sleep. Wakefulness is also commoner in babies and toddlers with adverse temperamental characteristics—those who, in the daytime, are more negative and intense in their expression of mood and more irregular in their habits.

Older children may fear a loss of control during sleep. They may, for example, be frightened they will pass faeces or urine and thus disgrace themselves. Others will be upset at the thought of missing television, curious about what their parents might get up to in the middle of the night, or determined to show their power to keep their parents running from one bedroom to another in the early hours of the morning. Lying in the dark or semidarkness, perhaps with the wind blowing the curtains through a half-open window, is often sufficient to stimulate anxieties in the older child of burglars, ghosts, giants, or other frightening phenomena.

In the fourth and fifth years of life, the need for naps is usually gradually reduced and then eliminated. Children are more likely to sleep through the night, though they may well wake earlier than their parents wish. Problems in getting off to sleep and wakefulness in the night sometimes persist, though nearly all children will sleep through the night once they start infant school. Bad dreams or nightmares become commoner and are often associated with a frightening experience, such as a television programme or video, seen on the previous day. Poor sleep and nightmares are less common in middle childhood, but as children move into adolescence, normal sleep needs may not be met because of increased social and academic demands. Difficulties getting up in the morning are common, and may be linked to late nights, drug and alcohol use, depressive or anxiety disorders, or simply unwillingness to face what promises to be a boring or difficult day.

4.3.2 SLEEP PROBLEMS

Sleep problems are common among children. Simonds and Parraga (1982) surveyed a population aged 5–20 years and found restless sleep (28%), sleep talking (13%), fear of the dark (10%), and bed-time rituals (8%) to be among the most frequently occurring difficulties. Anders and Eiben (1997) have provided a useful account of sleep disorders in childhood, based on the DSM-IV classification (American Psychiatric Association 1994).

Wakefulness at night

Wakefulness is by far the commonest sleep difficulty, with a peak frequency between 12 and 24 months of age (Richman 1981). About 20% of children of this age either take at least an hour to get to sleep or wake frequently or for prolonged periods during the night. About 10% of children show waking at night at 3 years; by 8 years the prevalence has dropped to 4% (Richman *et al.* 1982). In the young child, waking at night may be associated with adverse temperamental characteristics, maternal depression and anxiety, as well as stress in the family (Richman 1981). In most children with sleep problems, however, none of these factors is present, and the undue wakefulness cannot readily be explained by them.

Management
The management of difficulty in getting off to sleep and wakefulness at night (Richman *et al.* 1985) should begin with an assessment of the problem. An account should be obtained of the frequency and duration of the child's waking episodes over the previous week or fortnight. Enquiries should be made about the rituals at bedtime and what the parents actually do when, for example, the child wakes and comes into their room. Details of other possible areas of disturbance in the child—his social relationships, any feeding difficulties, etc.—should be obtained. The presence of depression and anxiety in either parent, and the social circumstances of the family, should be noted. Types of treatment already received, especially the previous use of hypnotics, should be identified, for, by 18 months, nearly a quarter of UK children have received hypnotic medication.

When, as is usually the case, the wakefulness is an isolated problem, parents can be reassured that the problem will pass and is of no serious import. Some sleep problems are, however, so exhausting for parents to deal with that they present a real threat to the stability of family life. Children with such problems can be treated, and successful therapy is likely to result in improvement in mother–child interactions during the day (Minde *et al.* 1994).

The treatment of choice is behavioural management (described below). Hypnotic medication, for example trimeprazine tartrate 30–60 mg last thing at night, may sometimes provide some temporary improvement, but is unlikely to result in lasting benefit.

A course of behavioural management should start with the parents charting the child's sleep pattern and their own response to it over a period of 10–14 days. The record thus obtained is very likely to show that parents are inappropriately rewarding the child for wakeful behaviour and failing to provide the best conditions for helping a child to get back to sleep after waking in the middle of the night. The father and mother may be spending up to a couple of hours in the child's room with the child calling out or crying if the parent attempts to leave. The child may be given quantities of sweet drinks if he wakes in the night and demands them. The parents may be alternately shouting at the child or taking him into their bed if he wakes.

Alterations in the management should then be discussed with parents. They should first be asked their own views on how they might change their behaviour. Cutting down on the length of bedtime rituals, replacing sweet drinks with water, and resisting the child's demands to get into the parents' bed will all prove helpful on occasions, provided that the parents can be consistent. If the child is old enough, a star chart marking nights when the child sleeps through and does not wake his parents can be kept. A minority of parents will be prepared to let the child 'cry it out', but many will not wish to do this. Some parents when faced with behavioural advice will turn out not really to be sufficiently motivated to change. Others will reveal levels of guilt or anxiety not originally detected and these may require more intensive counselling or psychotherapy.

Once a programme has been agreed, the parents should be encouraged to continue charting the child's sleep pattern and their own behaviour. A further two or three sessions to advise on continuing changes in management are usually sufficient to produce definite improvement, though often the child will still show minor sleep problems. It should be emphasized that this behavioural management approach, though effective in the majority of young children, is not likely to succeed where there are widespread emotional or behavioural difficulties, where parental anxieties or personality problems are thought to be a primary cause, or where social circumstances make it impossible for parents to institute a consistent programme.

The outcome of monosymptomatic sleep problems is good, and most do not betoken disturbance in the future. If they form part of a widespread pre-school behavioural disturbance, then they are much more likely to be followed by significant psychological problems at least in the middle school years.

Nightmares

Nightmares are frightening dreams that occur in the REM phase of sleep. The child will wake in an anxious state with slightly raised heart and respiratory rate, and then be fully orientated and able to recount his dream. The pattern of the nightmare and its underlying neurophysiological basis is, therefore, very different from a night terror (see below). Virtually all children experience at least occasional nightmares. Peak frequency is at about the age of 5–6 years, after which there is a decline in rate, though most people continue to experience them occasionally throughout childhood and in adult life.

A child experiencing frequent nightmares, occurring perhaps more often than once or twice a week, is a cause for concern. Most nightmares are stimulated by frightening experiences the previous day, such as watching a horrifying television programme or video. Parents whose children are having frequent nightmares will usually prohibit the watching of such programmes. A child having nightmares for some other reason is probably going through an unusually anxious stage and requires investigation, Enquiries should proceed along the lines described for other anxiety states (Section 4.4.2).

Night terrors, sleep-walking

Night terrors and sleep-walking are described together because they are both disorders of arousal, and have a common neurophysiological basis and genetic origin.

Night terrors are very upsetting for parents to watch. Usually about 2 hours after going to sleep the child sits up and appears terrified. He is likely to scream, shout, and moan, and sometimes tries to get out of bed. He may appear hallucinated and even deluded. The child does not respond when spoken to or attempts are made to calm him. There is a considerable rise in heart and respiratory rate. After a few minutes the child slowly settles and appears to go back to sleep. In fact, he has never really awakened.

A *sleep-walking* episode usually starts with the child sitting up 2–3 hours after going to sleep with a glazed expression on his face. He gets out of bed and walks mechanically, usually to his parents' bedroom or to the lavatory. Occasionally, he may wander around the house and, very rarely indeed, out into the street. He avoids objects and thus appears, at least to some degree, to be in contact with his surroundings. However, he does not respond to questions and is very difficult to wake. If he is guided back to bed, he will usually comply and go back to sleep. Often he will put himself back to bed within a few minutes.

Night terrors and sleep-walking each occur in about 3% of children, though one report has suggested that as many as 15% of 5–12 year old children have had at least one sleep-walking episode. The peak age for night terrors is 4–7 years and for sleep-walking somewhat older than this. The episodes occur in a period of arousal from EEG stages 3 and 4 sleep, so that the child is in fact quite deeply asleep when showing the behaviour. As many as 50% of sleep-walkers and children showing night terrors have a close family member who has shown one or other of these phenomena (Kales *et al.* 1980). The condition may be inherited in an autosomal dominant mode. Both conditions are likely to occur if, during the previous day, the child has experienced a stressful event, but, if they occur monosymptomatically, they are not in themselves an indication of emotional disturbance.

Management

Management of both sleep-walking and night terrors is similar. An account should be taken from the parents of the frequency and nature of the episodes, stressful events that might be upsetting the child, and the way the parents react when the episodes occur. Parents should be advised that it is unnecessary to wake the child. They should stay with the child while he is showing the behaviour, but beyond guiding the sleep-walking child back to bed, they need not take any other active measures. If parents are worried, and wish to take active measures, Lask (1988*a*) has described an apparently very effective procedure. This involves the parents keeping a record of the times at night when the child experiences night terrors, and then systematically waking the child up about 15 minutes before an attack is anticipated. If episodes remain frequent and persistent, occurring more often than once a week, but there is no evidence of unusual daytime anxiety, then it may be reasonable to try the effect of diazepam 2–5 mg last thing at night. This drug alters the proportion of stage 3 and 4 sleep, and has been reported to be helpful. Parents of sleep-walking children should be advised to secure external doors and windows, as, rarely, fatal falls from windows and dangerous wandering out into the street have been reported.

The outcome of both night terrors and sleep-walking is good, and usually they remit well before adolescence. A small minority of people continue into adult life.

Hypersomnias

The hypersomnias are disorders in which children or adolescents suffer from pathological excess of sleep. They are of two types: narcolepsy and the Kleine–Levin syndrome.

Narcolepsy

Narcolepsy occurs in 0.4–0.7% of early adolescents, and is therefore not uncommon (Anders and Eiben 1997). The patient experiences an irresistible desire to go to sleep, sometimes in the daytime. The sensation comes on very rapidly and usually lasts from 5 to 30 minutes. After the episode the child is usually fully alert within seconds. Usually attacks occur out of the blue, but sometimes they may be precipitated by unusual excitement. The subject may also at times experience *cataplexy* (sudden loss of muscular tone with a fall to the floor) or *sleep paralysis* (inhibition of muscle tone as the subject goes to sleep). Hypnagogic hallucinations may also occur. About 10% of patients suffer from epilepsy, implying that the condition is probably due to some form of brain dysfunction. The condition is probably largely neurophysioiogically determined, but experience of an emotional or stressful event can trigger attacks. A high proportion of adults with this condition have associated psychiatric disorders.

Narcolepsy is rare before the age of 10 years and more commonly occurs in late adolescence.

Kleine–Levin syndrome
The Kleine–Levin syndrome is a rare disorder occurring mainly in adolescence. Subjects show excessive somnolence during the day associated with markedly increased appetite, and other forms of behaviour disorder such as hypersexuality.

Management
Both these types of hypersomnia need to be distinguished from normal behaviour. It is, after all, common for people to take a nap in the afternoon, and many teenagers eat voraciously and seem, to their parents, to spend an excessive amount of time dozing in their beds. The distinction from normal behaviour lies mainly in the episodic nature of the disturbance, together with (in the case of narcolepsy) the rapid onset and recovery. The presence of epilepsy also needs exclusion. The main diagnostic feature, available only when a sleep laboratory equipped to carry out polysomnographic recordings, is accessible, is that the patient, when showing sleeping behaviour, can be demonstrated to have gone from the waking state straight to REM sleep. Normal sleep involves an initial period of non-REM sleep. Other psychiatric disorders, especially hysterical reactions, should also be considered in differential diagnosis (Guilleminault *et al.* 1974).

Treatment should primarily involve the encouragement of consistent bedtimes and rising times, with scheduled 20–30 minute naps during the day. Any precipitating factors such as emotional stress should be identified and, if possible, removed. The life of the child or adolescent should be altered to take account of the attacks. Teachers of a teenager with narcolepsy should be informed of the condition and encouraged to let their pupil withdraw from a class if there is warning that an attack is coming on. Older teenagers with narcolepsy should not be allowed to drive a car while attacks are still occurring.

Medication
Methylphenidate 5 mg in the morning and at lunchtime, increasing in older children to 10 mg in the morning and at lunchtime, is sometimes helpful in both these conditions. In older teenagers there is a danger of drug abuse with this medication, and, if prescribed, the drug should be administered only under strict control. Clomipramine 10–25 mg three times daily has been reported to reduce the frequency of narcoleptic attacks. The associated psychiatric disorders that may well be present (Dahl *et al.* 1994) will require psychological treatment, usually individual psychotherapy or family therapy. The Kleine–Levin syndrome has been reported to respond to tricyclic antidepressant medication and lithium (Pike and Stores 1994).

4.4 Emotional development and disorders of mood

Fear, anxiety, and depression occur in characteristic fashion during childhood. Their causes, the way in which they manifest themselves, and their adaptive function change as the child progresses from infancy, through childhood to adolescence. As most morbid or abnormal mood states are probably only extremes of normal mood, so the nature of mood disorders changes over this time.

In this section, fear and anxiety (both normal and abnormal) will be treated separately from depression, but it should be remembered that, in the individual child, there is often considerable overlap. The experience of one mood state is likely to be accompanied, at least to some degree by the presence of the other.

4.4.1 DEVELOPMENT OF FEAR AND ANXIETY

Definition

Fear and anxiety are intrinsic features of the human condition. Both are adaptive, but may become maladaptive if excessive or developmentally inappropriate. Some fears, such as *agoraphobia* (fear of open spaces), are not part of normal development, and are therefore regarded as pathological. The terms fear and anxiety are often used interchangeably, although some make a distinction between *fear* which is focused on a specific object or situation, versus *anxiety* which is diffuse and anticipatory. Both fear and anxiety have the same physiological manifestations.

Anxiety is defined as an emotion, an unpleasant feeling of tension or apprehension, accompanied by motor and physiological phenomena such as sweating, tremors, a dry mouth, and diarrhoea. It is a reaction to the perception of an imminent danger such as an animal or a doctor carrying a injection needle, or anticipatory such as a worry about a mother's health.

Anxiety shows developmental variations both in nature and in type of response, with some forms of anxiety declining and others emerging with increasing age (Campbell 1986; Marks 1987; Rutter and Garmezy 1983).

Anxiety in infants

Young infants show fear reactions to unfamiliar sounds, heights, falling, objects that approach rapidly or expand, and darkness. Because these fears occur without previous experience, it is argued that they are genetically programmed and adaptive, protecting the baby from possible harm. Infants are fascinated by new events and objects, but can also show fearfulness of them.

Stranger anxiety

By 4 or 5 months, and peaking in intensity at age 12 months, infants who had previously shown interest in any adult approaching them, now start to show anxiety reactions to unfamiliar people. Most infants will show anxious reactions to strangers by the age of 8 months, but their responses to unfamiliar people vary greatly and are affected by situation and context, including

- the presence or absence of the mother (with reduced intensity of fearful reaction to strangers while in the arms of mother)

- the strangeness of the overall situation
- previous experiences, such as positive experiences with strangers
- whether the stranger is an adult or a child (less fear towards a child)
- whether the stranger intrudes
- the degree of control of the infant over the situation (if the infant is mobile and has the possibility to approach mother, then the infant will show less distress when approached by a stranger) (Rutter and Garmezy 1983).

The blood relationship of the child to the stranger is not relevant, but a contrary belief explains why, for example, some grandmothers who see their babies for the first time at around a year of age are upset and angry when they are rejected.

The stranger reactions of infants contrast with the infant's curiosity about new situations. In the first months of life, the baby's attention is drawn by interesting new stimuli, including strangers. Later comes the recognition that some people are unfamiliar, followed by reactions of wariness or distress. The ability to detect someone's strangeness depends on the cognitive development of the child, especially the development of memory. Although in earlier infancy the infant is capable of recognizing familiar figures, especially the mother, by the time object permanence is established, the infant's memory is advanced to a point that it can recall what people look like rather than just recognize those who are familiar.

Separation anxiety
Related to stranger anxiety, but slightly later in development, is separation anxiety (Bowlby 1975). Infants will usually cry at the departure of the mother from age 8–24 months, peaking at 9–13 months. Separation anxiety decreases from about age 30 months onwards. Separation anxiety is a universal phenomenon reflecting the special evolutionary danger of being alone, a situation particularly hazardous in the young (Marks 1987). The type, duration, and intensity of separation anxiety is highly dependent on the age of the child, the quality of the mother–child attachment, the nature of the situation, and previous experiences with separation (Campbell 1986). Separation anxiety can occur when there are no strangers around, but it may be intensified by stranger anxiety if the infant is separated from the mother when a stranger is present. Long separations will lead to protest, despair, and then detachment (Bowlby 1975). Depending on the duration of the separation, the child may react with anger towards the caregivers after reunion, and may avoid or attack them. Separation anxiety keeps playing a role across the life span in the form of anxiety about loss, isolation and abandonment.

Anxiety in childhood and adolescence

Separation anxiety and stranger anxiety diminish during the pre-school period through maturation and experience. As children's cognitive abilities develop, and language, symbolic operations, and causal thinking emerge, typical fears change as well. Also, with increasing age, the child develops the capacity for anticipating events. For example, a child may worry about possible harm befalling the parents when they have gone out for the evening.

In the pre-school period, stranger fear may persist in the form of shyness. In this period, a number of new fears rapidly emerge, including fears of darkness, animals, imaginary beings, doctors, and storms. Some fears, for instance the fear of certain animals, may develop in children who had no such fears before and who have had no negative experiences with the feared animal. It is argued that these fears must be innate and developmental. Pre-school children may start worrying about rejection and abandonment by the parents, and many fairy tales have this as a central theme. Pre-school fears such as fear of darkness, burglars, and animals may be present in later childhood but diminish under the developing capacity to differentiate fantasy from reality. When children are ill or under stress, they often regress, and as a consequence fears that were forgotten may recur and disappear again as soon as the child is well.

During school age, the most common fears are for mysterious events, bodily injuries, and physical danger. School children may start to exhibit anxiety about personal adequacy and achievement, such as *test anxiety*. They have worries about friendships and bullying.

Adolescents may show anxieties related to social situations especially rejection (*social anxiety*), death, and major threats such as nuclear wars. Increased cognitive abilities in adolescents allowing abstract thinking, make them more vulnerable to fears about the future such as career choice, as well as religious issues. They may also develop fears about sexual matters.

Age and sex trends

During infancy and the pre-school years, there are no consistent sex differences in fearfulness. During the school years, reports by parents suggest girls have more specific fears than boys. Figure 4.2 shows the sex and age trends of parent reports on children's specific fears (except fear of school) in a general population sample of Dutch children aged 4–18 years (Verhulst *et al.* 1996). Very similar to the sex and age trends in a US general population sample (Achenbach 1991a), parents reported more fears for girls than for boys in middle school years and during adolescence, and a general decline in fears with increasing age. In contrast parents reported more worries for older than for younger children perhaps arising from increasing cognitive functions of the child. There were no sex differences in parent-reported worries.

Origins of anxiety

Anxiety, like pain, serves adaptation by its protective function. It not only protects the child from danger, but regulates social bonds, and, like pain, improves the chances of survival.

Some children seem more fearful than others. To some extent this variability in level of fearfulness is under genetic control. A number of fear stimuli (some animals, the dark, strangers) are thought to be innate, but experiences are also responsible for acquiring, increasing, or reducing fear reactions. A number of theories exist that try to explain the mechanisms through which anxiety is activated.

Fears of animals, situations, or places

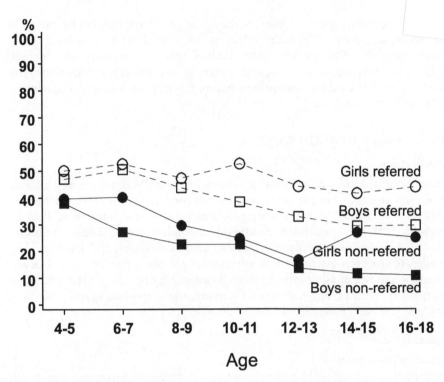

Fig. 4.2. Percentage of children aged 4–18 from the general population whose parents reported specific fears (Verhulst *et al.* 1996).

Psychoanalytic theory regards anxiety as a reaction of the ego to internal danger. This internal danger originates from (unconscious) wishes that are prohibited. As soon as the danger is recognized, the ego reacts by activating defence mechanisms. For example, a girl who has visited the doctor may, on returning home, start to play aggressively with her doll. By 'identification with the aggressor' the child tries to master her internal anxiety provoked by the physician's actions. Or, a boy who is angry with a newborn brother or sister may 'displace' his anger towards another person, or starts acting in an overfriendly way to disguise his anger. The child's hostile wishes cause anxiety which, in turn, set these defence mechanisms in action. Although psychoanalytic theory is helpful in understanding some internal mechanisms underlying the child's behaviour, its claims are not empirically tested, but may sometimes be helpful in explaining why a child is anxious.

Learning theorists regard anxiety as the result of conditioning. Certain stimuli are connected with anxiety, and avoidance of the feared object or situation reduces anxiety. By conditioning, fears can be both created and abolished.

Although the conditioning paradigm is certainly helpful for understanding and reducing some phobic behaviours, it does not explain all instances of fear acquisition.

Cognitive theory regards anxiety as the result of the recognition by the child of a discrepant event. When the infant is confronted with something unanticipated or unfamiliar, anxiety is the result. Cognitive therapists have focused on the misinterpretation of certain non-threatening events as fear provoking, and aim to correct these misinterpretations. Again, this approach to understanding is helpful in some situations.

4.4.2 ANXIETY DISORDERS

Classification

A number of anxieties arise in most, otherwise normally functioning, children. When such anxieties are excessive, and do not form part of a more generalized disorder, it is helpful to make a diagnosis using one of a number of ICD-10 categories that are specific to childhood and adolescence. These categories include separation anxiety disorder, phobic anxiety disorder, and social anxiety disorder. If anxieties in children or adolescents are not a part of normal development, a number of adult-type anxiety disorders may be categorized, including agoraphobia (with or without panic disorder), social phobia, specific phobias, panic disorder, and generalized anxiety disorder.

Clinical features

Pre-school (0–5 years)
It is normal for young children to show fears. If excessive, anxiety symptoms in young children can be categorized under the ICD categories that are specific to childhood. However, parents may also seek professional help for their child's anxiety, even if the symptoms are not so severe as to warrant a clinical diagnosis. These relatively mild conditions for which parents may seek help are:

- *Generalized anxiety and fearfulness.* Pre-school children with undue general fearfulness and anxiety will often show problems in even brief separation from their parents, especially their mothers. They will tend to follow their mothers around and scream if separated, even if this is for a short time and with a relatively familiar person. They are often generally miserable, whining children, who cry easily. Their general irritability and tension results in a tendency to have frequent temper tantrums. Specific problems of management, such as separation difficulties at night, when going to sleep, are common. Attendance at playgroup is an unhappy experience—the children take days or weeks to settle down and may never do so and have to be removed. They tend to mix poorly with other children, and not to want to go to other people's houses.
- *Specific fears.* Specific fears are very common in the pre-school period. Indeed this is a time when they are most frequently experienced and are most intense. In the first 2 years of life, the child has a special tendency to develop fears of

stimuli discrepant with normal experience. Thus, strange noises or an unfamiliar object in the room may produce fear. Fear of some strangers may be more pronounced than with others. Occasionally a child may develop a fear of a completely familiar person such as his or her father. This could be for an obvious reason that may be serious (the child has been hurt by his father), or trivial (the father has started to grow a moustache), or unaccountable. By 3 years, fear of animals (spiders, dogs, mice) is very common, as is fear of the dark and of ghosts. The abnormality of the fear can only be judged by its severity and persistence, and the social disability produced. Most normal fears in children of this age last at most only a few weeks or months, and do not interfere with the child's life.

Middle childhood (5–12 years)

Middle childhood is the developmental period in which generalized anxiety disorder, separation anxiety disorder, or phobias may evolve.

Generalized anxiety disorder

Children with generalized anxiety disorder are 'worriers' who suffer from excessive and unrealistic worries about their competence, past performance, or about the future. A key feature is the presence of 'free-floating anxiety', anxiety which is generalized and persistent and not restricted to any particular environmental circumstances. The following four broad features characterize the clinical picture:

- *Worries* about competence, past performance, future misfortunes, or future events such as school exams or sporting competitions. These children show excessive self-consciousness and a strong need for reassurance.
- *Restlessness, nervousness, inability to relax*
- *Physical symptoms:* motor tension, sleep disturbance, and symptoms due to autonomic overactivity, including light-headedness, sweating, tachycardia, epigastric discomfort, dizziness, etc.
- *Difficulty concentrating*
- *Irritability*

For a psychiatric diagnosis to be applicable, the symptoms should have been present most days for at least several weeks at a time. There are no specific laboratory or psychological tests as aids in making the diagosis. Interviews with the parents and with the child are usually sufficient sources of information to obtain a comprehensive picture of the anxiety symptoms.

Separation anxiety disorder

Distress and clinging behaviour may be appropriate and adaptive responses in young children when they are separated from their parents. However, when the child's anxiety over real or anticipated separation from people to whom the child is attached is of unusual severity for the child's age, and is associated with significant problems in the child's everyday functioning, separation anxiety disorder should be considered as a diagnosis. The anxiety symptoms are related to separation from people to whom the child is attached, and include:

- unrealistic worry about possible harm befalling people to whom the child is attached or fear that they will leave and not return
- unrealistic worry that some untoward event will separate him or her from those to whom the child is attached
- persistent reluctance or refusal to go to school because of fear about separation
- persistent reluctance or refusal to go to sleep separately from someone to whom the child is attached
- persistent inappropriate fear of being alone
- repeated nightmares about separation
- repeated occurrence of physical (anxiety) symptoms on occasions that involve separation
- excessive, recurrent distress (anxiety, crying, tantrums, apathy, withdrawal) in anticipation of, during, or immediately following separation.

The onset of separation anxiety disorder occurs before adolescence, although the disorder may continue into adolescence and even into early adulthood.

Specific phobias

Apart from school refusal (Section 4.4.3), handicapping specific fearfulness is somewhat unusual in middle childhood. Most common are fears connected with sleep. Children may be unwilling to enter their bedrooms by themselves or be too frightened to stay in bed. Lying in bed alone, the child may experience fears of abandonment by his parents or fears of burglars, ghosts, etc. An open window with a flapping curtain, or a creaky staircase, may enhance fearfulness. Fear will often lead the child to refuse to go to bed or stay in bed alone. As children with such fears are often taken into the parental bedroom or allowed to watch TV until well past their bedtime, the child is likely to come to perceive advantages in fearfulness, and this may lead to manipulative behaviour—the child insisting on privileges and claiming fear when none is present. Manipulative behaviour and fearfulness are often commingled. Other specific fears in this age group have usually arisen at a younger age. They include fear of dogs, other animals, and thunderstorms.

When a specific fear results in avoidance behaviour, and interferes with normal daily functioning, a diagnosis of specific phobia may be warranted. The phobic stimulus may involve certain objects, activities, situations, or persons. Examples of phobic stimuli are animals, heights, thunder, darkness, flying, dentistry, closed spaces, and open spaces (agoraphobia). Confrontation with the phobic stimulus results in a strong anxiety reaction and in avoidance of the situation, object, or person. The anxiety is indistinguishable from anxiety in other types of disorders. Parents find that telling their child that they do not regard the phobic stimulus as dangerous does not relieve the child from his or her anxiety. Children with phobias may develop anticipatory anxiety for the phobic situation.

Adolescence (12+ years)
A number of anxiety symptoms in adolescents may occur that may be severe enough to warrant professional attention.

- *Free-floating anxiety:* a sense of mental unease exists without attachment to any particular object, person, or situation. This is likely to be accompanied by a sense *of depersonalization* (a sensation of uncertainty about personal identity and bodily integrity) and *derealization* (a more or less acute sense of unreality).
- *Existential anxiety:* as well as an acute sense of depersonalization, a teenager may show anxious feelings related to an unusual concern for the reality of his own personal existence, his capacity to make real choices, and about the meaning of life.
- *Hypochondriasis:* headaches and stomach-aches with no organic basis are, at this age, likely to be replaced by a more adult form of hypochondriasis, with unusual concern over bodily health. Minor complaints are likely to lead to unnecessarily prolonged absence from school, college, or work. There may also be worries about personal appearance. Girls may be chronically anxious, for example, about the size of their breasts and buttocks. Exaggerated concern over bodily appearance in girls may also be more specifically linked to partial or full anorectic syndromes. Anxious boys may be unduly worried about their height, their acne, or the size or shape of their genitalia.

Further, a number of adult type anxiety disorders, such as social phobia and panic disorder, have their onset in adolescence.

Social phobia
Social phobia is present when adolescents have excessive anxieties concerning the possibility that they might do something or act in a way that will be humiliating or embarrassing. Commonly identified stressful situations include speaking, eating, and writing in public, going to parties, and speaking to authority figures. When confronted with the phobic situation, the adolescent will experience anxiety symptoms such as physical complaints (heart palpitations, shaking, flushing, sweating), and depersonalization and derealization. Adolescents may try to cope with anxiety by positive strategies such as cognitive coping strategies (such as telling themselves that there is no need to be nervous and that everything will be all right), or negative strategies such as refusing invitations or other forms of avoidance. The adolescent may feel embarrassed about the symptoms, and especially when the adolescent's coping strategies are rather subtle the problem may remain unnoticed by other people. Sometimes the avoidance is extreme and may result in almost complete social isolation. Socially phobic adolescents often

show negative thoughts about their performance and they have thoughts that others will negatively evaluate their social behaviour.

Panic disorder

Panic disorder is present when there are recurrent attacks of severe anxiety which are not restricted to any particular situation. These have a rapid onset and are unpredictable. A key feature is that the panic attack occurs out of the blue, with the typical physical anxiety symptoms often accompanied by a fear of dying, losing control, or going mad.

The existence of panic disorder in adolescents is well established. It is not clear, however, whether spontaneous panic attacks occur in prepubertal children. Adults with panic disorder often report anxiety symptoms in childhood, but it is not clear whether these patients really had panic disorder or other conditions such as separation anxiety disorder or specific phobias.

Prevalence

There are six relatively large scale community surveys with adequate sampling and assessment methodologies that provide prevalence rates for anxiety disorders (see Verhulst, in press).

In the majority of prevalence studies, the anxiety disorders were the most prevalent among all disorders. Few studies reported prevalences for the full spectrum of anxiety disorders. Most studies reported prevalences for separation anxiety disorder, overanxious disorder, specific phobia and social phobia. Differences between the studies mean that precise estimates of prevalence cannot be provided. An attempt to give rough estimates for disorders on which most studies reported, give the following results:

separation anxiety disorder   3%
overanxious disorder   3%
generalized anxiety disorder 2%
specific phobia   3%
social phobia   1%.

Few studies have examined the prevalence of panic disorder in children or adolescents. Verhulst *et al.* (1997) and Whittaker *et al.* (1990) reported prevalences of panic disorder of less than 1%.

Girls have somewhat higher rates of anxiety disorders than boys, and adolescents a higher prevalence of social phobia and lower prevalence of separation anxiety disorder than younger children.

Not every child with an anxiety disorder was severely handicapped in his or her daily functioning. In the Dutch prevalence study, 10.5% suffered from some kind of anxiety disorder based on the child interview (Verhulst *et al.* 1997). However, this prevalence figure dropped to 3.8% when only those individuals were counted who in addition to meeting the criteria for an anxiety disorder also showed probable general malfunctioning, and to 2.2% when only those were included who showed definite malfunctioning.

Background factors
- *Genetic and constitutional factors.* Anxiety runs in families, but from earlier family studies it is unclear whether the familial occurrence of anxiety is due to genetic factors or to upbringing. There are few studies on the genetic contribution to anxiety disorders in children. One twin study assessed the genetic and environmental influences on anxiety, and reported a significant genetic contribution for manifest anxiety, and overanxious disorder (which is very similar to generalized anxiety disorder), but not for separation anxiety disorder (Topolski *et al.* 1997). At this moment we know that genetic influences probably play a causative role in anxiety manifestations, but environmental influences are important contributors to the development of anxiety disorders too.
- *Temperament.* There are links between temperamental characteristics of children in the first years in life and later anxiety disorders. Children who are behaviourally inhibited, or shy and withdrawn early in life, have a predisposition to develop anxiety disorders later in childhood.
- *Parental behaviour.* Parental behaviour such as overprotection (often due to the parents' own anxieties such as separation anxiety), parental criticism, and punitiveness may be associated with anxiety in their children. Specific fears may be transmitted from parent to child.
- *Specific experiences and life events.* Excessive fears are sometimes triggered by unusually frightening events. A boy's fear of thunderstorms may begin after a severe storm when he thought his parents were not in the house. Most specific fears do not, however, seem to have their origin in such an event.
- *Cognitive appraisal of stressful events.* This is an important aspect in the emergence of anxiety disorders. Stressful or traumatic experiences, such as abuse, can lead to dysfunctional thoughts in some children who repetitively construe events as harmful or dangerous.
- *Social adversity.* Parents who are settled in their lives, without serious financial, housing, or marital difficulties, are more likely to be able to show sensitivity to their children's worries and anxieties, and thus help overcome them. Children living in homes where parents are pressurized by adversity are more likely to experience insecurity, and thus be predisposed to specific fears and anxiety.

Causative mechanisms
- *Biological and developmental.* Fear is an adaptive phenomenon. The experience of fear in the presence of danger encourages behaviour designed to achieve safety, especially proximity to protective figures. Young children, living as they do in a state of greater vulnerability and need for protection, naturally show a marked tendency to fearfulness. This gradually reduces with age. In some individuals, excessive or prolonged anxiety reactions can be seen as an overdevelopment of an adaptive mechanism.
- *Learning theory.* Children learn avoidance behaviour as a result of escaping from dangerous situations. The escape is associated with relief from the

unpleasant sensation of anxiety. Avoidance is thus reinforced or rewarded and is more likely to recur.

• *Psychodynamic theory.* Unacceptable aggressive or sexual impulses may be repressed so that the child is unaware of them. However, the focus of aggression may remain a stimulus for fear reactions, and the stimulus may become overgeneralized. Thus a boy with repressed aggression towards his father may show excessive fear not only of his father but also of other authority figures.

Assessment

Information on anxiety symptoms should be obtained from parents and child. Younger children have difficulty verbalizing their symptoms, and indicating the duration and frequency of their symptoms. Adolescents' self-reports are needed to reveal the internal and private symptoms of anxiety that may remain hidden from parents.

Information should be obtained on the duration of anxiety and fear reactions, and the degree to which they disable the child socially. It is important to establish the situations in which the anxiety is experienced, and the coping mechanisms the child uses to deal with the emotion when it occurs. The experience of anxiety reactions by other family members, especially the parents, is usually of considerable significance. Possible anxiety-provoking stresses both at home and school should be probed, even if they are not mentioned spontaneously.

Treatment

Generalized anxiety disorder

Although medication may produce some relief in case of severe anxiety in children and adolescents, the primary treatment modalities for generalized anxiety disorder are psychotherapeutic. The aims of treatment should be to reduce or remove unnecessary stresses producing anxiety, to help the child and family to understand more clearly the nature and function of experienced anxiety, and to enhance existing coping mechanisms.

• *Stress reduction and removal.* Where the child is responding to inevitable, ordinary stresses, it will not be appropriate or possible to remove them, but in some cases the child is in fact reacting to unnecessary stress. A child with a physical disorder may be fearful as a result of an unrealistic view of the likely outcome of his condition. A child fearful of sleeping alone can be moved temporarily into another bedroom shared with a sib. A child frightened that his mother is going to carry out a threat to leave home may be given reassurance.

• *Improvement in understanding the nature of anxiety.* Brief, focused counselling sessions with the family may enable insight to be gained into the way anxieties are transmitted from one family member to another. Alternatively, family members may be helped to see how tensions in the family are resulting in a child experiencing chronic insecurity.

• *A brief course of focused individual psychotherapy* (Section 9.2.2) may, with children over the age of about 8 years, enable insight to be gained into the way hitherto unexplained anxieties have arisen as a result of unacceptable impulses. In both family and individual sessions, a simple explanation of the way anxiety produces physical symptoms can be helpful.

- *Enhancing coping mechanisms.* The child is probably already using partially effective coping techniques to deal with the experience of anxiety. Encouraging the child to avoid unnecessary stresses, but to deal more effectively with necessary stress can be helpful. Relaxation techniques are sometimes useful in children over the age of about 10 years, as can the use of cognitive behavioural techniques (Ronan 1998) . Medication is not usually effective in dealing with anxiety states in childhood, and is only slightly more helpful in adolescence. In severe, generalized anxiety states, a minor anxiolytic agent such as diazepam may produce some symptomatic relief. The use of such medication should be limited to 2–3 weeks.

Separation anxiety disorder

Brief, focused counselling should be given to explain symptoms, course, and treatment possibilities. Behavioural treatment, including techniques such as systematic desensitization, exposure, and response prevention should be started. The approach is essentially the same as the one described for the treatment of school refusal (Section 4.4.3). A plan should be implemented for separation from mother. If necessary, family interventions can be used to support the child's autonomy, and to modify family functioning. Some authors advocate the use of tricyclic antidepressants, although the results of controlled clinical trials are inconsistent.

Other specific phobias

Behavioural methods should be employed in these conditions. Desensitization of *in vivo* type (Section 9.2.1) is usually effective. The child is encouraged to produce a hierarchy of feared situations, and then achieve relaxation, first with the least anxiety-provoking and then, when this has been achieved, with more severely anxiety-provoking situations. Operant methods can be used to reinforce or reward behaviour that retains the child in gradually increased contact with the feared situation. Alternatively, or in addition, the child can be encouraged to practice relaxation while imagining the feared situation or facing it in real life. If the feared situation is social, then it is often useful to get the child or adolescent to practise beforehand with parents or a friend how he is going to cope when the real situation occurs. Such role rehearsal can be useful, for example, when a child is frightened to go into a shop to make a purchase. A child may also be helped by a 'modelling' procedure—watching an adult or another child go through, in a relaxed way, an experience of which he is afraid.

Panic disorder

Although tricyclic antidepressants, benzodiazepines, and monoamine oxidase inhibitors are used in adults, no controlled trials of these medications have been carried out on children and adolescents with panic disorder. Case studies suggest that tricyclic antidepressants and benzodiazepines may be effective (Biederman 1987; Allen *et al.* 1995*b*).

Social phobia
Treatment involves the use of behavioural methods. Group psychotherapy and family interventions may also be indicated.

Outcome

In general, children with anxiety disorders have a reasonably good prognosis, although some may have remissions and exacerbations throughout childhood and adolescence, and even into adulthood. There are indications that children with separation anxiety disorder may show panic disorder or agoraphobia later in life.

4.4.3 SCHOOL REFUSAL

Definition

In school refusal an irrational fear of school attendance is the core symptom. Fear may be based partly or fully on fear of separation from home or from one or both parents (Bowlby 1975). It may, however, also be specific to school attendance or some aspect of it, in which case school phobia is an appropriate term to use. The condition is distinct from truancy in which children conceal their absence from school.

Clinical features

The problem usually shows itself first at a time of change of school or after a period of absence for some other reason, such as a minor illness. The onset may be acute, but is more often gradual with absences building up over a few weeks. Unwillingness to go to school may be expressed openly—the child, for example, saying that he dislikes a particular teacher who has been unpleasant to him, or that he has been bullied at school. Alternatively, the refusal may present with physical symptoms of tension and anxiety, more or less obviously linked to school attendance. Abdominal pain, headache, nausea, limb pains, attacks of palpitations, and a range of more unusual symptoms may be present (Hersov 1960). On questioning, it becomes clear that the symptoms are either absent at weekends or during school holidays, or present only in mild form at these times. The child may be able to go out in the evenings to play with his friends.

- *Previous personality.* The previous personality of the child is variable. Most have been rather 'good', quiet, conforming children who have never been in any trouble at school and are keeping up well with their work. A proportion, however, have been previously outgoing with many friends, and some have been having difficulties with their school work.
- *Family background.* There is characteristically a rather anxious and perhaps depressed mother who has, for some years, had an overly close relationship with the child in question (Skynner 1974). The child may be special because of being the last of a sibship (the 'Benjamin' syndrome) or for some other reason, such as a very premature birth. The father may be absent through

death or separation, or he may be a somewhat passive person who has difficulty in establishing his presence.

School factors

Although these have received little systematic examination, there may indeed be a stress at school which many of the children in the class are finding problematic—such as a very unsympathetic teacher. Alternatively, the school system may be rather lax in checking up on absences from school or there may be an overconcern regarding minor somatic illness amongst the school staff. Much more commonly, the teachers are aware of the irrational reasons for absence and have made sensible but unsuccessful attempts to get the child back to school.

- *Prevalence.* The condition is not a common one, occurring in less than 1% in the community (Last and Francis 1988). Severe school refusal occurs in less than 1 per 1000 children aged 10–11 years, although it is more common in 14 year olds (Rutter *et al.* 1976). Minor forms of school refusal with anxious reluctance to go to school for a few days, or chronic anxiety in a form that never actually causes the child to miss school, are much more common.
- *Age and sex.* The peak ages for occurrence are at the time of school transition, but there is also a peak in adolescence, so that 5 years, 11 years, and 14–15 years are the most common ages for presentation. There is no particular social class trend, and boys and girls are affected about equally.

Assessment

If the presentation involves a physical symptom, any necessary investigations should be rapidly carried out to exclude the presence of a physical condition. Usually the absence of physical pathology is fairly obvious, but just occasionally this may not be so. School refusal has been called the 'masquerade syndrome' (Waller and Eisenberg 1980) because its presentation may mimic so many other conditions. These include chronic viral infections, gastroenteritis, peptic ulcer, migraine, and cerebral tumour. In the remainder of this section it is assumed that these and other conditions have been excluded. It should be pointed out that school refusal for reasons of anxiety may coexist with any of these physical conditions as well as others.

Once the nature of the problem has been established, it is useful for whoever is dealing with the problem—such as the family doctor, paediatrician, educational psychologist, or child psychiatrist—to see the whole family, including the father if he lives at home. The way in which the problem has arisen should be discussed, and particular attention should be given to the possibility of a special relationship between the child and the mother, and any difficulties the father may have in asserting himself in the family. The attitudes of the family towards the real nature of any physical symptoms should be explored—are they seen as due to a physical condition or to anxiety? The nature of aggressive feelings that the child and mother might have for each other because of their mutual dependency might be examined. The child should be seen, at least briefly, separately, so that anxieties and worries that cannot be expressed in front of the family can be explored. It is also often helpful to see the parents together briefly, in case there are aspects of their own relationship that might be relevant. Finally, it is important for any health professional dealing with the problem to contact those in the school system—teacher, educational welfare officer, educational psychologist— who have been involved, to get their view of the situation.

At this stage the practitioner should have a view of the extent and severity of the problem, and the degree to which school or family relationship factors are relevant. Most commonly the problem can best be viewed as a combination of a disturbance of family relationships, and anxious personality traits in the child, sometimes associated with specific stresses in school.

Differential diagnosis includes truancy, depressive disorder in the child, an unusual and difficult-to-diagnose physical condition such as peptic ulcer (that may or may not itself be linked to stress or anxiety), and a stressful but well covered up situation in school, such as severe bullying, which might make any child reluctant to attend.

Truants, unlike school refusers, disguise their absence from school, are usually involved in other forms of antisocial behaviour, generally come from more disrupted families, and are often failing in school subjects. In older children, however, the distinction between truancy and school refusal is sometimes not easy to make.

Management

Return to school

In mild cases and those of recent onset, or where physical symptoms have been present for some time, but it has only recently been clarified that there is no physical condition present, the main aim of treatment should be to get the child back to ordinary school as soon as possible (Kennedy 1965; Blagg and Yule 1984). The practitioner should explain to the family how the problem is viewed, usually with emphasis on how this is not just the child's problem, but that of the whole family. The father may need to be encouraged to be firm with the child about school attendance and other matters. It is often helpful to sympathize with the mother concerning her feelings of being separated from her child while he is in school. The school should be contacted and a day agreed when a planned return is to be made. The assistance of the educational welfare officer may be invaluable. Indeed, most cases of school refusal are dealt with by educational psychologists and school welfare officers without any health professionals being involved at all. Some minor concessions may need to be made concerning attendance at assembly or PE classes. The use of short-acting anxiolytic medication on the morning of return may occasionally be justified. Using this approach a high proportion of mild cases and severe, but acute recently diagnosed cases will be resolved.

Chronic school refusal

Long-standing problems are not likely to recover so quickly. Referral to child psychiatric services is often indicated. The child may, for many months, have been enjoying a relaxed time at home with his mother during school hours, and it is not surprising that the prospect of a noisy school day produces overwhelming anxiety. The child may have a more deep-seated intrapsychic problem, or family relationships may have become seriously disturbed with little prospect of change. In some cases, parents develop an overvalued idea, almost amounting to a delusion, that their child has a physical problem making it impossible for him to go to school. It is especially important in these circumstances that there is good communication between health, education, and social services staff.

A variety of psychiatric and educational measures may be helpful in chronic school refusal. Some educational authorities run small units for disturbed children that can be attended first full-time, and then part-time while the child is integrated back into ordinary school. Pressure by parents to arrange home tuition should in general be resisted, as this merely results in the child being even more embedded in his home situation. Educational measures can be supplemented with individual psychotherapy for the child or a series of family interviews. Behavioural management, with techniques such as relaxation, and imaginal and *in vivo* desensitization can also be helpful.

In more intractable severe cases residential placement may be indicated, in a child psychiatry in-patient unit, in a residential school for children with emotional and behaviour problems, or in a boarding school taking a proportion of disturbed children. The admission needs to be carefully planned, but, if confidently handled, it can nearly always be successfully arranged. Once away from home, separation anxieties are often, at least temporarily, abated. A proportion of school-refusing children admitted to in-patient units will require long-term residential placement in schools for children with emotional and behaviour disorders.

Outcome

Most mild and acute cases resolve rapidly without further problem. More severe cases, especially those occurring in older children with widespread personality problems, do not have such a good outcome (I. Berg 1970). A proportion, about a third, go on to have significant psychiatric disorders of neurotic type in adulthood. Occasionally, school refusal develops into work refusal at school-leaving age, with features of the so-called 'inadequate personality' present (Berg *et al.* 1976). In women, school phobia may emerge into agoraphobia or fear of leaving home. A significant proportion of women with agoraphobia give a history of school refusal in their childhood. Nevertheless, most such children, even with severe school refusal, grow into healthy adults without serious mental health problems.

4.4.4 DEVELOPMENT OF DEPRESSIVE FEELINGS, BEHAVIOUR, AND BELIEFS

The concept of depression embraces a number of different components. They include depressive feelings, depressive behaviour, depressive cognitions or beliefs, as well as depressive disorders. Although both in normal development and in psychiatric disorders these are often linked together, they require separate description.

Depressive feelings

It is only by about the age of 6 years that children begin to use the language of emotional affect in adult fashion, referring, for example, to themselves and others as 'sad' or 'miserable'. It is reasonable to infer that younger children are experiencing such emotions when they look unhappy, but the knowledge of normal depressive feelings in very young children is limited because of lack of introspective information. By 10 years of age, 11% of boys and 13% of girls living on the Isle of Wight were reported by their parents to 'often appear miserable, unhappy, tearful, or distressed', and teachers of these children reported only slightly lower proportions to be affected in this way (Rutter *et al*. 1970*a*). In the same population, by 14 years of age, 21% of boys and 23% of girls reported themselves as often feeling miserable or depressed on a questionnaire, but nearly twice this proportion reported feelings of misery at a psychiatric interview (Rutter *et al*. 1976*b*).

Depressive behaviour

Characteristic depressive behaviour includes both non-verbal elements, especially crying and a sad facial expression, and verbal elements—usually expression of feelings of despair, hopelessness, and various depressive beliefs (see below). Not all crying is, however, a sign of depression.

Newborn babies cry in the first moments after birth, and subsequently crying from distress is frequent throughout the early years of life. The quality of cry varies according to its cause. Thus a sensitive mother can distinguish between the cries of hunger, pain, and discomfort, and indeed these three different types of cry can be distinguished electrographically. Normal infants may behave in a sad manner from the age of a few months, especially when they are separated from their mothers or other care-givers. Such separation may be physical or psychological, as when, for example, the mother is depressed and less sensitive to the needs of her young child. On these occasions the infant or toddler may become temporarily apathetic, refuse food, and generally lack vivacity and energy. Crying from pain and physical distress diminishes rapidly after the pre-school period.

Normal crying associated with mental distress persists, though to a diminished extent, throughout childhood and adolescence. Sadness may be present when a child temporarily goes quiet, does not want to play with his friends, or develops irritability in mildly frustrating situations that would normally be shrugged off.

Self-destructive threats and behaviour appear with increasing frequency throughout late childhood and adolescence. An American study found that 33% of 12 and 13 year olds had at least occasional thoughts of harming themselves, and 8% of Isle of Wight 14 year olds had had definite suicidal ideas over the previous year (Rutter *et al*. 1976).

Depressive cognitive beliefs

Unrealistically negative beliefs about oneself, one's future, and the world in general are a prominent feature of depressive disorders (Beck 1967). Transient thoughts of this nature appear normally during childhood. By the age of 7 or 8 years children can experience a devalued view of themselves as worthless, and not worth bothering about. By early puberty they can have views that their future holds little for them, and by mid-puberty that the world around them is rotten. In children with depressive disorders, such beliefs are held intensely and persistently.

Reaction to bereavement

Studies of children who have lost a parent by death reveal that characteristic reactions occur (Raphael 1975; van Eerdewegh *et al.* 1985). A relatively prolonged period of sadness, crying, and irritability lasting from a few days to several months may occur throughout childhood. Younger children are particularly likely to show bed-wetting and temper tantrums, and older children, especially girls, may show sleep disturbance and more clear-cut depressive reactions. School performance is often impaired, at least temporarily. Most children are not severely affected, and studies do not suggest that major psychopathology is at all common following early bereavement.

Reaction to bereavement is likely to be modified by the level of social support available to the family and the social and financial changes resulting from the death. The reaction of the surviving parent will be of major significance. The previous personality of the child and the coping mechanisms he employs will be relevant. A minority of young children blame themselves or the surviving parent for the parental death, but usually (though not always) communication within the family is sufficient to reduce the guilt and anger so produced. There is evidence that brief family interventions can improve the outcome in the bereaved child (Black and Urbanowicz 1987). There is a tendency for adults who have suffered bereavement in childhood to show slightly higher rates of psychiatric disorder, but the findings are somewhat inconsistent and, in particular, it is not clear whether the child's age at the time of parental death is of particular significance.

4.4.5 DEPRESSIVE DISORDERS

Definition and classification

Depressive disorders are conditions in which persistent lowering of mood (dysphoria) and lack of a sense of pleasure in life (anhedonia) are prominent and persistent features. The DSM-IV classification divides depressive disorders into major depression (which may have single or recurrent depressive episodes) and dysthymia. A depressive episode is made up of at least five out of nine symptoms of which either depressed mood or diminished interest or pleasure in everyday activities must be present. Others include significant weight loss or gain, insomnia, agitation or retardation, poor concentration, feelings of worthlessness, and recurrent thoughts of death. Dysthymia which, in children, must have been present for at least 1 year, involves depressed mood and two out of five symptoms including poor appetite, insomnia, low energy, low self-esteem, poor concentration, and feelings of hopelessness. The ICD-10 classification (see p. 19) makes similar distinctions, categorizing depressive symptoms into depressive episodes, recurrent depressive disorder, and dysthymia. Depressive psychoses and bipolar affective disorders are discussed in Section 5.6.3.

The meaning of depression

The classification systems described above reduce the meaning of the term 'depression' to a set of reasonably clearly defined symptoms. Although this is useful for research purposes, 'depression' has a set of wider and richer clinical meanings than the classifications suggest. The term can be used (Nurcombe *et al.* 1989) to describe

- an *affect or mood* ('I have felt really depressed over the last month')
- a *dynamic* ('He was depressed by the loss of his father')
- a *syndrome* (a cluster of behaviours and feelings demonstrably related to each other statistically)
- a *disorder* (a handicapping condition with a characteristic aetiology and course)
- a *disease* (a disorder arising from scientifically defined pathophysiological processes leading to rational treatment).

Too little is known about depression to think of it as a disease. The classifications aim to describe a set of depressive disorders but, in fact, there is little evidence that, in childhood, these different subtypes of disorder can be clearly defined from each other. It is likely that in childhood so-called 'dysthymia' merges imperceptibly into ordinary sadness and misery. In adolescents and very occasionally in younger children, dysthymia merges also, in its more severe form, into depressive syndromes more characteristic of adult-type depressive disorders of 'nuclear' type.

An important feature of depressive disorders in childhood and adolescence is the frequency of co-morbid disorders. In one study, over 90% of 8–16 year olds attending a clinic with a depressive disorder showed at least one additional disorder (Goodyer *et al.* 1997a).

Clinical features

Pre-school children

Although it is difficult or impossible to apply some of the features (such as low self-esteem, hopelessness, and recurrent thoughts of death) to classify depression in this age group, there is no doubt that babies, toddlers, and other pre-school children can appear depressed over a significant period of time and that it is meaningful to think of their psychological problems in these terms. Characteristically, when depressed, infants and toddlers are apathetic and refuse food. They are miserable, unhappy, and irritable, and may spend a good deal of their time crying and rocking. Such children are often referred to paediatricians because of failure to thrive. Growth failure is often accompanied by non-specific diarrhoea. On examination, no physical abnormality is found to account for the symptoms, but the child is fretful, insecure, and unhappy. There is often evidence of mild developmental retardation. The picture may occur as a result of gross and obvious neglect, or there may be more subtle reasons why the child is so disturbed.

Middle childhood

Depressive states at this age are often poorly differentiated from emotional disorders in which both anxiety and depressive features are prominent. It is unusual for children to be brought to the practitioner with depression of mood as the presenting feature. More commonly the depressed child presents with psychosomatic symptoms, especially headache or stomach-ache. Failure to make progress in school, with poor concentration and inattention, is also a common mode of presentation. Irritability, social withdrawal, and incapacity to cope with even minor frustration without a temper outburst may occur, but sleep and appetite disturbances are less common. Very occasionally, however, prepubertal children present with more classical features of depressive disorder—apathy, verbal and motor retardation, and loss of appetite. Feelings of low self-esteem can often be elicited by asking questions whether the child feels as good or worth as much as other children, or whether he thinks his parents like him as much as his sibs. Although deliberate suicide is extremely rare in this age group and even suicidal attempts are most unusual, depressed children do often wish they were dead and express this desire in response to questioning.

Children of this age may not admit to feelings of depression readily. They are more likely to complain of being 'bored' and of lack of interest in usual activities. Normal children tend to complain of boredom only in circumstances when they have nothing of interest to do, whereas depressed children are likely to say they feel bored most of the time. The depressed child nearly always looks miserable and unhappy and appears to lack vitality and energy.

As indicated above, attempts to distinguish major depressive disorder from dysthymia, and dysthymia from normal sadness and misery, although they may be necessary for administrative and research purposes, are not usually very helpful clinically in the preadolescent.

Adolescence

Depressive states in adolescence are more similar to those seen in adulthood. The teenager will often complain of feeling sad and apathetic, as well as lacking energy. Appetite and sleep disturbances are more common. There may be impairment of food intake, or the child may overeat to comfort himself. Difficulty in getting off to sleep at night and waking during the night may leave the teenager exhausted during the day. Bodily preoccupations are common, and the child may be taken up by worries over his appearance or symptoms of minor ill-health such as acne. A sense of futility and hopelessness may be experienced. Suicidal thoughts are relatively common, although suicide threats are much less usual.

Prevalence

The prevalence of depression in the pre-school period is uncertain, largely because of a lack of agreed criteria appropriate for this age group. In the preadolescent, although as many as 10–15% of children show depressed mood (Rutter *et al.* 1970*a*), only about 2% are diagnosable as depressed using DSM-III criteria. There is a sharp rise in the rate of depressive disorders in adolescence (Rutter *et al.* 1976). The prevalence of major depressive disorder in school populations of 11–16 year olds has been found to be a little above 3% for both diagnoses (Cooper and Goodyer 1993; Garrison *et al.* 1997).

There is little difference between preadolescent boys and girls in the rate of depressed mood and depressive disorder, but in adolescence depressed girls outnumber boys by about 2 to 1. The reasons for this may lie in hormonal or psychological differences. It has been found, for example, that the sexes are similar in their levels of perceived self-competence in preadolescence, but diverge during and after puberty. Low self-esteem may then act as a mediating variable, differentiating the sexes in their pre-disposition to depression (see below). Similar mechanisms may be responsible for the fact that depressive symptoms have been found to be more common in US population studies in young adolescents from minority race, of low socio-economic status, and with low school grades (Garrison *et al.* 1997).

Aetiology

Causes of depression can be divided into predisposing or vulnerability factors, and triggering or precipitating factors. A significant number of studies have been carried out in adults with depression to elucidate aetiological factors using this model (e.g. Brown and Harris 1978), but there are few relevant studies in childhood depression. Nevertheless, this is a growing area and more information is now available.

Predisposing factors

- *Genetic.* Most investigators (e.g. Strober and Carlson 1982) suggest depressive symptoms are raised in family members of seriously depressed children. The familial loading of depressed prepubertal children is higher than it is in adults (Neuman *et al.* 1997). The familial nature of depression leaves open whether the mechanism is genetic or environmental, and there are no clear-cut findings to elucidate this issue.
- *Temperament.* Studies suggest that quiet children with regular habits, slow to adapt to new experiences, are predisposed to emotional disorders if they become disturbed (Thomas *et al.* 1968). It is uncertain whether such factors also predispose specifically to depressive disorders.
- *Biological factors.* In adult depression there is some evidence that there are abnormalities of neurotransmitters, especially monoamine metabolism. There is also inconclusive evidence of cortisol hypersecretion. The evidence for neurotransmitter and endocrine abnormalities is weaker in children, but Goodyer *et al.* (1996) have found altered diurnal rhythms in cortisol levels in a group of depressed children and adolescents.

- *Chronic life adversity.* Babies and toddlers who are neglected and deprived of affection are at special risk for developing depressive states characterized by apathy and withdrawal. Older children with depressive conditions may also be living in circumstances where they are undervalued. The low valuation they place on themselves may be merely a reflection of the poor opinion held of them by members of their family, their teachers, and other children.

Depressed children are more likely to have mothers who have poor confiding relationships and high rates of distress themselves. They are more likely to come from broken homes. Parents rearing their children in conditions of serious social adversity, under financial pressure, poorly housed, or with marital problems, naturally find it difficult to provide sensitive, loving care for their children.

Various psychological mechanisms have been described, more especially in adults, to explain why these factors should predispose to depression. One helpful concept is that of *learned helplessness* (Seligman 1975): after several unsuccessful attempts have been made to escape from unpleasant circumstances, lack of motivation and apathy may supervene. A number of depressed children in what seem to them to be hopeless situations seem to fit this model well.

Triggering or provoking events
- *Undesirable life events* occur in excess in the 12 months before the onset of disorder (Goodyer *et al.* 1987). Although in depressed adults such life events are more likely to cause depression in predisposed individuals, the evidence for this in childhood is less certain. Nevertheless, it is probable that threats to a child's well-being that arise because of an event at home or at school will have a more powerful effect if the child is vulnerable because of his personality or because he has been sensitized by other previous adversities. It has been shown that child psychiatric attendees with depressed mood have more commonly previously sustained parental loss than disturbed children without such mood disturbance (Caplan and Douglas 1969). The onset of depression in children, as in adults, is commonly associated with the experience of loss, and a wide variety of experiences, often specific to the particular child affected, may be responsible.
- *Viral illnesses.* Lack of energy and mild depression of mood are common after febrile illnesses, especially measles and infectious mononucleosis. In a minority of children such postviral reactions are severe and may last weeks or months. It is uncertain whether these psychological reactions occur as a result of physiological or environmental factors. There is some evidence that, in adults, these reactions are accompanied by immunological changes, especially abnormalities of T-cell function (Hamblin *et al.* 1983).

Assessment

It is important to try to establish the nature and extent of depressive symptoms, and the degree of disability they are producing. Differential diagnosis of a depressive episode would involve exclusion of depressive psychosis, anorexia nervosa, a physical condition accompanied by mood change, and normal reactive feelings of sadness and unhappiness. Depressive symptoms may be present in a whole range of psychological disorders of childhood, and the diagnosis of a depressive condition should not rest merely on the presence of sadness of mood, but on the existence of a constellation of symptoms (the depressive syndrome) described above. The presence of *'masked depression'* (depression underlying other, usually physical symptoms) should be considered cautiously. With careful questioning, depressive symptomatology can be elicited from children and their parents if it is present and, in the absence of such symptomatology, the condition should probably not be diagnosed (Carlson and Cantwell 1980). An attempt should be made to identify the time of onset and events of possibly causative significance immediately preceding this point in time. Events involving a possible experience of loss are likely to be relevant, but physical factors, such as viral illness, should also be noted. A family interview may reveal the fact that the entire family is burdened by stress with the identified child acting for some reason as the only family member 'allowed' to experience distress. An interview with the child may elicit specific stressors, occurring for example at school, of which the parents may be unaware.

Treatment

Relief of stress

An attempt should be made to alleviate any stresses, such as family dysfunction and poor friendships, identified during the assessment procedure. Thus, the parents of a child depressed by a repeated failure in school can be encouraged to see if remedial help is available and to ensure that they and (if possible) the child's teachers, praise the child for even a very small improvement on previous performance. Such measures will often not prove sufficient on their own, but they are always worth taking, and there is good evidence to suggest that, if social adversity persists, the prognosis of a depressive disorder is significantly worse (Goodyer *et al.* 1997).

Improvement of communication

- The child may first be helped by individual counselling to become more aware of the factors responsible for depressed affect when this occurs. Some children, for example, become depressed whenever they are unable to express anger against those whom they feel are frustrating their wishes.
- Second, communication between family members can be improved in family interviews. The loss of a grandparent, for example, may have affected the whole family, but only the identified child may have shown prolonged symptoms. A family interview may clarify the degree to which all family members have suffered, thus allowing the identified child to share his burden of loss.

Cognitive behavioural methods

It has been pointed out that depressed individuals often have a distorted view of the way other people see them. Low self-esteem can be perpetuated if a child or adolescent misinterprets a remark as derogatory when, in fact, it was not intended to be so. Treatment of depression (Beck *et al.* 1979) can focus on encouraging patients to keep careful records of situations in which they feel their depressed view of themselves is confirmed. Using these techniques, in discussion of these situations with the therapist, a child may develop a more realistic view of the way he is seen by others. Cognitive behavioural methods have been found to have short term benefit in this condition, though longer term effects remain to be demonstrated (Harrington *et al.* 1998).

Other methods of enhancing the child's self-esteem may also be useful. A child who feels himself disfavoured by his parents in comparison to his sibs may well be misinterpreting their behaviour. Yet it can be helpful to suggest to parents that their depressed child has a (hopefully temporary) need for more affection and comfort than his sibs.

Physical methods of treatment
Medication should be reserved for the more seriously depressed child, as the risk of side-effects is likely to outweigh benefits in the mildly depressed. Further, even in the seriously depressed, a trial of psychological therapy should precede the use of medication. If psychological therapies fail, then antidepressants should be prescribed. Although a meta-analysis of controlled studies of the value of tri-cyclic antidepressants has failed to show benefit, they may still have a place in reducing co-morbid anxiety. More specifically effective are the selective sero-tonin reuptake inhibitors such as fluoxetin and fluvoxamine. Better evidence exists for their value (Emslie *et al.* 1997). Improvement should be expected within 10 days, and if this does not occur, the drug should be discontinued after 3 weeks. If effective, the drug should be stopped after about 2 months to determine if it is still effective. In mid- and late adolescence, electroconvulsive therapy should be considered for adolescents who have not responded to two adequate courses of antidepressant medication and remain severely depressed. The use of this form of treatment raises ethical issues, especially as there is inadequate evidence concerning possible medium-term adverse effects on cogni-tive function. However, in some circumstances, it may be life-saving (see p. 454).

Outcome

Most children (about two-thirds) with depressive disorders improve substantially following referral to a medical agency. This is probably because referrals are often precipitated by temporary crises and worsening of symptoms during the course of a fluctuating condition. The great majority of referred boys with major depression and dysthymia improve, though full recovery may not occur for several months or even years, and there is a considerably increased liability to further episodes of depression (Kovacs and Gatsonis 1989). The short-term outcome of major depression is strongly adversely affected by the severity of the original symptoms and by the presence of a co-morbid diagnosis of oppositional defiant disorder (Goodyer *et al.* 1997). There is also a substantially increased risk of adult depressive disorder in children and adolescents who have attended a psychiatric clinic with this disorder earlier in their lives (Harrington *et al.* 1990).

4.4.6 SUICIDE AND ATTEMPTED SUICIDE

Definition

Suicide involves a deliberate form of self-harm resulting in death. Attempted suicide is an act of self-injury, with a non-fatal outcome, that has some degree of suicidal motivation. Some who have completed suicide have not intended to do so, while others who have not died have genuinely wished to do so. Kreitman (1977) coined the term *parasuicide* to describe deliberate acts mimicking suicide, but not resulting in a fatal outcome. There are a number of risk-taking forms of behaviour that may have a self-destructive component.

Epidemiology

Suicide

The rate of completed suicide in the 10–14 year old age group in the UK is very low, at about 1 per million annually, and suicide in children under the age of 12 years is very rare indeed. In the 15–19 year age group, however, the rate is higher, at about 57 per million per year for males, and 14 per million for females in 1990 (McClure 1994). The rate of suicide in young males rose in the 1980s, but levelled out or declined subsequently. Rates vary considerably between different countries, but comparisons are made difficult by the different methods of recording deaths where the cause is undetermined.

Attempted suicide

Attempted suicide is a much more common phenomenon than complteted suicide. In the 10–14 year age group, it is less common, but in 15–19 year olds it occurs in about 500 per 100 000 per year, about 400 per 100 000 in males and over 600 per 100 000 in females. There is an excess in lower socio-economic groups. The rate of attempted suicide rose sharply in 15–24 year olds in the period 1985–1995 (Hawton *et al.* 1997).

Background features

Apart from the sex ratio, socio-economic status, and means of self-injury (see below), characteristics of those who commit suicide and those who deliberately harm but do not kill themselves are rather similar. These include:

- *Parental characteristics.* Parents often suffer from mental health problems especially depressive syndromes and personality disorders. Marital difficulties between the parents are often present.
- *Parental discipline.* This is likely to be inconsistent, but rigidly applied. Parents may be generally rather permissive, but then impose unreasonable restrictions.
- *Family communication patterns.* There is likely to be rather poor communication both of feelings and information within the family. Parents are often unaware of the suicidal ideas experienced by their teenage children (Monck and Graham 1988).

- *Social isolation of the child*. The child may be socially isolated and receive little social support from friends or family. Social support from friends may have been lost just before the suicide attempt. Some teenagers have run away from home before the attempt and are almost totally isolated.
- *Psychiatric state of the child or adolescent*. There is a high rate of depression (about 50%) among suicide attempters. Such depression is usually acute and reactive, but may be chronic. There may be a long history of disturbed behaviour including serious antisocial problems. In the older age group, drug and alcohol abuse are fairly commonly found.
- *Physical health*. Children with chronic physical ill health are particularly at risk for attempted suicide (Hawton 1982). In girls, the possibility of pregnancy should always be considered, especially as the discovery of pregnancy may have precipitated the attempt.
- *Contact with other suicide attempters*. There is a contagious component to attempted suicide. Youngsters engaging in this type of behaviour often have acquaintances or friends who have behaved similarly. Outbreaks of overdosing in schools have been described (Brent *et al.* 1988). This may explain why media programmes designed to reduce suicide in the young paradoxically appear to increase rather than diminish the phenomenon (Shaffer *et al.* 1988).

Characteristics of suicide attempts

- The great majority of those who attempt suicide do so by taking overdoses, usually of non-opiate analgesics such as paracetamol, but occasionally with psychotropic or other drugs. (Completed suicides involve a much wider range of methods with poisoning from vehicle exhaust fumes, hanging, shooting, and suffocation by other means as prominent causes.)
- The attempt itself may be only a trivial threat to the health of the child (swallowing half a dozen paracetamol tablets) or may require skilled intensive care in hospital over several days in order that the life of the child can be saved.
- Attempts are usually precipitated by crises in relationships, either with family or friends. A dispute over discipline is common, as is a row with a boyfriend or girlfriend. Bullying at school may have occurred.
- Attempts are often preceded by threats that have not been taken seriously. After the attempt, the teenager usually, but not always, communicates what he or she has done, often to the person towards whom most anger is directed.
- About half those who attempt suicide have attended a medical agency, usually the general practitioner, in the previous month. The visit is often connected in some way to the problem that leads to the attempt.

Assessment

This should be carried out as soon as possible after the suicidal attempt has been identified, and, if this has been necessary, the teenager has been successfully resuscitated. It should take place before the patient is discharged home. The involvement of a psychiatrist in the assessment is desirable, but not essential.

It is important, however, that it should be carried out by someone capable of assessing the risk of recurrence and the need for intervention on other grounds. For children under the age of 16 years it is preferable for assessment to be carried out on a paediatric ward. An appropriate form of assessment involves first an interview with the teenager, then an interview with the parent(s), and finally a family interview. Some professionals prefer to begin with a family interview.

Information of particular relevance that needs to be gathered includes:

- details of the attempt, number of tablets taken, was the attempt premeditated, was the patient alone, was anyone informed after the tablets were taken
- precipitating circumstances
- presence of emotional or behaviour problems in the months before the attempt
- quality of family relationships, especially in communication of feelings
- social network of the child
- previous involvement of helping agencies, general practitioner, social worker, etc.
- current suicidal intentions of the child
- present mental state of the child in other respects
- degree to which the attempt has altered the circumstances that precipitated it.

With this information available, the clinician should have a reasonably clear understanding of the reasons for the suicidal behaviour and of the action that needs to be taken. Where reasons for the attempt remain obscure, the possibility of sexual abuse should be considered. By the end of the assessment, the clinician should have information which enables the following questions to be addressed:

- Can the patient be allowed to go home?
- What is the risk of a subsequent attempt?
- What treatment is appropriate?

A useful mnemonic, PATHOS, is provided by Kingsbury (1996):

- Have you had Problems for longer than one month?
- Were you Alone in the house at the time?
- Did you plan the overdose for more than Three hours?
- Are you feeling HOpeless about the future?
- Were you feeling Sad for most of the time before the overdose?

It is suggested that those giving two or more positive answers are at high risk, and require psychiatric referral.

Treatment

The risk of recurrence is greater when the attempt has been seriously life-threatening, the child is depressed, the circumstances precipitating the event are unresolved, or the child's social supports remain poor. Follow-up is required if any of these conditions pertain, but otherwise this is a matter of clinical judgement. In particular, follow-up is less necessary if the attempt has been relatively trivial, and the precipitating circumstances appear to have been resolved.

The nature and intensity of treatment will depend on the circumstances and resources available. A small minority of attempters will be found to have obvious psychiatric disorders requiring admission to an inpatient unit. A further small number will require a few days' admission on the paediatric ward for observation. Most will be able to return home with follow-up appointments for treatment or to check on progress.

In cases where faulty communication has been responsible, family therapy sessions should be offered. Some teenagers will, however, benefit from individual counselling. Where school stresses have been significant, contact with the school should be made, together with an attempt to resolve the problems experienced there.

Outcome

A high proportion of suicidal attempters, in most studies around 25%, make a further attempt. Completed suicide also occurs, but the exact nature of the risk is not known. Boys and young men who are poor communicators, are living in circumstances of chronic stress, and are showing clinically significant evidence of depressive disorder are those at greatest risk for recurrence of further attempts, completed suicide, and other psychiatric disorders (Shaffer 1995).

4.5 Social development and antisocial behaviour

4.5.1 NORMAL SOCIAL DEVELOPMENT

Knowledge of normal social behaviour is helpful in understanding children and adolescents who show aggression and other forms of antisocial behaviour. Very early social development during infancy is described in Section 4.1.2.

As children move out of infancy, their social world extends beyond their immediate family. There are increased expectations for them to conform to social norms. Tantrums are no longer found amusing or even tolerated. They are expected to know the difference between what belongs to them and the property of others. Generosity and unselfishness become valued and rewarded.

The achievement of a reasonable degree of conformity requires the development of underlying skills and capacities. Where such development fails to occur, is slower than usual, or occurs in a deviant manner, one may expect socially difficult, antisocial behaviour to arise.

As children move into their third and fourth year, they gradually become more aware that other people have thoughts and feelings similar to their own. This leads to greater sympathy and empathy, and a greater wish to please others.

At the same time, they advance in their capacity to decide accurately when situations arise because of their own behaviour and when situations occur because of the behaviour of others. They make more accurate attributions. Some children have a tendency to blame others for events that occur (they are said to have an external locus of control), whereas others (with a more internal locus of control) tend to blame themselves.

The capacity to exert self-control in frustrating situations increases. Children gradually learn there are sometimes rewards for waiting and penalties for not waiting. If they cannot wait for a particular television programme to come on and insist on having the set switched on immediately, they learn they may finish up not watching the programme at all because they have been sent upstairs. Being able to delay gratification is an essential element in social development.

Emotional expression is also gradually brought under greater self-control. Temper tantrums become less frequent, as are prolonged bouts of crying. In frustrating situations, angry outbursts are replaced by the use of verbal rather than physical methods of persuasion.

These skills and capacities do not by any means always develop in a smooth, continuous fashion. An upset in the family or at nursery school may result in regression to an earlier phase. Nor do they develop in isolation. The style of parenting, for example, may promote or retard social development. Parents who notice when their children behave in a thoughtful way towards others and reward with praise will promote such behaviour more than where it goes unnoticed. There is also a range of normality. Some children will be more emotionally expressive than others. Some will have a greater tendency than most to blame others when things go wrong. These normal variations should not cause concern unless, over a period of time, they cause distress to others or to the child. If they do, however, they need to be taken seriously, for persistent transgression of social norms can result in serious social dysfunction and impairment.

When they are consulted about children who are disobedient and display other forms of difficult behaviour, family doctors, paediatricians, and mental health professionals are faced with controversial issues. First, should these forms of behaviour really be a concern of health professionals at all? Some, such as Goodman (1997a), think such problems should be left to parents, teachers and social workers, and dealt with as disciplinary, educational, or social in nature. Second, it is generally agreed that it is helpful to think of most psychiatric disorders as located within the child or patient. But is it reasonable to view antisocial behaviour in children in this way, when, especially in their early years, so much of their behaviour is reactive?

The section below on oppositional defiant behaviour deals mainly with children aged from about 2 to 8 or 9 years. It is suggested that, especially in the early years, this behaviour is best seen as arising from faulty interactions between the child and other family members. In the next section, the description of conduct disorders relates mainly to children and adolescents older than this. With neither of these disorders should it be assumed that a medical approach is the best one to take, but the fact is that health professionals are consulted about them, and need to have information enabling them to be helpful in these circumstances.

4.5.2 OPPOSITIONAL DEFIANT DISORDER (ODD)

Definition

A useful review of the whole field of behaviour problems in the early years is provided by Campbell (1995).

Clinical features

- *Control*. The child seems unusually intractable and difficult to manage. Foci of conflicts in the third and fourth year of life include bedtime and mealtimes. Food is refused and may be thrown around the room, and there are frequent temper tantrums. Frustration is poorly tolerated. The parents often say they cannot take the child out shopping because he shouts and screams when refused anything. Prolonged tantrums may occur several times a day. Later, in the early school years, conflict centres around getting ready for school, as well as behaviour at mealtimes and going to bed.
- *Aggression*. Once the child is able to speak, verbal aggression is almost invariably present. The child may also physically hit out, scratch or bite. Some children will physically attack their parents when frustrated but it is rare for them to hit other adults. Aggression towards parents is frequently triggered by conflicts over feeding, bedtime, or refusal of the parent to allow the child to have something he wants. Deliberate destructive behaviour, tearing down wallpaper or breaking furniture, may occur in the home. Away from home, aggression is commonly triggered off by situations in which the child wants something another child has, or is dispossessed of something he wants by another child. Frustration is followed by an immediate attack. This pattern of behaviour may well result in the child being found unacceptable in and excluded from a playgroup or infant school.
- *Activity*. The child is often reported to have been restless and to have had difficulty settling from birth or shortly afterwards. Feeding may have been difficult as a consequence. Subsequently, in the third and fourth year of life, there is a lack of concentration. The level of activity will, however, be variable, and when seen in the consulting room, the child may appear to concentrate reasonably well.

Inconstant features include:

- *Anxiety*. Although the child may be apparently rejecting parental control, it may be obvious that there is in fact a good deal of underlying insecurity. This may be shown by the child's unwillingness to be left with friends or familiar relatives even for a few minutes, or by his incapacity to let his mother out of his sight without a panic reaction.
- *Breath-holding attacks*. These are often a response to frustration, in which the child, usually aged between 18 months and 4 years, holds his breath at the culmination of a temper tantrum. In other children, breath holding occurs as an immediate response to pain or an anxiety-provoking experience.

In a minority of children, breath holding continues until the child goes blue before he takes his next breath, and, in a tiny number, the anoxia produces loss of consciousness and a brief convulsion.

Prevalence

Richman *et al.* (1982) in their study of 3 year olds in the general population found that 11% were definitely difficult to control, 9% were attention-seeking, 13% were active and restless, and 5% had frequent tempers (three or more a day or lasting more than 15 minutes). These problems are often associated. They occur more commonly in boys, especially in their more severe form. There is little association with social class. There are no satisfactory studies of the prevalence of oppositional defiant disorders, but about 20% of pre-school children have a significant behavioural or emotional problem. About 7% have a disorder of moderate or severe intensity (Richman *et al.* 1975; Jenkins *et al.* 1980). Approximately half of these are likely to show a diagnosable oppositional defiant disorder.

Aetiology

Social factors

Although social class measured by paternal occupation is unrelated, children with oppositional defiant disorder are more likely to be living in overcrowded circumstances, in high-rise buildings with inadequate play space. There is no clear-cut relationship with maternal employment. Some pre-school children benefit from a period apart from their mothers and others become more insecure. If the mother does go to work, the quality of substitute care is a major influence.

Child factors

Adverse temperamental characteristics may have been present from birth. Indeed it may be difficult to draw a distinction between these characteristics and the behavioural disturbance itself. The child has a definitely increased likelihood of developmental delay such as language retardation and night wetting beyond the expected age.

Parental factors

As this is often better seen as an 'adjustment' reaction, parental behaviour (see above) can be seen as part of the clinical picture rather than as an aetiological factor. Parents may, as a primary feature or a secondary reaction to a difficult child, be critical, rejecting, lacking in warmth, passive, and unstimulating. Mothers, in particular, may show high levels of depression and anxiety, and family relationships, especially the marital relationship, may be seriously disharmonious. Some parents, however, may show none of these adverse characteristics, retain warmth and affection for their children, and appear no more than understandably exasperated and irritated.

The mechanisms whereby these factors combine to result in a child with a severe behavioural adjustment problem are various. In some cases, adverse parental behaviour is obviously primary, in others it is mainly reactive. More commonly, a child with adverse temperamental characteristics and some developmental delay has been born into a family whose members are unprepared for social or personality reasons to cope with an unusually difficult child, though they might have managed well with a more placid, compliant one. As the child becomes increasingly rejected, more insecure, and thus more difficult to handle, so a vicious cycle may become established.

Assessment

A description should be obtained of the nature and severity of the various problems of which the parents complain, as well as other possible problem areas. It is necessary to establish the situation specificity of the various difficulties. With whom are they present, and in what circumstances? This will establish whether the problems are widespread or monosymptomatic, and often also whether the child's problems are related to underlying anxiety.

The level of disturbance in the parental personality and handling of the child should be assessed. How far are parents fixed in their behaviour, and how far open to possible changes? Finally, the child and parents should be observed together, to form a further impression of the parent–child relationship. Observation of the child is necessary to exclude other conditions such as the hyperkinetic syndrome and childhood autism, and to indicate the child's developmental level. The presence of physical symptoms, such as headache or stomach-ache, may suggest the need for a physical examination.

The condition may be differentiated from conduct disorders by the age of the child and from the hyperkinetic syndrome or attention deficit–hyperactivity disorder, by the lesser prominence of overactivity and poor concentration, and the marked presence of antisocial features.

Management

The management will depend on the severity of the problem, how widespread and handicapping it is, and to what degree the parents and child are motivated to receive help. Treatment of isolated feeding and sleep disturbances is described elsewhere, and, if the child is showing hyperactive behaviour, the section on the management of the hyperactive syndrome will be relevant (Section 3.4.2).

Parents of children showing primarily disobedient behaviour will benefit most from advice along behavioural lines. It will be helpful if the father can be involved in counselling sessions, but this will not always be possible. The focus should be on actual examples of difficult behaviour, and how the parents can change their own behaviour, so that they reward appropriate, 'good' behaviour and ignore or succeed in not giving attention to 'bad' behaviour. Regular charting of behaviour will enable the clinician to know when progress is being made, or when other approaches need to be tried. A cognitive behavioural approach to the management of pre-school problems has been described by Douglas (1998) and to oppositional defiant disorder in older children by Bailey (1998).

Family sessions involving other children may help to reveal that the identified child is in fact being 'scapegoated', and showing no worse behaviour than others, and may also improve communication between family members and establish greater consistency in matters of discipline. Parents may need to be helped to see how some of their behaviour, for example threatening to leave home if the child is naughty, may increase insecurity. Family sessions may also reveal that the child's behaviour forms a focus of conflict because the parents are unable to deal with other areas of disagreement or frustration in their own relationship.

Social measures involving, for example, an attempt to support parents in an application for more appropriate housing or to arrange a placement in a sympathetic pre-school facility, may be helpful.

Medication and individual psychotherapy for the child have little or no part to play in the management of this type of problem.

Outcome

It was once thought that behavioural disturbances occurring in the pre-school period had an excellent outcome. It has now been shown (Richman *et al.* 1982) that about two-thirds of children with definite pre-school behaviour problems remain disturbed at least into the early school years. Many will show conduct disorders. Boys in whom early restlessness is prominent appear to have a less good outcome than others. An amelioration of social or family circumstances does not necessarily produce an improvement in behaviour, though of course it is desirable for other reasons. Many children with oppositional defiant disorder go on to develop conduct disorder in adolescence (Biederman *et al.* 1996), and indeed, oppositional defiant disorder may well best be seen as an early form of conduct disorder.

4.5.3 CONDUCT DISORDER

Definition

All children show, at times, behaviour which contravenes social norms or personal or property rights. Most will go through brief periods of stealing and lying. A substantial minority go through phases when they bully other children, are aggressive in other ways, or truant from school. The child with so-called conduct disorder is different only in the extent and severity of difficult behaviour. There is therefore no sharp dividing line between normal and abnormal social behaviour.

Social norms are culture-specific. There are important differences between societies in their judgements as to when behaviour is antisocial. Chinese societies put much more emphasis on conformity than do western societies, though there are, for example, religious sects in the west that are highly demanding in this respect. In some schools, fighting among boys in the playground is regarded as a matter for serious concern: in others it will be taken for granted this will occur. The same behaviour may produce different reactions depending on who is responsible. Many people would feel differently reading about a group of university students turning over cars following celebration of a rugby cup victory, to reading of a group of black youths behaving similarly after being refused entry to a club.

Inevitably, the police, as well as professionals such as psychologists, psychiatrists, family doctors and paediatricians who are involved in assessing and attempting to help children with antisocial behaviour and their families, will be affected in their judgements of abnormality by values held by others in their society. These may change over time. The attitudes to bullying as an inevitable part of British school life changed during the 1990s, so that now bullying is much more likely to be seen as quite unacceptable by both parents and teachers.

Perspectives on antisocial behaviour
Doctors and nurses working in primary health care, mental health professionals, and those involved in different parts of the juvenile justice system such as the police and magistrates, are likely to view antisocial behaviour from different perspectives. For the police, magistrates and lawyers, punishment, as well as deterrence and rehabilitation, will be seen as a natural and desirable reaction to the detection of a young offender. For those working in the health professions, the main need is likely to be seen as understanding the reasons for the offence, with treatment as the priority in thinking about what to do about the problem.

Delinquency
Children who show antisocial behaviour may or may not be breaking the law. If they are, their behaviour may be considered as a form of juvenile delinquency. Delinquency is defined by the law. Thus legislation is always especially concerned to protect property, so that virtually any form of stealing is against the law. By contrast, lying, by itself, is not delinquent unless it occurs in court under oath. In fact, the great majority of antisocial acts are not detected. Antisocial behaviour can therefore be divided into that which is non-delinquent, undetected delinquent, and delinquent. For understanding causation, assessment and management, these legal distinctions are not particularly useful, but, of course, in determining what happens to a child who may or may not have broken the law, they may be crucial.

Classification

In ICD-10 (World Health Organization 1992) conduct disorders are divided into those confined to the family context, and into unsocialized, socialized, and oppositional defiant types. The last category is mainly used for younger children (see above). DSM-IV (American Psychiatric Association 1994) classifies conduct disorder and oppositional defiant disorders as two forms of disruptive behaviour disorders. Conduct disorders are divided into two sub-types, depending on age of onset—childhood onset and adolescent onset. Diagnostic criteria include the presence of three or more of the following: aggression to people and animals, destruction of property, deceitfulness or theft, and serious violation of rules. For oppositional defiant disorder to be present, there must have been a pattern of negativistic, hostile and defiant behaviour lasting at least 6 months. For all these diagnoses, there should be significant social, academic, or occupational impairment.

In the past, various attempts have been made to produce useful classifications of conduct disorder. In particular, the distinction between socialized and unsocialized disorders has been made, depending mainly on whether the behaviour has occurred in the company of others. *Socialized* delinquents are said to get on reasonably well with other children their age, and their offences might be seen as acceptable behaviour by other family members. They are more likely to show guilt over their misdemeanours and sympathy for their victims. *Unsocialized* delinquents, by contrast, offend alone and not in company, have poor peer relationships, and offend against their group norms as well as those of wider society. They show little guilt for their offences or indeed concern for other people in general. They are also said to show more neurotic traits. This distinction may be easily applied when looking at individuals at the extremes of the socialized/unsocialized continuum, but most antisocial children show features of both types. The distinction is probably most useful in adolescence.

More recently, Vitiello and Stoff (1997) have suggested, on the basis of statistical analysis of clinical samples that it may be useful to recognize two sub-types of aggression. There is overtly hostile, impulsive behaviour, often reactive to actual or perceived attack in an overaroused child, and there is covert, predatory, controlled aggression that is proactive and carried out to achieve some advantage to the individual. This division may be applicable to conduct disorders more generally. At this stage, although valuable to research activity, the classification of conduct disorder and its sub-types is of rather limited value to the clinician.

Clinical features

Middle childhood to early adolescence

Aggressive behaviour characterized by physical attacks on other children and, to a lesser extent, parents, is the most common form of antisocial activity. Verbal attacks, involving swearing and name-calling, are frequent accompaniments. Being thwarted by a parent or by another child is the most common precipitant of an aggressive outburst. However, at this age, more deliberate, premeditated aggression begins to occur. The child may plan to injure another either by himself or with a group. He may also be involved in deliberate cruelty to animals.

- *Stealing.* Before the age of 5–6 years, the concept of personal property is likely to be poorly developed, so that taking other children's possessions cannot meaningfully be regarded as stealing. After this age, stealing in a real sense does become possible, though many 6–7 year old children appropriate other children's belongings in what is often rather muddled territory between borrowing with permission, borrowing without permission, and deliberate stealing. By 7–8 years, children will sometimes be involved in stealing from shops, either alone or in groups. Stealing must be regarded as problematic if it occurs repeatedly, despite detection and reprimand, inside or outside the home. In younger children, stealing is most likely to result from a child's desire to comfort himself for feelings of deprivation. Older children's stealing is more likely to occur in gangs as part of marauding or 'self-proving' behaviour. Stealing is often followed by lying in order to cover up misdemeanours, and indeed the denial of stealing is probably the most common reason for lying in this age period. Whether stealing is followed by lying to cover up often depends on whether the parent or teacher, who knows very well that a child has been stealing, insists on the child owning up. Adults who do not do this often save the child from compounding his offence, but, perhaps misguidedly, it is often thought that it is important to give a child the opportunity to admit an offence in order to mitigate the seriousness of his behaviour.

- *Lying.* Less commonly, lying may take the form of spinning fantasies for no very obvious reason, but not to cover up offences. Children of this age may invent stories in which they have had accidents or illnesses that have in fact never occurred to them, or they may invent, for the benefit of their friends, a totally different set of family relationships from that existing in reality. Children who engage in fantasy production of this type may be seriously deprived of affection, but this is often not the case. They may lack social skills in making friends.

- *Disruption.* Antisocial behaviour in school may also take the form of disruptive activity not involving physical or verbal aggression. Some children may disrupt classes by frequent disobedience, wandering around, throwing things, and generally irritating other children and the teacher. Truancy is relatively uncommon in this age period, but can occur before puberty.

- *Fire-setting* is an uncommon form of antisocial behaviour, but does sometimes occur. It may arise as a result of experimentation with matches, or as a deliberate destructive activity. The latter occurs both as a group activity and in isolation. It is often accompanied by signs of other serious antisocial behaviour, and there is frequently a high level of disturbance in the home (Stewart and Culver 1982).

Other forms of antisocial activity in this age period include drug-taking, especially solvent abuse (Section 5.7.2).

Adolescence

Physical aggression as a sign of antisocial activity is less common in this age group though, when it occurs, because of greater physical strength, the outcome may be more serious. Gang-fighting in large cities is a common setting in which physical aggression occurs. Some individual children, however, show seriously aggressive behaviour at home or in the classroom. When frustrated, they may lash out against the person who has thwarted them. Sometimes such aggression may occur in a 'blind rage' with apparent lack of awareness of the surroundings. Such 'episodic dyscontrol' (Nunn 1986) may require differentiation from an epileptic attack, though usually there is a little good evidence for the presence of epilepsy.

Breaking into property and stealing is the most common form of offence for which youngsters of this age are charged, and in fact interviewing potential victims makes it clear that there are many more offences of this type committed (probably mainly by teenagers) than come before the courts. Stealing also takes the form of taking and driving away cars and motor bicycles. Vandalism of public property is a common occurrence, especially in some council housing estates, and this is also an offence mainly committed by teenagers. All these types of offence most commonly occur as a form of group activity.

During the final years of compulsory schooling, especially in inner-city schools, truancy becomes much more common. Persistent truancy is uncommon in primary school children. However, in the UK, as many as 20% of children in their last year of school are absent for unexplained reasons (Fogelman *et al.* 1980). Most truants spend the day out of school in groups, but in a minority it is an isolated activity.

Antisocial activity in adolescence may also take other forms, including drug-taking, and sexual offences, including sexual abuse of younger children. Sexual activity is common among teenagers in western society, and there is no reason to regard it as a form of antisocial activity. However, some girls (and a small minority of boys) who become involved in prostitution, and others whose sexual promiscuity puts them at risk of exploitation, can reasonably be regarded as engaged in a form of antisocial behaviour.

Associated problems

Although classification of child psychiatric disorders tends to make a sharp distinction between antisocial disorders and emotional disorders, many children who show antisocial behaviour are also unduly tense, anxious, and prone to anxiety and depressive feelings. In adolescence they also have a tendency to adult-type neurotic disorders, including hysterical reactions. Some are prone to feelings of hopelessness and make suicide attempts. The occurrence of co-morbid depressive disorder is common, and less frequently there may be co-morbid anxiety disorders. In younger children co-morbid hyperkinetic syndrome is common.

Background information

• *Prevalence.* The cut-off point between normal rebelliousness and conduct disorder is arbitrary, but can be reliably established. On the Isle of Wight, the 1 year prevalence rate of antisocial disorder was found to be about 3%, and in London the rate was found to be at least double this (Rutter *et al.* 1975). In Ontario, Canada, approximately 5% of boys and 2% of girls were rated by teachers to show conduct disorders (Offord *et al.* 1989). Delinquency rates vary very widely from place to place and from time to time. In the late 1980s, around 3% of 10–16 year olds in England and Wales were cautioned or sentenced for an offence in any one year. Not all boys charged with offences need necessarily be regarded as showing conduct disorders. For example, a boy charged with an isolated offence of shoplifting might well be considered within the normal range for antisocial behaviour. Conversely, self-report studies reveal that teenagers never before the courts have often committed dozens of offences in which they have not been detected and for which they have not been charged (Belson 1975).

- *Age.* The rate of physically aggressive behaviour declines gradually with age after puberty. Criminal activity, mainly offences against property, reaches a peak around 13–15 years and thereafter declines (Farrington 1995).
- *Sex ratio.* Boys are charged with offences 7–8 times as commonly as girls. There is a less marked sex difference for conduct disorders in younger children. Indeed, at 3 years there is little difference between the sexes: by 4 years the gap has begun to widen.

Social and neighbourhood factors

- *Social class.* Conduct disorders do occur more commonly in working-class than in middle-class children, but this is almost entirely due to differences between the social classes in family size, rates of overcrowding, and level of child supervision (Kazdin 1987). Similarly, once these factors have been taken into account, there is little or no difference between ethnic minorities and indigenous populations in their rates of conduct disorder. However, serious crimes, such as carrying offensive weapons, are much more likely to be committed by less privileged children. Even so, the police practice of selectively charging working-class children results in biasing the delinquency statistics. When detected in minor crime, middle-class children are more likely to engage the services of a solicitor and be warned and cautioned by the police (Palmai *et al.* 1967).
- *Ethnic status.* Currently in the UK, Asian children have somewhat lower, and West Indian children higher rates of delinquency than does the indigenous population, but it is quite uncertain if this arises from different policies on charging for offences. The rates among West Indian youths increased in the 1970s in line with unemployment rates, and this may reflect a causative association (Rutter and Giller 1983).
- *Schools.* Factors within schools can reduce delinquency rates even among children living in deprived urban neighbourhoods. Those schools where the staff are committed to educational values, set and mark homework consistently, and concentrate on rewarding good rather than punishing bad behaviour show lower rates of truancy and other forms of delinquency among their pupils (Rutter *et al.* 1979).
- *Other social factors.* Children living in inner cities, in poor overcrowded conditions, in neighbourhoods where there are high crime and unemployment rates, are at high risk for both conduct disorders and delinquency.

Familial factors

- *Communication.* Children living in families in which there is poor communication of feelings and a lack of awareness of and respect for the feelings of others, probably have higher rates of conduct disorder.
- *Family size and structure.* Children from large families are at particular risk. Those living in homes broken by divorce and separation are also at high risk.

If family relationships are discordant and disharmonious, this raises the risk of antisocial behaviour to a very significant extent (Rutter and Giller 1983).

- *Parental personality and health.* There is a relatively strong link between the presence of an antisocial personality in one or both parents and similar behaviour in the child (West and Farrington 1973). However, most young children showing conduct disorders do not have an antisocial parent. Depression in the mother is also linked to antisocial behaviour.
- *Parental child-rearing practices.* These effects are often difficult to distinguish from those of parental personality. Parents who are inconsistent in applying rules and regulations, disagree between themselves, and rely heavily on harsh punishment for bad behaviour rather than reward for good, are likely to have antisocial children (Patterson 1982).
- *Television and comics.* Children with aggressive tendencies have a special predisposition to watch violent television programmes and read violent material in comics, so the fact that aggressive children watch more violence does not necessarily mean that one can blame the media for violent behaviour, There is, however, some evidence that violence on television is responsible for promoting some degree of violent behaviour among boys (Huesmann 1986).

Personal factors

- *Genetic.* Twin studies suggest that, while genetic factors are of definite importance in adult criminality, they are of less significance in conduct disorders. Among adopted boys, the risk of juvenile delinquency is greater if the adoptive father has antisocial tendencies, and is raised less if the biological father has a criminal record but the adoptive father does not (Hutchings and Mednick 1974). Nevertheless, genetic factors do play a significant part in the causation of aggressive behaviour. They probably exert this effect by their influence on temperament and personality (see below). There is now good evidence that genetic and adverse environmental factors interact to contribute to cause antisocial behaviour (Cadoret *et al.* 1995).
- *Temperament and personality.* 'Difficult' babies are more likely to show aggressive behaviour problems later on. Hyperactivity/impulsivity, low autonomic reactivity, sensation seeking or risk taking, aggressivity, cognitive impairments, or executive planning deficits and problems in social cognition are all risk factors for persistent antisocial behaviour (Maughan and Rutter 1998). In particular, hyperactivity predicts the development of conduct disorders (Taylor *et al.* 1996).
- *Physical health.* Children with epilepsy and other disorders of cerebral function are at increased risk for conduct as well as for emotional disorders, though non-neurological disorders are much less closely associated (Howe *et al.* 1993). There is also a tendency for children with other physical disorders to show somewhat higher rates.
- *Educational retardation.* There is a strong link between conduct disorder and educational failure, especially specific retardation in reading ability. It is probable that many children who fail in school become discouraged and low in self-esteem, and take to delinquency to obtain rewards they are missing

elsewhere. It is also possible that underlying personality factors such as impulsiveness and excitability both impede learning and predispose to aggressive and antisocial behaviour (Maguin and Loeber 1996).

Labelling

Once a child has been labelled as antisocial, perhaps following a court appearance, the risk of further antisocial activity is increased (Farrington 1977). Delinquent children who have appeared in court seem to have a slightly worse outcome than those of a similar level of antisocial behaviour who have avoided a court appearance.

Assessment

Information should be obtained on the precise nature of the antisocial activity and the immediately precipitating circumstances. It is particularly important to know whether the behaviour involved is generally impulsive and preceded by frustrating experiences. It is also important to obtain systematic information on other aspects of the child's behaviour and emotional life, especially the presence of significant anxiety and depressive symptoms.

The developmental history, including experiences of illness and separation from either parent, is relevant. Particularly important is information on current family functioning, the quality of relationships in the family, the strength of positive and negative parental attitudes to the child, the way in which discipline is exercised, the attitude of other family members to the behaviour, and their view as to why it has occurred. Finally, it is important to know how the child and the family see the future in terms of the likelihood of recurrence, and whether they are motivated to receive any psychological help or think this could be useful.

The assessment of children with conduct or antisocial disorders is made more difficult by the fact that the person involved in assessment, whether this be a psychologist, doctor, probation officer, or social worker, is likely to be seen as an authority figure by the child and other family members. As one of the problems may be an antisocial attitude, obtaining information is often a tense procedure. It is therefore particularly important that the assessment is carried out by someone who can convey a sympathetic and understanding attitude, in a non-condemnatory manner. It is worthwhile spending time getting to know the child and family before embarking on obtaining precise details of antisocial behaviour.

Information about younger children with conduct disorders is often best obtained within the family setting, or at least with both parents and the child in question present. It is useful to acknowledge in the interview that the child would probably prefer not to be in the room hearing unpleasant facts about himself. The child may be asked right at the beginning whether in fact he wanted to come ɔ the consultation, and a sympathetic but firm attitude to this taken from the ɔutset. Very occasionally, parental attitudes may be so rejecting and negative it may be thought better to continue the interview with the child out of the room. However, if parental attitudes are of this nature, it is important to remember that the child is probably exposed to constant attack at home as well, so the experience of rejection is not likely to be a new one for him. Having seen the family members together, it is usually helpful to see the child separately and then the parents alone.

With older children and teenagers it will often be preferable to see the child by himself before seeing the parents, and to complete the assessment by conducting a family interview. If this is so, it is important not to transmit information the child gives in private back to the parents, without checking with the child that this is agreeable to him. The reverse is, of course, also the case.

Sometimes the child or one of the parents will not be willing to be interviewed at all. In many cases a useful service can be provided by seeing those family members who are motivated to receive advice and guidance. A situation that arises frequently is one where teachers are worried about a child's antisocial or aggressive behaviour, but the family shows no apparent interest in co-operating by going to a clinic or psychiatric department for an assessment. The options here are to conduct a school-based assessment, or to limit one's activities to obtaining further information from the teacher and providing advice on this basis alone.

Management

The form of treatment that should be offered will depend especially on the motivation of the child and family, the nature of the conduct problems, and the presence or absence of significant neurotic symptoms, especially tension, anxiety, and depression. A useful review of psychosocial treatments for conduct disorders is provided by Kazdin (1997). He describes the following approaches as most promising:

- *Cognitive problem-solving skills training.* This is based on the notion that children and adolescents with conduct disorders often have faulty cognitions, especially involving distorted attributions of aggressive intentions in other people and blame for actions they themselves have taken. In interpersonal cognitive problem-solving training, through diary-keeping, modeling and role play, they are encouraged to develop more accurate perceptions.
- *Parent management training.* The assumption here is that inconsistent, punitive child-rearing practices play a part in the development of antisocial behaviour, and may be changed, especially if there is sufficient parental motivation. Coercive interactions patterns are identified (Patterson *et al.* 1992; see Kazdin 1997), and work is undertaken either with the parent alone, or with the parents and child directly to modify these.
- *Functional family therapy.* The underlying hypothesis here is that the problem in the child is a reflection of the way all family members interact together.

The family members are seen together as a unit, and the aim is to improve positive reciprocity and communication patterns.

Multisystemic therapy
Multisystemic therapy involves a package of measures, especially functional family therapy and parent management training as described above. These are combined with individual counselling together with social and educational measures to improve the adolescent's capacity to function in the external world (Henggeler 1999).

Each of these forms of treatment has been shown to produce reasonable short-term results and some benefit in the medium term. However, success is limited and is less likely to occur if the problems are severe and widespread, and if the motivation of the child and family is ambivalent.

Medication has only a very small part to play in the management of children with conduct disorders. However, in a small minority of cases, where aggressive outbursts, though not epileptic in nature, appear to take the form of frequent 'blind rages' (Leicester 1982), haloperidol may be a useful treatment. A dose of 0.05 mg/kg body weight a day in two divided doses over a period of a few weeks or months may be helpful. The dose should be reduced if impairment of concentration, drowsiness, or dystonic symptoms occur.

As well as these specific techniques, management should include attention to ways in which family relationships can be improved and the child's energies channelled in more positive directions. Marital counselling may be indicated for the parents. Advice may be given to fathers as to how they might spend more time with their sons, or how different children in the family may be given more individual attention. Such advice may be helpful, perhaps by improving the self-esteem of children whose antisocial behaviour may be a sign of chronic discouragement and feeling of failure.

The management procedures described so far are likely to be helpful only where the child and family are motivated to receive help. In a substantial number of children this is not the case, and family members may even be unwilling to co-operate in assessment. Nevertheless, the lives of teachers, other pupils in the classroom, and other members of the community may be disrupted so that action may be indicated. In these circumstances a variety of interventions may be made, some by virtue of the powers held by juvenile court magistrates, others without such powers needing to be taken.

These measures include:

• Advice to teachers on ways of interviewing parents or applying behaviour modification programmes in the classroom. It is important for education authorities to develop behaviour support plans that determine provision for children with behaviour difficulties, and ensure good multi-agency working for such children.
• Supervision of the child and contact with the family by a social worker, court officer, or, where such exist, an education welfare officer, who is likely to be of particular help in cases of truancy.

- Court procedures such as the requirement for truants of regular reporting back to the magistrates on regularity of school attendance. Such procedures have been shown to be more effective in ensuring regular attendance than merely arranging for supervision without reporting back (Berg *et al.* 1978).
- Compulsory attendance at community-based centres for what has sometimes been known as 'intermediate treatment'—a variety of activities geared to the abilities of the child.
- Residential placement in special schools for children with emotional and behavioural problems, community homes with education on the premises (CHEs), or (for children at greater risk for violent or other serious antisocial behaviour) youth treatment centres.

Finally it is important to stress that, as the following section on outcome indicates, the prognosis for many children with severe conduct disorders, even with treatment, is not good. This means that it is important to place emphasis on preventive measures as described in Chapter 9.

Court reports

When a child has been charged with an offence, psychiatrists and psychologists may be asked to make assessments for the benefit of the magistrates to help them to decide how the child should be dealt with. In this case, it is important to make clear to the family at the outset why they are being seen and that anything they say may be put into the report. The information can be obtained in a similar manner to that described above.

In writing the report (Black *et al.* 1998) it is usually helpful to describe the circumstances of the offence and any precipitating factors. Relevant background information about the child's development, physical health, and mental state should be provided, as well as information about the child's family, including positive as well as negative factors. A statement should be made about the presence or absence of significant psychiatric disorder. Throughout the report one should carefully distinguish factual information from inferences. One should also distinguish information provided by the child, family, or other individual from that deriving from one's own observations. Jargon should be rigorously avoided, and any technical terms used should be explained. At the end of the report one should bring together the information one has obtained in a formulation. A recommendation may then be made at the end of the report about what would be a preferable line of action. If any form of treatment is recommended, it is important to check both whether this is available, and whether the child and family are motivated to receive it.

Outcome

The long-term outcome of children with conduct disorders varies considerably with the nature and extent of the antisocial behaviour (Robins 1978). Factors associated with good and bad outcome are reviewed by Maughan and Rutter (1998).

The problems that antisocial children develop in later life are diverse. They have an increased risk not only of antisocial or aggressive personality disorder, but also of neurotic conditions and schizophrenia. Their social lives are more likely to be disrupted by frequent job changes, and they may also show difficulties in establishing long-lasting relationships. Divorce rates are therefore high.

Although continuity of antisocial behaviour from childhood to adulthood is not high (most antisocial children do not grow up to be antisocial adults), the reverse is not the case. Nearly all seriously aggressive, antisocial adults have shown this pattern of behaviour in childhood. This means that the possibilities for prevention of antisocial behaviour in adulthood by taking action in childhood are, at least theoretically, very considerable. Reports of successful community-based preventive programmes for youth at high risk are relevant in this connection (Offord 1987).

4.6 Bowel and bladder control

4.6.1 NORMAL BOWEL CONTROL

In the infant, distension of the rectum with faeces stimulates periodic automatic voiding by relaxation of the internal and external anal sphincters. As the child gets older, the external sphincter and levator ani muscles that consist of striated muscular tissue come under voluntary control. In order to prevent faecal expulsion, the child learns to tense these muscles when he experiences a sense of fullness of the rectum. The internal sphincter (which is not under voluntary control) is probably triggered into a long-term contraction by this voluntary activity. The internal sphincter then operates until further rectal distension requires the child once again to exercise voluntary control.

Most normal bowel 'training' is, in fact, a co-operative achievement by mother and child, the 'potting couple'. Around the second half of the second year of life the child (now physiologically ready to achieve continence and able to sit still for a longer period of time) usually indicates he is about to pass a motion by making a characteristic sound, adopting a characteristic posture, or both. He may be eager to imitate adults or other sibs in their mode of defecation. Alternatively, the child's bowel habit is so regular that the mother knows when he is likely to pass a motion. In any event, at a promising moment, she encourages him to sit on the pot and, if he performs, shows great pleasure. Appropriate defecation is reinforced in the context of a mutually rewarding relationship, and 'training' usually occurs within a few weeks. It is usually more appropriate to think of the child as having matured sufficiently to gain a new skill, which his parents encourage him to use, rather than to conceive of the process as one of 'training' by parents.

4.6.2 CONSTIPATION

Definitions

• *Constipation* involves difficulty or delay in the passage of faeces.

- *Encopresis* is the passage of faeces of normal or near normal consistency into socially inappropriate places (including clothing).
- *Soiling* is the frequent passage of liquid or semisolid faeces into clothing (Agnarsson and Clayden 1990).

Clinical features

Constipation may present at any time from the first few weeks of life, but is an unusual presenting feature after 6–7 years. It usually, though not always, begins in infancy. The usual complaint is of failure to pass faeces except at infrequent or irregular intervals, and there may be associated pain, abdominal distension, and soiling. As constipation becomes more severe, it is likely to be accompanied by faecal soiling. Diarrhoea may also be a presenting feature. On examination, faecal masses are often palpable on abdominal examination and hard faeces are palpable on rectal examination. In older children, constipation may occur in association with encopresis (see below), and findings on examination may vary over time, with faeces palpable on some occasions, but not on others.

Aetiology

Physical factors

Constipation present from birth may be due to anal stenosis, other minor anatomical abnormalities, and Hirschsprung disease (a condition in which there is a failure of development of ganglion cells in the internal sphincter and a segment of rectum, so that the neuromuscular defecatory mechanism is deficient).

Infants may become constipated if they are not given enough to eat or drink, or because of overstrong artificial feeds. In older children, dietary factors (e.g. a diet low in fibre) may also be important. Very occasionally, constipation may be a presenting feature of organic disease, such as hypothyroidism or idiopathic hypercalcaemia. Other local physical causes include an anal fissure or fistula. These may make defecation painful so that the child withholds. Constipation may also sometimes follow a prolonged febrile illness.

Psychosocial factors

- *Parental factors*. Not so long ago, and this situation is probably little different now, it was not uncommon for mothers to begin to 'train' their babies to be clean in the first year of life (Newson and Newson 1963) by holding their children over the pot after meals. This is a futile exercise but, in itself, probably does no harm unless the mother becomes angry and frustrated when the child fails to perform. The 'training' of older children may also be adversely affected by parental behaviour. Mothers under stress because of tense family relationships, financial hardship, or overcrowded housing will have less time and patience to attend to their child's cues. If they react to the child's failure to achieve bowel continence by punitiveness, this is likely to make the child more anxious, and to achieve the opposite result to that intended (Woodmansey 1967).
- *Factors in the child*. The child may be poor at providing cues when he is ready to defecate. This may be because of global retardation, because he is generally

uninterested in pleasing his mother, or because he is using his capacity to control defecation in a battle for power with one or both parents. Younger children may have fantasies about their faeces and, once one is aware of these, the tendency to withhold faeces may become understandable. Thus, some children withhold faeces because they regard them as a necessary part of themselves they do not want to lose. They may therefore be worried about what happens to them after they are flushed away. Others regard faeces as a dirty part of themselves they do not want to have anything to do with, so they deny their rectal sensations and retain faeces.

- *Constipation and sexual abuse.* This is a complex and controversial issue. Children traumatized by sexual abuse may withhold faeces as part of a generalized response to stress. It is reasonable to assume that this is more likely if the abuse has involved anal penetration. The clinician should therefore consider sexual abuse as one possible explanation for intractable constipation and consider whether there is other evidence. If, on examination of a constipated child, on parting the buttocks, the anus is patulous, this is, in itself, not supportive evidence of abuse. It occurs in about 15% of severely constipated children (Clayden 1988). If the anus is initially closed, but then dilates (reflex anal dilatation), this is thought by some to be supportive evidence of abuse. It is, however, generally agreed not to be pathognomonic of abuse, and other evidence must be sought.

As a result of constipation, whatever its cause, a hard mass is formed in the rectum and lower colon. The internal sphincter becomes chronically stretched, and the child may have no sensation of fullness. Ballooning of the bowel above the mass can produce a functional megacolon. Liquid faecal matter accumulates, and oozes out around the sides of the constipated mass, producing intermittent soiling. Partial intestinal obstruction may occur, especially in young children, with abdominal pain and vomiting.

Management

An account should be taken of the development of the symptom. Constipation present from the first few days of birth suggests an organic cause. In other circumstances, the constipation is more likely to be functional. An account of early training practices should be obtained. The presence of associated behaviour problems is relevant, and the quality of parent–child interaction should be assessed.

Physical examination should include palpation of the abdomen for faecal masses, and examination of the perianal area for evidence of a fissure, as well as a rectal examination. In some centres, radiological investigation is routinely carried out and can provide an objective measure of the severity of constipation.

If constipation is present, it should be directly treated regardless of the level of psychological disturbance. Children cannot hope to achieve bowel continence if they have a large mass of faeces distending the rectum. Initially the mass should be cleared using a few doses of a simple but effective aperient such as liquid paraffin. If oral treatment is not effective, a brief course of enemas may be necessary, but prolonged courses of enemas or bowel wash-outs are unnecessary and undesirable. In any event, children should be carefully prepared for these potentially upsetting procedures.

Subsequently, to establish the bowel habit, it is usually necessary to continue with maintenance treatment for some months. This should consist of a diet high in roughage, fruit, vegetables, etc. and Senokot daily or every other day. A softening agent such as docusate (paediatric solution) is helpful initially for a couple of weeks, followed by an osmotic stool softener such as lactulose.

Associated with these physical forms of treatment, parents should be counselled to relax in their approach to the child's bowel problem. A positive approach with warm encouragement to the child to use the pot or toilet should be advised. The child should be praised initially just for sitting on the pot. Attention should be given to wider aspects of parent–child interaction with identification of more mutually enjoyable activities, so that there is less focus on the child's bowel problem. Children and families can be given 'bowel diaries' to record the frequency and consistency of bowel motions as well as where they are passed (potty, lavatory, or pants).

With this regime the great majority of children seen in primary care or in paediatric departments with constipation will improve considerably. Failure to improve should lead to a reconsideration of the possibility of a physical disorder with reference to a specialized paediatrician. If this is ruled out, more intensive psychiatric assessment and treatment along the lines described below in relation to encopresis are indicated. The possibility of sexual abuse should also be considered (see above).

Outcome

Constipation has a good prognosis. Given appropriate treatment, most will respond rapidly, though one study of children vigorously treated for chronic constipation found only two-thirds free of symptoms and off medication 4 years after discharge (Keuzenkamp-Jansen *et al.* 1996). A small proportion develop chronic constipation that persists into adulthood.

4.6.3 ENCOPRESIS

Encopresis involves the passage of faeces of normal or near-normal consistency in inappropriate places (including clothing). It may alternate with soiling—the passage of liquid or semisolid faeces into clothing.

By 3 years, 16% of children are still showing signs of faecal incontinence once a week or more, but by 4 years only 3% (Richman *et al.* 1982). By 7 years only 1.5% of children have still not achieved continence (Bellman 1966), and by 10–11 years this figure has decreased to 0.8%. Most children identified in surveys are probably showing soiling secondary to constipation, and only a minority true encopresis. Boys are affected 3–4 times as commonly as girls. There are no consistent social class differences.

Clinical features

Encopresis may be continuous from birth or may occur after a period of continence. It is unusual for it to begin after the age of 5–6 years. Mild constipation may be a constant feature, intermittent, or absent. Sometimes children with encopresis develop severe constipation with the clinical picture described above.

The soiling is often frequent, occurring several times a day. It may, however, not occur at school, but only when the child returns home. Parents will often interpret this as a hostile act on the part of the child, but, in fact, the soiling in the home setting may occur because the child feels more relaxed there.

The child's attitude to the soiling is variable. Some who soil their pants deny that it really occurs, or that they smell, and these have to be reminded to change clothing. They may have become habituated to the smell. Others are ashamed and embarrassed and go to great lengths to hide soiled pants. The faeces can be used to express aggressive feelings. Some children use them to smear walls and furniture, others deposit well-formed faeces in places likely to cause maximum distress—in glasses used for drinking, or in the parental bed. The soiling may represent one aspect of a child's attempt to retain the benefits of a younger child (regressive soiling). Despite normal intelligence, the child may be unable to cope with the increasing independence he is expected to show at school and elsewhere.

Associated psychological and psychiatric problems are almost invariably present, but, apart from the fact that the children are usually rejected by others because of their smell, are not of any very characteristic type. Children are usually of average or below average ability, though they may show significant educational retardation. They may be unduly anxious, show seriously aggressive behaviour, or neither of these. It is interesting that even 3 year olds who have failed to gain bowel control show an unduly high rate of behavioural problems (Richman *et al.* 1982). About a third of children who soil are also enuretic at night, and a smaller proportion are wet by day.

Aetiology

Encopresis, the passage of normal stools into inappropriate places, is never physically determined. A variety of factors in the parents, child, and in parent–child interaction have been identified as probably causative. None is invariably present, but there is a certain amount of consistency in the background factors usually in operation.

- *Parental factors*. These may seem to be of little significance. Alternatively, some parents of children with encopresis are quite unusually aggressive and punitive both in their general attitude and in relation to the child in question. They may also show unusually high standards of cleanliness and have expectations of conformity for their children's behaviour that are quite unreasonable. As a result of these characteristics, early bowel training may have been coercive and resulted in the child feeling himself a failure.

- *Factors in the child.* The child may be showing general developmental retardation with delay in achieving bowel continence as only one aspect of general immaturity. In children of normal ability, irrational fantasies about the faeces as described in relation to constipation (see above) may be present. These may result in a phobia of the pot or toilet. Encopresis is not uncommonly one manifestation of a generalized conduct or emotional disorder. Thus the child may be showing associated disobedience or aggressive behaviour, often linked with specific educational retardation. Children with associated aggressive problems are more likely to use their faeces for aggressive purposes, for example by smearing walls or windows. Less commonly the child may be generally depressed, fearful, or inhibited.
- *Family factors.* Family relationships may be characterized by a good deal of tension and disharmony. Communication may be poor. Not infrequently, the child with encopresis is scapegoated. There may be a constant battle for control, with the child using his capacity to control his own defecation as a weapon in the family conflicts.
- *Life stress.* Especially in children who have only recently gained bowel control, an unpleasant experience such as a frightening, acute illness, or an episode of bullying at school may precipitate the onset of encopresis.

Management

A combined approach involving both psychological and physical measures is desirable. In hospital practice this may be best achieved by a joint paediatric–psychiatric team.

- *General principles.* Whatever the specific approach used, certain general principles need to be followed. The child should be told he is not the only sufferer from this problem—it occurs in many other children. He should be given some idea, appropriate to his age level, of the mechanisms of defecation. The parents should be encouraged to ignore the child's soiling except at those times when they are involved in carrying out a behaviour modification programme (see below). In particular, parents should be discouraged from punishing the child for soiling. An attempt should be made to encourage activities which allow more positive parent–child relationships to be built up. While psychological treatments are in progress, the child should be occasionally checked for the development of constipation. Appropriate physical treatment should be given if this occurs (see above), and there is some evidence that laxatives should, in any case, be routinely employed (Nolan *et al.* 1991).
- *Behaviour modification.* As with other forms of behaviour modification, careful baseline monitoring, both of the undesired behaviour and of the reactions of the parents, is an essential first step (O'Brien *et al.* 1986). The most successful approach involves the shaping of an appropriate toileting habit. The child is encouraged to sit on the toilet for about 10 minutes after each meal. The behaviour is charted, and the child rewarded either materially or socially

(using stars, stamps, hugs, praise, etc.) for appropriate behaviour—first for sitting on the toilet and then for passing a motion into it (see Section 9.2.1 for a more detailed description of behavioural programmes). Behavioural techniques may be best discussed at family interviews, as their administration may give rise to parental disputes (the father, for example, thinking the child should be punished regardless). The presence of sibs is often helpful, but if the affected child is deeply embarrassed by his habit, he may not be willing to attend if they are present.

- *Psychotherapy*. As indicated, the child's encopresis may have an aggressive component or (in regressive soiling) be linked to a wish to be treated like a younger child. Understanding the reasons for these feelings and taking measures to help is usually best achieved in family sessions. Aggressive tendencies may, for example, be linked to a parent's lack of ability to show affection and concern. Aggressive behaviour may be covertly encouraged by the father. Family therapy offers an opportunity to explore issues such as these. Individual psychotherapy may also occasionally be indicated, especially when the problem appears part of an emotional disorder, or irrational fantasies appear to be present.
- *Medication* (e.g. imipramine) has been recommended as a treatment for encopresis, but there is no good evidence for its effectiveness.
- *Hospitalization*. Encopresis is usually managed on an out-patient basis. Failure to respond to an out-patient treatment programme over several weeks is an indication for admission. Encopresis may respond to behavioural management on a paediatric ward, but, if the facility is available, admission to a child psychiatric in-patient unit, where more intensive psychologically orientated treatment can be carried out, will often be desirable. In both settings, the work carried out will need to involve parents; otherwise symptomatic improvement will occur in hospital, but not be maintained in the home setting.

Outcome

Encopresis virtually always clears up by adolescence (Bellman 1966) and, although adult encopretics have been described, they are extremely rare. Treatment usually shortens the natural course of the condition, so that over 90% may be expected to improve over a period of a year (Levine and Bakow 1976). Outcome is better for those children who have a reasonably well-developed 'internal locus of control'—a sense of being in control of their fate. A short history and the presence of constipation are also good prognostic factors (Rockney *et al.* 1996). Although the encopresis disappears, associated symptoms, especially aggressive behaviour, may not, and here the outcome will depend on similar factors to those described in the discussion of the prognosis of conduct disorders (Section 4.5.3).

4.6.4 NORMAL BLADDER CONTROL

Children are incontinent of urine at birth because they do not have the necessary physiological maturity, the understanding to know what is required of them, or the motivation to achieve continence. By the second and third year of life, they have usually achieved all three of these requirements. Continence will occur if:

- The central nervous system has matured sufficiently. In babies reflex emptying occurs when the pressure inside the bladder reaches a certain point. Older children become able, as a result of maturation of the nervous system, to inhibit emptying by contraction of one or more of the bladder sphincters by day or at night when asleep. Maturation of nervous structures is partly genetically determined, and this explains why failure to gain bladder control at night often runs in families.
- There is no defect of the nervous system supplying the bladder and no congenital malformation.
- The parents can take a relaxed attitude to the achievement of dryness, and not make the child anxious about failure. Many mothers start toilet-training before the age of a year. Parents who begin at 18 months to 2 years and confine their 'training' to providing opportunities for voiding on the pot, especially when the child shows he is ready, and praising the child for a successful performance, are likely to see their children become dry earlier than those who punish for wetness or are upset by it (Brazelton 1962).
- The family is going through a settled time when the child is 18 months to 3 years old. There is evidence that if the family is under stress when the child is of this age, he or she will be slower to become dry.

4.6.5 ENURESIS

Definition

Enuresis can be defined as involuntary emptying of the bladder in the absence of an organic cause in a child over the age of 5 years. The term 'urinary incontinence' is usually employed if involuntary emptying occurs due to a physical cause. Enuresis may be nocturnal, diurnal (by day), or both.

Background information

At 3 years of age about 34% of children are still wetting by night, and 26% by day (Richman *et al.* 1982). By the age of 5 years, about 10% of children will be wet by night and about 3% by day (De Jonge 1973). By 8 years, 4% are wet by night and 2% by day (Richman *et al.* 1982). At 14 years about 1% of children are still wet by night. Boys are about twice as likely to wet as girls, and working-class children are slightly more likely to wet than middle-class ones.

Factors sometimes associated with wetting include:

- a family history of bed-wetting in parents or sibs
- unsettling events in the pre-school period, such as instability of family relationships, divorce, or separation (Jarvelin *et al.* 1990), or a history of unplanned separation of the child from his family
- the presence of behavioural problems in the child
- general developmental delay.

Enuresis may occur in any stage of the sleep cycle (Section 4.3.1).

Causation

Nocturnal enuresis is occasionally caused by physical disorders (see below). Much more commonly it is produced by an inherited delay in maturation of the relevant nervous structures, or less commonly, by an interaction between delay in maturation and environmental circumstances which, for one reason or another, fail to promote the acquisition of bladder control. Maturation delay may be shown by a small functional bladder capacity, as children with enuresis appear unable to retain as much urine in their bladders as non-enuretics before micturating. However, the fact that children with small functional bladder capacity have an increased tendency to show psychiatric disorders suggests that there is an interaction between psychological and physiological factors, rather than distinct groups of children with either physical or emotional disorders (Shaffer *et al.* 1984).

Long-standing environmental circumstances of significance include:

• A rigid approach to toilet training in which the child is expected to conform to unreasonable parental standards of toileting, fails to comply, is punished for failure, and is then made anxious and thus even more liable to wet himself
• Negative or indifferent parental attitudes that result in the child failing to care whether he wets or not, because he has such low self-esteem.

In addition to long-standing adverse circumstances, precipitating events may be of causative importance, perhaps by altering sleep rhythm. They include:

• Events that make the child anxious, such as sleeping in a strange house, seeing a disturbing TV film or video the previous evening, witnessing a parental argument, or having difficult schoolwork to do. Anxiety may also result in a child that normally wets having a dry night.
• Life situations that result in the child feeling more relaxed, for example the school holidays, may also affect the sleep rhythm so that the child is either more or less likely to wet at these times.

Finally, although this is unusual, some children deliberately wet the bed as a hostile or angry gesture towards their parents.

Clinical features

Most wetting is dealt with at the primary health-care level by general practitioners or health visitors. Those with physical pathology are referred for further investigation (see below). Other children referred to paediatricians and child psychiatrists have usually failed to respond to symptomatic measures, or show signs of emotional disturbance in addition to their wetting. Wetting may have been present from birth (continuous) or it may occur after months or even years of continence (onset enuresis). It may be present by day or by night, or only by night. The wetting may be regular and frequent, or intermittent. Causative factors, other than a presumed inherited failure of maturation of nervous structures supplying the bladder, are often absent.

Other urinary symptoms are also usually absent. Pain on passing urine (dysuria), blood in the urine (haematuria), or dribbling of urine, are all indications for full investigation and usually indicate an organic cause for the wetting. Girls are more prone to urinary infections than are boys.

Management

A careful history should be taken to elicit the onset, frequency of the wetting, and any precipitating circumstances. Enquiries should be made for possible signs of associated emotional or behavioural disturbance. Diurnal enuresis is more likely to be associated with emotional disturbance. Finally, the motivation of the child and parents to achieve change should be assessed, as this will affect management. For many children and parents, wetting is a trivial and unimportant symptom; for others it has come to dominate their lives. The possibility of nocturnal epilepsy producing enuresis can usually be excluded by the history. The presence of other urinary symptoms requires physical examination and further investigation. Otherwise, physical investigation should be limited to microscopic examination of a clean specimen of urine to exclude infection.

Management will depend considerably on the age of the child, the frequency of the symptoms, and the motivation of the child and family. However young the child or infrequent the symptom, if the parent is worried about the problem, the doctor or health visitor will need to take time to consider the problem seriously and provide helpful advice. The presence of associated emotional or behavioural problems is not a contraindication to a direct attempt to treat the enuresis. Indeed, sometimes such associated problems will improve if the enuresis is successfully treated. However, associated problems will occasionally need to be tackled initially. This arises if, for example, the child is too aggressive or inhibited to co-operate with a direct approach.

The first and often only important measure to take in monosymptomatic enuresis is the provision of reassurance about the nature of the problem, i.e. that it is not a symptom of disease, it is widely prevalent, and there is an overwhelming likelihood that it will clear up on its own, given some time. The child should not be regarded as lazy—he is doing his best. The information should be provided in a form that can be understood by the child as well as the mother. If the symptom is perceived as burdensome, then the doctor should sympathize with this and share the disappointment that the child is one of the minority to show the problem. A 5 year old child at school in a class of 30 can be told it is likely that at least two other children in the class have the same problem. The doctor should also sympathize with the mother's natural tendency to feel angry and irritated about the problem. In young children the doctor should suggest a return visit in a few months to check on progress.

In a child over the age of 5 or 6 years, it is reasonable to take a more active approach.

- First, it is sensible to find out *what the parents have already tried*. Usually parents have tried rather unsystematic rewards and punishment, as well as restricting fluids and lifting at night before they themselves go to bed. The last of these is indeed sometimes successful, but is unlikely to be so if the child is upset by being awakened and refuses to use the toilet.

- *Rewards*. Children may be helped by keeping a star chart or a chart in which they can stick in farm animals for 'dry nights'. Star charts emphasize the child's achievements rather than his failures, and they also ensure that a record of the child's progress is kept. This approach is more likely to be effective if the child and parents are motivated, and if the doctor or nurse show regular interest and enthusiasm.

- *Bladder 'training'*. Daytime wetting may be reduced if the child is encouraged, with parental supervision, to pass urine at gradually lengthening intervals. The assumption behind this approach is that some children have bladders of small functional capacity, and these need gradual expansion. (The basis of the treatment is of doubtful scientific validity, but nevertheless it is sometimes effective.) During a school holiday, the child is encouraged to pass urine (micturate) at intervals of $\frac{1}{2}$ hour on the first day, 1 hour intervals on the second day, $1\frac{1}{2}$ hours on the third day and so on, until there is an interval of 3–4 hours between voiding. Improvement in daytime wetting may be accompanied by an improvement in nocturnal enuresis.

- *Enuresis alarms*. This is the treatment of choice for children aged 6 years and over, living in good social circumstances, for whom reassurance and systematic rewards have proved ineffective (Dische *et al.* 1983). There are various types of alarm available, especially the bell and pad and body-worn alarms, and more recently developed mini-alarm systems. Using the bell and pad system, the child sleeps on two wire-mesh bed mats, connected to a bell or buzzer which goes off when electrical contact is made by the child wetting. When the buzzer goes off the child is awakened, if not already awake, and taken to the toilet. The machine is then reset. The body-worn alarm incorporates a tiny perineal wet sensor attached to a small alarm worn on the child's clothing. This is about as effective, and especially for girls, is more comfortable, but it is somewhat more likely to develop a mechanical fault (Fordham and Meadow 1988).

Both types of procedure require a co-operative child usually sleeping in a room by himself. Parents need to be motivated, and a doctor or nurse experienced in the use of the technique and willing to be in contact personally or over the phone at weekly intervals (or even more frequently initially) to advise over the mechanical problems that may arise. Given these conditions, about two-thirds of children respond favourably to this method of treatment. Some children relapse, but many of these respond to a second course of treatment.

Treatment failures may be due to failure of the parents to understand and follow instructions, false alarms, and failure of the alarm to wake the child (putting the alarm in an empty biscuit tin enhances the noise).

- *Medication*. Tricyclic drugs used in adults for treating depression do produce improvement in a significant number of children. Imipramine or amitriptyline

25–50 mg last thing at night may be prescribed for a 4–6 week period, the dose depending on the age of the child. The mechanism of action of these drugs is unknown. They may work by altering sleep rhythms or by an adrenergic or anticholinergic mechanism, though anticholinergic drugs prescribed alone are ineffective. Relapse usually occurs when the drug is stopped. Bearing in mind the danger of accidental overdosage by toddlers in the family, and the short-lived benefit obtained, most clinicians are reluctant to use drugs for this relatively benign condition, although in one trial they were found to be as effective as an alarm system (Fournier *et al.* 1987). They can be useful when it is important for the child to be dry for a short period, for example when going away on a school journey. Desmopressin has also been reported to be temporarily effective, especially when combined with an enuresis alarm (Bradbury and Meadow 1995).

- *Psychotherapy.* Monosymptomatic enuresis is not an indication for interpretive psychotherapy, though certainly children benefit from the support and understanding of a sympathetic doctor or nurse. However, if the enuresis is associated with symptoms of emotional disturbance, psychotherapeutic measures for the disturbance may also improve the wetting. Conversely, successful symptomatic treatment of enuresis as described above may sometimes reduce other signs of emotional disturbance, perhaps because the child gains generally in confidence and self-esteem.

Outcome

The great majority of children with enuresis will stop wetting before or during adolescence; 90% of children wetting at 7 years will have stopped by 14 years. A very small proportion do continue to wet into adulthood, and there are no well-validated methods of identifying these. Even they are sometimes helped by symptomatic measures applied in adulthood.

4.7 Prepubertal sexual development

4.7.1 NORMAL PREPUBERTAL SEXUAL DEVELOPMENT

Differentiation between the sexes begins in the first 3 months of fetal life. The presence of a Y chromosome in the normal XY male leads to the development of a testis which secretes two types of fetal androgen, up to the time of birth. One androgen promotes masculinization, and the other inhibits feminization. In the chromosomally normal (XX) female, the absence of these androgens results in normal feminization (Money and Ehrhardt 1972).

During the first 7 or 8 years of life, there is little secretion of sex hormones, and little further differentiation between the sexes. At about 7–8 years, there is an increase in pituitary gonadotrophin secretion, leading to a rise in androgen (in both sexes) and oestrogen secretion (in girls).

Psychosexual maturation involves the development of gender identity, gender role behaviour, and sexual behaviour.

Gender identity

Gender identity is the degree to which an individual perceives himself or herself to be male or female. By 3–4 years most children can correctly identify their own sex and that of other children, and have a strong sense of their own essential maleness or femaleness. From then on, gender identity usually remains firmly established.

Gender role behaviour

There are types of behaviour in which the sexes differ. Totally sex-specific behaviour is unusual in our culture, though certain characteristically feminine bodily mannerisms are commonly seen in girls by the age of 5 years, but rarely seen in boys at any age. Doll play, sewing, and cooking activities are much commoner in girls; rough-and-tumble games and play with guns and cars are more common in boys. But there is much overlap, and the differences are closely related to child-rearing practices. A more universal sex-typed characteristic is that, from about the age of 5 years, at least up to the onset of puberty and sometimes well beyond this time, boys prefer to mix and play with boys, and girls with girls. From an early age boys show more aggression and less prosocial behaviour than do girls (Maccoby and Jacklin 1980).

Sexual behaviour

Sexual drive, the wish to achieve sexual pleasure from stimulation of the genitalia, is present from birth and persists through early and middle childhood. As a result of increased androgen secretion, sexual drive increases sharply in early and mid-adolescence to reach a peak in late adolescence and early adulthood. Throughout childhood and adolescence there is a wide individual variation in the degree to which sexual drive is experienced. This variation is probably partly physiologically determined, but the presence or absence of sexually stimulating experiences is also of major importance. Such experiences may affect not only the intensity of sexual drive, but also the choice of sexual object.

Both boys and girls aged between 3 years and early puberty often show a good deal of curiosity about sexual differences and sexual behaviour. Secret games of doctors and nurses in which they examine and sometimes touch each other's genitalia are also common and part of normal behaviour. Children of this age may, however, also become involved in sexual games in which one child is victimized and sexually assaulted. This form of abuse is likely to be carried out by individuals or groups of children showing conduct disorders, and is obviously a cause of concern.

Masturbation

In infancy, occasional self-stimulation of the genitalia to produce pleasurable sensations (masturbation) is common in both boys and girls. It may occur from the first few months of life. Such self-stimulation can lead to orgasm-like phenomena in which the usually somewhat older child of 2–3 years can be observed to be in a state of acute excitement, with rhythmic pelvic movements, rapid respiration, and flushing of the face, followed by a sudden release and period of quiescence. Masturbation is somewhat more common, but is perhaps better concealed, in middle childhood. It is usually of no pathological significance whatsoever. Excessive masturbation may, however, occur and this is discussed below.

4.7.2 ANOMALIES OF GENDER ROLE

Increasingly in our society, boys and girls are encouraged to share activities and interests from an early age. Despite this tendency, sex-role behaviour remains rather sharply distinguished and, in middle childhood, most children prefer to mix in same-sex groups. Nevertheless, it is relatively common for both prepubertal boys and girls to show behaviour that is more common in the opposite sex. For boys this might involve playing with dolls rather than with toy cars, soldiers, and guns and perhaps occasionally dressing in girl's clothing, and, for girls, the reverse would be the case, with, in addition, a preference for rough-and-tumble play. Effeminate behaviour in boys and tomboyish behaviour in girls does cause concern in some parents and teachers. However, around 1 in 20 boys and 1 in 10 girls in a community sample sometimes or frequently behaved like the opposite sex, and, in itself, this is probably of little significance. It is somewhat less common, but again of itself probably of little significance if such boys and girls prefer to play with children of the opposite sex.

Parents and teachers who express concern about their children's behaviour in these respects can be reassured, although the clinician needs to be sure that the child in question does not show features of gender identity disorder (see below). Parents should be discouraged from rewarding the cross-sex behaviour by showing interest or playing along with it in a positive way. It is probably better to reward more conventional sex-appropriate behaviour, although some parents and teachers may object to this for reasons of 'political correctness.' Over time, it is likely that effeminacy in a boy or tomboyishness in a girl will gradually disappear, though in some cases the child may progress to develop a gender identity disorder.

Gender identity disorder

Gender identity disorder is present when, in addition to the cross-sex behaviour described above, a boy shows persistent and intense distress about being male, an intense desire to be a girl, preoccupation with female stereotyped activities such as cross-dressing and participation in girl's games, and repudiation of his own male anatomical structures (penis and testes) (World Health Organization 1992; American Psychiatric Association 1994). Girls show persistent and intense distress about being female, desire to be a boy, marked aversion to girl's clothing, and repudiation of their female anatomical form, often with fantasies of having a penis and testes. In both sexes, there is a wish to play with children of the opposite sex, rather than, as is usual at this age, children of the same sex. The prevalence of gender identity disorder is not known as there have been no population studies of its frequency, but it is probably a good deal less common than occasional cross-sex behaviour. This subject has been well reviewed by Bradley and Zucker (1997).

The aetiology of gender identity disorder is also unclear, though there are some suggestive pointers. Girls with congenital adrenal hyperplasia even though chromosomally male, are reared as girls by their parents. They nevertheless show an unusual amount of tomboyish behaviour. In the prenatal period they are exposed to high levels of androgen, and the possibility that this accounts for their later masculine behaviour is supported by animal studies of the effects of prenatal androgens. On the other hand, there is some evidence supporting psychosocial causation. Clinical evidence suggests that some mothers of children with gender identity disorders would have preferred a child of the opposite sex, and reinforce opposite sex behaviour by the way they dress and encourage cross-sex behaviour.

Management
Children with gender identity disorders should, if possible, be referred to a psychiatric clinic for a full assessment. The disorder may be one feature of a more widespread problem. For example, it is not at all uncommon for younger children with these disorders to show features of an insecure attachment, or older children to show an anxiety state. Some degree of family dysfunction may be present, and a proportion of children have been sexually abused within the family.

Treatment
The treatment will depend a good deal on the presence of other individual or family psychopathology, on the motivation of the parents and the child for change, and on the duration and severity of the disorder. Treatment may need to focus principally on the co-morbid problems. If the child does not want to change his or her sexual identity, but the parents are unhappy or distressed about the situation, a difficult ethical problem may arise. It is however always reasonable to offer parents suggestions about how they can best handle the problem. The removal of secrecy, at least within the family, may do much to remove tension. Subsequently, the school staff may need to be brought into the picture if the child insists on cross-dressing there.

Avoidance of any reinforcement of the cross-sex behaviour, together with gentle encouragement of more conventional activities, may make a difference in less ingrained cases. In more established cases, the parents may need to be helped to accept the child's orientation and the possibility that a homosexual outcome may occur (see below). They may also need help with their own marital difficulties or with the fact that they take different attitudes to the situation. If they are motivated to receive help, and often they are not, children may also benefit from counselling or individual psychotherapy. More formal behavioural methods will be helpful if the child is definitely motivated to change. No physical interventions, either hormonal or surgical, should be considered until well after puberty.

Outcome
In both boys and girls, there is a strong relationship between gender identity disorder and later homosexuality. It is distinctly less common for people who have

shown gender identity disorders in childhood to request operative treatment as part of sex reassignment in adulthood, indeed, only a minority do so. Further, some individuals, who have shown gender identity disorder in childhood, do later develop a heterosexual orientation, with or without treatment.

4.7.3 ANOMALIES OF SEXUAL BEHAVIOUR

Excessive masturbation of worrying degree in infancy and early childhood exists when it is occurring for hours in the day and interferes with the child's regular daily activity and sleep pattern. The child should be examined for the presence of local skin irritation on the penis or vulva, though the presence of sores is more likely to be secondary than primary. Occasionally, a primary lesion may be noted. In an infant, if a local lesion is present, the baby needs restraint to prevent further rubbing, while topical treatment is applied. In the absence of a primary cause, the presence of excessive masturbation should lead to the suspicion that the child is overly self-stimulating because it is generally understimulated. An alternative explanation that should be considered is that the child has been sexually abused. If understimulation is suspected, enquiry into the amount the child is left alone to its own devices should clarify the issue and, if deprivation is present, the implications for management are obvious. In infants where there is no evidence for deprivation, a behavioural approach to reduce the frequency of the habit is indicated. In older preadolescent children, excessive masturbation is very rare, and is usually accompanied by other signs of emotional disturbance. The possibility of sexual abuse should be considered. Assessment should explore wider aspects of the functioning of the child and family and, if sexual abuse is excluded, psychotherapeutic treatment for the child and family is likely to be indicated.

5

Adolescence and psychiatric disorders often beginning in adolescence

5.1 Adolescence

The word 'adolescence' is derived from the Latin *adolescere* (to grow up). The word 'adult' is derived from the same verb (*adultus*, to have grown up). Adolescence is therefore literally the period of growing up and becoming an adult. In western society the term is now mainly used to describe the period from about 12 to about 18 or 19 years, or the period of development from childhood to young adulthood.

Adolescence is marked by physical and social changes. Between 12 and 18 years marked bodily changes occur and, in all societies, the life that young people lead in this phase is eventful and changes considerably.

The physical changes involve:

• the adolescent growth spurt and the completion of physical growth
• sexual maturity.

Social changes in the adolescence of western society involve:

• Reduced dependence on the authority of parents and teachers, and increasing autonomy in decision-making.
• A gradual increase in the influence of others of the same age and a change from mixing in same-sex groups to mixed-sex groups.
• The occurrence of sexual relationships, usually heterosexual, but sometimes homosexual. The physical nature of these relationships may vary from the experience of physical desire with no physical contact to full sexual intercourse.
• Considerable educational demands, usually including the need to take tests and examinations. The results of these mark the adolescent as a high, average, or low achiever, and this often has considerable influence on subsequent career success and income.
• Entry to work and/or higher education, occurring towards the end or at the end of adolescence.
• Gradual achievement of legal permission to engage in adult activities such as buying alcohol and cigarettes, driving a car, and having a vote.

Both physical and social changes occur at varying points of the adolescent life span, so that, for example, in a mixed class of 14 year olds, there will commonly be a number of fully sexual mature girls, and a number of boys who have hardly entered puberty. Many authorities now find it helpful to distinguish between early and late adolescence.

5.1.1 PSYCHOLOGICAL CHANGES

It is much less easy to generalize about psychological changes in adolescence than about physical and social changes. A psychological stereotype of the 'typical' adolescent exists, but there is considerable controversy about the frequency with which the stereotype occurs and about how desirable it is when it does occur (Offer and Schonert-Reichl 1992).

The 'typical' adolescent is sometimes seen as bursting with sexual energy, moody and frequently depressed or even suicidal, prone to temper outbursts especially with parents, unruly, aggressive and untidy, reckless at the steering wheel, promiscuous in social and often sexual relationships, smoking, drinking alcohol, and using illegal drugs. This unattractive picture is barely relieved by adding that the typical adolescent is also seen as altruistic, idealistic, and deeply concerned about global issues such as the preservation of the natural environment. Although controversy about this stereotype exists, there are some points of agreement.

- Most adolescents do not fit into this stereotype. Adolescents have to cope with difficult physical changes in their own bodies, an increase in physical desire, and numerous social changes, but most are reasonably 'well-behaved', have reasonably amicable relationships with their parents, and get on reasonably well with a number of friends.
- Changes in autonomy inevitably bring a certain amount of friction between those in authority, especially parents and teachers, but usually the shift of power in decision-making is achieved reasonably amicably, with respect maintained on both sides.
- When seriously aggressive behaviour or emotional disturbance occurs in adolescence, this needs to be taken as seriously as it is at any other time of life. It is definitely not 'normal' for adolescents to be seriously aggressive or suicidally depressed. There is some evidence that rates of these problems has increased in western societies during the second half of the twentieth century.

Unanswered questions about the psychology of adolescence include:

- Is rebellion in adolescence with experimentation in relationships, clothes, hairstyle, music, drugs, etc. 'natural' and biologically determined by physical and hormonal changes, or are these phenomena socially determined, influenced especially by peer pressure, the media, and marketing forces? Is it 'natural' to have a rebellious adolescence, or is youth culture a manufactured phenomenon?
- Is it desirable to have a rebellious adolescence? Some authorities think this is the case, but others see it as undesirable, especially if it results in painful tensions for both parents and their adolescent children. Have people who go through adolescence without a good deal of experimentation 'missed out', or

have they been lucky? Does going through a rebellious adolescent phase promote later good adult adjustment?

These areas of controversy are important but unresolved. However, the practitioner will need to bear in mind that parents and teenagers themselves often have very decided views on them that may colour their behaviour towards consultation and the need for help considerably. A practitioner, who has a decided view on these issues should remember that not all adolescent patients or clients and their parents will hold the same views.

5.2 Sexual development in adolescence

Normal puberty begins in girls with breast development (between 8 and 13 years) and extends over about 4 years, with menarche occurring in western countries on average at about 13 years. In boys, the first pubertal changes to occur are in the size of the testis, though this is occasionally preceded by growth of pubic hair. Pubertal changes begin between 10 and 15 years, and last over about 5 years before full sexual maturity is reached. The first ejaculation occurs, on average, round about the age of 13 years. Although it is often assumed that puberty occurs much earlier than used to be the case, in fact, girls in the 1990s go through puberty only a month or two earlier than did those in the 1940s (Wellings *et al.* 1994). Changes in the age of menarche were much more marked in the nineteenth century.

5.2.1 EFFECTS OF EARLY AND LATE PUBERTY

There is a very wide range of ages over which normal puberty occurs. Within the normal range, there are certain characteristics associated with early and late maturation. Early-maturing boys are likely, on average, to be slightly more intelligent and educationally advanced, and to retain these advantages after puberty (Douglas *et al.* 1968). They are also likely to be more confident and assertive (Clausen 1975). Early-maturing girls are also likely to have some intellectual advantages, but positive personality characteristics are more likely to be linked to average, rather than to early, physical maturation (Tobin-Richards *et al.* 1982). In most societies, girls do not particularly like to be different from their peers, and either very early or late maturation may result in social discomfort. Early maturing girls are likely to be especially dissatisfied with the weight gain accompanying puberty and to show low self-esteem (Alsaker 1995). They may also show more behaviour problems. Adolescent boys do not wish to be conspicuous either, but early male maturation provides physical advantages relating to muscular strength that are particularly valued by boys.

Psychosexual maturation involves the development of:

- gender identity
- sex-typed forms of non-sexual behaviour (gender role)
- sexual behaviour.

5.2.2 SEXUAL BEHAVIOUR IN ADOLESCENCE

Masturbation

The great majority of adolescent boys masturbate at least occasionally to achieve sexual pleasure and relief of sexual tension, and probably most masturbate regularly. The habit is probably less common in girls, some of whom may masturbate only occasionally or not at all, though accurate estimates of prevalence are not readily obtainable. There is no evidence that the presence or absence of masturbation in either sex is of any pathological significance.

Problems involving masturbation in adolescence are of two main kinds. In some mentally handicapped teenagers, the habit is practised in public, often to the embarrassment and distress of parents. The teenager should be told to go to his own room when he starts to masturbate, and the parents can be encouraged to be very firm about this. Usually, but not always, this approach resolves the problem. If it does not, a behavioural programme should be instituted.

Some teenagers of normal intelligence experience severe guilt feelings in relation to masturbation. Reassurance about the universality of the habit usually does not resolve the problem, as the teenager has usually been reassured by others many times before. The guilt may be associated with obsessional preoccupations about pollution, and may be accompanied by depressive feelings. Alternatively, the teenager may be in a state of acute concern about religious issues, the nature of existence, etc., and persistent, distressing masturbatory guilt may be linked to worries of a much wider nature. In either event, if the youngster is motivated to attend, assessment of the psychiatric state followed by the opportunity for focused psychotherapeutic interviews or a cognitive behavioural programme may be helpful.

Heterosexual behaviour

The occurrence of sexual behaviour in prepubertal children is discussed briefly in Section 4.7.1. As soon as children enter puberty, the frequency of heterosexual behaviour increases rapidly, though many young people do, in fact, remain sexually inexperienced throughout their adolescence. The average age of first sexual experience of any type, such as kissing, cuddling, or petting is now around 13 years for boys and 14 years for girls. The average age of first full sexual intercourse is around 17 years for both sexes. The proportion of young women experiencing full intercourse before the age of 16 years increased from under 1% in the 1940s to around 20% in the early 1990s, with the increase in young men over this period being from around 5% to around 30% (Wellings *et al.* 1994). Although this change is often attributed to earlier sexual maturation, in fact the biological changes over this period have been quite small. For example, the age of menarche has only declined from around 13.5 years to around 13.4 years. Although information is less readily available on this subject, it is also likely that young people have more sexual partners than used to be the case. Problems associated with heterosexual behaviour include sexually transmitted diseases (not discussed in this volume), depression associated with loss of sexual partner, unprotected sexual intercourse and teenage pregnancy (see below) and parental concern about disapproved sexual behaviour in their children.

5.2.3 HOMOSEXUAL BEHAVIOUR IN BOYS

The frequency with which preadolescent and adolescent boys are involved in occasional or regular homosexual activity (usually mutual masturbation) is unknown. It is, however, fairly common and surveys suggest it probably occurs in about a fifth of the male population. It is more common in boys at single-sex boarding schools, and opportunity, or lack of it, for heterosexual activity is likely to play a considerable part. In that only about 3% of the adult male population is actively homosexual (Wellings *et al.* 1994), it is clear that only a small proportion of boys involved in homosexuality in childhood and early adolescence go on to show adult homosexuality.

Aetiology

Some studies using chromosome mapping suggest a genetic cause. Concordance for homosexuality is higher in monozygotic than dizygotic twins, again suggesting a genetic contribution. Studies of children with intersex conditions strongly suggest that both gender identity and sex-role activity are largely determined by child-rearing practices—the way in which the child is brought up—but the evidence for a biological, perhaps genetic contribution, is increasing.

Clinical features and management

Although homosexual behaviour is not at all uncommon in adolescence, it is an unusual presenting problem in both psychiatric and paediatric practice. More commonly, depression in adolescence is accompanied by fears of homosexuality that may or may not be realistic. Alternatively, parents may have justified or unjustified fears that their son or daughter is showing homosexual behaviour. In both these circumstances, the main task is to help the teenager or parents express their thoughts and feelings about the matter, and to provide relevant information. A non-judgemental approach with communication about the frequency of the problem and the degree to which it will realistically interfere with the individual's life will often be found supportive and helpful.

Parents who are concerned that their prepubertal sons are involved in homosexual activity can usually be reassured about the significance of the behaviour for later sexuality. Mid- and late-adolescent boys who show preference for sexual activity with other boys or men, when opportunity for sexual activity with girls is available, are more likely to be homosexual later. In earlier childhood there is probably little significance in homosexual or bisexual activity, unless it is part of a gender identity disorder (Section 4.7.2).

5.2.4 HOMOSEXUAL ACTIVITY IN GIRLS

Homosexual activity in girls is less common than it is in boys, probably occurring in about 10% of preadolescent girls in our society. Again, as homosexuality is only present in 1–2% of the adult female population, most girls involved in homosexual activity must grow up to be heterosexual or bisexual adults. A homosexual outcome is more common in girls who show marked a gender identity disorder of childhood, as well as in those whose homosexual activity persists into mid and late adolescence.

5.3 Early pregnancy

The rate of pregnancy in girls between 13 and 15 years has remained rather stable in the UK since the 1980s at between 8 and 9 per 1000 (Office of National Statistics 1996) Official statistics suggest that about half such pregnancies are terminated. The rate in 16–19 year olds is around 55–60 per 1000, with about one-third terminated. The UK has the highest teenage pregnancy rate in western Europe.

5.3.1 BACKGROUND INFORMATION

Most pregnancies in young teenagers occur in girls who have had relationships with the fathers for several months or even years, and are not the result of a brief promiscuous relationship. A significant number of such pregnancies are not seen as unwelcome by the girls themselves. A common problem is that the couple are in dispute with their parents about their relationship, and one or both may feel rejected. They are likely to be relatively ignorant about birth control methods. In a significant minority of cases, the pregnancy appears to be an unconscious attempt to achieve status and love in a girl with low self-esteem who feels unwanted by her parents.

There are strong health, educational and social disadvantages to such early pregnancy (NHS Centre for Reviews and Dissemination 1997):

- Pregnancy complications, such as toxaemia, and birth complications are more frequent.
- The girl's schooling is usually interrupted and may well terminate at this point.
- Her social relationships are often disrupted, both within the family and with her friends, and her employment prospects are impaired.
- Children of teenage mothers have a higher risk of sudden infant death syndrome and of prematurity.
- They are more likely to show developmental delays and have an increased risk of living in poverty.

The psychological aftermath of a termination may be very distressing. If the pregnancy is continued and the child adopted, this too is very upsetting, while if the girl continues to look after her baby, it will often receive inadequate care. It should be emphasized that these aspects of outcome are distinctly less prominent in girls who become pregnant in their late teens, though even here some social disadvantage to mother and child is likely to occur.

5.3.2 MANAGEMENT

Prevention of teenage pregnancy is discussed in Chapter 9. However, given that a high proportion of such pregnancies proceed to term, it is important to manage the situation in ways that will reduce the risks to mother and child as much as possible. Good antenatal care is sometimes difficult to provide in the early stages, as the pregnancy may be concealed. Once it has been identified, close monitoring, using a comprehensive approach with an attempt to provide psychosocial support and cut down smoking, will result in a better outcome. Home-based parenting programmes run by statutory services staffed by health visitors or by voluntary organizations improve parent–child interactions. Pre-school education and support should take into account the need of the young mother to continue her own education and training for employment. Many local authorities provide special centres for schoolgirl mothers. Mental health professionals should be aware of the availability of such facilities in their areas, and try to ensure that they take into account the psychological needs of both young mothers and their children, as early intervention may result in lower rates of psychiatric problems developing in this high risk group.

5.4 Anorexia nervosa

5.4.1 DEFINITION

Anorexia nervosa is a condition defined by the presence of significant, self-induced weight loss (or in the case of pre-pubertal children, failure to gain weight), body-image distortion, and a widespread endocrine disorder involving the hypothalamic–pituitary–gonadal axis resulting in delayed menarche or secondary amenorrhoea (World Health Organization 1992). The DSM-IV criteria (American Psychiatric Association 1994) comprise:

- refusal to maintain body weight
- intense fear of gaining weight
- disturbance in the experience of body weight, size, or shape
- primary or secondary amenorrhoea

Bulimia nervosa is characterized by preoccupation with eating and a craving for food. Overeating binges are followed by self-induced vomiting. This condition is not described in detail here because it mainly starts in late adolescence and early adulthood.

5.4.2 CLINICAL FEATURES

Age of onset

The age of onset of anorexia nervosa may be anything from 6 to 60 years, but the great majority of cases begin between 14 and 19 years of age. In one study of early-onset anorexia nervosa, age of onset varied from 7.7 to 13.7 years (Fosson *et al.* 1987). Dieting and loss of weight are the central, characteristic features of the condition. Onset of dieting behaviour may be sudden or gradual extending over weeks or months. There may be an obvious precipitating factor—commonly a group of girls has decided to lose weight together; most fail to lose any but a minority do lose weight and then stop dieting. One goes on to develop anorexia. Alternatively, a rather solitary, introverted girl may develop the condition following a chance remark about her appearance and need to lose weight. Girls who develop anorexia nervosa tend to have low self-esteem even before the dieting behaviour begins (Button *et al.* 1996).

Dieting

Initially dieting may be hidden from the rest of the family, or it may be overt. After a time it becomes apparent that there has been a marked reduction in food intake, and this leads to family arguments at meals. Frequently parents will press food on to the girl, and she will respond by eating less and less, cutting food up into small pieces, spending an apparently interminable time eating tiny quantities. Girls may enhance the effects of reduced food intake by taking drugs such as purgatives, appetite suppressants, or diuretics, or by self-induced vomiting, though this is unusual in the younger age group. Some girls also exercise in order to lose further weight.

Excessive dieting may alternate with episodes of binge-eating (bulimia). The bingeing may involve eating vast quantities of food, or quantities that the girl perceives to be enormous but are really quite normal. Again this is not a common feature in younger patients, though it is a central feature of bulimia nervosa.

The dieting behaviour is based on a morbid fear of becoming fat. Usually there are particular areas of the body the girl is particularly worried about, and these include especially the thighs, buttocks, breasts, and abdomen. The reasons why the girl has such an excessive fear of fatness are often, at least partly, unconscious, but occasionally a girl may attribute her desire to be thin to her wish to be attractive and popular. It is most unusual for girls to admit they are trying to avoid the biological changes of adolescence or womanhood.

Bodily misperception

Accompanying the morbid fear of fat, there is also frequently a misperception of bodily appearance—the girl overestimating the size of her thighs, stomach, etc. in comparison with other girls. As she genuinely perceives herself to be bigger than she really is, this misperception leads to further family conflict and arguments. It is also common for girls to misperceive the quantities of food they are given to eat, believing that their mothers are giving them excessive quantities, perhaps in order to make them fat.

The referral of the patient may occur for reasons other than loss of weight. It is quite common for girls to present to their family doctor with other symptoms such as constipation or amenorrhoea.

Other eating disorder syndromes

These include food avoidance, emotional disorder and selective eating (Lask and Bryant-Waugh 1993). In bulimia nervosa, the overeating or bingeing is a more prominent feature than undereating, but periodic dieting behaviour does occur, and the central psychopathological feature remains a fear of becoming fat (Russell 1979). Another characteristic picture, more commonly seen by primary care practitioners, is a marked preoccupation with physical appearance and constant ineffectual dieting, unaccompanied by amenorrhoea or even excessive loss of weight. Nevertheless, the condition is different from normal dieting in that the preoccupation with food and appearance 'takes over' the patient's life and causes a great deal of suffering.

Physical examination

In moderate or severe classical cases, this is usually negative, apart from the presence of signs of undernourishment. Parts of the body may be covered with lanugo or fine downy hair, but elsewhere the skin may be coarse and tough. Blood pressure may be reduced, and in severe cases hypothermia may be present. Laboratory investigations are usually also negative, though there may be a reduction of gonadotrophin levels, with low blood levels of oestrogens, luteinizing hormone, and follicle stimulating hormone. In contrast, there may be elevated levels of cortisol and growth hormone. The hormonal disturbance is of hypothalamic or suprahypothalamic type. A pelvic ultrasound scan reveals ovarian immaturity, and is increasingly undertaken as a measure of severity and progress following treatment. Gonadotrophin levels are also reduced in males. In adolescents who are severely affected, osteoporosis may occur, and cardiovascular effects include bradycardia and arrhythmias.

5.4.3 BACKGROUND INFORMATION

Prevalence

Anorexia nervosa occurs classically in about 0.1–0.2% of adolescent girls (Bryant-Waugh and Lask 1995). However, atypical mild forms occur more commonly than this in the age group at particular risk. The condition may be increasing in frequency, though there is some doubt about this (Fombonne 1995). It is extremely unusual in developing countries, though it is just beginning to occur among girls in westernized families living in large cities. The condition is more common among certain groups selected for thinness, such as ballet dancers, gymnasts, and models. However, girls in these occupations are much more likely to show extreme forms of diet control without other features of anorexia nervosa.

Family factors

There is a familial tendency to the condition, and sibs are affected more commonly than one would expect by chance. Twin studies suggest that there is a genetically determined element to the condition (Holland *et al.* 1988), and without this genetic predisposition the condition will not occur. It is more common in middle-class adolescents, and often in those who are regarded as unusually 'good' children, with a particularly high moral standard of behaviour, strongly influenced by the 'work ethic'. Mothers may be unusually critical of their daughters (Van Furth *et al.* 1996). Characteristic patterns of family functioning have been described in which there is overprotectiveness, linked to inadequate patterns of communication about feelings. Consequently, the overprotected girl is unable to establish her own individuality and autonomy, and, because of poor communication, she cannot protest and make her views and feelings known. Establishing control, at least over her food intake, is her means of achieving autonomy, but she only does this at tremendous cost to her physical health and social relationships. This pattern of family relationships, while certainly sometimes found, is not universal, and there is a wide variation of family pattern. It is important to realize that much family disturbance is secondary to the condition. Sexual abuse has been reported to be a common background factor, but appears to be no more frequent than in other psychiatric disorders (Vize and Cooper 1995).

Personality

Many, but not all, affected girls, have a history of unusually conforming behaviour. They tend to be quiet and somewhat compulsively altruistic, often wanting to train to be nurses or air hostesses, or attracted to other occupations in which service to others is a prominent feature. Again this is not universally found. What does seem more common in the psychopathology of patients is a lack of desire to enter the adult world of womanhood with its implications for independence, sexuality, and motherhood. The primary fear of fatness can, at least sometimes, be seen as a wish to avoid the rounded contours of female adolescence.

Societal factors

Probably societal attitudes to female appearance are of relevance. The condition is less common in societies where a rounded female figure is the desirable norm. In western industrialized countries, the 'perfect' figure (as evidenced by the vital statistics of pin-ups on magazine covers) has, at least since the 1970s, steadily approximated to a drainpipe shape.

   The endocrine changes that occur in the condition, such as the reduction in gonadotrophins, are probably secondary, although, once established, they may inhibit recovery. As discussed below, psychological improvement sometimes occurs rather rapidly once the physical changes produced by malnutrition are reversed. Physical factors may, therefore, be of little importance in primary causation but of major significance in the maintenance of the condition. The lack of primary importance of endocrine factors is confirmed by the occasional presence of the condition in classical form (apart, of course, from amenorrhoea) in hormonally normal males. Males are affected 10–15 times less commonly than females. However, in prepubertal children, sex differences in prevalence are much less marked with a female preponderance of only 3 or 4 to 1 (Fosson *et al.* 1987).

Neurochemical factors

Although most of the endocrine and metabolic changes are probably secondary to starvation, evidence for a primary neurochemical abnormality also exists

(Herzog and Copeland 1985). Increased endogenous opioid activity has been detected, and decreased levels of norepinephrine in cerebrospinal fluid persist after weight recovery.

5.4.4 ASSESSMENT

The form of the initial assessment will depend on whether this takes place in the general practitioner's consulting room, in a paediatric or general medical out-patient department, or in a psychiatric setting. In all settings, however, once the diagnosis is suspected, it is desirable to see both parents and the girl together so that the problems (including fear of fatness, dieting, binge eating, overexercising, etc.) can be identified within the family as openly as possible. Especially relevant are a description of mealtimes and the parental attitude to the girl's growing independence. Her previous personality and the means by which the family communicates and resolves problems more generally are also informative. Many girls are secretive about their dieting and exercise habits, and their statements cannot always be accepted at face value.

Some time should be spent with the girl alone, in order to attempt to establish her own view of the situation and attitudes to adolescence, sexuality, and womanhood. Other aspects of special relevance include her mood, the presence of any actual bodily delusions, as well as her level of weight and motivation for change. It is helpful to ask questions such as 'What would your ideal weight be?' and 'Are there any parts of your body you feel especially concerned about?' Physical examination should include obtaining an accurate height and weight (wearing only underwear), and noting pubertal status, and signs of malnutrition. If the latter are present, or a significant amount of weight has been lost, then further physical investigations will be required,

There are both physical and psychiatric conditions with which anorexia may be confused. Physical conditions include malabsorption syndromes and endo-crine disorders such as hypopituitarism. A careful history and physical examin-ation should allow exclusion of such conditions. It is important to remember that anorexia nervosa may coexist with physical syndromes. In particular, a link has been described with Turner syndrome and diabetes mellitus.

Psychiatric states that may be confused include depressive disorders and, much less commonly, schizophrenia. Many girls with anorexia nervosa do not suffer from a depressive reaction, and indeed their capacity to remain cheerful in the face of their apparently appalling predicament is rather characteristic. Neverthe-less, a significant number of girls are seriously depressed, and here the problem is to know whether the depression is primary with secondary loss of appetite and weight, or vice versa. The presence of other depressive symptomatology and attitudes to bodily appearance will usually clarify the diagnosis, but mixed pictures are seen especially in the younger age group. Depressed girls usually have a reduced appetite (normal in anorexia nervosa) and they usually wish to gain weight normally. Their activity level tends to be reduced. The presence of strongly delusional ideas related to bodily appearance may raise the possibility of schizophrenia. A small minority of girls presenting with apparently classical anorexia nervosa do develop unmistakable signs of schizophrenia. Males with anorexia nervosa share most of the features of the classical condition, except of course the amenorrhoea, but they are less likely to come from middle-class families.

5.4.5 TREATMENT

Once the diagnosis has been made, the nature of the condition should be explained to both the girl and her parents, if possible together. The condition is increasingly treated on an out-patient or day-patient basis, but loss of more than a few pounds in weight is an indication for in-patient assessment and treatment. A trial of out-patient treatment lasting a month or two can be followed by in-patient admission if unsuccessful. Earlier admission would be indicated if the weight loss worsened, there was evidence of definite metabolic disturbance or hypotension, or there was severe depression with risk of suicide.

Medication has only a small part to play in management. Appetite stimulants are unhelpful. The presence of severe anxiety and tension calls for the use of an anxiolytic agent, such as chlorpromazine. Tricyclic antidepressant medication may be used on a short-term basis if depressive features are prominent.

The mainstay of treatment, whether on out- or in-patient basis, is the use of a firm approach to weight gain followed by supportive and sometimes interpretive psychotherapy to the patient and family. Few girls accept admission to hospital easily. In most cases a family interview is necessary to point out to both the parents and the girl that anorexia nervosa is a life-threatening illness, and that, even if survival is not in question, the girl cannot be healthy or lead a normal adult life later on unless she is well nourished. By the time of presentation it is common for the patient to be dominating the family and to attempt to refuse admission. In these circumstances, the clinician should point out the inappropriateness of the child being in control, affirm the seriousness of the condition, and encourage the parents to assert their authority in the girls' best interest. With this approach, compulsory admission is very rarely necessary. Mild cases may be managed on an out-patient basis.

A target weight range should be established between 90 and 110% of the mean weight for the patient's height and age. The patient and family should be told that full health cannot be achieved until weight is maintained within this range. The girl should, in consultation with the dietitian, be given a diet on which she might expect to gain 1.5–2 kg (3–4 lb) a week. One or two food dislikes may be respected, but, in general, the girl should be expected to eat a full range of foods. Quarter- or half-portions may be presented for the first week or two, and the food should be presented in as palatable a way as possible. If weight loss has been severe, the patient should be nursed in bed until an agreed intermediate weight is reached, at which point limited, and then full, activity can be allowed. Tube feeding is very rarely required, and should not be employed except as a life-saving procedure. Twice-weekly weighing on accurate scales in underclothes is adequate to assess progress. Many patients are worried about becoming overweight, and these should be reassured that, at least while in hospital, nursing staff will see this does not happen. There are advantages if the criterion for progress is weight gain and not food intake, as the latter may be subject to distortion by the girl. Some authorities do, however, use food intake as a criterion of satisfactory progress. Improvement in food intake and weight gain may be accompanied by difficult behaviour, and it should be explaining to parents beforehand that this may occur and is indeed an encouraging sign.

Once the target range of weight is reached, it must be maintained; family meals in the in-patient unit, followed by weekends home, allow assessment of progress in this respect. During the period of weight gain and immediately afterwards, it is usually unwise to comment favourably on the girl's improved appearance. She may not regard herself as looking better, and such remarks can precipitate relapse. During this period of rehabilitation family interviews are particularly helpful, not just to allow exploration of feelings about the girl's eating habits, but also to discuss other issues concerning autonomy, decision-making, and communication in the family. Marital problems between the parents sometimes emerge at this point and may require separate sessions. If they are prepared to come, the presence of any sibs at these interviews can be additionally helpful. Once acceptable weight gain has been achieved, individual psychotherapeutic interviews also become more worthwhile, and it is often then possible for the first time to explore concerns about the meaning of adolescent bodily changes, sexuality, and adulthood with the girl. The girl can be helped to achieve more autonomy in decision-making, and to feel more in control of her life generally. Both family and ego-oriented individual psychotherapy can be helpful (Robin *et al.* 1994) though one study found that family therapy was more helpful with the younger patient (Russell *et al.* 1987). Even after full recovery in a prepubertal girl, height gain can be disappointingly slow. If periods fail to start when the girl has reached normal weight, clomiphene can be helpful to stimulate menstruation.

After discharge from hospital, contact with the girl and her family should be maintained to monitor weight and review general progress. A point of stability is usually reached after a few months in which it becomes clear that further intervention is not likely to achieve further change.

5.4.6 OUTCOME

With these measures, a proportion of girls, perhaps about a third, appear to make a full recovery (Hsu *et al.* 1979). Their attitude to their bodily appearance appears normal, and they no longer seem to have concerns about adolescent development. About a third retain a reasonable body weight, but they remain morbidly preoccupied with their appearance and often have other personality problems affecting especially their relationships with the opposite sex. Finally, a third, after perhaps failing to reach satisfactory weight, or after reaching it only with very great difficulty, fail to maintain it and may either be chronically underweight or develop periodic bingeing with consequent weight fluctuations. Girls in this group who have developed the condition before puberty may remain of short stature and never menstruate. Personality problems remain severe in this group. Suicidal attempts are not uncommon and about 5% do commit suicide. The mothering capacity of the intermediate group may be impaired, and they may have particular difficulties in feeding their babies and young children (Stein *et al.* 1994). The more severely affected will rarely marry. Full recovery may, however, be followed by a normal fertility rate and mothering capacity (Brinch *et al.* 1988). Poor prognostic factors in prepubertal children include early age of onset, depression during the illness, and disturbed family relationships (Bryant-Waugh *et al.* 1988). Severe cases requiring re-admission often do particularly poorly.

5.5 Adult-type psychiatric disorders

The major psychiatric classification systems distinguish between

- behaviour and emotional disorders with an onset usually occurring in child-hood or adolescence
- developmental disorders
- forms of disorder usually occurring for the first time in adulthood.

These last may occur in childhood and indeed, as knowledge has advanced, it has become clear that many of them do begin earlier than had been thought to be the case. Further, even though these adult-type disorders may not begin in full-blown form in childhood, recent studies have demonstrated that the adults suffering them have shown specific behavioural traits in childhood. The distinction between childhood-onset disorders and adult-onset disorders is therefore more blurred than the chapter headings of this book might suggest.

In neurotic, somatoform, and stress-related disorders, the child develops a maladaptive pattern of behaviour together with emotional disturbance. The pattern of behaviour may be very clearly related to stressful events or may appear to arise independently. More commonly the events that occur in the child's life are relevant to some degree, but the child's personality and early experience mould his response in a fashion characteristic to him.

Although in the major classification systems anxiety and depressive states are categorized as neurotic disorders, in this book they are dealt with in Section 4.4 as deviations of development. This is because, in childhood, maladaptive forms of behaviour and disturbances of emotional life seem more logically considered in terms of the child's development than as conditions arising *de novo*.

5.5.1 OBSESSIONAL DISORDERS

Definition

Normal children often show rituals in their early years. Particularly between the ages of 4 and 8 years, children may take great care to avoid the cracks while walking on pavements, hate to be parted from favourite toys, or line up their possessions in a very particular way. Such behaviour persists into adult life in the form of superstitious beliefs and practices. When irrational thoughts or behaviour of this type become handicapping, they form part of an obsessive–compulsive disorder.

- *Obsessions* can be defined as recurrent and persistent ideas that are experienced as senseless and which the individual tries to suppress.
- *Compulsions* are repetitive forms of purposeful behaviour performed in response to an obsession and aimed in some way at warding off the obsessive idea or some dreaded event (American Psychiatric Association 1994).

Clinical features

The onset may be slow and the disorder only gradually come to notice, or there may be a fairly rapid onset (Rapoport 1986). Children as young as 6 years may be affected, but the condition is commoner in mid-childhood and adolescence. Characteristically the child is noted to be spending a longer and longer time in the bathroom, repeatedly washing to prevent contamination. Homework may be repeatedly checked and takes an inordinate length of time. Bedtime rituals may be prolonged for hours while the child adjusts and readjusts the bedclothes or objects around him. At mealtimes the child may only be prepared to use certain utensils. There may be odd behaviour—for example, the child nearly always needing to go through a particular series of repeated movements with his feet before going through a particular door.

Obsessional thoughts are less common and may only be elicited on direct questioning. They are likely to take the form of unwelcome aggressive or depressive ideas (e.g. that the child's parents or he himself will die, or that he himself will harm someone) that the child cannot get out of his mind.

Attempts to change the child's behaviour by parents are met by resistance. There may be a transient improvement followed by a relapse. In severe cases the child will try, often successfully, to insist that family members alter their behaviour to fit in with his obsession. Manipulative behaviour may consist, for example, in getting the family to sit at table in a particular grouping.

The child is likely to be generally quiet and shy, as well as perfectionist. In some cases there is great variation in behaviour, the child being excessively neat and tidy in some respects, but slapdash in others. Children with tics, Tourette syndrome, and anorexia nervosa have high rates of obsessional symptoms (Rapoport 1986).

Associated anxiety, specific fears, and depression are relatively common. Such children do not usually show aggressive behaviour, but occasionally episodes when the child's obsessional behaviour is less prominent may be accompanied by increased rudeness and disobedience.

On examination the child may deny or attempt to minimize the extent of his ritualistic behaviour. He may also deny that he is in any way upset. Sometimes, however, there is considerable sadness and misery accompanying the child's feelings of helplessness in the face of his own behaviour. The child may be able to explain how his rituals arise—perhaps on the basis of superstitious thoughts that unless he carries them out, he feels some terrible event will occur. Feelings of 'internal resistance' (i.e. sensations of an internal struggle against obsessional thoughts or compulsive behaviour) which are often described by adults are not commonly expressed by children.

Prevalence

Relatively transient checking behaviour and bedtime rituals are common in childhood. Obsessional symptoms also commonly occur as minor features in emotional and depressive disorders. However, fully developed obsessional conditions are much less common. They have been described as occurring in American high school students at a rate of around 3%. A higher proportion, around 19%, have a subclinical condition with symptoms but little or no social impairment (Valleni-Basile *et al.* 1994).

Aetiology

Genetic and environmental influences

There is often a strong family history with about two-thirds of parents showing obsessional tendencies and about 5% obsessional disorders. Twin studies suggest a genetic influence in obsessional personality traits. Case reports suggest the condition may occur following brain injury or infection with the β-haemolytic streptoccus (Allen *et al.* 1995a). There is also, however, an environmental component, with parents of obsessional children having higher educational expectations and generally high standards of conduct.

Mechanisms

Obsessional symptoms have been seen as arising from brain dysfunction or from cognitive distortions especially relating to unresolved perceptions of threat (Bolton 1996). These are, of course, not mutually exclusive explanations, and cognitive distortion may arise as a result of genetically determined brain dysfunction. These symptoms can also be seen as exaggerations of adaptive behaviour, for repeated checking against danger is a form of behaviour with survival value.

Assessment

Particular attention should be given to the extent and severity of the obsessional symptomatology and the circumstances in which it occurs. Differentiation from normal forms of ritualistic behaviour needs to be made. The child's manipulation of other family members and responses of the family to the behaviour may be of great significance. Enquiry should be made as to the presence of associated symptoms of emotional disorder and aggression. The nature of obsessional thoughts should be probed to exclude the possibility of delusional beliefs. Obsessional symptoms may occur in emotional disorders and schizophrenia as well as in obsessional disorder.

Treatment

This can usually be carried out on an out-patient basis, though where the condition is well entrenched and severely handicapping, and the responses of family members are perpetuating the problem, admission to an in-patient psychiatric unit may be indicated. Admission often results in an immediate rapid reduction of symptoms, but these may recur when the parents visit or the child goes home for a weekend.

Counselling and support for the family are therefore indicated, either in family interviews or with parents seen separately. Parents should be encouraged to resist manipulation by the child. In established, severe cases this approach is unlikely to be effective in itself.

Behavioural approaches have been reported to have considerable success in adolescents (March 1995; Shafran 1998). The most effective technique is exposure and response prevention (Section 9.2.1). Following a baseline period, the child is encouraged to reduce compulsive behaviour by a self-imposed graded regime. Parental co-operation in cutting down the behaviour is also required. External constraint by nursing staff on an in-patient basis may be necessary in severe cases that fail to respond to out-patient treatment.

Medication
The use of the tricyclic drug clomipramine has been recommended as of specific value in obsessional disorders. There is evidence for its effectiveness in adolescence and it is worth using as an adjuvant to other therapy (DeVeaugh-Geiss *et al.* 1992). Fluoxetine has also been shown to be of value (Riddle *et al.* 1992).

Individual psychotherapy
Insight-orientated individual psychotherapy has been reported to produce good results (Hollingworth *et al.* 1980). Probably neither individual nor family therapy alone is as effective as behavioural approaches combined with counselling and medication, but they can be useful adjuvants.

Outcome

Reports of treated series of cases suggest that the condition is often persistent over time, though symptomatology may vary (Rettew *et al.* 1992). In one series of children followed for 2–7 years, three-quarters persisted, and those treated with clomipramine did no better than those untreated with this medication (Flament *et al.* 1990). Many severe and intractable cases of adult obsessional disorder have begun in adolescence, so clearly there are a significant number of early-onset cases that have a chronic course.

5.5.2 PSYCHOSOMATIC SYMPTOMS AND SOMATOFORM DISORDERS

There is a sense in which all disorders are or may be psychosomatic, but some are more psychosomatic than others! The psychological and the physical can interact in a number of different ways. For example:

- *Stressful events* can impinge on an individual who has a vulnerable organ system to produce physiological changes. These then result in physical symptoms. Thus in an individual who has a vulnerable bronchial system, excitement or disappointment may produce physiological changes which result in an asthmatic attack. This type of interaction occurs in some cases of peptic ulcer, abdominal pain, and migraine. Indeed, these are sometimes called psychosomatic disorders. However, some children with asthma and peptic ulcer have no psychological reasons for any of their symptoms, others may have some attacks that are 'psychological', and others attacks that occur for different reasons such as infection or allergy. So it is better to refer to *psychosomatic interactions* than to psychosomatic disorders.

- Some psychiatric disorders are accompanied by physical symptomatology. For example, girls with anorexia nervosa may, in severe cases, develop hypothermia or amenorrhoea. The psychiatric disorder itself is likely to occur as a result of a combination of constitutional and environmental factors.
- Some lifestyles predispose to physical or psychiatric illness or disability. Thus a sedentary lifestyle or an unhealthy diet may predispose to obesity. Excessive alcohol consumption may result in gastritis or alcohol dependency. Some types of psychiatric disorder predispose to a risky or unhealthy life style. For example, children with attention deficit hyperactivity disorder are at unusual risk of road traffic and other accidental injuries.
- Illnesses or disabilities, such as Down syndrome or diabetes mellitus, that are entirely physical in nature, may impact on the life of a child in such a way that they cause psychological distress or psychiatric disorder. This type of interaction is sometimes termed *somatopsychic*.
- Finally, physical symptoms may occur that have no organic basis. Such medically undiagnosed physical symptomatology is grouped together in the official classification systems as *somatoform disorder*. Types of somatoform disorder include conversion disorders, chronic fatigue syndrome (also known as myalgic encephalopathy), pain syndromes, hypochondriasis, and somatization disorder. The last two of these are little described and probably very unusual in childhood and adolescence (Fritz *et al.* 1997). The first three, conversion disorder, pain syndromes exemplified by headache, and chronic fatigue syndrome, are dealt with in this section. The other types of psychosomatic interaction described above are dealt with elsewhere in the book.

Conversion disorder

In conversion disorder physical symptoms (such as paralysis), or mental symptoms (such as loss of memory), which usually signify physical disease are present in the absence of evidence of such physical disease. Conversion disorders (which used to be called *hysterical disorders*) are classified in ICD-10 (World Health Organization 1992) as a form of *dissociative disorder*, and in DSM IV (American Psychiatric Association 1994) as a *somatoform disorder*. *Conversion* and *dissociation* are terms used to describe unconscious psychological mechanisms.

- *Conversion* is said to occur when an emotional conflict is transformed into a physical disability. This may occur in a way that has obvious symbolic significance, for example weakness of the hand in a conflict over aggression, or it may merely allow the child to avoid an unwanted situation (secondary gain).
- *Dissociation* occurs when one part of mental life is split off from another.

These concepts are often difficult to apply because, not infrequently, conversion symptoms are present, yet convincing evidence for these psychological mechanisms is lacking.

Conversion disorder can usually be seen as a type of 'abnormal illness behaviour' occurring when a child develops a need to be a patient when he is not physically ill even when he has to suffer inconvenience and disability (Mechanic 1978). Being ill can be seen as a pattern of behaviour. A physically ill child behaves appropriately when he goes to the doctor, takes time off school, acknowledges sympathy, etc. The child can be seen to be enjoying the benefits of the 'sick role' (Parsons 1951). Many clinicians now find this framework of 'illness behaviour' the most helpful, but in a minority of cases, it still seems necessary to invoke unconscious mental processes as important in causation.

Prevalence
Conversion disorders are unusual throughout childhood, and very rare indeed before the age of 7–8 years. Their precise prevalence is uncertain because of problems of definition, but is probably less than 1 per 1000 children. The rate increases in adolescence. The sex ratio in childhood is equal, but, by adolescence, more girls than boys suffer from the condition. There is no particular relationship with social class. The condition is much more common in some economically less developed countries than it is in western societies (Fritz *et al.* 1997).

Clinical features
Children or teenagers may suffer from 'active' symptoms such as pain in a limb, pseudoseizures, or other abnormal movements. Alternatively, they may show a deficit of function. Types of deficit include aphasia, aphonia, visual or hearing defects, and unilateral or bilateral limb weakness and stupor. The symptoms may have come on after a particular stressful situation or when the child is about to face a stressful event. It may also arise during or following a minor physical illness, such as a viral infection. The child may show other signs of emotional or behaviour disorder, especially depressive features, but more commonly this is not the case. Indeed the adolescent may be apparently indifferent to his problem (*belle indifference*). More commonly there is distress and at least an apparent wish to be rid of the symptom.

The family background may show obvious signs of disturbance, but this is not invariable. There is likely to be undue parental concern over physical complaints, and, if the disability is chronic, the parents may well be attached to the notion that there is an underlying physical disorder. Alternatively, family functioning may be chaotic and disorganized (Grattan-Smith *et al.* 1988).

Related conditions
- *Tension headache and abdominal pain.* Headache and stomach-ache are common non-organic symptoms and are discussed elsewhere (Sections 3.8.4 and below). In a minority of cases, the function of these symptoms (especially the benefits of the sick role) may mean that it is helpful to manage them along the same lines as conversion reactions.

- *Physical disease accompanied by excessive disability.* Some children are more disabled by a physical condition than one would expect on physical grounds alone. Occasionally a conversion or 'hysterical' reaction appears to follow on a fully physical illness, symptoms persisting when the organic cause is no longer present.
- *Symptoms referable to various psychophysical interactions.* Asthmatic attacks, diarrhoea related to anxiety, and palpitations are all examples of symptoms in which psychophysical mechanisms, sometimes related to autonomic nervous system activation, are implicated. It is usually not appropriate to regard these as conversion reactions.
- *Epidemic 'hysteria'.* A number of reports have been published of groups of children or teenagers (especially girls), who have, *en masse*, succumbed to symptoms such as faints, dizziness, and headaches. Characteristically the episode begins with symptoms such as these, thought to be due to some infectious disease or toxic agent, often occurring in a girl of high status in her group. Other girls, especially the more anxious in the group, then experience similar symptomatology. Isolation of the affected girls, and strong suggestion to the remainder that the epidemic has now passed its peak and will gradually subside, is usually sufficient to bring it to an end. Intensive investigation is likely to prolong the problem and is unnecessary, as the true nature of the problem is usually clear after the first two or three girls have been examined.

Assessment and management

The history, together with observation of the child and physical examination, may reveal obvious inconsistencies in the child's disability, making it highly improbable or impossible that the child is suffering from a physically determined condition. It may be possible to demonstrate muscular power in some situations but not in others. Children with conversion blindness may show inconsistent performance on charting their visual fields. The pattern of signs elicited will not correspond to any known neurological lesion.

If a psychiatric diagnosis is obvious, then unnecessary further investigations should not be embarked upon, as these will only prolong the disorder. On the other hand, where real doubt exists, physical investigations should be thorough, as a significant number of childhood conditions diagnosed as hysterical ultimately turn out to have organic pathology (Caplan 1970). Conditions most commonly missed are epilepsy, maculoretinal cerebral degeneration, spinal tumours and abscesses, and (in the case of postural symptoms) dystonia musculorum deformans. Epilepsy is not infrequently missed as many children with pseudoseizures also suffer with epileptic fits (Section 3.8.2).

Further discussion may reveal the meaning and purpose of the physical symptoms. They may allow the child to avoid a painful situation by adopting the role of a sick person. Symptoms may have been inappropriately rewarded with undue attention—not only by parents and the family. Doctors who find the child's symptoms puzzling and challenging may also reward the child for his abnormal behaviour with the attention they provide. The symptoms may be necessary for family adaptation, allowing the parents to focus on their child's symptoms, and thus avoid talking about their marital problems. They may also reflect deep-seated conflicts of which the child is unaware. Finally, the symptoms may be a sign of another form of mental disorder, such as severe depression or schizophrenia.

Treatment

Once the diagnosis of conversion syndrome has been made, the initial discussion with the parents and child needs careful planning (Schulman 1988). The clinician should first be sure he fully understands how the parents and child see the problem. Do they acknowledge the possibility of a psychological cause for the disability? If they do, the task of the clinician will be that much easier. Having established existing family attitudes, it should be explained to the family that there is no evidence for any current physical cause for the condition. The physical investigations that have been carried out should be gone over carefully with the family and the reasons for not making a physical diagnosis fully explained. Nevertheless, there is obviously something very wrong. It is important to explain the genuineness of the symptoms—the child is definitely not 'putting it on'. It can be explained too that, in some children, upsets of one sort or another sometimes produce physical symptoms, and this provides an opportunity for discussion of the role of stress in the child's life. This may or may not be apparent.

The principles of treatment, described below, can then be explained to the parents. In cases where parents are 'stuck' with the notion that the child's symptoms must be physically determined, then it may be best for the clinician to accept the parents' view that this may be the case. However, the clinician needs to go on to suggest that, as no physical diagnosis has been made and therefore no physical treatments can be applied, unless the child is to remain crippled, some form of 'rehabilitation' needs to be applied.

It is wise to give a good prognosis early on, and to suggest strongly that recovery will occur over a few weeks or months. The child can then be told to expect to gain greater control over his symptoms. How this is to be achieved will become apparent as treatment proceeds. It is important to arrange follow-up appointments to monitor progress and ensure the child is not taken elsewhere for yet more investigations. If a child is under the care of a family doctor or paediatrician, and the symptoms are not improved with this form of management within a few weeks, then referral to a child or adolescent psychiatrist for transfer of care should be arranged. A joint interview with the family involving both the paediatrician and the psychiatrist is helpful as an initial step.

A range of treatments may be applied to children with conversion disorders, some of which will require admission to an in-patient psychiatric unit. Some children benefit considerably from physiotherapy, enabling them, for example, gradually to regain power in paralysed limbs without losing face (Dubowitz and Hersov 1976). Family interviews may be required to improve communication between family members or to help family members to become more aware of maladaptive functioning. The child may benefit from individual psychotherapeutic interviews. Suggestible children may improve with hypnosis.

The details of treatment will vary depending on the nature of the problem, but the principles remain the same. An attempt is made to understand why the child has developed such abnormal illness behaviour so that he can be helped to achieve a more adaptive solution to his problems (Goodyer and Taylor 1985). During the treatment, previously unsuspected stresses at home or school may be revealed, but quite often improvement occurs without obtaining full understanding why the problem should have developed in the first place.

Outcome

Most children with conversion disorders improve symptomatically with suggestion and active treatment, such as that described above (Leslie 1988), but a significant proportion remain resistant to treatment (Grattan-Smith *et al.* 1988). The subsequent personality outcome of these children is unknown, however, and may not be so favourable. Good prognostic signs include an acute onset and the presence of parents prepared to consider psychological factors seriously.

Recurrent non-organic abdominal pain

Clinical features

This type of abdominal pain usually presents in children aged between 5 and 12 years. Pain is usually diffusely experienced in the abdomen and may be accompanied by headaches and pains in other parts of the body, especially the limbs and joints. It may be accompanied by nausea and vomiting. Sometimes the pain may come on in direct relationship to stress, such as at the beginning of a new term at school, but more often there is no such obvious relationship. The child may, however, be generally tense, anxious, or depressed. Often the child has had a rather tense personality since early childhood.

Physical examination reveals a lack of definite, localized tenderness or rebound tenderness. If physical examinations are carried out, they prove negative. The pain tends to last a few hours and then remit, but it may be more persistent than this and relapses are common. In a small proportion of children with this condition, abdominal pain occurs in regular association with vomiting, headache, and low-grade fever. This constitutes the so-called *periodic syndrome*, a poorly defined condition possibly related to migraine (Section 3.8.4) or to emotional disturbance (Apley and MacKeith 1968). If vomiting is present, this condition is usually referred to as *cyclical vomiting* and, in these circumstances, headache and fever are absent. Usually attacks of cyclical vomiting last only a few hours and the child is unwell for a day or so. Very occasionally the vomiting is persistent and produces life-threatening dehydration.

Background features

Recurrent abdominal pain is a common feature of growing children and occurs in 10–15% of the population (Garber *et al.* 1990). Boys and girls are roughly equally affected, and there is no specific link with social class. Both the children and their mothers have increased rates of depressive and anxiety symptoms. It is possible that these psychological symptoms are a reaction to the presence of chronic pain, but comparisons with children with organically determined pain suggest this is unlikely to be the case in most circumstances. Family patterns of illness behaviour seem to reinforce or reward complaints of pain and lead to withdrawal from everyday activities when it occurs. (Walker *et al.* 1993). The recurrent abdominal pain is often associated with pain experienced elsewhere in the body, especially headaches.

The mechanism of pain production is these cases is unknown. Pain may be due to muscular tension, but undue sensitivity to normal abdominal sensations is a more likely explanation, and is better backed by systematic investigations (Fritz *et al.* 1997)

Assessment
Chronic or recurrent pain in the abdomen in childhood can occur for organic and non-organic reasons. Among the non-organic group are those where the aetiology is psychogenic, and others where the cause is unknown.

Identifiable organic causes account for only about 10% of cases of children with recurrent abdominal pain, the remainder being either of psychogenic or unknown cause. Renal tract infections, mesenteric lymphadenitis, chronic pancreatitis, peptic ulcer, Crohn's disease, and ulcerative colitis are the most common organic conditions found, but none of these occurs frequently. A host of other conditions, such as gastro-oesophageal reflux, gastritis, duodenitis, and carbohydrate malabsorption have been described (Murphy 1993), but are also uncommon. Follow-up of cases of recurrent abdominal pain reveals a very low rate of missed organic diagnoses (Walker *et al.* 1995).

Clinical features distinguishing organic and non-organic pain
Pain of organic cause is likely to be well-localized and restricted to the abdomen. Non-organic pain is more likely to be diffuse and accompanied by pain elsewhere in the body, especially the head and limbs (Table 5.1). Severity of the pain and the presence of associated vomiting are not good guides to its aetiology. In non-organic pain there are often signs of associated emotional disturbance—especially anxiety, depression, and a tense personality. Organic pain is more likely to be linked to tiredness and pallor.

Table 5.1 Abdominal pain

	Organic pain	Non-organic pain
Frequency (%)	10	90
Type of pain	Localized	Diffuse
Pain wakes child at night	Often	Rarely
Pain elsewhere in body	Unusual	Common
Vomiting	May be present	May be present
Emotional state	Usually normal	Usually anxious, tense, depressed
Abnormalities on examination and investigation	Present	Absent

Physical examination is the best single indicator, with localized tenderness and rebound tenderness indicating an organic cause. Even severe non-organic pain is usually unaccompanied by tenderness on palpation. Physical investigations, especially examination of the blood, urine, and radiological tests, may be useful in excluding organic causes.

The quality and time relationships of the pain therefore, together with the presence of nausea or vomiting and other abdominal symptoms, should be identified. Are there associated aches and pains in other parts of the body? Has there been any loss of weight? What is the association of the pain to stressful events and, in general, how anxious and tense has the child's emotional state been? What potentially upsetting events have there been at home or at school at the time the pain started? Indeed, is the abdominal pain really a presenting sign of school refusal? Do other family members suffer from stomach-aches or headaches?

Physical examination should be carried out with particular concern for the degree of abdominal tenderness. Physical investigations may be indicated, but in most cases of recurrent abdominal pain these will not need to extend beyond examination of the urine.

Treatment

In those rare cases where there is vomiting producing dehydration, medical management may require intravenous therapy and antiemetic medication. Stemetil, diazepam, or chlorpromazine may be helpful. Subsequent management should, however, proceed along the lines described below for non-organic abdominal pain.

Assuming organic causes have been virtually excluded, it is helpful to explain to parents and child that no serious physical condition is present and that the child has a relatively common problem that can be expected to get better over the next few weeks or months. It can then be explained that often, though not always, the type of pain and other symptoms the child is experiencing can be due to tension because of emotional upset. Have the parents or child thought this possible in their case? Has anxiety about school been considered?

The response to this question will enable parents and older children to express their present understanding of the problem in psychological terms. They may have already come to this conclusion and be ready to discuss psychological management. Alternatively, they may be indignant at the suggestion.

Once this information is available, it is likely that the clinician will be able to conclude that the non-organic pain experienced by the child falls into one of three groups:

- somatic symptoms part of a wider emotional disturbance with anxiety, depression, etc.
- monosymptomatic response to stress in the child's circumstances
- pain of uncertain aetiology in which psychological factors may or may not be playing a part.

When abdominal pain forms part of a generalized emotional disorder characterized by anxiety, treatment should proceed along the lines described in Section 4.4.2. If the pain is monosymptomatic, but due to tension, then a course of cognitive behaviour therapy in a family context is indicated (McGrath and Goodman 1998). Such treatment has been evaluated and found to be more effective than standard paediatric care (Sanders *et al.* 1994). In cases of uncertain aetiology, the child and family should be reassured that, although the cause is unknown, the pain is very likely to disappear. Follow-up should be arranged to check on progress and, if the pain continues and the family members are motivated, to consider what stress factors might now be operating to maintain it. It is important in these cases to ensure that usual activities are continued as far as possible, and invalidism avoided.

Outcome

With the type of management described above, most paediatricians describe an excellent short-term outcome in 60–80% of their cases. No controlled trials of psychological management have been reported, so it is impossible to know whether this makes a difference to outcome.

Follow-up studies of children with this syndrome suggest that between a third and a half continue to suffer abdominal pain in later childhood and adulthood (Apley and Hale 1973). Children of parents who continue themselves to suffer abdominal pain are especially likely to show pain persistence (Christensen and Mortensen 1975). This suggests either that the persistent form of the symptom has strong genetic loading, or that family patterns of responding to stress by somatic symptoms are learnt within certain family systems.

Chronic fatigue syndrome (myalgic encephalomyelitis)

The diagnosis of chronic fatigue syndrome is controversial. Some clinicians would see it as a form of depressive disorder, and would not think it warranted a separate category. Others would be dismayed and even angry to see it classified under the heading of psychosomatic symptoms and syndromes and would think it more appropriate for it to be classified as an infectious disorder. In this book it will be treated as a reasonably discrete clinical entity, probably with multiple causation though often of unknown aetiology, usually responding best to a combination of psychological and physical management.

Clinical features

Chronic fatigue syndrome occurs in both children and adults. Symptoms are often, but by no means always, preceded by symptoms of a viral illness. It is unusual for the presence of a virus to have been confirmed by laboratory investigation. The child, or more often adolescent, fails to recover completely from what appears to have been a bout of influenza, and starts to complain of the cardinal symptom, extreme tiredness with any sort of physical effort. Physical fatigue is felt as lack of energy or strength in the muscles, but there is also mental fatigue, characterized by lack of energy, alertness, and ability to concentrate. Accompanying symptoms include pain or aching in the muscles (myalgia), and sleep disturbance. There are also often signs of mood disturbance, especially depression with apathy and lack of interest in activities that are normally enjoyed. There may also be anxiety symptoms and irritability. Mood often deteriorates if the disorder progresses.

These symptoms are not unusual after a viral illness, and usually disappear within 2–3 weeks. However, in a minority of children and adolescents they persist. It has been suggested that, for research purposes, the diagnosis should not be made unless the symptoms last 6 months (Sharpe 1991), but bearing in mind that a child with these symptoms is very likely to be missing school, it seems reasonable to be concerned if they persist beyond a couple of weeks.

The prevalence of the disorder is unknown, but there are wide differences between countries and between different regions in the same country. It is a relatively frequent cause of attendance at paediatric facilities in the UK, but much less so in the US. It is equally common in boys and girls, though girls are more frequently affected in adolescence. Suggestions that the condition is more common in higher socio-economic groups arise because of referral bias. In adults, at any rate, in primary care studies, there is no particular relationship with social class.

Management

The clinician should exclude known physical causes of fatigue, including anaemia and chronic infectious disease. Viral studies should be carried out, though often the results will be difficult to interpret. In addition, a psychiatric assessment should be undertaken, both because the symptoms may be part of a psychiatric disorder, and because there may be serious secondary emotional disturbance. The possibility of a school refusal syndrome should be considered, and this will involve knowing something of the child's recent attendance pattern, performance, and behaviour in school.

Before embarking on a management plan, the clinician should clarify the parental attitude to the symptoms. Do they see this as an entirely physical problem, or are they open to examining possible psychological factors? If the condition has been present for some time, the parents may have already joined a self-help group, and this may have encouraged a negative attitude to examining emotional aspects of the problem. It should also be emphasized that some self-help groups encourage open-mindedness on this matter.

Assuming this is acceptable to the parents, the clinician should be guided by the following principles (Marcovitch 1997):

- Once the initial investigations have been carried out and proved negative, further physical tests should be avoided.
- It should be acknowledged that the exact cause of the problem is likely to remain uncertain. Nevertheless it should be emphasized that a great deal is known about the best methods of achieving improvement.
- The importance of understanding what is going on by looking at mind–body interactions should be emphasized.
- The genuineness of the symptoms should be acknowledged.

- Family and social issues should be explored if this is acceptable to the parents.
- Close liaison should be maintained with the school, and home tuition should be avoided in favour of part-time attendance at school or a tutorial unit.

A systematic programme of graded exercise (Fulcher and White 1997), or cognitive behaviour therapy (Deale *et al.* 1997) should be undertaken. Both of these have been shown to be effective in adults and are probably so in children. More informally, the child and parents should be encouraged to try and do a small additional amount of exercise each day to try to build up strength and confidence. This may be problematic, as the parents may have been told that all exercise should be avoided. If this is the case, argument should be avoided, but gentle physical rehabilitation should still be encouraged from time to time. Various additional forms of therapy may be helpful, including more formal physiotherapy and antidepressant medication.

The outcome is usually good, but a minority of children remain disabled, some seriously so. For these a period of rehabilitation in a paediatric or psychiatric unit may be helpful.

5.5.3 POST-TRAUMATIC STRESS DISORDERS

Definition

Children who are exposed to chronic stress, such as sexual abuse within the family, or acute, unexpected, overwhelming stress in the form of a natural disaster or a major trauma such as an earthquake, or being raped or seeing their parents forcibly taken away, may react in a characteristic way. In both major classificatory systems, this is categorized as a post-traumatic stress disorder (PTSD), and in both systems the reactions children show are not considered separately from those of adults.

Clinical features

The characteristic reaction (American Psychiatric Association 1994; Eth and Pynoos 1985) involves intense fear at the time of the event, re-experience of the traumatic event as a recurrent, distressing recollection in the waking or dreaming state, sudden acting or feeling as if the event was recurring in a 'flashback', and intense psychological distress when events (such as anniversaries) occur that symbolize the original trauma. The child persistently avoids stimuli associated with the trauma, for example by making efforts to avoid recollecting them, experiencing a feeling of detachment from other people, and may regress in feeding or toileting habits. There may be symptoms of increased arousal, including sleep disturbance, irritability, difficulty in concentrating, and hypervigilance.

In childhood, this pattern of symptomatology is probably most likely to occur after sexual abuse, but a similar picture has been described after different forms of disaster, including bush fires (McFarlane 1988) and civil war (Sack *et al.* 1997).

Vulnerable children, already predisposed to psychiatric disorder by family disharmony, school failure, or other stresses, are those most likely to be affected, but previously normal children can also show the characteristic picture.

Management

In natural disasters affecting large numbers of people, this needs to be considered at a community level, as well as at a family and individual level. Indeed, there is some evidence that the length of time it takes the child to adjust is closely related to the time it takes the community in which the child lives to reorganize (Galante and Foa 1986). The effectiveness of relief workers in promoting self-help activity among victims and keeping family members together is therefore a major factor in outcome. In addition, children seem to benefit if they are encouraged (but not forced) to recount their experiences individually, with a group of peers, or with other family members. Play material, drawing, and painting may be useful adjuncts if the child is being seen individually. Smith *et al.* (1998) have described an evaluated cognitive behavioural approach to PTSD arising as a result of a variety of different traumatic experiences.

The value of a diagnosis of PTSD in children who are victims of political violence has been questioned on two main grounds (Richman 1993):

- First, the symptoms are non-specific. Children and adolescents who have, for example, seen their parents forcibly removed, tortured, or even murdered may show a wide variety of problems such as depressive states and somatic complaints.
- Second, the medicalization of the reaction of victims of violence with its consequent emphasis on therapy or treatment may distract attention away from the need for appropriate political action.

In these circumstances, Richman (1993) counsels against psychological therapies, and in favour of giving priority to the provision of basic material needs, health and education services, community services, etc. Nevertheless, in these circumstances children may still benefit from the opportunity to talk about or re-enact their experiences in play.

The outcome of children with PTSD will vary depending on a number of factors. Children who are victims of a natural disaster, such as a flood, fire or earthquake, but whose families remain intact, will obviously fare better than children who are victims of political violence whose parents have been forcibly removed, who may have to migrate or endure months or years in dreadful social circumstances in a refugee camp. In general, children who, after their traumatic experience, continue to live with familiar figures, in good social and emotional conditions, will usually gradually lose their symptoms. On the other hand, where the trauma has been at the hands of family members, as is often the case in sexual abuse, the outcome may be far less positive, with disabling symptoms persisting well into adulthood.

5.6 Psychoses

5.6.1 DEFINITION AND CLASSIFICATION

Definition

The psychoses are conditions in which there are major abnormalities of thinking (shown by the expression of incoherent and illogical thoughts), beliefs, and perception (shown by delusions and hallucinations). Such abnormalities are usually accompanied by gross behavioural changes.

In psychotic disorders there is a loss of contact with reality and a lack of insight on the part of the patient that there is anything wrong, whereas patients suffering from neurotic disorders, though they may be severely handicapped, are in touch with reality and realize they have problems. The distinction has been encapsulated in the aphorism 'neurotics build castles in Spain whereas psychotics live in them'. The distinction is not clear-cut, and is less frequently made than used to be the case, but it still has value, especially in the older child and adolescent.

Psychotic disorders appear less commonly in infancy and childhood than in adolescence and adulthood. This is probably because their actual prevalence is lower, but diagnostic difficulties may also be responsible. Especially in very young children, the identification of abnormalities of thinking and perception presents major problems.

Classification

Psychotic disorders can be divided into:

- schizophrenia
- bipolar affective disorder
- organic psychotic states
  — unaccompanied by intellectual deterioration/dementia
  — accompanied by intellectual deterioration/dementia
- atypical psychoses.

Until recent times, childhood autism was regarded as a form of childhood psychosis, but it is now realized that this condition has more in common with disorders and delays of development such as developmental aphasia and mental retardation.

Aetiology

Apart from organic psychotic states, the underlying pathophysiological bases of psychoses are not known. Information is, however, available on both genetic and environmental risk factors. The lack of a known organic causation for schizophrenia and bipolar disorder has led to their being labelled as 'functional', i.e. caused by disturbance of function rather than physical structure. This term is not very helpful, and is likely to be less used as the aetiology of these conditions becomes clearer.

5.6.2 SCHIZOPHRENIA

Definition

Schizophrenia is a condition with characteristic disorders of thought, perception, mood, and sometimes posture.

Clinical features

The condition most commonly presents for the first time in adolescence or early adulthood. It may, however, present in characteristic form before puberty (Green *et al.* 1992).

Characteristic features are:

* *Thought disorder.* The child or young person is likely to have difficulty expressing his thoughts, and be incoherent and apparently illogical. 'Loosening' of thought associations may involve moving from one word or idea to another in an apparently random manner.
* *Delusions.* These are false beliefs impervious to reason. They usually take a paranoid form, i.e. the child or young person believes those around him are hostile and threatening. Primary delusions, which are characteristic of schizophrenia, are those that arise directly out of normal experience and are not secondary to hallucinations.
* *Hallucinations.* These are false perceptions without sensory stimulation. In schizophrenia they are usually of auditory type—voices outside the person's control, talking to him directly or referring to him in the third person.
* *Disorders of motility.* Catatonic behaviour in which the young person takes up abnormal postures or enters into an unresponsive state or 'stupor' may occur.

In addition to these central features of schizophrenia, other less specific symptoms may also occur. These include disturbances of mood, acute excitement, depression, and anxiety, as well as mannerisms, stereotypies, and inappropriate social behaviour.

The condition may present in an acute or insidious manner. In the latter case, it may be many months before the child is realized to have a serious mental disorder, being regarded in the meantime either as lazy or as showing a less serious psychological problem.

Prior to onset the young person may have been normal, or, more commonly, have shown some degree of developmental delay (Zeitlin 1986). Early language delay is common, and other developmental abnormalities such as clumsiness may have been present (Asarnow *et al.* 1995). Other neurodevelopmental anomalies such as muscular hypotonia have been described. There may have been difficulties with information processing, deficits of attention, signs of minor neurological abnormalities, autonomic hyper-responsiveness, social difficulties, and emotional lability (Neuchterlein 1986).

Following an acute phase, the young person may return to normal or enter into a 'negative state' in which active symptoms such as delusions and hallucinations are absent, but he is apathetic and lacking in motivation. Such a negative state may be followed by another acute attack, and recurring cycles of this nature may persist for years or throughout the individual's life.

Aetiology and background features

The exact nature of the aetiology of schizophrenia is unknown.

Genetic factors

There is strong evidence that genetic factors are involved, as:

- First-degree relatives have a substantially increased risk. The child of a parent or sib with schizophrenia has about a 12% risk compared with 1% in the general population. There is also increased risk in relatives of schizotypal disorder—a personality disorder with many of the features of schizophrenia, for example remoteness, inability to make friends, and oddities of speech, but without adequate evidence to make the full diagnosis.
- Monozygotic twins show distinctly higher concordance rates than dizygotic. The exact difference in rates is uncertain, but that there is a difference seems clear-cut.
- Fostered and adopted children of parents with schizophrenia have a similar risk of developing the condition when compared with those brought up by their schizophrenic parents (Heston 1966).
- Children with schizophrenia have an increased rate of developmental abnormalities in their early lives (Hollis 1995). Indeed, some now regard schizophrenia as a developmental disorder (Murray 1994). Considerable efforts have been made to identify neuroanatomical, neurophysiological, and biochemical abnormalities in schizophrenia. Ventricular size appears increased, and the volume of some mesial temporal structures is reduced. There are specific neuropsychological deficits affecting attention as well as verbal and spatial memory. Children with schizophrenia have been shown to have similar anatomical and neuropsychological deficits to adults (Hendren *et al.* 1995). The fact that symptoms of schizophrenia are specifically improved by drugs that block dopamine receptors suggests that abnormalities of these receptors may play an important part in aetiology.

Other organic factors

Many other organic factors may, in an individual case, play an important part. Perinatal trauma may have predisposed the child to develop a psychosis. Other trauma, encephalitic infections, neoplasms, and irradiation may also precipitate an apparently typical attack of schizophrenia with 'organic' features (see below).

Environmental factors

Various characteristic patterns of family interaction have been described as having aetiological significance. The 'double-bind' hypothesis suggested that schizophrenia may be precipitated by communication of inconsistent messages from parent to child, but now appears discredited (Leff 1978). However, parents of children with schizophrenia do show more overt criticism of their children than parents of depressed children, perhaps because they are frustrated by their children's tendency to drift off the point (Asarnow 1994). It does seem clear that if a teenager with schizophrenia is in contact with parents with high emotional involvement (expressed emotion), this is likely to precipitate relapse. Such emotional involvement might sometimes precipitate the onset of the schizophrenic illness in the first place.

In older patients, the role of other non-specific 'life events' in precipitating relapse has also been demonstrated (Birley and Brown 1970), and these are probably also of importance in children and adolescents predisposed to the condition.

Prevalence

Schizophrenia occurs in 0.5–1% of the adult population, but is much rarer in the prepubertal period. The rate in late adolescence is about 3 per 10 000. In this younger age group, boys are more commonly affected than girls. There is a link with low social class, and this may be because the effects of the illness reduce social competence, and result in downward social drift.

Assessment

As well as obtaining as clear a history as possible from parents and child or young person, with emphasis on the pre-morbid personality, suspicion of schizophrenia should lead to a formal psychiatric examination, a request for psychological testing, and a neurological assessment.

In most cases of schizophrenia, diagnosis presents little difficulty. In young children, however, establishing the presence of thought disorder, delusions, and hallucinations may be difficult. The fact that a child or young person mutters to himself and appears preoccupied should not, for example, be regarded as evidence that he is hallucinated, though certainly such behaviour should arouse this suspicion. Further, the presence of hallucinations need by no means always indicate a diagnosis of schizophrenia. Instead, other psychotic or neurotic disorders (Garralda 1984) or a drug-induced state may be responsible. It is important to exclude organic disease. The presence of disorientation or clouding of consciousness (again sometimes difficult to detect in young children) should raise the possibility of an organic condition. The presence of epilepsy should be carefully considered. Epileptic attacks may be followed by confusional states with psychotic features. Further, children and adolescents with long-standing temporal lobe epilepsy are at special risk for developing schizophrenia. A full neurological examination should be carried out, and positive findings will require further investigation.

In children who have abnormalities from the pre-school period, childhood autism should be considered, though very occasionally autism may be followed by a schizophrenic state (Petty *et al.* 1984). In affective psychosis (manic–depressive disorder), delusions and hallucinations may also occur, but their content will be different (see below). Mixed pictures (schizoaffective states) with features of both types of psychosis, have been described in adulthood.

Treatment

In general, this should follow lines used to treat schizophrenia in the adult patient, but the educational needs of the child and his family situation are likely to require special consideration.

Acute phase
Psychotropic medication (Section 9.2.5) such as chlorpromazine or haloperidol is indicated. The child or adolescent is likely to require admission to an in-patient unit. The family members require support to understand the nature of the illness and its likely outcome.

Chronic phase
If the child or adolescent enters a state of low motivation with a continuing predisposition to future acute attacks, continuing close supervision is required. Maintenance phenothiazines given orally or by depot injection will reduce the risk of relapse, but the use of chlorpromazine or haloperidol on a long-term basis is reducing because of the serious risk of tardive dyskinesia. Clozapin and risperidol are now more frequently employed. The use of electroconvulsive therapy should be limited to cases where catatonic stupor is a prominent feature. In these cases, excessively rare in childhood and adolescence, it is usually highly effective.

Counselling of family members to reduce emotional overinvolvement should be combined with supportive psychotherapy for the child. In children of school age, special educational facilities are likely to be required, possibly in a special day or residential setting. Genetic counselling should be made available, if appropriate, to the patient himself, as well as to the parents or sibs.

Outcome

The outcome will depend on the nature of the illness. The insidiously developing form with previous developmental and personality abnormalities has a poor outcome, with the risk of subsequent prolonged dependency. On the other hand, a single, acute attack in a previously normal child or adolescent may have no significant sequelae. The distinction between affective and schizophrenic psychosis in adolescence is not easy, and a teenager apparently suffering from schizophrenia may have later episodes more characteristic of manic–depressive psychosis (Zeitlin 1986).

5.6.3 BIPOLAR AFFECTIVE DISORDERS

Classification

The psychiatric classification of disturbances of mood or affective disorders is complex, but two main groupings are described in DSM IV (American

Psychiatric Association 1994). The ICD-10 (World Health Organization 1990) classification is in most respects similar.

- *Unipolar or bipolar disorders.* In these there are reasonably clear-cut episodes of hypomania and/or severe depression often with psychotic features.
- *Depressive disorders.* These consist particularly of depressive episodes and recurrent depressive disorders and are described elsewhere (Section 4.4.5).

The distinction between uni- and bipolar disorders and depressive disorders is blurred, but they are described separately here because, unlike depressive disorders, bipolar disorders cannot easily be seen as arising as extremes of normal development. Consequently, in this book, while depressive disorders are described in Section 4.4.5, bipolar disorders are described as one of a number of adult-type psychiatric disorders.

In unipolar disorders there are single or recurrent episodes of either hypomania or depressive disorders (but not both). Children with bipolar disorders have recurrent episodes of both depression and hypomania.

Clinical features

In contrast to schizophrenia, in general, the personality of children and young people who suffer from bipolar disorders is excellent with good school attainment and peer relationships (Quackenbush *et al.* 1996). However, bipolar disorders may be preceded by co-morbid conduct disorder (Kovacs and Pollock 1995).

In depressive episodes, there is gradual or sudden marked lowering of mood and loss of energy. Mood may be lowest in the morning. Appetite and weight may be lost. Sleep disturbance is usually absent in this age group, but may occur. There is often retardation of movement and speech, though occasionally agitation and pressure of talk are present. The teenager may express thoughts of unworthiness, guilt, hopelessness about the future, and desire for death. Suicidal behaviour may occur. Delusions and hallucinations are usually absent and, if present, their content appears to arise from the youngster's mood. Thus he may hear voices accusing him of crimes he imagines he has committed, or believe that his body is rotting.

In hypomanic episodes, there is elevation of mood with excitement and pressure of talk. Irritability is a prominent feature. The teenager will be unduly energetic and require less sleep than usual. Disinhibited behaviour may lead to financial extravagance or sexual misdemeanours (Geller and Luby 1997). The youngster may have inflated ideas of his own capacities that may reach a delusional level. Hallucinations may occur, but are uncommon.

Prevalence and background factors

Bipolar disorders are rare before puberty, but increase in frequency of presentation during adolescence. The condition occurs with equal frequency in boys and girls, though, at the upper end of this age group, females predominate.

Genetic factors

Evidence in favour of a significant genetic contribution arises mainly from studies of older patients. The risk of bipolar disorder is much increased in the offspring of parents with this diagnosis (Todd *et al.* 1996). Studies of twins and adopted children support the genetic hypothesis, though no clear-cut pattern of inheritance has been determined.

Other organic factors
Major depressive disorder sometimes follows head injury, viral infections such as influenza or infectious mononucleosis, and cerebral disease. Various metabolic abnormalities have been identified in this condition, particularly affecting mono-amine neurotransmitters (especially 5-hydroxytryptamine), and cortisol metab-olism, but no clear-cut physiological basis has emerged.

Environmental factors
In older sufferers from this condition it has been demonstrated that predisposing or vulnerability factors include early parental loss and separations. Precipitating factors include life events that could be construed as posing a threat to the well-being of the patient. The study of life events in childhood and adolescence is still sketchy, but it seems plausible to suggest that environmental factors operate similarly in this age group, producing low self-esteem, a sense of help-lessness, and an inability to think other than pessimistically.

Assessment
The severely depressed child or adolescent requires a full assessment with par-ticular attention given to the family history and possible precipitating events. In assessing the mental state, it is important to consider carefully the likelihood of suicidal behaviour. Organic disease should be excluded by physical examination and, if necessary, further investigation. Differentiation from depressive or dys-thymic disorder is often difficult but, in any case, the practical implications of making the distinction are often not clear. If psychotic symptoms do not appear to arise directly from the patient's mood, a diagnosis of schizophrenia should be considered. However, misdiagnosis of schizophrenia in adolescents with bipolar disorder is common, and an accurate diagnosis may only be possible after a period of follow-up (Werry *et al.* 1991).

Treatment
Acute depressive phase
- *Counselling or supportive psychotherapy.* Although it may be difficult to conduct interviews with a very depressed and mute, or unduly excited, over-active teenager, every effort should be made to form a relationship. Relatively brief but frequent sessions for this purpose are indicated. This will allow an opportunity for examining the onset of the illness, with a view to preventing recurrences. The development of a trusting relationship also probably reduces the risk of suicide. The family as well as the teenager will benefit from a counselling approach.
- *Securing the safety of the patient.* Youngsters with this condition may attempt to harm themselves, and admission to a psychiatric unit may be necessary for this reason.

- *Medication.* In depressive disorders of this severity, antidepressant medication should be prescribed. Tricyclic antidepressants may be tried initially, but evidence for their effectiveness is weak. There is increasing clinical evidence that the selective serotonin reuptake inhibitors are more effective and safer in children and adolescents (see Section 9.2.5).
- *Electroconvulsive therapy (ECT).* If, after two 6 week courses of different types of antidepressant medication there has been no improvement, and the patient remains severely depressed, consideration should be given to the use of ECT. The presence of depressive stupor and severe motor or verbal retardation are the main positive indications. In general, ECT seems less effective in the younger age group than in older patients, but the indications for its use are similar (Bertagnoli and Borchardt 1990) (see also p. 454).

Acute hypomanic phase

The principles of counselling and securing the safety of the patient and others around him will again form a major component of the treatment plan.

Haloperidol in dosage up to 0.05 mg/kg body weight per day in three divided doses is likely to be effective. Long-term treatment with this treatment should be avoided if at all possible because of the risk of tardive dyskinesia. Clozapin may be a safer alternative.

Chronic phase

In teenagers subject to recurrent attacks of acute disorder, lithium carbonate is usually, though not always, an effective prophylactic (Kafantaris 1995). The existence of a relative who has responded to this medication is a useful indication for its use (Delong and Aldersdorf 1987).

Outcome

Recovery from the acute phase of the condition nearly always occurs in a few weeks. An acute onset with a precipitating factor and a complete return to normality usually indicates relapse will not occur. Absence of a precipitating factor, family history of recurrent illness, and a failure to return to normality indicate likely relapses. If psychiatric disorder recurs in adult life, depressive features are again likely to be prominent. A severe disorder of apparently affective type in childhood or adolescence may, however, recur later with more obviously schizophrenic features.

5.6.4 ORGANIC PSYCHOTIC STATES

Delirium

Delirious states are not uncommon in young children with acute infections. Clouding of consciousness with diminished response to external stimuli, misperceptions, visual hallucinations, and disorientation can also occur after the ingestion of excess quantities of certain drugs such as ephedrine, atropine, and tricyclic antidepressants, as well as non-prescribed drugs such as solvents and amphetamines. Delirious states also, although rarely, occur as part of epileptic attacks in the ictal or postictal phase.

Organic psychoses without dementia/intellectual deterioration

Non-progressive cerebral conditions are occasionally associated with psychotic reactions. These are usually of acute or subacute schizophrenic type (see above). Underlying conditions include cerebral infections, especially in encephalitic conditions, withdrawal states from certain drugs (especially alcohol and amphetamines) and epileptic attacks.

Suspicion of an organic cause for an acute schizophrenic illness should be raised if there is a history of epilepsy or drug ingestion, if the psychotic symptoms are accompanied by disorientation in time and space, and if hallucinations are of visual type.

Dementia

Dementia involves irreversible deterioration of intellectual skills, and is often accompanied by change in behaviour or personality.

Clinical features
In infancy and childhood dementia is shown first by a loss of recently acquired skills. A young child may stop speaking and develop incontinence of urine and faeces. Autistic features may also occur, but the condition is differentiated from autism by the fact that there is continuing deterioration, sometimes leading to death. In older children, handwriting may deteriorate, and this may be followed by the child being unable to read at a level previously attained. There may also be a psychotic reaction, most commonly of schizophrenic type. Non-psychotic behavioural changes such as undue fearfulness or aggressive behaviour may precede the psychotic symptoms and intellectual deterioration (Corbett *et al.* 1977).

These psychotic features are usually accompanied by other evidence of organic disease. Such evidence depends on the nature of the condition, but is likely to include especially epileptic fits and involuntary movements. Sometimes, however, these obvious signs of organic disease are absent. In these circumstances, it is quite common for the condition to be treated as purely psychiatric, the evidence for intellectual deterioration having been overlooked (Rivinus *et al.* 1975). This situation may persist for several years.

Aetiology
There are a large number of causes of dementia in childhood, all of which are rare. For a full description of these progressive conditions see Brett (1983). They include:

- infections, especially subacute sclerosing panencephalitis
- neurometabolic disorders, for example the gangliosidoses, leucodystrophies, and mucopolysaccharidoses
- Huntingdon's chorea

- chronic poisoning, for example with lead
- neoplastic conditions (especially from leukaemic infiltration of the meninges and as a complication of treatment of leukaemia, methotrexate-radiation leucoencephalopathy)
- other conditions of uncertain aetiology such as Rett syndrome.

Management

- *Assessment.* The physical investigation of these conditions is outside the scope of this book. Psychological assessment of children with dementia is often helpful to establish a baseline for intellectual functioning, to monitor progress, and to advise on educational approaches.
- *Treatment.* Most of the conditions described above are progressive, with death occurring after several months or years. The terminal phase is often extremely distressing, partly because of its protracted nature. Many of the conditions have genetic implications, sometimes clear-cut, often rather uncertain. This means that anxiety not infrequently hangs over younger children in the family for a number of years, and decisions over further pregnancies are difficult.

Such stressful circumstances mean that it is particularly important for strong emotional support to be provided by the paediatric and primary health care team involved. Support and practical advice from a medical social worker, and the use of hospital or hospice care to provide respite for the family can produce considerable relief (Section 7.7).

5.7 Drug use and abuse

5.7.1 DRUG USAGE

Drugs play an important part in the group culture of children and adolescents. In particular their use:

- promotes the individual's identity with the group: a child who takes up smoking or glue sniffing may feel he is drawn closer to a group where this is normal behaviour
- marks an individual child's entry into the adult world: a teenager who goes into a pub for the first time has undergone a rite of passage
- reduces group anxiety: alcohol at parties removes social inhibitions and thus promotes enjoyment
- results in enhanced, shared experience: small groups of teenagers smoking cannabis achieve an extension of normal experience which they regard as valuable and enjoyable. The fact that, in most countries, cannabis is an illegal drug, may enhance the enjoyment even further.

Unfortunately, all drugs, except when taken in small quantities, damage health and impair social functioning. When taken in large quantities they all can and sometimes do lead to marked social or physical impairment and occasionally to death. Measures taken to reduce their use, whether directed towards individuals or society, need, however, to take into account the positive social functions already mentioned, for otherwise such measures are likely to be ineffective.

Prevalence of drug use

The use of alcohol, tobacco, and illicit drugs varies from country to country and, within countries, between regions. Further, the legality of certain drugs varies between countries, so that, for example, while cannabis consumption is illegal in most countries, this is not the case in the Netherlands. The figures that are given here (Miller and Plant 1996) are for 15 and 16 year olds in the UK, but are typical of those found in most westernized countries.

Nearly all had consumed alcohol at some time in their lives, and over three-quarters had been intoxicated at some time. Half had consumed more than five drinks in a row in the last month. About two-thirds had smoked cigarettes at some time in their lives, and about one-third had smoked in the last month. About two-fifths had used cannabis at some time, and this was, by far, the illicit drug most commonly used. However, glues and solvents had been used by one-fifth, amphetamines and LSD by about 1 in 10. Ecstasy (MDMA) had been used by about 1 in 12, but the numbers involved with this drug may have increased since the survey was carried out in 1995. Heroin, cocaine, and crack were each used by less than 2.5% of those surveyed. There were remarkably few differences between boys and girls, except that girls smoked cigarettes rather more.

These figures make it clear that consumption of tobacco, alcohol, and cannabis is widely prevalent by mid-adolescence. Further, while it used to be considered that tobacco and alcohol were 'gateway' drugs leading on to more dangerous drugs, the pattern now is that alcohol and illicit drugs are regarded by young people as alternatives rather than one leading to the other.

5.7.2 DRUG MISUSE

Factors influencing the excessive use of drugs

Social factors
- *Cost and availability.* Use is strongly related to expense. There is good evidence that, as the relative cost of alcohol has gone down in relation to the cost of living, its use has increased. Further, in many countries, the amount of available income to children and young people has significantly increased. Drugs more readily available in large cities, such as cocaine and heroin, will be used less frequently in rural areas.
- *Pattern of use by adults.* The use of certain drugs, such as solvents, has grown up relatively independently of use by adults. The use in childhood of more socially acceptable drugs, such as tobacco and alcohol, is however heavily influenced by the degree they are used by adults.

- *Media effects.* Portrayal in the media of cigarette smoking and alcohol consumption as glamorous has an influential effect, especially among the disadvantaged. Lyrics of popular songs not infrequently sound the attraction of drugs, particularly cannabis.
- *Legal status of use.* Banning a drug legally may enhance its attractiveness to anti-authority teenagers, but illegality also discourages use by affecting availability. In many places however, cannabis and ecstasy are as freely available as alcohol. The example of cannabis usage (see below) makes it clear that this is not a universal rule.
- *Health education measures.* There is, so far, little evidence that traditional health education measures (lectures and group discussions on harmful effects of drugs, etc.) have any effect on drug use, though they may affect knowledge and attitudes. Children and teenagers do, however, need and deserve information about alcohol and other drugs to enable them to make sensible choices.

Personal/individual factors
- *Sex.* There are now remarkably few differences between boys and girls in the amounts of alcohol and other drugs they consume. .
- *Genetic factors.* With some drugs, for example alcohol, there is evidence that genetic factors may predispose an individual to addiction once a pattern of regular use is established (Bohman 1978), but social factors are of far greater importance in determining the level of consumption within a population.
- *Domestic circumstances.* Poor housing, overcrowding, and disharmonious family relationships are likely to encourage teenagers to spend more time out of the house and thus increase contact with other drug users.
- *Pattern of drug use in the family.* Youngsters who see their parents and sibs smoking, drinking alcohol, etc. are likely to take up similar habits. Teenagers whose friends use drugs are likely to be even more heavily influenced.
- *Personality characteristics.* The teenager who is extrovert in personality, impulsive, and more inclined to take risks than his contemporaries, is also more likely to be a heavy drug user. Low self-esteem and depression are also related to drug use.
- *Educational and occupational failure.* An individual denied these sources of self-esteem will seek other ways to boost his morale.

The importance of social and cultural factors overrides that of personal factors. Most drug users do not have significant adverse psychosocial factors in their background, but this is not the case in those who misuse drugs.

Substance (alcohol and drug) use, abuse and dependency

Although, especially in the case of illicit drugs, many parents and teachers will become concerned long before this point is reached, substance abuse can only be diagnosed when the pattern of drug or alcohol use is affecting the young person's life and causing impairment. The effects may be physical, psychological, or social. Drug dependency is said to exist when an individual suffers physically or psychologically if the drug is withdrawn over a short period of time or there is loss of control over use. Tolerance, a capacity to be able to cope with larger and larger quantities of the substance without ill-effects, is another sign of dependency, but is often slow to develop in adolescents.

General principles of assessment and management

The clinical features of alcohol and other drug abuse will depend on the substance in question, and these are described in the following sections. However, there are general principles of assessment and management that are common to all types of substance abuse.

The most striking common feature is that the young person himself or herself does not perceive that a problem exists. The problem usually presents in one of three ways.

- Probably most commonly the youngster comes to attention because of a co-morbid (accompanying) disorder. This is often some feature of a conduct disorder, such as stealing, or repeated fighting or other aggressive behaviour, but there may also be signs of depression or an anxiety state.
- Second, the young person may present with a problem directly arising out of the drug or alcohol abuse, such as serious intoxication requiring attention in an Accident and Emergency department, or an acute psychotic state following consumption of a drug such as amphetamine or LSD.
- Finally, the problem may present when a parent appears depressed or in a chronic anxiety state, the cause of which turns out to be concern about drug use in their child.

Parents are often slow to realize that their teenage children are taking drugs or alcohol in excess, but finally recognize that this is a possible cause of changes in behaviour such as slowed movements, lethargy and lack of motivation, slurred speech, drowsiness, and irritability. There may be a decline in school performance due to absence from school and lack of concentration. Sudden, increased demands for pocket money or petty thefts within the home may also be indicative.

Where a clinician suspects or diagnoses alcohol or drug abuse, the following information will be a minimum requirement before a plan for management can be formulated (Royal College of Physicians 1995):

- an account of the current consumption of the substances involved
- the circumstances of consumption, e.g. alone or in the company of others
- the psychological needs met by consumption, e.g. relief of anxiety and depression
- general physical health, including where appropriate, laboratory investigations of liver function, etc.
- psychiatric state, including any other significant behaviour and emotional difficulties

- family structure and function, especially the quality of relationships with other family members
- educational and/or employment status
- personality strengths, interests, hobbies, etc.
- motivation for change, insight into present problems.

Much of this information will need to come from parents, teachers and others who have been involved with the child or young person.

General principles of treatment

Often the greatest challenge in management is to succeed in increasing the motivation of the youngster concerned so that he or she actually wants to receive help. The skills of motivational interviewing (van Bilsen and Wilke 1998) with emphasis on initial acknowledgement of the adolescent's concentration on themselves, the creation of an atmosphere of collaboration, and the adoption of a non-moralizing attitude can be helpful in this respect.

If motivation can be achieved, then the use of techniques such as individual psychotherapy and counselling, communications skills training with the family, family counselling or therapy, group work along the lines employed with older problem drinkers and drug abusers, and finally rehabilitation with attention to the finding of opportunities for continuing education or employment will become relevant. In addition, attention should always be given to treatment of any accompanying or co-morbid condition, and to support for other family members. In some cases, it is so difficult to raise the motivation of the young person concerned that support for other family members, especially parents, may be the most valuable form of help the clinician can provide.

Volatile substance misuse

Pattern of use

Solvent misuse, most commonly glue sniffing (Sourindrhin 1985) occurs most commonly in boys aged 11–17 years, with a peak age of 13–15 years. Adhesives, cleaning substances, petrol, and lighter refills are the most common sources. Substances are inhaled from paper bags or saturated rags, or direct from the containers themselves. Inhalation usually though not always occurs as a group activity, often in derelict houses in inner-city areas. Mostly glue sniffing is a transient form of behaviour, engaged in as a risk activity by bored youngsters. Occasionally it fulfils a more important psychological need, relieving anxiety and depression. In this minority of cases, a progression to more dangerous drug usage is more likely.

Clinical features and complications

Inhalation of solvents is usually followed by a short period of intoxication with light-headedness and slurring of speech. Physical symptoms following sporadic usage include nausea, vomiting, headache, abdominal pain, and tinnitus. Clouding of consciousness and visual hallucinations may also occur as a transient toxic psychosis (Skuse and Burrell 1982).

Chronic usage of these substances in higher concentration can produce serious effects. Chronic encephalopathy and fits have been reported in children (King *et al.* 1981), and older users have suffered kidney and liver damage. Death is not uncommon, with around 70 deaths a year recorded in England and Wales between 1985 and 1995 (Taylor *et al.* 1998).

Treatment

Children and teenagers with this habit are most unlikely to come to attention at health clinics merely because they are glue sniffing. Most will never appear at health agencies. A minority will be referred to child guidance or child psychiatry units because of associated psychiatric disorders, or attend hospitals or accident and emergency departments because of physical complications.

Disturbed children and adolescents with glue sniffing as one of their problems will require full psychiatric assessment and appropriate treatment depending on the nature of their psychiatric disorder. This may include consideration of ways in which they can be helped to find alternative ways of relieving anxiety and depression, or to find alternative group activities.

Physical complications such as fits and renal damage will also require appropriate treatment. Again, during and after such treatment, consideration needs to be given to ways in which the youngster can be rehabilitated and helped to avoid re-involvement in the habit.

Prevention

There are legal measures to restrict the sale of solvents to children in many countries. Early detection by parents and teachers can be achieved if they are aware of the signs. The finding of empty containers, the presence of children in an intoxicated state, and the appearance in a child of erythematous spots around the mouth and nose can all suggest that glue-sniffing is occurring.

A Department of Health campaign directed towards parents in the early 1990s, stressing the need to discourage the activity while finding alternative occupation for children involved without making martyrs or heroes out of them, seems to have been reasonably effective in England and Wales, in that it was followed by a reduction in deaths.

Cigarette smoking

Pattern of use

In 1995, 33% of 15 and 16 year old boys and 40% of 15 and 16 year old girls in the UK had smoked in the previous month, with about 1 in 20 smoking more than 11 cigarettes a day. There is strong continuity between smoking in childhood and adulthood. About 1 in 3 of those who become regular smokers in adulthood have begun before the age of 9 years, and 80% of all regularly smoking children in the UK remain regular smokers in adulthood.

Various studies have established that children are more likely to smoke if they are boys, come from working-class families, are educationally failing, are extrovert in personality, go to schools where teachers themselves smoke (Bewley 1979), and (of overriding importance) their parents and close friends smoke.

Clinical features and complications
Children who smoke are more likely to suffer from upper and lower respiratory infections, and indeed they are more likely to suffer from these conditions if their parents smoke, even before they begin to smoke themselves. (As they get older they are predisposed to chronic respiratory disease, lung cancer, and myocardial infarction.)

There are no established direct, psychological ill-effects of cigarette smoking in childhood, but secondary problems sometimes occur. Thus teenagers involved in stealing money from their parents are not infrequently stealing to obtain money to buy cigarettes.

Treatment and prevention
It is most uncommon for teenagers to request help to overcome a smoking habit. More frequently, boys with antisocial problems referred because of some aspect of their conduct disorder turn out to be heavy smokers. It is unusual for them to want help with the habit.

Over recent years, modestly successful preventive measures have been developed (Royal College of Physicians 1992). Lectures and small group discussions emphasizing the dangers of smoking are ineffective. By contrast, the use of role-playing techniques in which, for example, a youngster is given skills to refuse a cigarette at a party when offered one, are more successful (Botvin *et al*. 1980; Telch *et al*. 1982). Health professionals involved in dealing with children and teenagers suffering from conditions such as hypertension and cystic fibrosis, in which smoking has a particularly deleterious effect, should remember to provide advice about smoking even though they are dealing with a young group of patients. The advice may be more relevant than they may suspect.

Cannabis

Pattern of use
Smoking an extract made from the flowers and leaves of the Indian hemp plant, *Cannabis sativa*, is a widespread practice throughout the world, though illegal in the UK. About a third of people in their mid-teens and early twenties in the UK are occasional smokers and about 10% smoke regularly. Many who begin the habit in adolescence continue it intermittently into adulthood.

Clinical features and complications
There is no evidence that intermittent, moderate usage is harmful, though users often report that the sense of relaxation and mild euphoria for which they smoke in the first place may persist over 1–2 days, producing a state of generally low motivation over this time. More prolonged usage may result in mild chronic apathy.

Heavier intermittent or regular usage is sometimes associated with clear-cut adverse reactions. Acute intoxication with gastrointestinal symptoms may result. Episodes of perceptual distortion and occasionally frank though transient psychotic reactions may also occur (Naditch 1974). Psychological though not physical dependence has been reported. Regular users may withdraw from the challenges of the external world into a state of chronic low motivation. Such individuals then become at risk for entering into more dangerous drug-taking activities.

Treatment and prevention

Adverse psychological reactions other than reduction in drive and motivation are rare, and in any case do not usually come to medical attention. If they do, withdrawal from the drug is sufficient to produce improvement. An apparently prolonged reaction of psychotic type is unlikely to result from the effects of the drug alone, and is more probably a response to a constitutional predisposition to psychosis, though this issue is controversial.

Preventive action is of doubtful validity in a drug that apparently has fewer adverse effects than tobacco smoking, but teenagers and parents should be better informed of those adverse effects that do occur.

Alcohol

Pattern of use

About 5% of men and 2% of women in the UK are problem drinkers. As alcohol consumption virtually always begins in childhood and adolescence, and as problem drinking in young people is increasing in frequency, there has been increased interest in and concern about the alcohol consumption of children and young people.

The average age at which UK children have their first alcoholic drink is 10–11 years. By 15–16 years (Miller and Plant 1996), about half the population of both boys and girls will have had more than five drinks in a row within the last month. At this age about a quarter of the teenage population have had a hangover in the previous 6 months and about 1 in 20 have had a drink in the morning to steady the nerves or get rid of a hangover. About 1 in 3 boys and 1 in 5 girls will have got into a fight after drinking (Royal College of Physicians 1995). About 3% have missed a day's schooling due to drinking.

Evidence is lacking, but it is probable that heavy drinking is associated with characteristics similar to those occurring with other heavy drug users (see above). In general, social and cultural factors outweigh personal factors in importance in defining those at greatest risk.

Clinical features and complications

The picture of acute alcohol intoxication is well known and requires no description. Probably the main danger of acute intoxication lies in proneness to accidents (especially road traffic accidents) and predisposition to violent behaviour.

Chronically heavy alcohol consumption is, even in adolescence, likely to lead to problems that are:

- *social:* financial difficulties, educational failure, problems in obtaining employment (due to unpunctuality, irritability, etc.)
- *psychological:* confusion, memory lapses, irritability
- *physical:* especially chronic gastritis.

True alcohol dependency, with inability to cease alcohol intake without withdrawal symptoms and a tendency to relapse, is unlikely to occur until early adulthood, but does occasionally occur in teenagers. It is much more common in the mid to late twenties in young people who have begun to drink heavily in adolescence.

Treatment and prevention

A discussion of the treatment of alcoholism is beyond the scope of this book. Good accounts may be found elsewhere (see Ritson *et al.* 1993). The prevention of alcoholism by conventional health education methods does not seem effective. It is likely that social skills training directed towards individuals in helping them to refuse drinks would have more success. Evidence does suggest that fiscal measures raising the relative cost of alcohol would also reduce the rate of alcohol consumption in the young population.

Other drugs

Young people may also use a variety of other drugs. These include:

- *Amphetamines.* Taken by teenagers because of its euphoric effect, this drug can produce a state of acute excitement with overtalkativeness, insomnia, raised pulse, and blood pressure. On withdrawal, a paranoid psychosis with delusions and visual hallucinations has been described. Ecstasy (3,4-methylene-dioxymethamphetamine, MDMA) is closely related chemically to amphetamine, and has similar euphoriant effects. A number of deaths have been reported either from overheating, or from fluid overload resulting from excessive fluid intake taken to avoid overheating.
- *Barbiturates.* These may be taken orally or intravenously. Young users are usually on multiple drugs. Periodic drowsiness, slurred speech, and depressive mood are common.
- *Cocaine.* This is usually taken by sniffing, but also by injection, for its euphoric effect. Psychological dependence occurs early in its use. Withdrawal may be followed by a paranoid psychosis and characteristic 'formication'—a feeling of ants underneath the skin. *Crack cocaine* is a crystalline form of cocaine, taken by playing a flame on a crystal and then inhaling the smoke.
- *Heroin* (acetyl morphine). This is the most commonly abused narcotic drug of morphine type. It is usually taken by injection for its euphoriant effect, followed by relaxation. Again psychological dependency occurs early, and withdrawal is extremely unpleasant. *Methadone,* a drug used for maintenance therapy in heroin addicts, has similar effects, and has become quite widely available for illegal use.
- *Lysergic acid diethylamide* (LSD). This is a synthetically manufactured hallucinogen, taken in tablet form because of its intensifying effect on sensory perception. Other effects include acute excitement, panic, and unpredictably aggressive behaviour. The effects generally last up to about 12 hours.

The treatment and prevention of abuse of these drugs is described elsewhere (see Schechter 1978). Addiction to cocaine and heroin is particularly dangerous.

The expense of maintaining an adequate supply is likely to lead to stealing and other offences. Lack of money for food results in malnutrition with proneness to infection. Although natural recovery can occur, the risk of death from suicide or infection is considerable. Needle-sharing leading to HIV infection remains a common hazard in many large cities. Teenagers addicted to these drugs, especially if motivated to receive help, require urgent referral to specialist centres. Parents need support whether or not their children are motivated to receive treatment. Illegal drug use in adolescence puts the individual at risk for major social problems later in life (Kandel *et al.* 1986).

5.8 Personality disorders

Both major classification schemes express some reservations about using the concept of 'personality disorder' in children. Thus the glossary to ICD-10 (World Health Organization 1992) states that it is unlikely 'that the diagnosis of personality disorder will be appropriate before the age of 16 or 17 years'. DSM-IV (American Psychiatric Association 1994) is less discouraging. It states that personality disorder categories may be applied to children or adolescents in those relatively unusual instances in which the individual's particular personality traits appear to be pervasive, persistent and unlikely to be limited to a particular developmental stage. To diagnose a personality disorder in a person under the age of 18 years, the features must have been present for at least a year, and, using DSM-IV a diagnosis of antisocial personality disorder cannot be made in an under-18 year old. In fact clinical experience suggests that all types of personality disorder (paranoid, schizoid, schizotypal, antisocial, borderline, histrionic, narcissistic, avoidant, dependent, and obsessive–compulsive) may be seen in under-18 year olds, in a form that makes it extremely likely that they will persist into adult life.

However, because the diagnosis of personality disorder implies a chronic disability, clinicians are understandably and appropriately reluctant to apply what might be regarded as such a damning label to a child or adolescent (Wolff 1984).

Although, therefore, some children do show early signs of enduring personality characteristics, especially of obsessional, histrionic, antisocial, schizoid, and borderline type, it is not generally regarded as desirable to refer to such children as showing personality disorders. More commonly, they are described as showing unusual patterns of personality development without a firm diagnostic statement being made.

6

Child–adult continuities in psychiatric disorders

6.1 Introduction and definitions

Knowledge about the continuity of psychiatric disorders into adult life is relevant to all child health professionals. Parents wish to know what the future holds for their disturbed offspring. Professionals may need such information in order to evaluate their own therapeutic and preventive efforts. For example, if all children with a particular condition, left untreated, do badly when followed into adult life, then even a small degree of professional success would be worthwhile. On the other hand, adult outcome should not be regarded as the only criterion of success. Even if all children suffering a disorder were eventually to get better untreated, treatment in childhood might still be worthwhile if it reduced the length or severity of the problem in childhood.

There is now a considerable amount of information concerning both adult outcomes of childhood mental problems and childhood precursors of adult psychiatric illness (Robins and Rutter 1990). It is clear that there is considerable continuity of psychiatric disorder even from the pre-school years to early adulthood (Caspi *et al.* 1996), with even greater continuity over shorter periods, such as from early adolescence to young adulthood (Ferdinand and Verhulst 1995). The interpretation of such information is, however, complicated in a number of ways:

- Continuity of a disorder may be simple (*homotypic*) or transformed (*heterotypic*). An individual may show the same problem in adulthood as in childhood (*simple continuity*), or a childhood diagnosis may be followed by a different, adult diagnosis (*transformed continuity*). Alternatively, of course, the disturbed child may grow into a mentally healthy adult (*discontinuity*).
- Continuity of service is a poor criterion of continuity and discontinuity. For example, only a relatively small proportion of adult neurotic patients have attended child psychiatric departments as children, but this is at least partly because such a small proportion of emotionally disturbed youngsters attend clinics. This issue highlights the need for long-term epidemiological studies examining total population samples.
- Quite different levels of continuity may be found, depending on whether one starts with a disturbed childhood group showing a particular diagnosis and follows forwards, or starts with an adult group showing the same diagnosis and looks backwards. Most children with a particular diagnosis may improve, but if one looks at adults with the same diagnosis, nearly all of them may have shown the problem in childhood. This is in fact the case with conduct (antisocial) disorders: see below.

If diagnostic continuity is present, the processes underlying such continuity need to be understood if rational preventive action is to be taken. Here again, there are various issues to be considered. For example:

- Continuity may be present because the psychopathological process is internalized and impervious to external changes.
- Continuity may be present but only because the risk factors leading to a disorder, especially adverse social circumstances, are almost invariably stable. Continuity of diagnosis may merely be a reflection of continuity of adversity, and, if circumstances do change, discontinuity may occur. Further, continuity can also be considered in relation to the presence of risk factors in childhood and the subsequent likelihood of disorder in adulthood. For example, it has been found that the presence of multiple adversities in childhood predicts virtually all forms of non-psychotic adult psychiatric disorders (Kessler *et al.* 1997).

6.2 Findings

Child-to-adult and adult-back-to-childhood continuities will be considered separately in this section. Information in this section can be supplemented by reference to the relevant sections of the book dealing with different diagnoses.

6.2.1 CHILD-FORWARD-TO-ADULT CONTINUITY

- *Simple (homotypic) continuity.* Autism and schizophrenia generally persist relatively unchanged into adult life. Similarly, although they have a better prognosis and many more cases improve than is the case with autism and schizophrenia, when anorexia nervosa, Tourette syndrome, and obsessional disorders persist into adult life, as they not infrequently do, there is strong continuity of diagnosis.
- *Mixed simple and transformed continuity.* Most children with conduct disorders do not grow up to be adult criminals, but when they do have problems in adulthood, they are likely to show a mixture of conduct (aggressive personality) and affective disorders (Quinton *et al.* 1990).
- *Transformed (heterotypic) continuity.* Children with the hyperkinetic syndrome or attention deficit hyperactivity disorder (ADHD) often show conduct disorders in adult life (Gittelman-Klein and Mannuzza 1989). However, they may also show an adult form of ADHD (Toone and van der Linden 1997).
- *Discontinuity.* Unless they show co-morbid depressive disorder, children with anxiety disorders are generally well adjusted in adulthood (Last *et al.* 1997). The great majority of children with nocturnal enuresis do not show this symptom in adolescence or adult life, and there is no evidence that they show a higher rate of other disorders later in life. Encopresis also usually remits by adolescence, but there is less certainty about whether this symptom is a risk factor for other disorders in later life.

The mechanisms underlying child–adult continuity probably vary considerably from diagnosis to diagnosis. For example, in schizophrenia and autism, the underlying psychopathology appears largely intractable to environmental change. This may also be true for the severe conduct disorders of childhood and, to a lesser extent, the hyperkinetic syndrome. In contrast, continuity shown by children with less severe conduct disorders and emotional disorders may be much more a result of the persistent nature of the family and wider social adversity they are likely to experience.

6.2.2 ADULT-BACK-TO-CHILDHOOD CONTINUITY

- *Simple continuity.* Most but by no means all cases of adult autism, obsessional disorder, Tourette syndrome, agoraphobia, and anorexia nervosa begin in childhood or, much more commonly, in adolescence.
- *Transformed continuity.* Only a small minority of cases of schizophrenia begin in childhood or adolescence. However, when information about the childhood of those adults who develop schizophrenia later is available, it suggests that they have tended to show other personality features. These pre-schizophrenic precursors include antisocial behaviour restricted to the family setting, and social isolation arising from rejection by peers, perhaps because of odd, incongruous behaviour (Zeitlin 1986).
- *Discontinuity.* Although there is rather inconsistent evidence that they may have suffered traumatic experiences in childhood such as loss of a parent, most adults with either major or minor affective disorders have not shown significant emotional or behaviour problems in childhood. This is, of course, not true for the not insubstantial number of adults with affective illnesses who have suffered anxiety states or depressive disorders in childhood or adolescence. It is likely that as further information accrues, this view of the pattern of adult–child continuity in affective states will need to be modified, for example by considering chronic disorders separately from episodic.

Finally, it should be emphasized that information in this section on continuity relates entirely to probabilities. For most diagnoses, there are many individuals who do not show the characteristic pattern of continuity and discontinuity described here.

7

Psychosocial aspects of
physical disorders: general

An important distinction has been made (World Health Organization 1980) between *impairment* (loss or abnormality of physical or psychological structure or function), *disability* (the consequence of the impairment), and *handicap* (the social disadvantage of a disability). Thus a child may have an apparently small impairment, such as a chronic disfiguring skin rash on the face, causing little disability, but a considerable degree of handicap (unwillingness to go to school). Obviously the reverse may also be the case.

In the UK 3–3.5% of children suffer from one or more disabilities. Of these, about 10% are severely disabled (Office of Population Censuses and Surveys 1989). This level of prevalence is likely to be similar in other westernized countries. Behaviour disorders are the commonest cause of all disabilities, but severe mental retardation (learning disability) is the commonest cause of severe disability, in terms of its impact on the capacity to participate in ordinary activities and live independently.

Of the chronic physical conditions from which disabled children suffer, asthma is the most common, affecting 2% of all children of school age, though some studies have found higher rates. Eczema occurs in about 1% of children, so that illnesses with an allergic component account for a large proportion of chronic childhood physical disability. Neurological conditions are the next most common types of disorder—epilepsy occurs in about 8 per 1000 and cerebral palsy in about 2–3 per 1000. The remainder consist of a wide range of other physical disorders, of which the most common are sensory defects, congenital heart disease, diabetes mellitus, and orthopaedic disorders.

As medical treatment improves, and the period of survival for many conditions increases, although *incidence* (numbers of new cases) remains the same, the *prevalence* (numbers in the population) of disabling disorders rises (Newacheck *et al.* 1986). Further, the nature of an illness may be transformed by a new treatment. The 5 year survival rate of children with leukaemia has improved over three decades from around 0% to around 60%. For parents, the stress of bereavement has been replaced by the stress of uncertainty. For children, a relatively brief and painless illness has been replaced by a prolonged series of hospital visits and treatments with many unpleasant aspects such as painful procedures and alopecia. Doubtless for most such children the new technology has had positive results, but for many it has not. Similarly, new forms of operative procedure, including cardiac transplantation, have transformed the picture in congenital cardiac disease, and new antibiotics and other forms of treatment have markedly prolonged survival in cystic fibrosis.

A broad account of prevalence gives a rather misleading picture of the pattern of disability, because it takes no account of the severity of disorders. Although asthma and eczema are common, and each is occasionally extremely disabling, most children who have asthma and eczema are able to lead normal lives. Some of the less common disorders such as cerebral palsy are usually much more disabling. Further, consideration of the pattern of physical disability in isolation fails to take account of the fact that most severe disability in children with physical disorders arises from associated handicaps, especially mental retardation and psychiatric disorders. Thus, cerebral palsy is frequently associated with mental retardation and specific learning disabilities which hamper the child's life and impair development to as great a degree as the physical condition. The allergic conditions are not, in general, accompanied by associated serious learning difficulties. In order to obtain a true picture of the pattern of physical disability, it is therefore necessary to consider the severity of different conditions and the other problems with which they are associated.

7.1 Psychosocial causes of chronic physical disease

Psychosocial factors may be important in aetiology, either of the development of the physical condition in the first place, or of its maintenance and persistence. Thus, brain damage associated with cerebral palsy sometimes occurs as a result of injuries inflicted by parents on the child in infancy (Diamond and Jaudes 1983). Asthma is an example of a condition which is produced by an inborn lesion (hyper-reactivity of the bronchi), but in which persistence often depends on the presence of psychological triggering mechanisms. In other conditions, such as the various forms of childhood cancer, social and psychological factors are probably of little importance, either in primary aetiology or in maintenance.

Socio-economic factors are generally of less importance in the aetiology of chronic physical diseases than is the case with mild mental retardation and some behavioural disorders. Some chronic conditions, such as failure to thrive, obesity, and recurrent upper respiratory tract infections are, however, commoner in the more deprived sections of the population, and injuries, both accidental and non-accidental, are much commoner. Inappropriate diet, difficulty in maintaining hygienic conditions, and chronic financial stress leading to parental depression are probably the most important reasons for the association between these physical conditions and low socio-economic status.

In considering causation, it is usually unhelpful to think of some conditions occurring in children as 'psychosomatic' and others as 'non-psychosomatic'. In any particular condition (cerebral palsy and asthma are examples), stressful life events may be prominent in aetiology in some children but absent in others (Goodyer 1992). It is often very difficult to determine whether, in a particular child, a life event is the cause of a disorder or a result of its impact. For example, poor achievement in school and consequent disciplinary action might precipitate an attack of juvenile arthritis or might be the first sign of its presence.

7.2 Impact on parents

The effect on parents of the discovery that their child has a chronically handi-capping condition depends on a variety of factors including the nature and severity of the condition (especially the amount of physical care the child needs), the age at which the condition is diagnosed, the presence of associated handi-caps, the personality and previous experience of the parents, the temperament of the child, the amount of help available from relatives and friends, and the quality of health, social welfare, and educational services available.

When a child is born with a handicap, or develops a serious condition after a period of good health, parental reactions tend to follow a characteristic course (Drotar *et al.* 1975). Perhaps surprisingly, these reactions, although they may be severe, do not appear to influence the attachment of the physically handicapped child to a significant degree (Wasserman *et al.* 1987). The reactions are akin to those following bereavement and indeed, although the child remains alive, the parents have suffered the loss of the normal child they expected to rear. Initially there is a stage of shock during which parental feelings are numbed, and a sense of unreality is experienced. The parents are in such a state of anxiety that they find it difficult to absorb information given to them even when it is presented repeatedly and in a very simple form. There may be then a stage of denial when the seriousness of the condition is questioned; the parents may have fantasies that the child will be magically cured, or take the child to a variety of different phys-icians. This is followed by a stage of sadness and anger when depressive feelings and sensations of guilt predominate, but parents may also rage against fate, each other, the child with the handicap, or the physicians who have been involved. Sometimes their anger may be justified—often it is not. Finally, the parents go through a phase of adaptation to the situation and reorganize their lives accordingly. They are able to see the child and his future in more realistic terms, and make plans for his care, education, and future that accord with his real potential.

Not all parents go through these various stages, and there is no reason to think that there is anything amiss if they reach the stage of adaptation by some other route. Some parents, for example, appear never to go through a stage of shock or denial. The absence of a period of sadness is, however, a cause for concern. There is evidence that women who are widowed who do not go through a period of mourning suffer more psychological and physical complaints later on (Raphael 1975), and, by analogy, one would expect parents who do not experience depres-sive feelings after the loss of their normal child to be similarly at risk.

The speed at which parents reach a stage of adaptation varies considerably. Usually this takes a period of several months, but it may occur more rapidly than this, and the process may also take several years. Some parents get stuck at the phase of denial or anger, and spend the whole of their lives either pretending to themselves and others that the child's handicap does not exist, or raging against the supposed (or actual) people responsible for producing the handicap in the first place. The doctors or midwife present at the delivery may be blamed, for example, for congenital defects.

As a disability becomes chronic, so parents' longer-term coping mechanisms come into play. Coping has been defined as 'the effort to master, reduce, or tolerate the demands arising from a stressful transaction'. A useful tool, the *Coping Health Inventory for Parents* (CHIP), for the measurement of coping by parents of children with chronic illnesses has been developed by McCubbin *et al.* (1983). Coping is made possible by physical resources (such as money and employment), social resources (such as friends and relatives), and psychological resources (such as beliefs, problem-solving skills, and personality). It is preceded by appraisal of the situation (Lazarus and Folkman 1984), which may be more or less realistic. Various ways of coping have been defined. They include recourse to practical measures, wishful thinking, stoicism, the seeking of emotional support, and passive acceptance. Clearly, some of these are more likely to be successful than others. Coping strategies are discussed further below in relation to children's reactions.

Although positive coping responses are perhaps the most striking feature of parental reactions, there is a cost. Mothers of children with severe disability do, as a group, show high levels of psychological distress. Some parents with strong personalities become more vulnerable to other stresses, and life may be made more difficult by financial demands arising from meeting the needs of the disabled child (Sloper and Turner 1993).

7.2.1 PARENTAL RELATIONSHIP

Parents often do not pass through the period of initial adjustment at the same pace. Characteristically fathers are likely to spend more time in the phase of denial, perhaps protecting themselves against depressive feelings by preoccupation with the medical details of the handicap. They are likely to be particularly deeply affected by having a handicapped male child. Mothers are more likely to suffer protracted periods of guilt and sadness. The capacity of the parents to communicate and share their feelings affects the pace at which each of them will complete the 'mourning' process. Thus, if a mother is experiencing deep and incapacitating feelings of sadness, her husband may come to believe that he cannot afford to feel sad, or the care of the family would break down. In fact, if a father can admit to his depression and discuss it with his wife, this often leads to a reduction in intensity in her sad feelings. The opportunity to share sad feelings may enable a woman to experience a lightening of her mood. In non-communicating or poorly communicating families, this is less likely to occur.

The rate of marital breakdown in parents of children with physical and mental handicaps is either the same as that in the general population or very slightly raised (Eiser 1993). These findings are at first difficult to reconcile with clinical impressions that the presence of a physically handicapped child has a profound effect on the marital relationship. The reason for the inconsistency probably lies in the fact that while, in some marriages, the child's problem is something about which the parents take quite different attitudes and cannot communicate, thus producing a rift between them, in others the child's difficulties act as a focus of shared concern and bring the parents closer together than otherwise they might have been. Apsley Cherry Garrard wrote 'The mutual conquest of difficulties ... is the only lasting cement of marriage'. The presence of a child with a handicap will alter the functioning of a marriage in a variety of ways (Sabbeth and Leventhal 1984). The closeness of the couple, decision-making processes, and patterns of communication may all be affected. The effects of these changes may, however, be positive as well as negative. Nevertheless, studies examining the quality of the marital relationship in the parents of chronically ill children overwhelmingly show higher levels of marital distress and dissatisfaction than are found in the general population (Eiser 1993).

7.2.2 IMPACT ON PARENTAL SOCIAL LIFE

The effects of having a handicapped child on social life have been well documented. For a minority of parents of children with serious handicaps, leisure activities are curtailed, mothers cannot go back to work when they want to, and there is a restriction in the number of additional children. Nevertheless, when comparisons are made with families without a handicapped child, surprisingly few differences may be noted. Many families with handicapped children would have a rather restricted social life even if their child had been normal. The financial costs of handicap may include loss of the mother's income, visits to hospital, purchase of aids, and alterations to the home to meet the needs of the child. These may be considerable, even with a condition as apparently as innocuous as eczema (Su *et al.* 1997), and the financial effects, though mitigated by the availability of benefits, may seriously affect the life of the family. Financial hardship is likely to be particularly great in single-parent families, when there is only one wage earner and the burden of care cannot be shared.

7.2.3 ATTITUDES TO THE CHILD

Most parents eventually develop a warm and loving relationship with their handicapped child, though inevitably they are sometimes irritated, perhaps by the child's slowness to learn, by behaviour problems, or by the extra demands upon them which the presence of the handicap may entail. However, a minority of parents show attitudes that are less helpful in the promotion of their child's development. The child may be unrealistically perceived as more vulnerable than he really is (Green and Solnit 1964), and this may result in the child being overprotected and infantilized. Alternatively, the child may be rejected and treated with indifference or neglect. For most parents, the healthy appearance and normal development of their children is a source of self-esteem. For some, especially those whose self-esteem is vulnerable for other reasons, the presence of a handicap is a severe blow to their pride, and marked negative reactions develop. Morbid reactions of parents to their handicapped children are not common, but when they do occur, they are often characterized by ambivalence with a mixture of overprotection and rejection.

7.3 Impact on the child

Like children without handicaps, those with chronic disability can be viewed as requiring to gain gradually increasing mastery of their environment (skill acquisition). To achieve this, as well as acquiring skills, they need to be able to enjoy mutually satisfactory relationships with others and a realistic view of themselves as worthwhile people (a positive self-concept). In considering the impact of handicaps on children's development, it is useful to think of these interrelated areas (skill acquisition, self-concept, and emotional development and relationship formation) separately.

7.3.1 SKILL ACQUISITION

Some physical handicaps almost inevitably result in delay in the acquisition of particular skills. Motor handicaps of cerebral-palsied children and the language deficits of deaf children are examples. However, there is also the possibility that failure to acquire skills may arise indirectly, not as a result of the physical disability itself, but for a variety of other reasons—such as lack of stimulation from parents, inadequate schooling, repeated absences from school, or low self-expectations on the part of the child himself.

Most children with physical disabilities do not suffer from the indirect consequences of their handicap in this way. Language development, reading ability, and non-language skills usually develop normally. However, there are exceptions. In the Isle of Wight study (Rutter *et al.* 1970*a*) it was found that children with physical disabilities had 2–3 times the rate of specific reading retardation of children in the general population. They found that 14% of physically handicapped children were more than 28 months behind their expected reading ability, compared with 5% of the general population. A variety of other studies have produced similar results (Schlieper 1985). Children with epilepsy and other brain disorders are particularly likely to be affected in this way (see below), but it is not just these who show educational disabilities. In children with other physical disorders, absence from school and low educational expectations, both from the children themselves and from their teachers, as well as other factors already mentioned, may be responsible (Charlton *et al.* 1991). Repeated absence from school is likely to be especially important in those subjects, such as arithmetic, where new knowledge is often acquired in steps, each of which depends on a previous skill having been learned. In middle-class families parents are likely to ensure that a child has not missed out on a particular important step, but in working-class families—where communication with the teacher may be less satisfactory—ground may not be made up in this way.

7.3.2 SELF-CONCEPT

There are three important aspects to self-concept in the child with a physical disability—the child's body image, his self-esteem, and his view of the cause of his disability.

Body image

The handicapped child's view of himself, if it is to be realistic, needs to take account of whatever it is that is wrong with him. In some children this may be a visible physical deformity such as a skin lesion. In others there may be an invisible physical defect such as a leaky heart valve; in yet others, such as children with epilepsy, the child may be anatomically intact, but have a functional disability.

As in the case with non-disabled children, the disabled tend to see themselves as they believe others see them, so if they are led to think, by what a parent says, that a large birthmark on the face is hardly noticeable, or that a tiny blemish is grossly disfiguring, this will certainly have an impact. As children get older the effect of other children's comments on their disability may become as important as their parents' views.

Self-esteem

There are two components to the degree to which an individual values himself—cognitive and emotional. Thus a child can see himself as brighter or less bright, more or less attractive than he really is. Independently of the cognitive self-appraisal, a child can feel unduly sad or negative about himself and have a tendency to self-criticism, or he can view himself positively and with confidence. It is quite possible for a child to recognize his own perhaps quite severe limitations as a scholar, and yet feel he is a person who really matters in the world. Children with physical handicaps vary considerably in both these components of self-esteem. Most have a realistic cognitive self-appraisal and a positive view of themselves. However, some do show evidence of low self-esteem. In the early years, the problem is likely to arise from the depressed and negative feelings that their parents may have about them, but in later years, the views of other children grow in importance to the disabled child.

Both perception of body image and self-esteem are likely to become of greater emotional importance in adolescence, when there is increased concern about identity, future career, and attraction to the other sex. Just as normal children who have not shown any particular worries about their appearance may become preoccupied with it soon after puberty, so children with physical handicaps may, at this stage of life, become acutely concerned about their disability for the first time in their lives. Despite this possibility, low self-esteem is not a frequently occurring characteristic in adolescents with chronic illness.

Perception of causes of disability

There is a characteristic development of the way in which children see the cause of illness (Brewster 1982). In the pre-school years (aged 4–6) they are likely to see their disability as inflicted on them by others, perhaps as a punishment for misbehaviour. In middle childhood, the notion of contagion becomes more important, and they may see their problem as something they have 'caught' from another child or adult. Only by about the age of 10 years have they developed more mature concepts of personal vulnerability, with more or less appropriate ideas of physiological or anatomical causation. However, this notion of children gradually becoming more advanced, by stages, in their understanding of illness, fails to take into account the degree to which a child's experience of his own illness or the illness of others can influence his perceptions. This can sometimes make a considerable difference (Eiser 1989).

7.3.3 EMOTIONAL DEVELOPMENT AND FORMATION OF RELATIONSHIPS

Prevalence of psychiatric problems

Most children with physical problems develop a satisfactory relationship with their parents, sibs, and other children, are able to control their aggressive impulses as well as other children their age, and do not suffer from undue anxiety, depression, or other symptoms. However, most studies (e.g. Cadman *et al.* 1987, in a total population study carried out in Ontario, Canada), though not all, suggest that children with physical disabilities do have a somewhat higher rate of behavioural and emotional problems than do children in the general population. In the Isle of Wight survey (Rutter *et al.* 1970*b*) children with physical disorders had about double the rate (12% versus 6%) of psychiatric problems than did normal children, and the rate was higher still in those with epilepsy (about 28%) or other evidence of cerebral dysfunction (40%). Breslau (1985) has confirmed that children with brain dysfunction are at increased risk for psychopathology, and that the quality of family environment does not modify this risk (Breslau 1990).

The long-term adjustment in adulthood of physically disabled children suggests that most regard the quality of their lives to be good (Query *et al.* 1990). However, in terms of educational achievement and behavioural difficulties, those who have been brought up in economically and socially disadvantaged circumstances do less well than others more favoured (Pless *et al.* 1989).

Family factors

As in children without physical disorders, the emotional development of the physically disabled child will depend very considerably on family factors. To a considerable degree the mechanisms whereby family factors produce a childhood disturbance are likely to be very similar in the handicapped to the non-handicapped child. However, in the child with a physical problem, adverse parental attitudes may be particularly focused on the disability. Thus a parent who would have been somewhat overprotective anyway may become much more so with a physically vulnerable child. Children who are treated as fragile may come to see themselves as such and become unduly anxious, for example, about physical contact with other children. Alternatively, they may react against parental overprotection and become unnecessarily reckless. A child who is rejected by his parents will often take over the low valuation his parents have of him. Thus, a handicapped 13 year old child who eavesdropped and overheard his parents say that it would have been better if he had never survived, developed a depressed view of himself and made a suicide attempt.

Individual coping and defence mechanisms

A child with a physical disorder is subjected to a specific stress and an unusual cause for anxiety. The way in which individuals deal with anxiety-provoking stresses can best be viewed as a mixture of mainly conscious behavioural strategies (*coping behaviour*) and mainly unconscious psychological *defence mechanisms*. These interact with each other (successful coping can reduce the need for an unconscious defence), but it is easier to consider them separately.

Coping behaviour

People who deal successfully with stress tend, among other strategies, to:

- Ration the amount of stress they cope with at any one time. Very bad news is absorbed bit by bit. Thus a child may say to himself: 'I am just going to think about my operation tomorrow. I don't want to think further ahead than that.'
- Try to obtain information about their problems from a number of different sources.
- Rehearse to themselves behaviour that is going to be difficult for them. Thus a coping child with a scar who is frightened of teasing will rehearse what he is going to say before the teasing occurs.
- Try a variety of ways of dealing with a problem, rather than stick to an unpromising approach.
- Construct buffers against disappointment. For example, a coping child having an operation would prepare himself beforehand for the failure of the operation as well as its success.

These various coping mechanisms are, of course, used by parents as well as children in dealing with the unpleasant facts of a physical disorder (Hamburg and Hamburg 1980).

Defence mechanisms

A child faced with unacceptable aspects of a physical disorder whose coping behaviour is unequal to the task may use unconscious psychological mechanisms to deal with problems he is unable to accept at a conscious level. He may:

- *Deny* the problem exists. 'I do get badly teased at school, and I don't know what to do about it.' = 'I don't get teased at school.'
- *Rationalize* the problem. 'I feel miserable about how short I am.' = 'Everyone feels miserable from time to time.'
- *Project the emotion* on to someone else. 'I feel angry with myself for not being able to stop having fits.' = 'My mum feels angry with me because of my epilepsy.'
- *Regress.* 'If I were 3 years younger, it would be all right for me to want my mum around more, so I'll act younger.' = 'I just like my mum around a lot of the time.'

- *Repress* the problem. 'I feel very sad because I think no girl will ever want to have sex with me because of the way I look.' = 'I don't have any sexual feelings.'
- *Displace* the emotion. 'I feel guilty about my eczema and I don't know why.' = 'My room is in a mess and I feel guilty about not clearing it up.'

Commonly, children show a mixture of at least partially effective coping strategies and defence mechanisms. As coping improves, so the need for unconscious processes is diminished. The use of defence mechanisms may be healthily adaptive, and occur while coping mechanisms are being strengthened.

7.4 Impact on the sibs

The brothers and sisters of children with physical problems may themselves develop behavioural disturbances. For example, though most sibs of children with chronic epilepsy and Down syndrome do not have problems, some studies have shown them to have significantly more disturbance than one would expect by chance (Breslau *et al.* 1981). The sib may be relatively neglected, feel unable to bring friends home because he is frightened of what they will think of his handicapped brother or sister, or show emotional reactions for a variety of other reasons. Some girls with a younger, handicapped sib may suffer severe limitations of their social lives because they are expected to spend a great deal of time looking after the handicapped child. As time goes on, sibs of chronically handicapped children have been shown to suffer an increase in depression and social isolation (Breslau and Prabucki 1987). There may also be benefits to sibs in having a handicapped brother or sister. These include an increased capacity to cope with stress, and an enhancement of their caring, altruistic tendencies (Horwitz and Kazak 1990).

7.5 Principles of psychosocial management of physically handicapped children and their families

7.5.1 COMMUNICATING A DEPRESSING DIAGNOSIS

Bad news comes in various forms in paediatrics. In some cases, such as myelomeningocele, a diagnosis of serious import can be made immediately after birth. In others, such as diabetes mellitus, the diagnosis is usually made over a period of 1 or 2 days when the child is much older. Some diagnoses, such as cystic fibrosis, may be preceded by a long period of ill-health and uncertainty, but may also be made at or shortly after birth, especially if there is a previously affected sib. In yet others, such as asthma or epilepsy, the seriousness of a diagnosis may only be realized after routine treatment measures have failed to improve what is usually a relatively benign condition. The principles of imparting the diagnosis (Taylor 1982) will be similar in all these circumstances, although the details will vary considerably (see also p. 103 for discussion of communication of diagnosis of mental retardation). Principles include:

- The doctor involved in imparting information of serious import should be the most senior and experienced in the team.
- If at all possible both parents should be present, even if this means a delay of a few hours or a day or two and (if the mother is a single parent and agrees) even if the parents are not living together. The greatest support parents receive will be from each other, and they should be able to share the burden from the start.
- It is useful to start by spending some time finding out about the parents' current state of knowledge. 'I wonder what you yourselves have thought might be wrong with X.'
- Aside from the above provisos, the news should be broken as early as possible, and the practitioner should be as open and honest as possible about it. It is usually helpful to begin by listing the symptoms and investigatory findings, and then give the diagnosis before pausing to give the parents the oppportunity to ask questions and express their feelings. The use of simple language to explain the problem without shirking technical labels, if this seems appropriate, is helpful.
- After receiving the diagnosis, parents will often ask a large number of questions. This will usually enable the clinician to give information about causation, outcome, forms of treatment available, and genetic implications. As parents are likely to be in a state of shock, they will not take all this information in when it is first imparted. They are likely to need a number of opportunities to ask the same questions. If a team of people are involved, it is important that they decide beforehand who can take responsibility for communication of information (junior doctors, nurses, etc.), and ensure the same message is put over by all concerned. If parents, after a session or two, have not asked questions about a particularly important aspect—causation, outcome, etc.—then the subject should be raised with them to give them an opportunity to discuss it further. They may or may not be ready to do so.
- The positive as well as the negative aspects of outcome should be presented. 'In the UK, all children are able to receive education. It should always be possible to control pain effectively', etc.
- Emotional responses to the information should not be discouraged. If a parent starts to cry, then one can say 'I know this is terribly upsetting. It is very natural you should show your feelings.' It does no harm for the doctor, nurse, or social worker involved to admit they themselves feel sad or worried about the situation.
- When the initial interview with the doctor is over, it may be helpful for the parents to have someone (nurse, social worker) with them to continue to talk to. This person ought also to be sensitive to the parents' wishes to be alone at this point.

The child may be of an age to understand the diagnosis and its implications. In these circumstances, it is usually sensible to see the parents first and discuss with them how and in what form information is to be given to the child. There are many views on how much information should be given to children of different levels of understanding, and this is discussed further below.

When parents of disabled children are asked about their satisfaction with services, the lack of skill and sensitivity with which bad news has been imparted is high on their list of aspects of care they found unsatisfactory and most upsetting (Milner *et al.* 1996).

7.5.2 CONTINUED COUNSELLING

The family with a physically handicapped child is likely to require continuing medical advice, but also continued counselling. The social and personal needs of the child and family will change with age. Inevitably the doctor with ongoing responsibility for medical care will find himself aware of parental attitudes, and discussing educational and other aspects of the child's life. For many families who would be reluctant to seek help for non-medical or psychiatric reasons, the medical consultation to review a child's needs provides the only opportunity for wider discussion of social and psychological factors. As the well-being of the child may depend at least as much on these as on his physical state, and the two are probably closely related anyway, it is important that doctors dealing with physically handicapped children on an ongoing basis have reasonably well-developed counselling skills.

The principles of ongoing counselling include:

- An opportunity, built into the system, to discuss social and psychological development and related problems. Right from the start, families should feel this opportunity is not just an extra service available on demand, but something they are expected to require. For this to happen, either the doctor must make routine enquiries along these lines and have time to deal with issues raised, or there should be someone available, such as a social worker or psychologist, with whom he or she works closely, who can take this responsiblity. Counselling does not, however, merely, or even mainly involve giving advice. It includes being able to listen to anxieties and, on occasion, respond with sympathy without attempting to offer solutions.
- As with the breaking of depressing news, continuing counselling is more likely to be effective if both parents are present.
- It is important to make sure that the clinician is aware of new skills the child has acquired since last seen. These are as important as any problems that may have developed.
- When considering how to advise concerning problems that may have arisen, it is helpful to focus particularly on what the parents and child are getting right at the present time, rather than on what they are doing wrong. It may be easier to build on existing coping skills rather than to eradicate faulty practices. A mother may be generally rather overprotective, but allow her child to spend the night with relatives or friends. It may be more useful to spend time on working out with her how the night spent away from home enhances the child's confidence and independence than focusing on what she will not let the child do.

- It is best not to give blanket advice, but to be as specific as possible. If a father is emotionally distant from his child, working out a particular activity the two might do together is more useful than just suggesting that father spends more time with the child.
- Some doctors are discouraging to the expression of emotion in parents because they are embarrassed by it or fear that dealing with it will be too time-consuming. The expression of emotion and understanding its cause often clarifies issues and saves time in the long run. Once a doctor gains confidence in dealing with the expression of emotion, embarrassment is usually no longer a problem.
- When parents differ about an issue, for example letting a child go to a special school, it is usually better not take sides. By contrast, working out with each parent why they feel the way they do will often result in the parent with the more irrational view ceding the point.
- Families change over time. It is dangerous to stereotype a family or family members and forget that they may have undergone considerable development since last seen.
- Communication with others working with the child and family is an important part of the job. It is very rare for people such as schoolteachers to feel they have too much information and often teachers are surprisingfy unaware of the implications even of relatively common conditions (Eiser and Town 1987). There may be difficulties in knowing whether to transmit information that is relevant, and yet might be shameful or embarrassing to the family. It is often sufficient in these circumstances to indicate that there are serious domestic problems affecting the child without being explicit about a father's alcoholism or a mother's depressive illness. Often teachers know about these matters from what even quite young children write in their essays. It is important to ask permission from parents before communicating with other agencies, and to explain what information it is intended to communicate. If in doubt whether to communicate a particular piece of information, then it is always sensible to check with parents what their views are on the matter. The most useful communication is two-way, and this is easier face to face or on the telephone than by letter. Teachers and social workers often have information concerning, for example, compliance with medication, that is of great relevance to medical management.
- Many children with chronic physical disorders have multiple medical problems and require a team of professionals to assist them. In these circumstances it is useful for one of the team to be nominated as co-ordinator for each family, and for other specialists not to attempt to take over this role. If the child's needs are complex, it is likely that this co-ordinator will be a member of the hospital team rather than the family doctor, but if this is the case, it is still vital that the family doctor, who is likely to be the first port of call in emergencies, is kept fully in the picture.
- Health professionals are likely to be the counsellors that families see least of, although, because of their status and sometimes their expertise, their influence is likely to be disproportionate to the time they spend. However, many parents

obtain great help from discussion with relatives outside the family, friends, teachers, and other non-health professionals. Of course, such people can sometimes be unhelpful, as can doctors, but, on balance, their supportive value far outweighs their negative effects.

- Doctors may have a special part to play in introducing parents to others who may be especially helpful, including parents of children with similar problems. Regular parent groups organized by social workers (Bywater 1984) or other professionals, can be practically helpful and emotionally supportive. Parent organizations, linked to particular disabilities, provide a most helpful forum for information-sharing and mutual support, and often doctors or social workers can indicate how these can be contacted. In the UK, 'Contact-A-Family' (1998) provides a useful list of addresses. A small minority of parents seem to manage to avoid facing their own problems by putting all their energies in these organizations, leaving nothing for themselves and their own families, but the overall positive contribution of these bodies is considerable. When health professionals are in the early stages of counselling parents of a child with a chronic illness, perhaps they should not ask themselves 'Should I put these parents in touch with a self-help organization?', but rather 'Which self-help organization shall I recommend?'.

- It is often difficult for paediatricians to know when to refer problems to psychologists and psychiatrists (Graham 1984). Obviously not all emotional, behavioural, relationship, and learning problems can be referred. Relevant factors in deciding on referral include the availability of interested mental health professionals, the severity and persistence of the psychological problems, and the motivation of the family. When paediatricians, psychiatrists, and psychologists meet regularly at ward liaison meetings or on psychosocial rounds (see below), there are usually few real problems over referral. Absence of communication between paediatricians and child psychiatrists is the most common reason for non-referral by the former group (Oke and Mayer 1991).

7.6 Hospitalization

Admission to hospital is a common experience for children. In the UK about 6% of children are admitted each year and, by the age of 5 years, about 1 in 4 children has been admitted at least once. The mean duration of admission is about 6 days, and the majority of children have relatively short admissions of 3–4 days or less. In the UK, about 1 in 7 children is admitted to adult wards rather than to special children's facilities. The commonest causes for admission are acute respiratory infections, but other infections, injuries, and ill-defined conditions without a definite diagnosis are also very frequent causes of admission.

Although most admissions to hospital for illness are short term, about 4% of admissions are for more than a month, and some children remain resident in long-stay hospitals, on a more or less permanent basis, usually because of a combination of severe mental retardation, sensory impairment, and physical disability.

7.6.1 SHORT-TERM EFFECTS OF HOSPITALIZATION

The reaction of young children admitted to hospital varies considerably, and will depend particularly on whether separation from parents occurs, and on how discrepant the hospital environment is from the child's everyday experience at home. Thus, if a child is not separated, retains familiar toys, is given food he likes to eat, is called by the same name as he is at home (perhaps Jamie and not James, for example) and is able to continue to watch his favourite television programmes, the reaction to hospitalization may be minimal (Brown 1979). On the other hand, young children separated from their parents into new surroundings are likely to show distress that is much more marked. Initially they often show a wary approach to their new environment. At the point of separation from their parents, an angry protest with crying, sometimes leading to uncontrollable sobbing, is relatively common. Eventually, this active distress will give way to an expression of general misery, often with food refusal and sleep disturbance. Subsequently, the child will apparently become resigned to the situation. When the mother visits, he will, however, be likely to show angry feelings towards her for apparently abandoning him, and the cycle of protest, despair, and detachment (Bowlby 1975) will be repeated when she once again leaves him. This pattern of behaviour may last for several days or even weeks. Many young children, however, do become adjusted to ward life, make special relationships with particular nurses, and lose their tendency to distress when their mother leaves, with the realization that she will indeed return before too long.

Older separated children of school age are also likely to be wary on admission, but are distinctly less likely to show anger and despair to the same intense degree. They may, however, become preoccupied with reunion with their parents, counting the hours or minutes until the next visit. Both older and younger children are likely to develop fear reactions to specific nurses or technicians who have been involved in administering painful procedures. Again, younger children are likely to show these reactions more intensely.

After discharge from hospital, younger children in particular may show unusually difficult behaviour with their parents, apparently testing them out to see if they are still loved or likely to be sent away again. Feeding and sleeping problems are relatively common. There may, however, also be positive effects arising from hospitalization. Sick children, and those around them, may gain valuable experience and knowledge from a hospital admission in terms of a sense of generosity and concern for others (Parmelee 1986).

7.6.2 LONG-TERM EFFECTS

Children who have been repeatedly admitted to hospital in early and mid-childhood are slightly more likely to develop behavioural and emotional disturbances in adolescence (Quinton and Rutter 1976). The effects are particularly likely to be present if the admissions are for long periods and if the children come from disadvantaged homes. The reason for this is unclear, and it is possible that, with improvements in hospital practice, this adverse effect may be minimized or disappear altogether (Shannon *et al.* 1984).

7.6.3 FACTORS MODIFYING DISTRESS

The short-term effects of admission to hospital will depend on a variety of factors including especially:

- The *age* of the child. Above the age of 1 year, the younger the child, the more severe the distress is likely to be.
- The *social circumstances* of the family, for example the degree to which they are already financially stretched, and the relationship between the parents.
- Adequacy of *preparation* for hospitalization (see below).
- The *condition* for which the child is admitted. Children whose illness produces greater distress and discomfort will be more disturbed.
- The necessity for frequent *painful procedures* (Saylor *et al.* 1987).
- The presence of *familiar figures*, especially the parents, during the admission. Thus, if rooming-in facilities are available, this will markedly cut down short-term distress.
- *Previous experience* of hospitalization.
- The *parent–child relationship*, and especially the level of anxiety of parents and the degree to which their anxiety is communicated.
- The *temperament or personality* of the child.
- The *coping style* of the child in the face of stressful medical procedures. This may be active (information-seeking) or avoidant (information-denying) (Peterson 1989).
- The availability of adequate *play and education facilities*.
- The attitudes of *hospital staff*.
- The degree to which *ward organization* is child-centred.

7.6.4 PREVENTION OF ADVERSE EFFECTS OF HOSPITALIZATION

Distressing reactions to hospitalization can be reduced by a humane and thoughtful policy towards child care (Vernon *et al.* 1965). If, in addition, extra resources are available for staff and equipment, distress can be reduced still further. The following measures have been demonstrated to have a beneficial effect:

- *Preparation for the admission.* For planned admissions the hospital should provide a booklet describing what will happen when the child is admitted, ward routines, and procedures, etc. Parents of young children can be recommended suitable storybooks to read to their children. If at all possible, parents and children should visit the ward beforehand—perhaps immediately after the admission is decided upon in the out-patient department.

- *Rooming-in facilities* should be available for parents of all children under the age of 5 years, and for older children who are very ill, or likely to be unusually upset by the admission.
- *Visiting* by parents and sibs should be permitted at all times and should be actively encouraged. Parents should be particularly encouraged to visit on critical days, for example days when an operation is to be performed or the child is to have an important investigation. Parents should be made to feel welcome on the wards, and a sensitive, practical attitude taken to the fact that some may well be bored, angry, distressed, and manipulative at different times. The advantages of involving parents in the care of their children far outweigh the dangers of attempting to exclude them.
- Children should be adequately *prepared for all painful or unpleasant procedures* by discussion and, with young children, suitable play material. No attempt should be made to disguise the fact that a procedure is unpleasant. Specialist wards will need special equipment for this purpose. It is particularly important to prepare children for postoperative discomfort and procedures.
- *Nursing and medical staff* working on children's wards should receive adequate instruction in procedures necessary to reduce distress. In particular, an attempt should be made to increase their awareness of distress and its likely causes, so that they can take action accordingly. They should be aware of the developing child's changing concepts of illness.
- The presence of *trained teachers* is necessary to provide appropriate education for children fit enough to receive it. Trained play staff should also, if at all possible, be available to assist in preparation for procedures, enable anxieties to be expressed and understood more generally, and to occupy children, especially those young children whose parents cannot be available all the time.
- The ward atmosphere and organization should be *child-centred*. Thus, as far as possible, mealtimes, waking and sleeping times, etc. should be geared to the needs of the children and families rather than those of the staff. Children should, if possible, have nurses specially allocated to them so that they have the opportunity to develop trusting relationships.
- *Social work, psychological, and psychiatric back-up services* should be available to all ward staff. If at all possible there should be a regular psychosocial meeting once a week to discuss both psychosocial aspects of ward organization and procedures, and specific children causing concern. Such psychosocial meetings can have a therapeutic effect and also provide an educational experience for paediatric medical and nursing staff. Educational goals can include the encouragement of a developmental approach to emotional and psychosomatic reactions, and greater psychosocial understanding of illness in relation to children's cognitive level and coping techniques. The meetings can also assist in earlier recognition of emotional and management problems, especially those concerning severely ill children as well as anxious or manipulative parents.
- In addition, the conduct of joint paediatric *psychiatric work* with families of sick children in which physical or emotional problems interact will prevent tendencies to see children and family problems in either/or (physical/psychological) terms (Bingley *et al.* 1980).

- Medical and nursing staff working with sick children and their families or in a special-care baby unit are often under severe *stress* themselves. They may benefit from a regular opportunity to discuss their own feelings in relation to their work, and provide emotional support for each other. The sharing of feelings of anger or depression that often arise in relation to paediatric care can benefit not only junior nurses and medical staff but also more experienced professionals. Such regular staff support groups may be initiated by, and involve, mental health professionals, or be organized entirely by the paediatric, nursing, and social staff themselves. Staff on wards where there is a relatively high level of mortality or chronic disability among patients are particularly likely to benefit from such group activities.

7.6.5 EFFECTIVENESS OF PREVENTIVE MEASURES

There is evidence that the measures described above are indeed effective in reducing short-term distress due to hospitalization as well as emotional disturbance after discharge (Wolfer and Visintainer 1979). The long-term effects of hospitalization appear to have been reduced following the introduction of more liberal visiting and admission policies in the 1960s (Quinton and Rutter 1976). In well-run units, the level of distress is now a good deal less than it used to be (Shannon *et al*. 1984).

7.7 Care of the dying child

The death of a child is an uncommon event in the developed world. In the UK just under 6 per 1000 pregnancies end in stillbirth, the psychosocial aspects of which are discussed in Section 8.1. After birth about a further 4% die in the first 4 weeks of life—mainly of very low birthweight and congenital anomalies. Subsequently, the death rate, still mainly due to congenital anomalies, is about 2 per 10 000 for the rest of the year, remains at about 3 per 10 000 for 1–4 years, and declines to about 2 per 10 000 from 5 to 15 years (Platt and Pharaoh 1996).

After the first year of life, injuries are the most common cause of death, accounting for about a quarter of the total mortality. Deaths from injuries are much commoner in lower socio-economic groups. After injuries, congenital anomalies and neoplasms (cancers) are responsible for most deaths from 1 to 5 years, and neoplasms remain the second commonest cause throughout the rest of childhood. The remaining deaths are caused by a wide variety of conditions, especially respiratory and cardiac disorders.

Although the experience of death is a quite frequently occurring event for those working in specialized centres dealing only with serious or complicated children's disease, for most other health professionals dealing with children it is fortunately not a common experience. For the family of a child with a fatal illness, the experience is made even more harrowing by the infrequency with which death nowadays occurs in the young. Because the event is so unusual, family members, friends, and people at work may feel uncertain how to behave or show sympathy, and leave family members isolated and unsupported.

7.7.1 PHASES OF GRIEF

Parents

Parents of children with chronic illnesses with a frequently fatal outcome, such as leukaemia and cystic fibrosis, first experience grief when they are told the diagnosis and realize they have lost part of the future of their child. The term *anticipatory mourning* is sometimes used to describe the grief reactions they experience at this time. Subsequently the parents experience a second phase of mourning, *terminal grief*, when the child dies. If the illness is acute, or the first phase of parental mourning is protracted, the second phase may supervene before initial mourning is completed.

The process of parental grief is similar to that described above in relation to reactions to the diagnosis of chronic physical handicap, but, of course, the emotions of parents faced with the death of their child are likely to be more intense (Burton 1974; Gyulay 1978). The period of shock when the parents hear the news may be accompanied by denial ('This can't be happening to me') and guilt ('What could I have done to make this happen?'). Somatic complaints such as dizziness, palpitations, weakness of the legs, and ringing in the ears are common. Subsequently, over the next few weeks, parents feel a variety of other emotions. Irrational fear and anger predominate. They may withdraw from relationships with others. Inability to accept the news may lead to internal 'bargaining' ('If I pray then this terrible thing won't turn out to be true'). Eventually the reality of the situation is more or less accepted and the parents are, for the first time, able to experience appropriate sadness.

Communication between parents may be difficult during these phases of grief, for mourning often proceeds at a different pace for the two of them. Pre-existing tensions may be worsened. A mild drinking problem may turn into a more serious one. Parents already on the verge of separation may stay together 'for the sake of the child', but their resentment towards each other and towards the child may increase. In contrast, some parents may genuinely be drawn closer together. These are likely to be the parents whose coping mechanisms in the face of stress (see above) are effective, and who find they cope better when they share the tasks placed on them by the child's illness.

Children

Young children develop mature concepts of death much earlier than is generally appreciated, so that by the age of 5 years, about two-thirds of children in the general population have complete or almost complete understanding of the finality of death (Lansdown and Benjamin 1985). The concept of death may be more advanced if the child has experienced the death of a pet or of an elderly relative in the family. The development of a mature concept of death is a gradual process, which may be speeded up in children who spend a good deal of time in hospital because they are inevitably made more aware of its implications.

The fears of the fatally ill child are usually less to do with death than with fears of separation and painful procedures. Older children also experience these fears, but their reactions to the situation are usually much more complex. Although they need their parents for security, support, and information about their predicament, parent–child communication is often poor. Children see their parents to be anxious, upset, and perhaps angry. They may not wish to upset them further by expressing their own anxieties, and may indeed feel protective towards their parents. The child's own anger, perhaps stimulated by inability to lead anything like a normal life, may be directed towards the parents and inhibit communication further.

In the terminal phase, children may lose interest in their surroundings. With older children, it is often clear to those around them that they are aware of their predicament, even if there has been no discussion of the outcome. Fears of pain and discomfort become more prominent. In many cases the blurring of consciousness that precedes the final moments of death produces brief agitation before coma and death supervene.

7.7.2 MANAGEMENT

The above account should make it clear that families respond in very different ways to the fatal illness of a child, and the main task of professionals involved with them is to ensure that family members feel supported, well informed, and understood whatever their particular reactions may be (Burton 1974). This is much more likely to occur if there is a *key worker*, usually a social worker, whose task it is to co-ordinate the psychosocial aspects of care provided by nursing, medical, and play staff, and mental health professionals. This key worker may also take responsibility for linking the local community support network, including the primary health care team, school teachers, and local hospital staff with the specialist team.

During the initial grief phase, family members may wish to go over the details of the condition a number of times before they can absorb the information. Angry responses may elicit resentment in staff, but need to be seen as understandable. Parents who are involved in their child's care, and made to feel their contribution is important, will find it easier to cope.

Some parents, lost in their own grief reactions, may benefit from having the needs of the ill child and his or her sibs gently indicated to them. The needs of the sibs are often similar to those of the patient. Parents who feel discouraged and rejected by their children need particular support. Formal or informal groups of parents with children suffering from similar conditions may be helpful.

The problem of what to tell the child with a fatal condition is not easily resolved. Most of those experienced in the care of dying children now feel that openness concerning the outcome, linked to reassurance about the ability of nursing and medical staff to control pain and discomfort, is the policy of choice. However, parental views on this matter have to be paramount and, in a number of cases, the child will make it clear he is not ready to discuss the matter. A flexible approach is therefore desirable. If children are given information by professionals, it is important that parents are present at the time. Often parents will prefer to communicate information themselves.

Whether the final terminal phase is in hospital, at home, or as is very occasionally the case, in a hospice for dying children, strong support from professional staff is particularly important over this period. Requests for autopsy, procedures for allowing the parents privacy in which to show their feelings, permission for donation of organs for transplantation, explanation of the information on the death certificate—these matters need to be planned beforehand so that parents do not suddenly feel abandoned by familiar staff after the death of their child. Most hospitals dealing with children with fatal illnesses arrange a routine post-bereavement visit with paediatric staff at 4–6 weeks after the death, so that issues concerning the final stages of illness and the genetic implications of the disease can be further discussed. Some hospitals and children's units arrange post-bereavement counselling for parents who think they would find this helpful.

8

Psychosocial aspects of specific physical non-neurological conditions

8.1 Stillbirth and neonatal death

Prevalence

In England and Wales stillbirth (late fetal mortality) occurs at the rate of about 6 per 1000 live births. Death *in utero* is usually associated with the presence of a condition of the placenta or umbilical cord, or a congenital abnormality in the fetus. However, a range of other factors may be responsible. Death in the first 4 weeks of life (neonatal mortality) occurs in about 4 per 1000 live births. Congenital abnormalities, the respiratory distress syndrome, infections, and complications of delivery are responsible for most such neonatal deaths.

Psychological reactions

A comprehensive review of parental reactions to perinatal loss is provided by Zeanah (1989). Parental reactions to the unexpected death of the baby they have anticipated vary in severity. Severe emotional shock is the commonest immediate reaction, and this may be followed by feelings of numbness, preoccupation with thoughts of the dead baby, and difficulty in accepting that the baby is dead (Forrest *et al.* 1982). A mourning reaction is likely to persist for several months, and may normally last up to about a year. During this time recurrent feelings of sadness and thoughts of the dead baby are likely to recur. Significant factors affecting the severity and resolution of grief include the overall physical health of the mother, the gestational age at the time of the loss, the quality of the marital relationship, and pre-loss mental health symptomatology (Toedter *et al.* 1988). Induction of delivery within 24 hours of death *in utero* and ensuring the family has a token of remembrance of the baby, such as a photograph, reduce subsequent anxiety symptoms (Radestad *et al.* 1996). Occasionally more prolonged reactions occur with longer-lasting implications for the marriage and family life, but this is probably unusual, though there is a lack of systematic follow-up data.

Psychosocial aspects of management

Arrangements made following stillbirth need to be sensitive to parental feelings (Forrest *et al.* 1981). The issue of a certificate of stillbirth or death certificate may be distressing. Arrangements for the funeral need to take into account parent's wishes. Mourning may be facilitated if the parents are encouraged to see, touch, and even perhaps hold their dead baby. A photograph of the baby may help parents to remember and come to terms with the death. Parents should be encouraged to attend the funeral and the baby's grave should be properly marked. Results of necropsy should be communicated to them by the paediatrician or pathologist with concern for their anxieties about future pregnancies. Parents appreciate open and honest discussion with the paediatrician and nursing staff after the loss, and are very sensitive to attempts staff may make to ignore or avoid talking to them. They do not appreciate advice from doctors to have another baby so as to 'get over' their loss, but value information about future risks to enable them to make their own decisions.

Brief counselling for bereaved parents to help them come to terms with their loss does not seem to have an effect on mental health outcome, though it is often much appreciated at the time (Lilford *et al.* 1994). Most anxiety and depression has remitted by 8 months after the event (Vance *et al.* 1995).

8.2 Sudden infant death syndrome (cot death)

Definition

Sudden infant death syndrome involves the sudden and unexpected death of an infant that is not linked to any clear-cut cause.

Clinical features

Babies involved are almost always between 1 month and 1 year of age, with a peak incidence between 4 and 6 months. The baby is usually found dead by the parents either first thing in the morning or after a period, sometimes quite brief, of being left unattended. There is a story of mild respiratory symptoms in the previous 2 or 3 days in about a third of cases. 'Near-miss' cot deaths in which a baby is suddenly noted not to be breathing, and is resuscitated by shaking, also occur. There may be no serious after-effects, but in some cases anoxic brain damage sustained may result in severe mental retardation.

Prevalence

Sudden infant death syndrome occurs in about 2–3 per 1000 live births. In the UK, it is the most common cause of death in the period from 1 month to 1 year. Its prevalence in the UK reached a peak in 1988, and subsequently fell from from about 2.3 per 1000 to about 0.7 per 1000 in the early 1990s, probably as a result of a public campaign to reduce the practice of putting infants sleeping in the prone position (Gilbert 1994). It occurs in all social classes, but is more common in babies living in deprived circumstances. It is distinctly more common in families where there are adverse social circumstances and the father is unemployed or absent (Taylor and Emery 1988), and someone in the family smokes (Gilbert 1994). Large families and young single mothers are also risk factors. There is a slight male preponderance. There is an increased risk of the condition in babies where a sib has previously died of it. The risk in these children is about 1%.

Aetiology

Basically the aetiology of sudden infant death syndrome is not understood, but it is thought that sudden respiratory arrest occurs as a result of a wide range of different infective, circulatory, biochemical, and immunological abnormalities, sometimes possibly aggravated by an inappropriate sleeping position or passive smoking. In a minority of cases (probably a small minority) deliberate and concealed suffocation by parents is the cause of respiratory arrest (Emery 1985), and this possibility should be considered more carefully where there is a recurrence.

Usually, affected babies have had a normal development, but in a minority there have been previous apnoeic episodes or other, less obviously related abnormalities of the pregnancy and neonatal period.

Psychosocial aspects

Parents' reactions to the sudden and unexpected death of their young infant are, not unexpectedly, very severe. There is usually a period of disbelief, then shock, followed by an acute bereavement reaction. Mourning for the dead infant usually lasts several weeks or months, but may be further prolonged. Some parents, though by no means all, experience a sense of guilt for inadequate care and failure at not being available to their baby in his terminal moments. Parents may express anger towards each other, the dead child's sibs, or professionals who have previously seen the child. The grief experienced by older siblings may go unnoticed, but it is often as prolonged as that of their parents, and may show itself as a behaviour problem (Hutton and Bradley 1994).

Compared to controls, mothers who have experienced such a loss continue to show high levels of anxiety and depression, and fathers show increased alcohol consumption as long as 30 months after the event (Vance *et al.* 1995).

Immediate management may be complicated by police enquiries which may, even if sensitively carried out, add to the distress of parents. Inquest proceedings may also exacerbate guilt and anger.

Counselling

Families where an infant has died in this way will be helped if strong, unequivocal emotional support is available from members of the primary health care team, especially the health visitor and family doctor. Additional help can be provided by the paediatrician, especially if he has already been involved in the care of the child. A full explanation about the nature of the condition, with some idea of the various possible causes, should be given. Parents should be reassured about their own responsibility, except in cases where this is definitely in question. Continued support, at least over several weeks, will be necessary and, if mourning is prolonged, referral to a psychiatric or counselling service is desirable. All parents should be given a leaflet providing information about the condition and availability of counselling. A description of a children's hospital-based bereavement counselling service for parents who have lost a child in this way is provided by Woodward *et al.* (1985).

Home monitoring

In a proportion of babies who have had a 'near-miss' cot death, who have been observed to have apnoeic attacks in hospital, or who have been born as sibs to babies who have died in this way, alarm systems to wake parents if the child develops respiratory arrest can be installed. False alarms, with enhancement of anxiety, are common with this apparatus. The impact on family life may be considerable (Wasserman 1984), with marital breakdown apparently a not infrequent occurrence. Other factors may have affected family relationships, but such alarm systems should not be instituted without due consideration of their benefit and possible adverse effects. There is, however, no evidence that adverse cognitive or emotional effects on the child persist, when children monitored in this way are followed up several years later (Kahn *et al.* 1989).

8.3 Malformations

8.3.1 CLEFT LIP AND PALATE

Clinical features

The baby is born with a defect of the lip and/or palate, resulting from failure of the normal process of fusion of embryonic tissues during fetal development. If the defect involves the lip, it will be obvious at birth, and indeed may now be diagnosed antenatally by ultrasound screening. Isolated defects of the palate may only be identified when the palate is examined during routine physical examination of the newborn, or when the baby begins to feed. Occasionally an isolated defect of the palate is covered with mucous membrane (submucous cleft), so that the defect is not identified until the child's speech is noted to have a nasal quality. Cleft lip and palate are associated with other congenital abnormalities, especially congenital heart disease, in about 10% of cases.

The condition is surgically correctable, and, in skilled hands, the cosmetic results are excellent with little obvious deformity. Depending on the nature of the defect and the practice of the surgeon, operative procedures may be carried out in one or two stages. Surgical repair of the lip is now generally carried out at 1–3 months of age and of the palate at 6–12 months. Consequently, if the palate is affected, the baby will require a dental plate and/or a special teat for feeding for the first few months of life. Babies whose cleft is confined to the lip can usually be breast-fed.

Apart from the minor cosmetic defect, the outcome may be complicated by recurrent ear infections leading to hearing loss. Articulation defects may also arise either as a result of the structural abnormality or the hearing loss.

Background factors

Cleft lip and palate syndromes occur in about 1.4 per 1000 births, cleft lip alone being rather more common than cleft palate. The condition is mainly genetically determined with a risk of 1 in 25 for children born to an affected parent. The concordance rate is 40% in monozygotic twins, but 5% in dizygotic twins and sibs. The administration to the pregnant mother of certain drugs, including lithium and phenytoin (Epanutin), also increases the risk.

Psychosocial factors

Cleft lip or palate is one of the commonest congenital abnormalities, and there is extensive information on psychosocial aspects (Lansdown 1981; Tobiasen 1984). Parents naturally respond with severe shock to the first sight of their deformed baby, but this usually dissipates in a few days. Feeding difficulties are common, not just for the obvious practical reasons, but because many mothers are made anxious by the child's defect, and this anxiety is transmitted to the baby. Speech and language problems develop in as many as 75% of affected children.

The later psychological adjustment of children with repaired clefts is usually good, assuming that the surgical repair has been effective. However, even minor physical defects attract teasing at school, and this is especially the case with deformities of the mouth and teeth (Lansdown and Polak 1975). The great majority of children have intelligence and educational attainment within the average range, although the mean level of ability is somewhat lower than average. However, teachers tend to underestimate the intelligence of children with unsatisfactorily repaired clefts (Richman 1978), and the presence of undetected hearing problems may also lead to a misdiagnosis of mental retardation.

Psychosocial aspects of management

Following a warning about the baby's appearance with an explanation that the defect, although apparently seriously deforming, is surgically correctable, the baby should be shown to both parents, preferably together, as soon as possible. However, it is misleading to suggest that this is simply an anatomical abnormality that can be cured surgically. The care of the child with cleft lip and palate requires the services of a multidisciplinary team, available from birth to adulthood. The parents will need continuing emotional support and explanation, especially over the first few days, and they should be put in touch with a member of a specialist multidisciplinary team very shortly after birth. Before-and-after photographs of children with repaired clefts are usually very reassuring. It is, of course, important that other congenital defects that may be associated are identified, so that the implications of these can also be discussed with parents.

Procedures and advice concerning feeding should take into account the fact that mothers may often find the situation upsetting as well as practically extremely difficult. However, the great majority are able to cope and become very deft in helping their children to feed. It is important that parents are given full details of the nature of the operation with information about how the baby is likely to look immediately postoperatively and during the subsequent weeks.

The advice from infancy of both an audiologist and a speech therapist is important in the detection of hearing impairment and remediation of speech defects. These professionals are likely to be able to give good advice on how to talk to the child about the nature and cause of his defect. It is usually possible for parents themselves to help children cope with teasing at school through discussion with the child's teachers. Referral to a psychologist or psychiatrist will be necessary only if psychosocial problems are persistent, and, in this case, factors other than the cleft deformity are likely to be of significance. Psychiatric problems may centre around feelings of inferiority and an exaggerated sense of feeling rejected, with low self-esteem. Counselling with behavioural advice to improve social skills will often be effective, but a minority of affected children, usually those who have experienced additional family problems, may require more formal psychotherapy. As children reach their teens, it is important for parents to explain to them the genetic nature of the defect and the risk of inheritance.

8.3.2 HYPOSPADIAS

Hypospadias is a congenital deformity of the penis found in about 1 in 350 male babies. The cause is unknown, but there is a familial, probably genetically determined transmission. The external meatus (orifice) is on the undersurface of the penis rather than at the tip, and this is often associated with bowing of the penis (chordee). Treatment is surgical, but surgical practice is variable. There is now a tendency to operate in single-stage operations between 6 and 12 months. Results are usually good for appearance and function, and depend mainly on the severity of the deformity. Postoperative complications requiring reoperation are not at all uncommon. Unless there are special reasons, later operation is not recommended (American Academy of Pediatrics 1996).

Psychosocial aspects

Parents are often particularly anxious about this condition and the operation necessary to correct it, for a number of reasons. They are likely to be concerned (with some reason—see below) for the later sexual competence and fertility of their sons. The condition is one that many parents feel embarrassed about, and secrecy can mean it is more difficult for them to receive emotional support from family and friends.

Operative procedures need careful explanation to both parents and children well before surgery. The child is often in considerable discomfort following operation, and the appearance of bandages and tubes is anxiety-provoking, especially if unexpected. The postoperative course is sometimes accompanied by an excess of aggression or withdrawn behaviour in the child.

Despite apparently normal endocrine function, a usually relatively normal appearance of the penis, and a normal capacity to achieve erection, there is an increased risk of sexual and psychological maladjustment of the adult who has had a hypospadias repair in childhood. Many will not have such problems, but follow-up studies of variable quality summarized by Schultz (1983) suggest that, as a group, they experience intercourse later and less frequently than controls (Berg *et al.* 1981). They are less likely to marry and have children. Both in adolescence and in adult life, the self-perception and psychosexual adjustment of hypospadias patients is related to the cosmetic result and to their feelings of satisfaction and dissatisfaction that go with it. Many would like re-operation to produce cosmetic improvement (Mureau *et al.* 1995, 1997).

The apparently unsatisfactory sexual and personality outcome of a number of affected children suggests that counselling both in childhood and adolescence might have a beneficial preventive effect. It is important that youngsters who might well believe themselves still to be deformed or inadequate should have an opportunity to express their feelings and thoughts on this matter, and that adults who have required the operation in childhood should have access to sexual counselling if they are experiencing difficulties in this sphere.

8.4 Injuries to children

In developed countries injuries are the major cause of death in the 1–14 year age group. The term 'accident', with its implication that random forces outside human control are responsible, is inappropriate to describe the events producing injuries. In fact, much is known about the factors involved in injury occurrence, and the behavioural characteristics of injury victims and their families have been found to be of significance.

Prevalence and background factors

In England and Wales, injuries cause over a tenth of deaths in the 1–14 year age group and about half the deaths in the 15–19 age group. Road traffic accidents are responsible for about half these deaths. Drowning and burns also produce significant mortality. Injuries producing less serious results are very common. In the UK, about 1 child in every 6 presents to a hospital Accident and Emergency department with an injury at least once each year. Boys are injured about $1\frac{1}{2}$ times as commonly as girls, and in the 15–19 year age group they have a much greater vulnerability to road traffic injuries. There is a strong social class link with fatal injuries, in that children of manual and unskilled workers are much more likely to sustain fatal injuries and burns at all ages. Children in social class 5 are five times more likely to sustain a fatal injury than those in social class 1 (Roberts and Power 1996). Social class trends for less serious injuries are much less marked, and some studies have failed to find any social class differences at all.

Personality and behaviour

Boys who are aggressive, competitive, impulsive, and overactive are prone to injury, and temperamentally 'difficult' children are especially at risk. Children who have had repeated injuries in the pre-school period are several times more likely to continue to suffer repeated injuries during school than those without such an early history (Bijur *et al.* 1988), but persistent adverse social circumstances may be as important in explaining this finding as childhood personality.

Family type and functioning

Children living in single-parent or reconstituted families, and children of less well-educated mothers are at extra risk (Matheny 1986; Roberts and Pless 1995). In addition, maternal depression is associated with the occurrence of injuries to children (Brown and Davidson 1978). Children are more liable to injury at times of family crisis and change, as when another family member is suffering a physical illness or the family is involved in a house move. All these factors are likely to exert their effect by reducing the level of supervision.

Psychosocial aspects of management

When a child sustains an injury, physical assessment and appropriate medical treatment must take immediate priority. However, where resources in terms of time and available staff permit, psychosocial considerations can contribute significantly to management.

Assessment

Psychosocial factors need consideration because of:

- relevance to medical management: a child of distressed and panic-stricken parents may need to be admitted because supervision of care at home will be inadequate
- the possibility that injuries have been non-accidentally caused: the nature of the injuries and mode of presentation may provide clues (Section 2.1)
- the circumstances of the injury, which may give rise to serious parental guilt and self-blame: the quality of parental supervision at the time of the accident may need attention if recurrences are to be avoided
- the possibility that behavioural disturbance in the child or emotional problems in other family members may have made an important contribution to the occurrence of the injury.

Management

Again, emergency physical treatment must take precedence. In deciding whether further management measures need to be taken in the light of the injury, it is necessary to:

- establish whether the injuries could have been caused non-accidentally— if this is the case, further management is described in Section 2.1
- enable parents to express feelings of guilt and anger with themselves, their child, or someone else thought responsible for the accident
- provide treatment for children with behavioural and emotional problems which have come to notice as a result of the injury.

Occurrence of an injury may, even if the injury is 'accidentally' caused, indicate that the quality of parental supervision or level of family conflict and non-communication require further attention.

8.4.1 PSYCHOLOGICAL AND PSYCHIATRIC OUTCOME FOLLOWING INJURY

General

The majority of injured children do not develop any long-lasting significant behavioural or emotional sequelae. In the short term, about 1 in 7 children show symptoms of post-traumatic stress disorder (Di Gallo *et al.* 1997). In a small group, injury to a limb can be followed by a hysterical reaction in which the disability is much greater than the extent of the physical injuries would warrant. Other forms of neurotic disability following accidents appear to be uncommon in childhood (Lishman 1987). The nature as well as the severity of the injury is likely to be of significance in determining seriousness of behavioural and emotional outcome. Thus head injuries (see below) may have a direct effect on subsequent cognitive and behavioural development, owing to interference with brain function. Burns (see below) may have specifically deleterious effects for other reasons, for example the necessity for repeated painful procedures and the prolonged hospitalization required to achieve rehabilitation. Severe, multisystem injuries to children are likely to have profound psychological and social effects on the survivors and their families, lasting for years after the injuries occurred (Harris *et al.* 1989).

Head injury

Cognitive outcome

The best indication of the severity of a head injury lies in the duration of post-traumatic amnesia—the period of time from the occurrence of the injury to the point when memories again become continuous. The relationship between the severity of injury and psychological sequelae has been thoroughly investigated by Klonoff *et al.* (1977) and by Rutter *et al.* (1983).

In children with post-traumatic amnesia lasting less than 2 weeks, cognitive impairment does not appear to occur. The child's intellectual status following the injury can be expected to remain the same as before it. When the post-traumatic amnesia lasts 2–3 weeks, transient or persistent cognitive impairment occurs in virtually all children, and persistent impairment is the commonest outcome if the period of amnesia is longer than 3 weeks. Visuospatial and visuomotor skills are impaired to a greater degree than verbal skills. The pattern of cognitive functioning following injury does not provide a clear guide to the site of the damage, although academic attainment may be more affected following left-hemisphere lesions. In children with severe injuries most cognitive improvement takes place in the first year, though minor improvements can continue into the second year, or even longer than this (Klonoff *et al.* 1977). Rather surprisingly, the age of the child is not a good predictor of outcome (Oddy 1984).

Psychiatric outcome

The rate of subsequent behavioural and emotional problems does not appear raised in children with a post-traumatic amnesia of less than 1 week. Thus, if a child with an injury of this level of severity shows a behavioural or emotional problem after the injury, it is improbable that this is a direct result of the brain injury. The functioning of the child and the family before the injury is the best predictor of psychosocial functioning 3 years after the injury (Rivara *et al.* 1996).

In children with post-traumatic amnesia lasting longer than a week, the rate of psychiatric disorder rises sharply, whether or not cognitive impairment has occurred. Such psychiatric disorder is present in excess even in those children without obvious neurological sequelae. In general, the behavioural sequelae that occur are rather non-specific in type, except that marked social disinhibition (undue cheekiness and proneness to make embarrassing remarks) is especially common. The type of symptom is unrelated to the site of the lesion, except that depression appears more common when the lesion is in the right frontal or left posterior region.

Although age and sex appear little related to psychiatric outcome, the intensity of family reactions and the number of social problems in the family do appear to have a modifying effect. Children whose parents react least intensively and those from families living in advantaged circumstances appear to have the best outcome.

8.4.2 ACCIDENTAL POISONING

Epidemiological findings

In the UK about 9 in every 1000 children under the age of 5 years require attention in Accident and Emergency departments each year because they might have ingested a harmful substance. However, of these a significant number (perhaps two-thirds) turn out not to have swallowed anything harmful (Calnan *et al.* 1976). Over 30 child deaths a year occur in the UK as a result of accidental poisoning. The peak age is between 2 and 3, with boys somewhat more at risk than girls. Drugs and household products together account for over 95% of substances ingested (Wiseman *et al.* 1987). Analgesics, anxiolytics, bleaches, and detergents are most frequently involved.

Social and family factors are often prominent in the background of accidentally poisoned children (Shaw 1977). The children tend to come from overcrowded homes in which there have been a number of changes of accommodation. Their families are characterized by high rates of marital disharmony and other types of family conflict (Sobel 1970). Rates of mental ill-health in parents are high. Surprisingly, there is rather little relationship between the degree of care over storage of drugs in a safe place and the risk of the child being poisoned. The personal characteristics of the child, however, are relevant. Poisoned children are more likely to show high levels of overactivity.

The outcome of children who have been accidentally poisoned does not suggest that the poisoning itself is likely to have long-term adverse effects. Intellectual status and rates of emotional disturbance have not been found to be significantly different than in matched groups of children. However, the adverse psychosocial factors so often found in children who have been poisoned are themselves likely to have long-term consequences on behaviour.

Non-accidental (deliberate) poisoning of children is discussed in Section 2.2.

Prevention of injuries and accidental poisoning: psychosocial aspects

There is increasing evidence that, with an active injury prevention policy, a decline in the rate of injuries can be achieved. (Child Accident Prevention Trust 1989). Preventive measures that appear effective include:

- *road safety precautions*: compulsory use of seatbelts in cars and compulsory use of helmets for motorcyclists.
- *domestic equipment design*: careful design can make paraffin heaters, ovens, saucepans, etc. more childproof.
- *protective barriers for windows* in high-rise council or municipal property.
- *teaching children to swim* reduces drowning accidents.
- *design of playgrounds*, for example use of impact-absorbing surfaces.
- *child-resistant containers* for drugs, both prescribed and non-prescribed.
- the use of *smoke alarms* to reduce the risk of domestic fires and burns.
- *drug safety*: encouraging family doctors to provide antidepressants, etc. in small quantities and to give warnings to mothers of their dangers to children.

In theory, all these measures require back-up by an active health education programme with instruction to parents on how to help their children avoid injuries from domestic equipment, drugs, and other dangerous or poisonous substances. In practice, evaluation of such health education appears to have disappointing results, whereas the practical environmental measures listed above are more successful (Gatherer *et al.* 1979).

Although there are various correlations between adverse background psychosocial factors and occurrence of injuries, there have so far been no clear-cut implications for prevention arising from these findings. For example, it would probably not be cost-effective to direct health education programmes to those at high risk for psychological reasons. Nevertheless, attention to psychosocial factors in the management of these children found to be subject to repeated injury (see above) might well have an impact on the risk of subsequent re-injury.

8.4.3 BURNS

Burns and thermal injury present specific psychosocial problems. Children living in socially deprived, overcrowded circumstances where accident control is more difficult are more likely to be involved, as are those with certain physical conditions and behavioural states, such as epilepsy and the hyperkinetic syndrome. Burns may be inflicted non-accidentally, for example by lighted cigarettes.

In the acute phase, after the burn has been sustained, there will be acute pain and, if the burn is extensive, intensive care for life-saving procedures. Subsequently the child may require numerous grafting operations with prolonged hospitalization.

Parents are particularly likely to experience guilt after their child has been burned. The extreme suffering of the child, and the fact that the injury may indeed have been preventable, will exacerbate guilt feelings. Mothers who were socially stressed before their child was burned and where the thermal injury is severe, are at particular risk for mental health problems subsequently (Mason and Hillier 1993). Parents may find it very difficult to accept the scarred appearance of their child and respond by rejection or overprotection. Parents (preferably both fathers and mothers together) will benefit from counselling sessions to ventilate their feelings and to ensure that they are understood and emotionally supported. Group sessions of parents of burned children are also helpful, especially if attended by nursing staff who can provide practical advice, as well as emotional support.

The level of development and maturity of the burned child will influence the type of reaction that occurs (Sawyer *et al.* 1982). Many children regress in their behaviour and become more clinging. There are often intense fearful reactions to the painful procedures involved in changing dressings, and phobic, over-anxious behaviour may persist after recovery from the burn (Stoddard *et al.* 1989). Low self-esteem and antisocial behaviour are relatively common in older children and teenagers. Burned children will benefit from careful preparation and explanation in relation to painful procedures. Allowing the child an element of control in the procedure will also reduce distress. Hypnotic procedures (Section 9.2.6) may be helpful in the older child and teenager. Children will also benefit from the opportunity for discussion of their feelings about their appearance. Before return to school, it is useful to arrange a visit by a nurse or psychologist to the school, so that teachers can be helped to prepare other children for the changed appearance of the burned child as well as the child's likely sensitivity to teasing.

8.5 Infectious diseases

Infectious diseases, particularly respiratory and gastrointestinal illnesses, are easily the most common reason for child consultations with family doctors and admission to hospital. There are important psychosocial risk factors for these frequently occurring disorders, and these will be briefly discussed. In addition, a number of infectious diseases directly or indirectly affect brain function, either in the acute phase or subsequently as a result of chronic brain damage. These may produce cognitive deficits and behavioural and emotional changes. These will also be described.

8.5.1 PSYCHOSOCIAL RISK FACTORS FOR COMMON INFECTIOUS DISEASES OF CHILDHOOD

The likelihood of a child developing an infection will depend on factors related to exposure to the infective organism (especially the intensity of exposure and the virulence of the organism) and factors related to the child (especially the level of immunity and specific host response). Both broad social and specific environmental factors have been demonstrated in population studies to be of importance in susceptibility and probably exposure to infection.

Social factors

There is a definite tendency for children from lower social class families to suffer more from respiratory infections and gastroenteritis. The reasons for higher rates of bronchitis in UK working class children probably lie in the higher rates of parental smoking and large family size in the lower socio-economic groups (Colley and Reid 1970). A large number of siblings will usually mean overcrowded accommodation and greater likelihood of exposure to infection. Parents in lower socio-economic groups are also more likely to suffer from lung disease themselves, and their children are more likely to be exposed to environmental pollution, especially smoke from domestic fuel and industrial waste.

Working-class children are less likely to be immunized against infections such as whooping cough and measles, both of which have significant postinfective morbidity. They are more likely to face stressful circumstances in their lives (see below).

Stress

Stressful circumstances may predispose to infection. For example, β-haemolytic streptococcal infection has been found to occur more often after a period of family stress (Meyer and Haggerty 1962).

There are modest associations between measures of psychosocial adversity and child health status, including respiratory illness. But these are not just associations; the stress contributes in some way to the development of the infection. A stress that carries a negative connotation, involving loss or disappointment, is likely to be responsible. A number of studies have illuminated the processes whereby such stress leads to infection. There may be activation of the sympathetic adrenomedullary or of the hypothalamic–pituitary–adrenocortical axes. Alternatively, the endogenous opioid system may be altered by stressful circumstances. Any of these, may involve a decline in immune function, and thus lower resistance to infection. There are considerable individual differences determining physiological responses to stress, and this must explain, to some degree, variations in vulnerability to exposure to infection (Barr *et al.* 1996).

As well as contributing to the causation of infectious illness, psychosocial factors may, if the disease process affects the brain, have an effect on subsequent psychological functioning. The psychological and psychosocial impact of infectious disease is particularly affected by whether it occurs in the intrauterine period or after birth.

8.5.2 FETAL INFECTION

Human immunodeficiency virus

The human immunodeficiency virus (HIV), a slow virus belonging to the subgroup of retroviruses, produces loss of T4 lymphocytes with consequent loss of resistance to infection. Acquired immune deficiency syndrome (AIDS) is the endstage of the condition, in which chronic degenerative neurologic disorder with recurrent opportunistic infections progresses to a fatal outcome. Children usually succumb to opportunistic infections without going through a stage of chronic neurologic disorder. Groups at particular risk are

- children with haemophilia (infected before 1985 with contaminated blood, (and therefore now unusual in the paediatric population)
- children who have been sexually abused
- adolescent male homosexuals and their partners (including adolescent girls in the case of bisexual men)
- drug abusers using contaminated needles.

Vertical transmission may occur to the fetus via the placenta in infected, pregnant women. This is now the most common form of infection in children, but is preventable by antiretroviral drugs if the mother's condition is diagnosed in pregnancy.

Psychosocial aspects: prevalence, background factors and presentation
The psychosocial aspects of HIV/AIDS vary, depending on the mode of acquisition.

Children infected by vertical transmission
The prevalence of paediatric HIV infection and AIDS varies considerably from country to country and within countries by region. For example, in England and Wales, 30 new cases of AIDS were reported in 1994 and it is estimated that there will be 55 in 1999, whereas in the USA, 700 new cases were reported in 1992, with the prevalence rising year by year. The social composition of those infected by the virus also varies considerably. For example, in London there is a heavy preponderance of babies born to mothers from ethnic minority groups, often with fathers who have visited or migrated from African countries where the disease is endemic. This is not the case in Scotland, where most cases have arisen from needle sharing among drug-abusing, indigenous young people. However, in most situations, vertically transmitted cases are most common amongst the most socially deprived sections of the population suffering from poor housing, poverty, and poor employment prospects.

Vertically transmitted HIV infection may be suspected at birth when the mother is known to be infected. However, because of the passage of maternal antibodies, the condition cannot be firmly diagnosed until the child has reached 18 months, when a significant number will be found to have contracted the virus, but others will not. Many infected children will not be diagnosed until they present at an older age with unexplained recurrent infections, loss of skills or generalized lymphadenopathy. The diagnosis will then, of course, carry devastating implications for the parents.

The course of the condition is again very variable. Some children rapidly succumb to opportunistic infections, while, less commonly, others develop a dementing illness. Yet others remain well at least into adolescence and early adult life. In one study (Grubman *et al.* 1995), a quarter of infected children aged 9–16 years were asymptomatic. In symptomatic children, early development may be marked by delay in expressive speech and subsequent cognitive impairment arising as a direct result of brain damage. Indirect effects arise as a result of the multiple stresses to which infected children are exposed. They may include aggressive behaviour, depressive and anxiety symptoms, withdrawal, and school failure.

Children affected by sexual abuse

HIV infection is an uncommon complication of abuse, but should be borne in mind by those investigating the problem. It may occur at any age and should be especially considered when the abuse has involved anal penetration, and the perpetrator is a male homosexual.

Infection in adolescence

HIV infection in adolescence may arise as a result of sexual activity or needle sharing among drug abusers. The prevalence of infection among adolescents is unknown, but it may be assumed that a number of cases of AIDS arising in young people in their twenties have been contracted during this phase of life. Again a preponderance of cases come from deprived sections of the population, with high rates among homeless young people, prostitutes, and those living in poverty. However, there is a much wider social spectrum among homosexual males. The presence of a homosexual orientation is a risk factor, as is risk-taking behaviour which may form part of a psychiatric disorder. The condition may present at a clinic for sexually transmitted diseases, when the young person presents with signs of another infection, or with opportunistic infection, or with signs of dementia—intellectual deterioration, loss of concentration, and confusion.

Psychosocial aspects of management

Once diagnosed, the management of these HIV cases is always complex, and requires the services of a multidisciplinary team in a specialist centre, but health care professionals not working in such centres will also find themselves involved. An excellent extended account of different psychosocial aspects of management has been written by Krener (1996).

When a baby is born to an infected mother, the uncertainty concerning the HIV status of the baby will be extremely stressful. Although most babies will be able to remain with their mothers, where care is thought to be inadequate the infant may require substitute parenting. Placement of the baby suffering from HIV infection will produce a need for support for the new carers. If the baby stays with the mother, as will usually be the case, the mother will herself need help in dealing with guilt reactions as well as reactions relating to her own fatal or potentially fatal disease.

Young people at risk of infection and those already infected will often require counselling and the opportunity for peer group support. The presence of psychiatric disorders arising from indirect effects of the infection will indicate the need for treatment. Psychiatrists and paediatricians may be involved in health education (including sex education), and in the development of outreach programmes and other social measures for drug abusers and other young people alienated from their families. Parents may themselves require counselling to cope with their own grief at the predicament in which their children find themselves.

Congenital rubella

Congenital rubella occurs in the UK in about 1 per 50 000 live births, but more frequently when epidemics occur. The fetuses of women who contract the condition in the first 2 months after conception are most at risk (95%), but the risk has diminished very substantially by the end of the fourth month of fetal life.

Commonly occurring sequelae are ophthalmic conditions (especially cataract), a wide range of neurological disorders, microcephaly, heart defects, sensorineural deafness, and enlargement of the liver and spleen. Mental retardation occurs in about 50% of cases.

Among mentally retarded children affected by congenital rubella, autism (Section 3.5.1) is a particularly common complication (Chess and Fernandez 1980). Autism is usually present from birth, but may occur after a period of apparently normal development, perhaps because the live virus may continue to survive after the birth of the child.

Identification of rubella as a cause of mental retardation or autism in an older child depends on the presence of the characteristic associated defects. Antibody tests are of value in excluding the diagnosis but, if they are positive, this is not necessarily significant, as the child may well have contracted a postnatal infection. The great majority of children with rubella-induced autism have been identified as suffering from rubella at birth.

Prevention of congenital rubella is possible with existing vaccines, and, in many countries, the routine immunization of young children with measles, mumps, and rubella vaccine (MMR) is achieving increasing success, so that, in many countries the birth of children with this condition has become rare. Termination should be offered, after explanation of the risk of fetal infection, to women contracting the condition early in pregnancy.

Cytomegalovirus (CMV)

CMV infection is also a mild condition in adults, but may produce serious defects if transmitted from pregnant mother to fetus. In the UK about 1 in 200 babies is born showing evidence of active infection (excreting virus in urine), and about 10% of these show subsequent evidence of damage. The child may be born with low birthweight, enlargement of liver and spleen, purpura, and eye defects, but most are normal at birth. There is no good evidence that CMV causes mental retardation or learning difficulties in the absence of other characteristic clinical features. In one study (Ramsey *et al.* 1991) 45% had neurological impairment, most showing gross motor or psychomotor abnormalities, but some sensorineural deafness. The remaining 55% were neurologically normal at follow-up. The presence of neurological signs in the neonatal period predicted a poor prognosis.

Other infections

Other infections, such as herpes simplex and syphilis, may also impair fetal development and, if they do not result in fetal death and abortion, may be followed by severe developmental retardation.

8.5.3 POSTNATAL INFECTIONS: MENTAL STATES ASSOCIATED WITH INFECTION

Acute and subacute confusion (delirious states)

Confusional states may occur as a result of toxic or metabolic processes without invasion of brain tissue during any infectious illness, but occur most frequently in young children and when transient or persistent encephalopathy or meningitis are present. During the course of the infection the child may first become irrationally angry, irritable, or miserable. This is usually rapidly followed by episodes of drowsiness or reversal of sleep rhythm. Hallucinations, especially of visual type, are quite common. Generalized convulsions, sometimes prolonged, may occur. A child may misperceive other people to be objects, and vice versa, and be disorientated in time and place. Sudden irrational fearfulness or depression may occur. A marked feature of delirium is its variability and transience. Very occasionally, depending on the underlying condition, the cerebral involvement may result in coma, which can be irreversible, but usually marked and rapid improvement in the child's mental state occurs as the child recovers from the underlying condition.

The differential diagnosis of delirium includes especially drug-induced states following accidental or non-accidental ingestion of toxic substances, or other forms of intoxication, closed head trauma with frontal lobe confusion, hypoglycemia, and an acute psychotic state. A careful history should clarify the diagnosis. Epilepsy may also present with acute or subacute confusion. Again the history, together with careful observation of the child to exclude non-convulsive status, and investigations, especially an EEG, will be helpful here.

Postinfective psychiatric and psychological sequelae

Depressive states
Postinfective feelings of apathy, mild malaise, and depression are not uncommon, and usually last no more than a few days. Much more rarely, prolonged depressive reactions of considerable severity and sometimes associated with school refusal may occur. These usually follow influenzal-type illnesses and infectious mononucleosis, but may occasionally follow other infectious conditions. The reason why some individuals are affected in this way is unclear, but it has been suggested that, in infectious mononucleosis, psychological reactions are associated with specific T-cell phenomena (Hamblin *et al.* 1983). Affected children are often living in adverse psychosocial circumstances, so that an interaction between this immunological phenomenon and environmental factors is probable.

Management of these severe postinfective depressive states will depend on the presence of associated family and school problems and the personality of the child. As with other depressive states, psychological treatment of family or individual type should be instituted, and antidepressant medication may be indicated. Viral infections may also be followed by the chronic fatigue syndrome (Section 5.5.2).

Dementia

Progressive intellectual deterioration following infection is extremely rare, but occurs particularly in *subacute sclerosing panencephalitis*. Children with this condition usually present between 3 and 18 years, with a mean of 10 years. It is four times as common in boys as in girls. The onset is often characterized by a fall in school performance, thought to be due to laziness or some environmental stress. Deterioration in speech and handwriting is common. The child may become irritable and moody. The presence of an organic rather than a psychologically determined condition should be suspected when there is actual loss of skills rather than merely failure to make progress.

The condition is thought to be due to the measles virus, and follows several months or years after an apparently typical measles infection. A characteristic form of myoclonic jerk occurs in the more advanced stage of the condition. The diagnosis is made by a sustained rise in measles antibody titre in serum and cerebrospinal fluid. There is also a pathognomonic EEG pattern with bursts of high-voltage spike waves occurring on a background of slow activity. The disease is almost always fatal, though there may be a very prolonged period of chronic illness with slowly progressive dementia.

Dementia may also occur towards the terminal stage of AIDS infection, and as a feature of other progressive, non-infective brain disorders.

Learning deficits

Children surviving meningitis (e.g. of tuberculous type) and encephalitis (e.g. mumps, measles, chickenpox, etc.) may not fully recover and show long-term general and specific deficits, though the prognosis of encephalitis is generally good (Rantala *et al.* 1991). Specific deficits of visuospatial and visuomotor abilities have been reported in a group of children as long as 6–8 years after an attack of *Haemophilus influenzae* meningitis (H. G. Taylor *et al.* 1984). However, other studies (Tejani *et al.* 1982) suggest that low IQ may not be a feature of children who have previously suffered from *Haemophilus* infections. There is some evidence that children contracting meningitis or other CNS viral infections before the age of 1 year are at risk for later learning deficits (Lawson *et al.* 1965; Chamberlain *et al.* 1983). In one follow-up study of children suffering from bacterial meningitis in the first year of life and then followed up 6–16 years later, about 10% had some degree of mental retardation, and about 15% had language delay, often linked to hearing loss (Sell 1987). Viral meningitis in the first 3 months of life may be followed by subtle deficits in receptive language (Baker *et al.* 1996).

Parental reactions

A severe infection, particularly in a baby or young child, is an extremely frightening experience for parents. Even parents who are professionally qualified as nurses or doctors find the experience of coping with a somnolent child with high fever very stressful. Parents whose children suffer febrile convulsions often believe that their child is about to die (Baumer *et al.* 1981).

Reassurance of parents whose children are suffering from acute infection is emotionally supportive and reduces unnecessary anxiety. In those uncommon cases where infections lead to serious sequelae, there is often a long period of uncertainty before it is clear whether the child has suffered permanent brain damage. In these circumstances, sharing of uncertainty rather than unrealistic reassurance is likely to be more helpful. Specific psychological intervention may be indicated in some families, but long-term benefit of such intervention has not been established (Kupst *et al.* 1983).

8.6 Metabolic disorders

A very large number of metabolic disorders occur in infancy and childhood. Most are very rare and occur as a result of inborn errors affecting the metabolism of amino acids, carbohydrates, protein, lipid, purine, and other compounds. Psychosocial aspects of a small number of the less rare disorders with particular psychiatric or developmental significance, are described here.

8.6.1 PHENYLKETONURIA

Definition

Phenylketonuria is a disorder of amino acid metabolism in which there is a deficiency in phenylalanine hydroxylase, the enzyme responsible for converting dietary phenylalanine to tyrosine.

Aetiology

The condition, which occurs in about 1 in 15000 births, is an autosomal recessive disorder. The enzymatic defect results in excessive production of phenylpyruvic acid, phenylacetic acid, and phenylacetylamine. There is consequent interference with maturation of grey matter, defective myelination, and cystic degeneration of white matter in the central nervous system.

Clinical features and treatment

If untreated, children with phenylketonuria are usually markedly developmentally delayed and become severely or moderately mentally retarded. Normal intelligence has, however, occasionally been reported in untreated cases. Epileptic fits, eczema, and behavioural disturbances (especially hyperkinesis and autism) are common accompaniments.

The condition is treatable if diagnosed within the first few days of life. Universal screening from day 5–8 of life now ensures that virtually all children born with the condition are identified. Treatment involves a low-phenylalanine diet, with close monitoring of blood phenylalanine levels throughout the first 7–8 years of life. Subsequently, a relaxed diet with some restriction of phenylalanine intake is usually advised until mid-adolescence (but see below).

Dietary treatment should be instituted in a specialized centre. Specially manufactured low-phenylalanine milk substitutes provide the main source of nutrition in the early years, and other foods have to be severely restricted. This means that the child is unable to lead a normal social life. In the pre-school years this is not usually problematic, but in older children conflict over the diet may occur, especially if family relationships are tense for other reasons, or if the child is temperamentally difficult (Kazak *et al.* 1988). Counselling can be helpful in preventing and managing these kinds of difficulties.

Treated children are usually within the normal range of ability in adulthood (Schmidt *et al.* 1996), though their mean IQ is lower than that of the general population (Beasley *et al.* 1994), and they have an increased likelihood of minor neuropsychological anomalies in adulthood. Relaxation of diet in mid-childhood results in a small but definite decrement in intelligence (Holtzman *et al.* 1986). Rates of behavioural deviance are raised in treated children with phenylketonuria (Smith *et al.* 1988) when compared with classroom controls. Affected children show more mannerisms, fidgetiness, restlessness, and poor attention, as well as being more anxious, solitary, and miserable. Behavioural deviance is inversely related both to IQ and to the quality of biochemical control in the early years. Residual abnormality of phenylalanine metabolism, or the effect of having to take a rather unpalatable diet, may be responsible for high rates of behavioural deviance. Genetic counselling is an important component of family management.

Outcome

The outcome of early treated cases is usually good and, in adulthood, a normally independent life is to be expected. Unless they return to a diet before conception affected women are, however, likely to give birth to children with congenital abnormalities and mental retardation as a result of the exposure of the fetus to high levels of maternal phenylalanine. (Brenton and Lilburn 1996). Phenyl-ketonuric women planning to have a baby should therefore go on a carefully monitored low-phenylalanine diet, which should be monitored from before conception to delivery. If this is achieved, one can be cautiously optimistic about a normal outcome for the child.

8.6.2 GALACTOSAEMIA

Galactosaemia is a rare disorder of carbohydrate metabolism in which there is a deficiency of the enzyme galactose 1-phosphate uridyl transferase. Insulin production is stimulated so that the brain is exposed to persistent hypoglycaemia and other metabolic abnormalities, producing brain damage and dysfunction. Damage to the liver, spleen, and eye (with cataract formation) also occurs. It is transmitted as an autosomal recessive condition. Brain damage can be largely prevented by the administration of a galactose-free or low-galactose diet, but this is highly restrictive and is necessary for the whole of the individual's life.

Intellectual development in treated cases is satisfactory in the first decade, but subsequently declines (Schweitzer *et al.* 1993), so that a high proportion of adolescents and young adults have an IQ less than 85. However, it may be that recent methods of management produce better results.

Studies of emotional and behavioural development have found that treated children have high rates of problems (Fishler *et al.* 1966). Younger children tend to be fearful and anxious, and older children are more aggressive and anti-authority in their attitudes. It is likely that these difficulties arise partly as a result of residual brain dysfunction, and partly as a reaction to social problems arising both in the family and outside from the need to persist with an unusual diet.

8.6.3 MUCOPOLYSACCHARIDOSES

The mucopolysaccharidoses are a group of disorders affecting storage of carbohydrate. They are classified according to the precise type of enzyme deficiency that is present. The terms *Hunter syndrome* and *Hurler syndrome* and, more descriptively, *gargoylism* were used to describe varieties of the condition before the metabolic defects were identified.

The conditions are normally identifiable by the characteristic facial appearance at or shortly after birth. In all the mucopolysaccharidoses there is a normal early development for about 6–12 months, followed by a failure to develop further and subsequent mental deterioration. There are associated skeletal and other organ defects. No particular emotional or behavioural difficulties are associated with the condition. Sufferers may die in childhood or survive into early adulthood. A precise metabolic diagnosis is desirable, as different variants have different genetic implications—the conditions may be inherited in an autosomal or sex-linked recessive form.

High rates of behaviour problems have been found in children with this group of disorders, especially those with Hunter or Sanfillipo disease aged 5–9 years. These include destructiveness, restlessness, aggressiveness, and sleep problems. Parents find children with these problems extremely distressing and often lack any form of support. Behavioural interventions can be helpful in reducing their impact (Bax and Colville 1995).

8.6.4 LESCH–NYHAN SYNDROME

The Lesch–Nyhan syndrome is a very rare disorder of purine metabolism in which there is a defect of the enzyme hypoxanthine-guanine phosphoribosyl transferase. It is of particular psychiatric significance because of the association with mental retardation, which ranges from mild to moderately severe (Matthew *et al.* 1995), and severe self-abusive behaviour. It is a sex-linked condition, and all reported cases have been boys.

Affected children show choreoathetosis and moderately severe mental retardation as well as self-destructive behaviour. Self-mutilation is of a different order from that occurring in other forms of mental retardation and autism. Biting of the child's own lips and cheeks produces loss of tissue with sinus formation. The fitting of dental prostheses can be useful here. Severe head banging can produce further brain damage.

Treatment of the self-mutilation can be extremely difficult. External restraint is nearly always necessary. Behavioural modification with removal of attention from the undesirable behaviour has produced short-term improvement (McGreevy and Arthur 1987). The use of carbamazepine has produced a reduction in self-mutilation (Roach *et al*. 1996).

8.7 Endocrine disorders

8.7.1 THYROID DYSFUNCTION

Hypothyroidism

Deficiency or abnormality of thyroid hormone secretion occurs for a large number of reasons, of which by far the most common is incomplete development of the thyroid gland. If the gland is absent or virtually absent at birth, severe hypothyroidism (*cretinism*) ensues. If some function in the gland remains, mild hypothyroidism occurs. In some children, deficiency of thyroid secretion only becomes apparent in later childhood (*juvenile myxoedema*).

The clinical features of untreated hypothyroidism (coarse facial features, neonatal jaundice, early feeding difficulties, and constipation) are associated with mental retardation. The degree of mental retardation depends on the severity of the hormonal condition and may therefore range from mild to severe.

Prevalence

Congenital hypothyroidism is relatively common, occurring in about 1 in 4000 births. Screening for the condition has now been widely introduced, and is commonly carried out 4–6 days after birth. Once the diagnosis is confirmed, treatment consists of a daily dose of thyroxine. This should not impose a significant burden on children and families.

Studies of children treated with thyroxine following identification shortly after birth suggest that their mean intelligence is within the normal range, but somewhat below that of matched controls (Murphy *et al*. 1986). Those with very low pretreatment thyroxine concentrations have a mean deficit of around 10 IQ points, but those with lesser involvement are likely to have an IQ within the average range (Tillotson *et al*. 1994). Minor neurological problems may be present, especially motor inco-ordination and other motor disorders (Murphy *et al*. 1986). Infants with high plasma thyroxin levels in the first year may show difficult behaviour (Rovet *et al*. 1989). Later in childhood, they have a raised rate of psychiatric deviance, and this tends to be of neurotic type, although there may also be raised levels of activity and attentional deficits.

Thyrotoxicosis

Thyrotoxicosis may occur in the neonatal period or in later childhood (*juvenile thyrotoxicosis*), but is very rare. As in adults, psychological changes may be among the presenting features. In particular, there may be anxiety symptoms, lack of concentration at school, and restlessness. The associated loss of weight and goitre (swelling in the neck) make it unlikely that the physical condition will be missed, but sometimes the child is thought initially to show a primary psychiatric disorder.

8.7.2 DIABETES MELLITUS

Definition

Diabetes mellitus is a condition in which there is a failure of production of insulin, the hormone responsible for clearing glucose and ketones from the blood. There are two types:

- In *juvenile-onset diabetes*, the patient is dependent on insulin for survival. The onset of this condition is usually between 3 and 15 years of life, but it may occur later.
- In *maturity-onset diabetes*, which usually comes on much later in life, a different pathological mechanism, independent of insulin production is involved.

In this section, only juvenile-onset diabetes will be considered.

Background features

Diabetes mellitus occurs in about 2 per 1000 schoolchildren in the UK and North America, though its frequency varies in different parts of the world. The cause of the condition lies in a failure of the islet cells in the pancreas to produce insulin, but the reasons for this failure are unknown. An immunological defect is probably involved, involving autoimmune destruction of the islet β cells. Chromosome studies have provided further evidence of a genetic cause. Animal experiments suggest that a virus infection may, at least sometimes, be responsible. In addition, twin studies and the familial incidence of the condition make it likely that there is an inherited predisposition or vulnerability to environmental agents such as viruses. The more remote possibility that emotional stress may be a precipitant is discussed in more detail below.

Clinical features

Children who suffer from diabetes mellitus are likely to present with abdominal pain, excessive thirst, and polyuria (excretion of excessive quantities of urine). The development of nocturnal enuresis may be a very early symptom. Sufferers tire easily and their appetite, though initially increased, is later reduced. Symptoms develop from onset to a state of serious metabolic disturbance over a period lasting a week to a month. As the disease progresses, severe vomiting occurs and the child gradually enters a comatose state. Without rapid and competent medical treatment, the condition is fatal. Death is, however, now extremely rare in developed countries.

Treatment of the acute diabetic condition or *ketoacidosis* is followed by a period in hospital in which the child is treated with an appropriate diet and regular insulin injections. After initial adjustments, it is usually possible to achieve very satisfactory stability of the condition with one or two daily injections administered by the parents, or, in children over the age of 10–12 years, by themselves. More flexible regimes with injections before meals and a longer acting injection at night are now available and are popular with children.

Glucose levels are monitored by blood-testing, using test-strip readings of blood glucose, usually carried out by the parent or child. More accurate assessment of control is possible by measurement of glycosylated haemoglobin. Some children with diabetes, however, remain unstable, and psychological factors, discussed below, are of definite significance in some, perhaps most, of these cases. In unstable diabetes the danger of coma from low blood sugar due to an excess of insulin is greater than the risk of coma from excess glucose in the blood. Insulin coma is often entered rapidly, but the child or parent will usually have sufficient warning from feelings of dizziness to prevent it occurring with a sweet drink or lump of sugar. Dietary management is also important.

Links with psychological factors

Onset

There is no good evidence for the existence of a specific diabetic type of personality—a suggestion made in the 1950s. There is weak, retrospective evidence that children who have had adverse experiences in the first 2 years of life are prone to develop the condition later (Thernlund *et al.* 1995). There have also been suggestions that external stress factors, either of a non-specific nature or specifically related to loss of a parent, might precipitate the illness. It does seem established that there is an excess of life events in the few months preceding the onset of the condition, particularly in older children. It is, however, possible that the events that occur may not be independent of the early symptoms. If, for example, the child's resistance to infection or tolerance of stress is reduced in the early stages of diabetes, then the child might be admitted to hospital or put down a class in school for this reason. An investigation limited to the study of events preceding the diagnosis of diabetes might wrongly imply that the hospitalization or school difficulty was the cause rather than the result of the condition.

If external stressful events are of significance in precipitating the onset of the condition, they might exert their effect either through their influence on pituitary secretion and catecholamine production, or by reducing resistance to virus infection. In the present state of knowledge, it seems improbable that they play an important contributory part in the onset of the condition, although, as seen below, they may well exert an important influence on its course.

Diabetic control

Although the majority of children with diabetes achieve very satisfactory control with minimum inconvenience to themselves and their families, a minority present control problems and, in a smaller proportion still, these difficulties produce a major disruption in the child's life, requiring frequent out-patient visits, hospitalizations, and absence from school. Such 'brittle' or 'labile' cases of diabetes may be due to specific metabolic or endocrine factors, but they are more likely to be due to the direct or indirect influence of stressful factors operating on the child.

- *Direct factors*. Laboratory studies have demonstrated that the production of pituitary hormones and catecholamines induced by stress can lead to a decrease in insulin production and an increase in free fatty acids in the blood. A stressful interview has been shown, for example, to produce an increase in urinary epinephrine. A β-adrenergic blocking substance administered before the stress interview prevents these physiological changes. It has therefore been suggested that the effect of stress on diabetic control is mediated by endogenous catecholamines acting on adrenergic β-type receptors. However, as exposure to stressful situations does not result in changes in circulating levels of glucose, ketones, or free fatty acids (Kemmer *et al.* 1986), it seems unlikely that stress has a direct physiological effect producing hyperglycaemia.

• *Indirect factors*. The success of diabetic control depends on the compliance of the patient and family with treatment—diet, injections, and urine-testing. Compliance can be affected by the quality of organization of care in the home. It is likely to be poor in those families where, for reasons of financial hardship or personality conflicts between the parents, or a combination of the two, the home care is relatively disorganized (White *et al.* 1984). The confidence and self-esteem of the parents is an important key factor (Grey *et al.* 1980). Some parents react to their own anxiety about the diabetes by becoming more overcontrolling and rigid, or alternatively rejecting and neglectful.

The control of the diabetes also provides a ready-made focus for parent–child conflicts. Diabetic children are expected gradually to take over their own care as they move into adolescence. If the child is having difficulty in achieving separation from his parents smoothly, he may, consciously or unconsciously, use the threat of refusal to comply with treatment as a means of manipulation. Failure to comply may also occur in depressed children who have lost interest in their own survival. Such low self-esteem may occur because of neglectful behaviour on the part of parents preoccupied with their own problems.

Studies of poorly controlled diabetic children show high divorce rates in the parents, frequent chronic family conflict, and generally inadequate parental care (White *et al.* 1984; Marteau *et al.* 1987). The children themselves are often depressed, angry, and low in self-esteem, and show learning and disciplinary problems in school. Major psychiatric problems may be associated with suicidal attempts. Family relationships have been found, albeit in uncontrolled studies, to be characterized by overprotection of the children, lack of flexibility, and poor resolution of conflict (Minuchin 1974).

Learning problems

Children with diabetes show an increased rate of learning problems. This probably occurs as a result of mild, chronic metabolic disturbance, as cognitive impairment in younger children is related to time since diagnosis. Children diagnosed before 5 years are more likely to show specific visuospatial problems. Later-onset diabetes is more likely to have an effect on verbal, left hemisphere performance.

Behaviour and emotional problems

Rates of psychiatric disturbance in children with diabetes have been extensively studied, and most investigators find increased rates (Johnson 1988). A wide range of problems is described, and there is no particular behavioural profile. High rates of anxiety, depression, low self-esteem, anger, obsessive–compulsive symptoms, hyperactivity, and schizoid traits have all been found by different workers. Although in poorly controlled diabetes there are high rates of individual and family disturbance (see above), those who have looked at general population groups of children find that, if anything, it is the more rigidly controlled who show higher rates of problems (Fonagy *et al.* 1987), though the reverse has also been found.

Psychosocial aspects of management

After a period of initial adjustment, most children with diabetes and their families will cope well with the social and psychological stresses imposed by the illness (Northam *et al.* 1996).

Coping behaviour in these well-functioning families can be enhanced by early and repeated full explanation of the illness and its implications. Practical advice over diets, perhaps with the suggestion that the whole family should modify its nutritional intake to some degree, will be helpful.

The implications of the condition for the child and family will alter as the child grows into adolescence (Cerreto and Travis 1984). Advice on insulin management should include discussion of ways in which children can gradually become responsible for their own injections and urine- and blood-testing, certainly as they move into their early teens and usually earlier. Both children and parents often find it useful to experience a deliberately induced minor hypoglycaemic attack in hospital so that they can learn to recognize the signs and gain confidence in how to deal with it. Parents and children should be encouraged to think that diabetes is quite compatible with a normal, active life, and there are a number of helpful booklets available describing how this can be achieved. Adequate knowledge of the condition predicts a better psychosocial adjustment (Sullivan 1979).

The psychiatric appraisal of poorly controlled diabetes requiring repeated hospitalization for recurrent ketoacidosis can be a crucial aspect of management of these difficult cases. It has been estimated that physical factors such as intercurrent infection are responsible for only a minority of these problems (White *et al.* 1994), though it remains possible that there are metabolic reasons why some children rather than others go out of control so rapidly when faced with stressful situations.

Assessment, which may be carried out by the paediatrician, social worker, psychologist, or psychiatrist, should involve, at least at some point, a whole family interview, an interview with the parents, and an interview with the child or teenager. The focus should mainly be on aspects of family life other than the diabetes and its control, for it is here that the key to the problem usually lies. A home visit, especially in families where co-operation is poor, will also often be helpful.

Three psychological approaches to treatment in cases of poor diabetic control have been found helpful. Psychoanalytically based individual therapy has been shown to be effective in a carefully controlled clinical trial (Moran *et al.* 1991). Good results have also been claimed for family therapy (Ryden *et al.* 1994). The focus in family sessions is likely to be on the way in which the parents find it difficult to allow the child autonomy, and on achieving better ways of reaching resolution of conflicts. Behavioural methods of treatment, with the setting of short-term goals for the child and family, have also been found to be useful. Principles of behavioural management are described elsewhere (Section 9.2.1). A combination of family and individual approaches is likely to be most effective. Although most children with difficult to control diabetes requiring hospitalization can be managed on a paediatric ward with psychiatric input, a minority with serious behavioural problems may be better managed in a psychiatric unit (Kroll and Shaw 1994).

8.8 Blood disorders

8.8.1 HAEMOPHILIA

Definition

Haemophilia is a condition in which excessive bleeding occurs because of deficiency of one of the factors (factor VIII or IX) necessary for blood clotting to occur. The type of haemophilia depends on which factor is deficient.

Clinical features

- In *mild* cases of haemophilia, in which the level of the deficient factor is between 5 and 50% of normal, unusual bleeding only occurs when the child is exposed to serious trauma, as, for example, with a serious accident or surgical operation such as tonsillectomy.
- In *moderate* cases (1–5% of the deficient factor present), bleeding occurs with mild trauma or dental extraction.
- In *severe* cases (deficient factor less than 1% of normal), spontaneous bleeding occurs.

In the severe form, abnormal bleeding may occur from superficial skin cuts. Bleeding into soft tissues and muscle may produce painful bruising, and such bruises (haematomata) may occasionally prove dangerous if they put pressure on vital structures. Nosebleeding and haematuria (blood in the urine) may occur. Bleeding into joints may result in swelling and pain requiring immobilization. If this occurs frequently, or is inadequately treated, the immobilization may result in atrophy of muscles because of disuse.

Treatment consists of stemming the bleeding and replacement of the deficient factor with a plasma concentrate. Such treatment can now be carried out on an out-patient basis or in the home.

Aetiology

Haemophilia is a sex-linked recessive disorder and the defective gene is carried on an X chromosome. Women who are carriers are clinically unaffected, but

50% of their sons develop the condition. All the daughters of affected males are carriers. Sons of affected males are unaffected except in the highly improbable circumstance that their mothers are carriers. The condition occurs in about 1 in 15 000 males. There is no particular link with social class, and psychosocial factors are of no importance in primary aetiology, though they may influence the course of the condition (see below).

Psychosocial aspects

Haemophilia of mild or even moderate severity usually has rather little impact on the psychosocial life of the child and family. Occasionally, where there are pre-existing factors contributing to vulnerability, the presence of a disorder, even with relatively minor implications, will have a significant effect on the child's personality development and family life, but this is unusual. Severe haemophilia more frequently has a major impact (Markova *et al*. 1980*a*).

Parents of severely affected children are generally well-adjusted in the degree to which they protect their children from hazards such as sharp objects. Some, however, are markedly overprotective, and take unnecessarily strict precautions. Such parents are also those most likely to show guilt, as well as bitterness and resentment over the child's development of the condition. Rates of marital distress are high (Cairns and Lansky 1980). Many parents, however, successfully cope with their children's vulnerability by denial, apparently experiencing little anxiety about the possibility of injury or excessive bleeding. Fathers are generally quite highly participant in child care, but if complications of the condition become frequent or severe, this may put strain on the parental marriage, and the couple may find themselves in frequent disagreement over how the child should be managed. However, children with this condition are not at high risk for the development of psychiatric disorders and their social lives are usually not socially impaired (Logan *et al*. 1993).

Severely affected children are usually outgoing in personality, experiencing only relatively brief periods of sadness and withdrawal after a bleed. Although unable to participate in contact sports, they are often fascinated by such activities and may become preoccupied with them. Young affected children may be unusually clumsy in their use of sharp objects such as knives and scissors because they have been prevented from using them. School performance is usually within the average range, even though the children almost inevitably miss an unusual amount of school because of their condition. With modern forms of treatment, the great majority, even of severely affected children, are able to attend normal school (Markova *et al*. 1980*b*).

In the mid-1980s, a number of children with haemophilia received blood products infected with the HIV virus and contracted AIDS. Most of these have now passed through the paediatric age period. The psychosocial management of HIV infection is discussed in Section 8.5.2. Unfortunately, a new problem of uncertain dimensions has now arisen with blood products contaminated with hepatitis C.

Emotional factors may have an influence on the likelihood of bleeding. Usually bleeding is precipitated by minor trauma, but apparently 'spontaneous' bleeding sometimes occurs. In a minority of children this may occur just before some exciting event such as an outing or party. The mechanism may involve an autonomic response to emotional stress altering the integrity of the capillary wall (Mattson and Gross 1966).

Differential diagnosis of the condition may include non-accidental injury (Section 2.1). The occurrence of spontaneous bruising may mean that parents of mildly or moderately affected children have been wrongly suspected of injuring their children. The crisis that this may have produced has occasionally had long-lasting effects on family functioning.

Specific psychosocial effects of management

- *Genetic counselling.* The genetic aspects of the condition are not easy to grasp, and both parents, and, as they get older, affected children and their sibs, need frequent opportunities to discuss this issue. Decisions about further children must, of course, be left to parents following provision of full information. In the early 1990s antenatal detection of this condition is becoming increasingly possible.
- *Good communication* between family and paediatrician is vital. Parents and children should have a feeling of confidence that they know precisely what to do if bleeding occurs, and have clear advice on the level of protection the child really needs.
- That minority of *parents who suffer adverse emotional reactions* need continuing counselling. Their children are likely to be overprotected. Professionals should encourage as normal activity as possible. The supervised use of sharp tools such as knives and scissors when the child is still quite young (4–5 years) is helpful in preventing clumsiness (Markova *et al.* 1984).
- *Teachers* in the normal schools these children now mainly attend need adequate information about the nature of the condition, necessary protective measures, and what to do if bleeding occurs. The fact that many boys prevented from participating in sporting activities nevertheless enjoy play-fighting with their friends often exasperates teachers, who need opportunity for discussion.

8.8.2 LEUKAEMIA

Leukaemia is a cancer or neoplastic condition of the white cells of the blood. It is the most common form of malignancy in childhood, accounting for about half the total number of cancers in this age group. About 5 in 100 000 children are affected. Acute lymphoblastic leukaemia is the most common form of the condition.

Clinical features

The condition can occur at any time during childhood, but it is most frequent between 2 and 4 years of age, and is unusual after puberty. There may be an acute or chronic onset. Usually there is a period of several weeks of ill-health with susceptibility to infection and general malaise. The child will often be pale and look unwell. Then an episode of bleeding or some other traumatic event may make it clear something serious is amiss. Clinical examination may reveal bruising, an enlarged liver and spleen, and bone tenderness. The diagnosis is made by examination of a blood film and sample of bone marrow.

Aetiology

The cause of the condition is unknown, although in a minority of cases genetic factors or exposure to irradiation may be relevant. The incidence is raised in Down syndrome. A viral cause has been suspected, but not confirmed.

Treatment and outcome

Treatment is usually carried out in specialist centres. After initial acute treatment, it consists of chemotherapeutic drugs to induce a remission of the neoplastic process, and cranial irradiation to prevent the spread of the condition to the central nervous system. With this treatment a considerable majority of the patients go into a remission, although a proportion relapse. Children who relapse may be treated with bone marrow transplantation (Section 8.14). If persistent response to treatment occurs, currently the chemotherapy is stopped after about 3 years. Because the treatment suppresses body immunity, even the common childhood complaints such as chickenpox and measles can produce a fatal outcome, so if the child is in contact with these and other conditions, immune globulin is given. Over the past two decades, treatment has gradually improved the prognosis. The condition used to be universally fatal, but now the 5 year survival rate is in the region of 60% and, although inevitably some uncertainty remains, it is anticipated that many children have been permanently cured.

Psychosocial aspects

Initial diagnosis

Because the initial presenting features are often so non-specific, the diagnosis is quite frequently missed in the first few weeks by the family doctor. Once suspected, however, the diagnosis can be rapidly confirmed. Consequently, the parental reaction is likely to be one of severe shock, coupled sometimes with anger at the family doctor. Parents are likely to be unable to absorb complex medical information at the first interview with the physician. This is particularly the case with this condition because of the complexity of medical treatment required and the wide range of uncertainty about prognosis, with a real possibility both of death and of complete cure. Parents are not unnaturally bewildered, and require repeated interviews for clarification. They sometimes believe that the illness has been precipitated by some stressful event. The evidence in favour of a precipitating role for stress in the condition is poor.

Active treatment phase

During the initial active phase of treatment, frequent visits to hospital are required. Bone marrow investigations are painful and may be the aspect of the condition and its treatment most feared by the child. Adequate preparation linked to the availability of play facilities in the out-patient department to divert the child before the procedure will reduce distress. Short-term side-effects of treatment, including nausea and vomiting, mood changes, and constipation, are relatively common. Hair loss is a complication of radiotherapy which makes the child conspicuous at school and almost inevitably leads to embarrassment and sometimes teasing from other children. Older children can be offered a wig or prefer to wear a cap to cover their baldness.

The susceptibility of the child to infection causes a great deal of parental anxiety. The danger is a real one, yet the quality of the child's life can be greatly impaired if exaggerated precautions are taken to keep the child out of contact with others who just might be infected. Direct communication of parent with head teacher and class teacher to explain the situation and request information where infectious diseases are reported in classmates can be backed up if necessary by direct doctor–school contact by telephone. Active concern by all professionals involved with psychological and social problems is usually found helpful at this stage.

Later phase
While children are in remission on maintenance treatment, anxiety is usually, but not always, reduced. Parents usually maintain a more optimistic attitude than the physicians concerned, and children are generally more optimistic still. Many families cope well with the chronic stress and anxiety (Kupst and Schulman 1988). However, rates of depression, anxiety, and sexual problems in parents have been reported to be high, and many parents are reluctant to disclose such problems, so that their professional advisers may be unaware of them (Maguire 1983). Factors associated with good coping include harmonious family relationships, a supportive network of family and friends, lack of other stresses, open communication, and an attitude of living in the present (Kupst and Schulman 1988). Successful coping is achieved with a range of processes and what suits one family may not suit another. Some mothers find talking about the problem with other people is helpful, but with others this is most unhelpful. Some may function well with full acceptance of the problem, others by the strong use of denial. Fathers more commonly cope by not talking about the condition. Some families, perhaps most, are drawn more closely together by the stress; some find it distances them. Most help is obtained from family members and friends. Communication with the child should not be forgotten, and children even as young as 3 years can understand a surprising amount of apparently technical information (Eiser *et al.* 1993).

School problems are relatively common. As a result of the irradiation, children who are diagnosed and receive treatment before the age of about 5 years may develop specific cognitive deficits, especially loss of short-term memory and poor concentration (Smibert *et al.* 1996). These problems do not seem to affect children irradiated at an older age. Younger children, however, tend to find difficult those school subjects such as arithmetic which involve sequential learning. It is currently uncertain to what degree special remedial help can overcome these deficits; nor is it known for how long they persist, but extra educational help is often indicated.

Not unnaturally, teachers are inclined to allow children with leukaemia extra leeway, and avoid putting even the normal amount of pressure on them to do homework and conform in the classroom. Good physician–school communication can ensure that teachers are aware that children with leukaemia tend to thrive best when they are treated like others and normal pressures are applied. School refusal has been reported in children with this condition, and this is likely to be related to parental anxiety (see Section 4.4.3).

Relapses terminating in a fatal outcome still do unfortunately occur in about 30–40% of children with leukaemia, even with the best available treatment. Psychosocial aspects of terminal care, including communication with the child in these circumstances, are discussed in Section 7.7.

8.8.3 THALASSAEMIA

Thalassaemia is an inherited disease caused by a failure of synthesis of normal adult haemoglobin. It is commonest among people living in the eastern Mediterranean, but also occurs in other countries. It is inherited as an autosomal recessive with the homozygote suffering from the major form of the disease. The heterozygote carrier shows minor haematological abnormalities, but is usually clinically normal.

It usually presents in the first 6 months of life with pallor due to anaemia, and failure to thrive. The facial appearance is often unusual, because of skull deformities. Treatment is symptomatic and involves frequent blood transfusions, but eventually organ failure from chronic iron overload results in premature death.

The psychosocial aspects of this condition have been little studied, but are of considerable significance. Anaemia can be prevented by subcutaneous injections of desferrioxamine, and young children especially may develop phobic reactions to the medical procedures involved. Short stature and failure to enter puberty are not infrequently associated with low self-esteem and withdrawal reactions. Children are likely to be especially vulnerable when a sib or other close relative has died of the condition. There is a high rate of psychiatric disorder in children with this condition (Aydin *et al.* 1997), and their sibs may also be adversely affected (Labropoulou and Beratis 1995).

Discussions in groups of parents of children with this condition have revealed (Tsiantis *et al.* 1982) that communication about the disease within the family is often poor. Parents may show maladaptive denial and express a good deal of guilt about their responsibility for the condition, though the presence of the condition may have a binding effect on the marriage (Tsiantis *et al.* 1996). It is uncertain how far this is a general phenomenon, but certainly parent groups would seem to offer an opportunity for the provision of mutual support and the improvement of family communication. Genetic counselling is of major importance, as identification of the heterozygous state and antenatal detection of the homozygous condition, either by amniocentesis or, in the first trimester, by chorionic villus sampling, with the possibility of therapeutic abortion, has now become possible.

8.8.4 SICKLE CELL DISEASE

Sickle cell disease is a blood disorder found almost entirely in Africans and people of African descent. An inherited defect of haemoglobin results in the red cells becoming sickle shaped and prone to clumping together. As a result, they stick in small blood vessels and vaso-occlusive complications occur because these become blocked. The most important consequences are anaemia and acutely painful episodes arising from the death of tissues which are starved of oxygen. These episodes often begin in early childhood when acute pain is experienced most often in the hands and feet, but also in the arms, legs, back, and abdomen. Treatment of the pain includes analgesics and fluids by mouth. Exchange blood transfusion may be necessary. In the homozygous form of the disease, there is a not inconsiderable mortality in the first 5 years of life from complications such as pneumonia and renal failure. However, subsequently expectation of life is only slightly reduced.

Children and adolescents with this condition do not have raised rates of psychological disturbance when compared to general population samples (Cepeda *et al.* 1997). The episodes of pain occur on average once a fortnight, and are highly disruptive of schooling and recreational life (Fuggle *et al.* 1996). Most episodes are managed at home, and a community-based focused pain management service, involving and supporting other members of the family as well as the affected child, can enhance children's resilience and improve their quality of life (Fuggle *et al.* 1996).

8.9 Respiratory disorders

8.9.1 ASTHMA

Definition

Asthma is a condition in which there is intermittent, reversible obstruction of the respiratory airways due to hyper-reactivity of the airway lining to a variety of stimuli. The characteristic wheeze is produced by forced exhalation through narrowed bronchi.

Background factors

Asthma occurs in between 5 and 15% of the population in childhood, with quite marked variability between different countries (Gergen *et al.* 1988). It often begins in the first 2 years of life, when distinction from 'wheezy bronchitis' is difficult. Occasionally, first attacks occur later in childhood. There is no clear-cut link with social class. In young children, in whom infection is prominent as a causative factor (see below), working-class children are probably more commonly affected, whereas in the older age group it is more frequent in middle-class children. There was an increase in the prevalence of asthma in many countries in the 1980s and early 1990s (Rona *et al.* 1995). The cause of this increase is uncertain.

Causation

A family history of allergic disorder is common, and it is likely that a genetic predisposition to asthma is inherited as part of a general tendency to allergic illness. Children who develop asthma have often previously suffered from infantile eczema, and may show other atopic manifestations.

Attacks are precipitated in vulnerable children by a variety of environmental agents or events. Allergens may be inhaled or ingested. They include pollens, housedust (in which the house mite may be the principal causative agent), feathers, and animal fur. A variety of foods, including eggs, shellfish, and cow's milk, may induce attacks. Attacks may also be precipitated by upper respiratory tract infections of a bacterial or viral nature, so that often asthma occurs when the child gets an ordinary cold. Prevalence is higher in children of parents who smoke.

In addition to these allergic precipitants, attacks are also produced by non-allergic factors. Of these, psychological stresses, to be discussed in more detail below, are amongst the most common, but physical exercise and cold weather also fall into this category.

Links with psychological factors

Psychological factors are often of major importance in the precipitation and maintenance of asthmatic attacks, but earlier-held views that the condition is primarily of psychological nature were largely incorrect. There is no evidence that major life events play a part in aetiology, and no specific personality profile characteristic of asthma. However, the condition does have some specific effects on family relationships. In children with a strong family history of asthma, early parenting difficulties predict an early onset of asthma (Mrazek *et al.* 1991).

Direct psychological precipitants

In vulnerable children any event likely to produce an emotional reaction may also precipitate an attack. Events causing anxiety, anger, and anticipatory excitement are most commonly responsible, and, in these circumstances, the attack often occurs as the emotion is experienced. Situations about which the child may reasonably be worried (such as a separation from one or both parents, or school tests and examinations), those which might induce anger (such as any sort of frustration), and the onset of pleasurable activities (such as Christmas or a birthday) may all therefore be responsible.

The mechanisms whereby emotional states produce asthmatic attacks are not well understood, though there is no doubt that intense emotion can reduce pulmonary flow rate. It is likely that the hypothalamic–limbic–midbrain circuits are activated following appreciation and interpretation of a psychologically meaningful stimulus at cerebral level. The activation of these circuits is known to influence immune systems. Presumably there is a final common pathway, involving the release of chemical mediators immediately preceding the asthmatic attack, and this may be reached either by direct influence of neuroregulatory pathways from the brain in arousal states produced by emotion, or as a result of hypersensitivity to allergic substances. It is also possible that the various forms of respiratory behaviour associated with emotional expression—laughing, crying, etc.—may sometimes act as specific triggers of attacks.

Indirect psychological contributory factors

Indirect factors include those that affect the child's likelihood of experiencing emotional states productive of attacks as well as those that affect the child's vulnerability to allergic stimuli, for example by non-compliance with medication.

Family factors

Family factors are probably the most common and important psychosocial influences. Mrazek *et al.* (1987) have shown that insecure attachment is more common in severely asthmatic pre-school children, in comparison with healthy controls, and Kashani *et al.* (1988) that parents of asthmatic children are indeed unusually anxious. Asthma in its acute form is a very frightening condition for anyone to observe, and for parents it is often terrifying, because death may seem so near. It is therefore only natural that between attacks parents should show a great deal of anxious and protective behaviour towards their asthmatic children. Such anxiety is readily communicated, and the child is then more likely to experience an attack. Family studies of children with asthma, in comparison with healthy and diabetic children, have demonstrated that the families of asthmatic children tend to rigidity and overinvolvement or enmeshment in their relationships (Gustafsson *et al.* 1987).

   The occurrence of the attack provides a further reason for parental anxiety, and the cycle is complete. The circular chain of events may be temporarily broken by medical treatment, and admission to the safe environment of a hospital ward is often a considerable reassurance in these circumstances. However, if the child is admitted to hospital every time a minor attack occurs, a pattern of unnecessarily frequent admissions may be established. The way in which contact with parents can elicit asthma has been well demonstrated in an experiment in which parents of selected asthmatic children were encouraged to spend 2 weeks away from home while their children were looked after by substitute parents. The design of the experiment meant that the children were still exposed to the same allergens in the domestic environment. In a sizeable number of the children, there was a marked reduction in asthmatic attacks, followed by an increase when their parents returned (Purcell and Weiss 1970). In contrast, a small minority of parents can also show marked denial of the presence of the condition in their child and fail to ensure adequate medical care. Such rejecting behaviour may result in the child becoming aggressive, and also at risk of unnecessary invalidism or even death as a result of medical neglect.

Psychological factors in the child

• There is no specific *type of personality* associated with asthma. Nevertheless, a proportion (about 10%) of asthmatic children show significant emotional and behavioural problems of different types, and asthmatic pre-school as well as school-age children show higher rates of disturbance than healthy controls (Mrazek *et al.* 1987). Although such disturbances may be caused by factors unrelated to the asthma, for example family disturbances, school stresses, and adverse temperamental characteristics, the asthma or some aspect of treatment may be used by the child as a means of expressing anger or frustration, or of gaining attention. Severely asthmatic children show the greatest levels of emotional disturbance, aggression, and anxiety (McNichol *et al.* 1973). Further, the presence of depression in severely asthmatic children is associated with increased asthma mortality and requires skilled attention (Mrazek 1992).

• *Illness-related abnormal behaviour.* The occurrence of an attack may allow a child to avoid a stress he would otherwise have to face. Some children develop the capacity to induce attacks deliberately with this in mind. Children may not take medical measures they know will abort an attack, if the occurrence of an attack will bring them advantages. Non-compliance with medical treatment may also occur in children unable to face the fact that they do have an illness. By 'forgetting' or refusing to take their prophylactic medication, they are able to deny the fact that there is anything wrong with them. Some parents who cannot cope with the idea that they have an ill child may also behave in this way. Asthmatic children, depressed and discouraged for a variety of reasons, including parental neglect and rejection, may fail to abort attacks because they have such a low self-image that they do not see themselves as worth troubling about. Parental neglect has in these cases encouraged self-neglect. There is some evidence that children who are low in allergic potential are generally more likely to have asthmatic attacks in which psychological mechanisms are prominent.

Assessment

Assessment first involves the establishment of the diagnosis and of precipitating factors leading to attacks. A broad approach to assessment from the beginning is desirable. Parents and children should be asked if they have observed the effects of the various substances breathed in or eaten that are known to induce attacks. In addition, they should be asked about the possible effects of other factors such as exercise and psychological stresses in precipitating and maintaining attacks (Matus 1981).

It should be possible to assess the attitudes of the child and family to the asthma. Is the degree of worry and concern commensurate with the severity of the disorder? Is there overconcern about a relatively minor problem or denial of a serious disorder?

Where psychological factors appear prominent, either at the onset of the condition or once it is well established, an account of the quality of family relationships and the child's experiences at school should be obtained. The possibility that factors unrelated to the asthma are affecting the way in which the illness is experienced or reacted to should be borne in mind.

Treatment

Treatment of asthma in childhood first involves competent medical management, both in acute episodes and between attacks. As well as appropriate medication, this should include advice on the avoidance of allergens. The attitude of the child and other family members to the asthma should be monitored. It is often helpful to encourage the child and parents to express anxieties they may have about the recurrence of acute attacks and the possibility that the child may die in one of them. In fact, the mortality from asthma is low, and the physician can be reassuring in this respect. Some forms of medication such as theophylline may occasionally have an adverse effect on behaviour and learning, but this side-effect is uncommon and probably represents an idiosyncratic reaction (Weldon and McGeady 1995). Steroids, however, do not appear to affect psychomotor adaptation as has been suspected (Bender *et al.* 1987).

The child should be encouraged to lead as normal a life as possible and, in most cases, no restrictions at all other than those related to diet and avoidance of allergens need be imposed. Some children have exercise-induced asthma, however, and these should be discouraged from provoking attacks by exercising to the degree that produces one. Normal school attendance should occur as far as possible. There is evidence that asthmatic children are, as a group, of average or a little above average ability, but may develop educational retardation probably due to prolonged school absence (Hill *et al.* 1989). Counselling of children themselves is beneficial in its effect. A systematic educational training programme for children with asthma aged between 8 and 13 years has been shown in a controlled trial to have positive medical and psychological effects (Colland 1993).

In cases where there is non-compliance with medication or allergen avoidance, or the child seems to be deliberately inducing attacks, there needs to be a more intensive investigation of the child and family. It needs to be understood, for example, why the child prefers to have an attack rather than to go to school, or why it is so important to a child and family that he denies the fact that he has an illness to such a degree that he forgets to take medication.

The management of psychological factors leading to exacerbation of asthma will depend on the formulation of the problem. When a child is clearly gaining more from having attacks than he would if he did not have them, an operant behavioural approach is often helpful. Where there is a problem within the family in the communication of feelings and perceptions of the asthma, family therapy may be effective. There is evidence that brief family therapy designed to improve family communication produces a modest but definite improvement in lung function (Lask and Matthew 1979). When the child's pattern of behaviour suggests internal conflicts resulting in self-destructive tendencies or ill-understood outwardly directed aggression, brief, focused individual psychotherapy is indicated. If, however, the child is generally anxious, but there is no good evidence that deep-seated conflicts are responsible, a course of relaxation may be helpful. It is in these circumstances that hypnosis is likely to have an effect, though there are no controlled trials demonstrating its efficacy in asthmatic children. In a small minority of children where asthma is severe and protracted, and there is evidence from the effects of repeated hospitalization that the child fares better away from home, residential schooling will be indicated. With more effective medication, the need for such special schooling has decreased.

Outcome

Most children with asthma (about three-quarters) improve considerably at or before early adolescence (Blair 1977). A minority of those who remit do, however, relapse in late adolescence and early adulthood. There is no evidence that the prominence of psychological factors has either adverse or benign influence on the course of the physical condition.

Psychological aspects of the condition may, however, have a long-lasting impact both on the personality of the child and on the life of the family. In particular, because of the fact that emotional arousal provokes attacks, some children become emotionally constricted and frightened of the experience of powerful feelings. This may lead to the development of a rather introverted and inhibited personality. Most children with asthma will, however, develop normally, and there is no evidence that they are especially prone to psychological problems later in life.

8.9.2 CYSTIC FIBROSIS (MUCOVISCIDOSIS)

Definition

Cystic fibrosis is an inherited condition which affects the function of all exocrine glands—those glands that discharge their secretions directly into the body. The secretions of these glands are abnormally viscid and pathological effects occur due both to deficiency of the secretions and to obstruction of the various ducts. The most seriously affected organs are the lungs and pancreas, but other organs such as the liver, sweat glands, and intestines are also involved.

Clinical features

Universal neonatal screening has now been introduced experimentally in a number of centres. Depending on the severity of the condition in the individual, cystic fibrosis may present at any time of life, but most commonly the first signs occur in infancy or early childhood.

At birth the intestine may already be obstructed by secretions—a condition known as *meconium ileus*. This condition, which can be treated successfully, requires early surgical intervention if the infant is to survive. In early and mid-childhood, chronic respiratory infections and failure to thrive, caused by malabsorption, are the most common presenting features. However, cystic fibrosis may also present in other ways, including diarrhoea due to intestinal malabsorption, or prolapse of the rectum. The diagnosis is confirmed by testing the patient's sweat for salt concentration.

Usually the most serious and prominent symptoms are respiratory. The child becomes chronically infected with both common and uncommon organisms (especially *Pseudomonas*). Eventually these become more and more difficult to control, and death occurs due to respiratory failure. The patient may, however, survive for many years following diagnosis, and many treated with antibiotics, regular physiotherapy, and vitamin supplements now live on into adulthood. The prognosis depends on the severity of the condition, the availability of treatment, and treatment compliance. There has been a marked improvement in survival rates in this condition since the 1960, so that a majority of children now survive until at least until mid-adolescence, and many into adulthood.

Causation and incidence

Cystic fibrosis is genetically determined as an autosomal recessive, so that the risk for future births after the birth of an affected child is 1 in 4. It occurs in about 1 in 2000 births, and there is a roughly equal sex ratio. The affected gene was cloned and sequenced in 1989. On the basis of prenatal investigation of gene markers, it is now possible to give accurate information to parents about the likelihood of their child being affected. It is also possible to identify carriers of the condition.

Psychosocial aspects

Psychosocial aspects of cystic fibrosis have been extensively reviewed by Lask (1995). There are a number of specific psychosocial features of this condition which complicate its management (Burton 1975). The outlook for patients is very variable, so that it is difficult for both parents and children to develop firm expectations for the future. Often, before a decline sets in, the child will remain relatively well for several years, requiring only intermittent treatment for respiratory infections. With other children the progress is much more rapid. The terminal phase of the condition is also variable in length, with some children experiencing a rapid deterioration leading to death, and others suffering from apparently overwhelming infection, but then recovering and returning to a life of good quality for several more months or even years. The introduction of heart–lung transplantation in children and adolescents nearing the terminal phase of their illness has improved life expectancy for some, but—though the view expressed here is controversial—it is at present uncertain whether the quality of life after the operation justifies its performance.

The demands of treatment made upon the child and parents are very considerable. Thus parents, especially mothers, are likely to be involved in physiotherapy (postural treatment to drain the lungs) 2 or 3 times a day, to a total of several hours a week. The need for replacement enzymes, antibiotics, and vitamins adds further to the burden of treatment. The daily active involvement of the parents with treatment of the condition means that the risk of child and parent becoming emotionally overinvolved with each other and totally preoccupied with the illness is considerable. Heart–lung transplantation brings problems of compliance because of the difficult post-transplantation treatment regime, and the unpleasant side-effects of the medication.

Parental understanding of the nature of the condition is often limited, and this impedes communication with the sick child and sibs. A significant proportion of parents remain unaware of the genetic implications and the risk of further affected children, perhaps partly because they are not adequately informed, and partly because they may have difficulty absorbing the information.

Family relationships

Although family functioning in families with a child with cystic fibrosis has been found to be normal in terms of adaptability and cohesiveness (Cowen *et al.* 1986), and such families do not perceive themselves to be under particular stress (Walker *et al.* 1987), there is no doubt that family life is greatly affected by the birth of such a child. Parents often treat the child with cystic fibrosis more indulgently than their other children (Burton 1975). They set fewer demands for independence and conformity. This is particularly likely to be the case if they have previously lost a child with cystic fibrosis. Not infrequently this leads to jealousy between the affected child and non-affected brothers and sisters. Other behavioural problems, such as temper tantrums, disobedience, and problems with other children, may also arise for similar reasons.

Despite these various special stresses, the evidence from controlled studies (Gayton *et al.* 1977; Bywater 1981; Drotar *et al.* 1981) suggests that the rate of behavioural and emotional disorders in children with cystic fibrosis is not higher than that of children with other non-cerebral physical disorders. Some investigators (e.g. Cowen *et al.* 1986), however, have found rates of disturbance to be high in uncontrolled studies and have pointed particularly to rates of aggressive behaviour in young children. Further, while eating disorders are relatively common in children with this condition (Steinhausen and Schindauer 1981), adolescents and adults are more likely to show depressive and anxiety states (Pearman *et al.* 1991). Mothers are more likely to be depressed the more severe they perceive their child's illness to be (Walker *et al.* 1987). The level of disturbance in affected children is related, to some degree, to the amount of social support the family receives (Frydman 1981). Although the children do miss school because of their condition, and sometimes have less educational pressure placed upon them than they might otherwise, their educational standards are usually not retarded.

The sibs of children with cystic fibrosis are also exposed to especially stressful circumstances (Cowen *et al.* 1986). Parents often do not explain the nature of the affected child's condition to brothers and sisters, who may consequently feel confused and uncertain how to react. Older children tend to be solicitous towards and make allowances for the younger affected child, but where an unaffected child is younger than the affected sib, this occurs less often and negative reactions are much more common (Burton 1975).

Reactions of the affected children to their own illness are various. Most, despite being inadequately informed about the nature of their condition, come to terms with their disability and cope with the symptoms of their illness and demands of treatment with great fortitude. Many affected children particularly enjoy sporting and other outdoor activities when they are well. A small proportion react to their disability with denial and refusal to accept their treatment—physiotherapy or tablets. Usually denial or compartmentalization in the child is linked to a similar attitude in parents, who are likely to have difficulty in talking with the child about the nature of the illness.

Management of psychosocial problems
Ensuring that both parents (fathers as well as mothers) of children diagnosed as suffering from cystic fibrosis are well informed about the nature of the condition and its genetic implications will prevent much misunderstanding both between parents, and between parent and child. Parents should also be encouraged to have the same level of expectations for behaviour and self-help for their affected child as for their other children.

There is evidence that children are better adjusted if parents can communicate with children about their illness and its implications (Burton 1975). The same holds true for non-affected sibs. This does not mean that parents should emphasize the fatal outcome of the condition from the outset, but it does mean that children should know they have a chronic condition, and it is not their fault or that of their parents. They should know that they will always be likely to have symptoms, and that these are likely to become more severe as time goes on. They should have the opportunity of sharing their feelings of disappointment, grief, and anger with their parents, who will themselves adjust better if they (the parents) can share their own feelings with others, relatives, friends, and professionals. Management of the psychosocial aspects of terminal stages of illness are discussed in Section 7.7. However, it should be emphasized that, with modern treatment, many patients survive with a good quality of life well into mature adulthood.

8.10 Genitourinary disorders

By far the most common urinary tract disorder of psychological significance is enuresis (Section 4.6.5). However, a number of other urinary tract disorders also raise some specific psychosocial issues, and these will also be briefly discussed in this section.

8.10.1 CONGENITAL MALFORMATIONS

Severe congenital malformations of the urinary tract are relatively uncommon and, when they occur, are not infrequently incompatible with survival. However, relatively recent surgical advances have improved the prognosis for some conditions. The least uncommon is the presence of posterior urethral valves, occurring in boys, usually presenting in the first year of life. The valves obstruct the outflow of urine and this leads to distension of the bladder, ureters, and kidneys. Surgical treatment is often fully successful, but partial success may require further hospitalization, for example for implantation of the ureters into the colon. Such procedures often understandably raise anxieties in parents concerning matters such as the subsequent sexual function of their children.

8.10.2 URINARY TRACT INFECTIONS

These infections are relatively common throughout childhood, and occur more frequently in boys during the neonatal period but subsequently more commonly in girls. In the first year of life, failure to thrive with irritability and poor feeding may be caused by chronic or recurrent urinary infections. In babies from socially deprived backgrounds, it may be unclear to what degree failure to thrive is due to an infection or to relative neglect. Young children presenting with failure to thrive and identified as having urinary infections which are then successfully treated should therefore be carefully followed up to assess whether other factors might be responsible for growth failure.

The occurrence of a proven urinary infection in a child is an indication for physical investigation to determine whether there is a structural or physiological abnormality such as reflux. In the absence of such abnormalities, aetiology of psychosocial significance should be considered, though this will not frequently be present. Poor social circumstances linked to inadequate hygiene may be relevant. Aspects of the history or examination of the external genitalia may raise a suspicion that the girl is subject to sexual abuse.

8.10.3 CHRONIC RENAL FAILURE

Failure of kidney function is usually caused by chronic glomerulonephritis, pyelonephritis, or congenital abnormalities, but sometimes by a variety of other conditions. Progressive renal failure results in uraemia and death unless modern treatments, particularly haemodialysis and renal transplantation, are available. The general indications for haemodialysis and transplantation are outside the scope of this book. However, some paediatricians regard instability of the family and the presence of psychological disturbance in the child as relative contraindications to these procedures. Psychosocial appraisal has not reached a stage where successful prediction of compliance is possible, though there is some evidence for the importance of particular adverse factors.

Studies of psychosocial aspects of children with chronic renal failure have been reviewed by Postlethwaite *et al.* (1996). Technical improvements in haemodialysis, which mean that home-based treatment is now possible, have reduced the stress on children and families, Nevertheless, psychological problems occur more frequently than normal in children with chronic renal failure on dialysis (Garralda *et al.* 1988). The more severe the physical problem, the more likely is the child to show emotional difficulties, particularly anxiety, loneliness, and overdependency on parents. There is a reduction in levels of behavioural disturbance after dialysis has been established, probably arising from alleviation of parental anxiety. Nevertheless, the stress on family life remains considerable. Treatment takes 12–18 hours a week, diet has to be restricted, and complications are not uncommon. Nevertheless, children are usually able to attend normal school on a reasonably regular basis.

Renal transplantation is a preferable form of treatment, but is not always available. About two-thirds of transplants are successful. Organ rejection is therefore fairly common and is associated with high rates of depression and anxiety in the children and adolescents concerned. Aggressive and hostile reactions may also occur in this age group. Psychiatric problems in children with renal transplants occur at about twice the rate of those in healthy children (Klein *et al.* 1984). The children are preoccupied with their short stature—an almost inevitable complication of the renal disease and steroids used to suppress organ rejection. Girls are particularly upset by the bloated facial appearance produced by steroids, and this and other factors not uncommonly lead to non-compliance with medication. Good preparation for the various procedures and for operation, with warning of the side-effects, as well as involvement of the adolescent patient in the decision to transplant, may reduce subsequent non-compliance, so that transplantation may be expected to result ultimately in overall psychological improvement. Nevertheless, adolescents with chronic renal failure frequently fail to reach a satisfactory level of independence by early adulthood (Rosenkranz *et al.* 1992). Mental health professionals may have a useful part to play in this aspect of management.

8.10.4 UNDESCENDED TESTIS

Undescended testis is a fairly common condition occurring in about 1 in 50 boys and may be diagnosed either at birth, on school entry medical examination, or by parents at any time. The testis may have failed to descend or may have descended to an abnormal position. In either event, if natural descent does not occur in the first year, surgical treatment is necessary for various reasons (risk of malignancy, preservation of fertility, cosmetic reasons, etc.) and is usually carried out before the age of 2 years. Surgery is generally successful.

Because of anxieties that both parents and professionals experience when talking to children about their genitalia, preparation is often inadequate. Adequate preparation of the child for the procedure is, however, particularly important because boys often have fears about being permanently mutilated in the genital area. Anxiety about castration, which used to be thought a common fantasy, is probably less common than fears of mutilation of the penis. There is no good evidence that boys undergoing this operation, if adequately prepared, need suffer long-term adverse psychological consequences, nor is there evidence that the timing of operation has long-term psychological significance (Cytryn *et al.* 1967).

8.10.5 INTERSEX DISORDERS

In intersex disorders, sexual appearance is ambiguous or there is inconsistency in features of sexual differentiation. The criteria for sexual differentiation include

- chromosomal structure
- internal morphology
- external morphology (the appearance of the external genitalia)
- pattern of sex hormone secretion
- gender identity (the degree to which individuals perceive themselves as male or female)
- gender role (pattern of sex-typed behaviour)
- choice of sex object.

Although chromosomal or gonadal sex are sometimes suggested to be the indicators of 'true' sex, there is no logical justification for this, and indeed gender identity and role might just as reasonably be regarded as the best indicators.

In so-called 'true' hermaphroditism the gonads contain both ovarian and testicular tissue. Conditions of this type are extremely rare. More common are male and female pseudo-hermaphroditism in which chromosomes and gonads are clearly differentiated, but the external genitalia are ambiguous. Thus in male pseudo-hermaphroditism the chromosome structure is XY, and testes are present, though there is cryptorchidism and the external genitalia have a female appearance.

Congenital adrenal cortical hyperplasia, when it occurs in chromosomal females, causes female pseudo-hermaphroditism and is by far the most common intersex condition. It results from an inherited (autosomal recessive) enzyme defect, usually of 21-hydroxylase. This affects steroid production and there is excessive androgen excretion *in utero* and subsequently. In boys this produces precocious puberty. Girls present at birth with ambiguous genitalia. A salt-losing syndrome is often associated. The condition is diagnosable after birth and treatable with steroids.

Decision as to which sex the child should be reared should be taken as soon as possible after birth when the condition has been investigated and the diagnosis made. Decision-making should involve parents, paediatricians, and the paediatric surgeon, and a psychological or psychiatric input is often helpful. At this stage, the most relevant consideration is the likely external appearance after plastic surgery.

Issues of reassignment of sex after a period in which the child has been brought up in one sex-role require very careful consideration with strong psychological or psychiatric input. In general, reassignment of sex after 2–3 years of age presents very considerable problems and involves a major family crisis, as gender identity and parental perceptions are relatively fixed by this time (Money and Ehrhardt 1972). Reassignment has been described at puberty with five α-reductase-deficiency males brought up pubertally as females, but this occurred in a closed community where the condition is relatively common and accepted by members of the community.

Although the physical outcome of congenital adrenal cortical hyperplasia is usually satisfactory, given early diagnosis, psychosocial outcome may be much less so (Hochberg *et al.* 1987). Chromosomal girls raised as females tend to be tomboyish in manner and, postpubertally, have a higher than expected rate of homosexuality (Money *et al.* 1984). Chromosomal girls raised as males usually have a small penis even after surgical reconstruction, and show poor peer relationships and later low sexual potency. If early reassignment of chromosomal females with congenital adrenal cortical hyperplasia who have been raised as boys is possible, this should be discussed with parents.

Children with intersex conditions and their parents are likely to benefit from continued psychological and psychiatric counselling (Money 1975). Practical advice concerning how to deal with situations in which, for example, the child's genitalia may be seen by other children will be helpful. Information about the future can be presented in a positive manner. For example, parents and, as they get older, children, can be told marriage will be possible as well as child-rearing, though this may need to be by adoption. Self-esteem is often closely linked to a clearly defined sexual identity, and children with intersex conditions may need special encouragement for their performance in school or in recreational activities so that they can maintain a good self-image. Counselling for children and families should not be discontinued after the prepubertal years, but should continue well into adolescence, when new difficulties may need to be faced.

8.11 Organic gastrointestinal disorders

8.11.1 PEPTIC ULCER

Duodenal ulcers are not common, but occur occasionally in childhood. As in adults, the pain is likely to be epigastric, but there may be little relationship with mealtimes. Episodes of pain are periodic, and the pain may wake the child at night. The condition often presents with an attack of gastrointestinal bleeding. There is often a positive family history.

Psychological factors are usually not prominent, but sometimes the pain may be precipitated by stress. Peptic ulceration has been reported as occurring in association with school refusal. Children with the condition have also been reported to be shyer and more tense than controls, with an increase in school difficulties (Christodolou *et al.* 1977). Early separations from parents and parental loss have been reported to occur in excess.

Attention to stress factors and family tensions should form part of management, which will otherwise consist mainly of dietary advice, antacids, and possibly other specific medication. Many ulcers occurring in childhood do become chronic, and it is possible that attention to stress factors improves the prognosis.

8.11.2 CROHN'S DISEASE

Crohn's disease is a chronic, inflammatory condition, most commonly occurring in the ileum, but also appearing at times in other parts of the alimentary tract. The condition runs a chronic course and, when it occurs in childhood, often produces significant social disability and growth failure.

Psychological factors are not thought to be of importance in aetiology. Children suffering from the condition have a high rate of associated behavioural and emotional problems (Engstrom and Lindqvist 1991), with high rates of psychiatric disorder linked to greater disease activity. Stress may precipitate relapses. Paediatric management of the condition is often highly complex. It is therefore important for the clinician and others involved with the child and family to be aware of the family circumstances and school progress to a degree which allows monitoring of these factors and, occasionally, intervention to reduce impairment which may be considerable (Rabbett *et al.* 1996). Psychiatric referral may occasionally be indicated if associated emotional problems become prominent.

8.11.3 ULCERATIVE COLITIS

Ulcerative colitis involves chronic inflammation of the colon and rectum. It is uncommon in childhood, but can occur in children as young as 7–8 years. The symptoms, especially pain and the passage of mucus and blood in the stool, usually continue over several years with frequent remissions and relapses.

Partly because of the risk of cancer in parts of the bowel affected over very long periods, surgical treatment with creation of an ileostomy is now more readily undertaken. Most, but not all, children adjust well following stoma surgery, but careful preparation is required, giving the child and family the opportunity beforehand to meet others who have had the operation (Lask 1988*b*). Adverse psychological factors should not delay operation if the medical condition of the child suggests this is necessary.

Psychological factors are thought to be of little importance in aetiology (Feldman *et al.* 1967), but they often play a part in the maintenance of the condition and in the precipitation of relapse. The rate of psychological disturbance among childhood sufferers is high (Engstrom and Lindqvist 1991) and is not of any particular type, though obsessive–compulsive symptoms occur more commonly than in other physical conditions (Burke *et al.* 1989). The presence of disturbance is not related to the severity of the condition or to specific physical features other than growth failure.

Psychotherapy has been recommended as an adjuvant to surgical and medical treatment (McDermott and Finch 1967), but attention to psychological factors is probably best provided by the clinician responsible for medical management. His long-standing acquaintance with the family will enable him to be sensitive to likely stresses operating on the child. Psychiatric referral should be limited to those cases where there are associated persistent behavioural and emotional problems or non-compliance with treatment.

8.12 Congenital heart disease

About 1 in 150 children is born with a congenital heart defect, and this is therefore the commonest type of congenital malformation. The defect may vary from the trivial (e.g. a small ventricular septal defect) to a defect incompatible with life even if skilled surgery is available. About 1 in 10 children with congenital heart defects has an associated defect elsewhere in the body.

The condition is usually polygenically determined. However, children with some chromosomal abnormalities (e.g. trisomy 21, Down syndrome) have high rates of heart defects, and some defects arise because of abnormalities in the pregnancy (e.g. maternal rubella).

Detection of the condition may occur at a routine postnatal examination or during a medical examination for some other reason in an older child. Occasionally an abnormality may be suspected antenatally following ultrasound scan. In the majority of children who present in the neonatal period or early infancy, there is cyanosis, slow feeding, breathlessness, failure to thrive, or other symptoms.

Many cardiac lesions can be confirmed by non-invasive echocardiography but a significant proportion of children will proceed to cardiac catheterization, a procedure not without risk. Subsequently, many affected babies will receive surgery, but a few will have conditions too severe for successful operation. These receive symptomatic treatment but have a fatal outcome. Surgery is often remarkably successful, but a number of children require re-operation, either as a planned procedure or because the initial operation was only partially satisfactory.

8.12.1 PSYCHOSOCIAL ASPECTS

Trivial heart conditions

In a number of children with 'innocent' murmurs, follow-up reveals that the detection of the murmur and subsequent parental anxiety have led to overprotection and invalidism. The same outcome occasionally occurs with minor heart conditions of no functional significance. In these children, great anxiety may occur every time the child has a minor procedure or operation such as a dental extraction, because of the need for antibiotic cover. The danger of overprotection is unrelated to the seriousness of the cardiac condition (Garson *et al.* 1978). The mother's perception of the seriousness of a heart condition is a much more powerful predictor of child adjustment than is the actual medical severity (DeMaso *et al.* 1991). Once it has been decided that a murmur is of no pathological significance, review appointments are likely to raise unnecessary anxiety. Complete reassurance with discharge from the out-patient clinic is more likely to avoid overprotection and invalidism.

Inoperable defects

Some children are likely to have a relatively brief life. Parents will require considerable support over this period and after the death. They may be particularly upset because they will often be attending clinics where the prevailing mood is one of optimism, with most children doing well. For a discussion of psychosocial aspects of terminal care, see Section 7.7.

Operable lesions

With advances in paediatric cardiac surgery, children with operable lesions now form the largest group. All such children and their parents have to face cardiac catheterization, a major operation, and a period of postoperative uncertainty. A proportion have to face further operations and, in a minority, operative procedures fail to correct the lesion adequately and a fatal outcome ensues. Specific psychosocial aspects that need to be considered in the care of these children include:

- Awareness of the fact that the heart is often regarded by parents as the most vital organ the child possesses. A defect of the heart is particularly frightening even if, to the clinician, the lesion seems rather minor.
- The possibility that mothers will have greater difficulty interacting with their infant in the early months than would be the case with an unaffected child.
- The anxiety-provoking nature of the procedures. Parents need full explanation of the procedures before they occur. The nature of the catheterization should be fully explained with a prior visit to the catheterization room. Parents need to be given details of the cardiac lesion, the likely site and extent of the incision, and the likely appearance of the child after the operation. They should have the opportunity of a prior visit to the intensive care unit where the child will be nursed postoperatively and should be given a description of the likely rate of progress subsequently. They should be given

an honest account of the risks of the operation and the rates of the various complications.

The introduction of heart and heart–lung transplantation requires special consideration. Children who are put on waiting lists for transplantation are usually extremely ill and impaired in their functioning. Their expectation of life without transplantation is often limited to 1–2 years or even less. Parental anxiety is usually high, and there is often poor communication between parents and children. Some children die while on the waiting list, and there is a low, but significant operative mortality.

Postoperatively, the results in terms of physical function are usually good, though obviously time-limited. Compliance with medication is important for survival. Family dysfunction before operation does predict treatment compliance postoperatively. DeMaso *et al.* (1995) found reasonably good functioning post-transplantation in nearly 80% of children and young people. However, other centres, perhaps less selective on social grounds in their assessment of suitability for operation, have obtained a less encouraging psychological outcome. In any case, the stress associated with the operation and subsequent course is so significant that it is especially important there should be good communication between medical and nursing staff and between them and the family members.

The nature of the preparation of the child will depend on his age. Much surgery is now carried out with neonates and children under the age of 18 months, for whom no verbal preparation is possible. Good preparation of parents will ensure that the anxiety reactions of such young children are minimized (Glaser and Bentovim 1987). For older children, a coping skills training model has been shown to bring benefit (Campbell *et al.* 1995).

Older children require explanations appropriate to their cognitive level. It has been shown that good preparation of young children can reduce anxiety and increase co-operation during cardiac catheterization (Cassell and Paul 1967). Children over the age of about 2 years need some verbal explanation and the opportunity to visit the place in which they will be nursed after operation. From a slightly older age, children need explanations of the nature of the defect, the site and extent of the incision, as well as the likely degree of postoperative pain and discomfort and the steps that will be taken to alleviate these. They need to know for how long they will be in hospital and what their condition is likely to be on discharge.

Many operative cardiac procedures are so well established that the risks of operation and uncertainty concerning outcome are very low. With other procedures this is not the case. Parents and children need extra support, advice, and explanation in these circumstances.

Children with congenital heart diseases have about twice the expected rate of behavioural and emotional problems compared with children in the general population. Because of the extra risk of unnecessary invalidism in cardiac patients, it is important at follow-up to check carefully on school attendance and the degree to which the child is allowed independence outside school hours. Where over-protection is a problem and fails to improve after reassurance and advice, referral to a social worker or psychiatric facility will be desirable. The presence of psychiatric disorder may be unrelated to the cardiac lesion, and a wider assessment of the family may be helpful.

Behaviour and emotional problems

The rates of behaviour and emotional problems in operated children depend to some degree on operative success (Kramer *et al.* 1989). Asymptomatic children do not, as a group, have higher rates of problems than healthy controls. On the other hand, children with physical conditions following surgery do appear to have higher levels of anxiety and impulsiveness as well as a greater sense of inferiority when compared with physically fit children and healthy controls (Kramer *et al.* 1989). Children with complex cardiac problems and those with chronic family difficulties are most at risk (Spurkland *et al.* 1993). Parents may not be aware of underlying concerns that children experience. The increasing numbers of survivors into adolescence present additional problems (Utens *et al.* 1993). Even 25 years after operation, survivors remain under undue psychological stress (Brandhagen *et al.* 1991).

Cognitive development

Although very occasionally an operative disaster can lead to permanent brain damage, the intelligence of the great majority of children with operated congenital heart lesions is within the average range, though their mean IQ is somewhat lower than that of their sibs. Cyanotic patients function definitely less well than children with functional murmurs (Wright and Nolan 1994), but again, most are within the average range. There has been some concern that the profound hypothermia and cardiac arrest procedures commonly used in corrective cardiac surgery may affect intellectual outcome. Follow-up studies have, however, been reassuring in that mental retardation and neurological sequelae have been found to be very uncommon. The mean IQ of children subject to such procedures in infancy is about 10 points below average, but the great majority have abilities within the normal range.

8.13 Skin disorders

8.13.1 ECZEMA (ATOPIC DERMATITIS)

Eczema is a common skin condition in which there is dryness and scaling of the skin with associated itching and scratching. It usually begins in the first 18 months of life in children in whom there is a familial disposition. The condition is probably caused by an inherited immunological dysfunction, and most patients have elevated IgE levels and T-cell abnormalities. It may start at the time of introduction of artificial milk or mixed feeding, but other potential allergens may also be important. Treatment involves mainly the use of soap substitutes and emollients, as well as creams and ointments, with antihistamines at night for sedation. The use of wet wraps can reduce scratching. The condition is nearly always benign, clearing up in the first few years of life. It is, however, often very distressing while it is present and, in a minority of cases, it is both severe and persistent at least into the middle school years.

Psychosocial aspects

In the early years, the presence of severe, widespread eczema may lead to problems in the development of attachment (Rauch and Jellinek 1988), as one or both parents may be repelled by the condition and have problems in cuddling or even holding the child. Later, particularly in children in whom the condition runs a chronic course, psychological problems may be involved in the maintenance of the condition. In some children, stressful situations appear to exacerbate the condition. In others, the need for very frequent bathing and bandaging, tasks often performed by the mother, leads to resentment on the part of the child, and this may distort the mother–child relationship (Wittkower and Hunt 1958). The mother may come to feel that she alone knows how to care for her child and be unwilling to share the tasks involved. This may make her feel hostile and resentful towards the child. Conversely, the child may become extremely dependent on his mother and angry and irritable with her. The parents may well feel the child could do more to stop himself scratching, and this too can lead to mutual irritation and arguments between the parents. However, these parent–child relationship problems are only present in a minority of cases. Behaviour problems, especially sleep difficulties, are prevalent in young children with eczema, but security of attachment is not usually affected (Daud *et al.* 1993).

Although in adults there is work to suggest that individual psychotherapy can be helpful in eczema (Brown 1972), this may not be the case with children. Here it seems more probable that, in those cases where psychological factors are prominent, family sessions designed to improve communication between family members and allow more sharing of the child's physical care, would be valuable. An educational approach to parental counselling directed towards more effective limit-setting and self-understanding of ambivalent feelings may be helpful (Koblenzer and Koblenzer 1988). Associated sleep problems, which are sometimes prominent and exhausting to both children and parents, may respond to behavioural management programmes (Section 4.3.2).

8.13.2 NEURODERMATOSES

The neurodermatoses are conditions in which both the skin and nervous system are affected.

Tuberous sclerosis

Tuberous sclerosis is a condition in which there is abnormal proliferation of nerve cells giving rise to benign and occasionally malignant tumours in the brain. There may also be tumours of the heart, liver, and other organs. A characteristic skin lesion, producing a butterfly-shaped rash over the nose and cheek, is usually present. The condition is often inherited as an autosomal dominant.

The condition may present with epilepsy (infantile spasms, partial or generalized seizures) or developmental delay, and is usually diagnosed in the first 3–4 years of life. As well as mental retardation, there may be intellectual deterioration caused by repeated, uncontrolled epilepsy or the development of single or multiple cerebral neoplasms. There is a very high rate of associated psychopathology in this condition. Hyperactivity is common. The rate of autism and autism spectrum disorders in children with tuberose sclerosis has been estimated to be over 80% in one population-based study (Gillberg *et al.* 1994). The rate is highest in those with mental retardation, and can also be predicted by the location of the brain lesions (Bolton *et al.* 1997).

Treatment is symptomatic and involves anticonvulsant medication to control the attacks and often special education. Autistic syndromes and hyperactivity will need treatment along the lines described in Sections 3.4 and 3.5. It is important to provide genetic counselling, although the existence of *formes frustes* (partial syndromes in which only one or two features of the condition are present) means that some uncertainty concerning the genetic risk is inevitable.

The outcome is variable, and depends on the spread of lesions and whether malignant changes occur. A chronic rather than a rapidly deteriorating course is usual.

Neurofibromatosis (Von Recklinghausen disease)

Neurofibromatosis is caused by a spread of cells from nerve sheaths to other parts of the body, where they may form tumours, usually benign, but with a risk of malignant change. One form of the condition occurs in infancy and early childhood. It is inherited as an autosomal dominant.

The clinical features of the condition depend on the site and spread of the lesions. A variety of cognitive deficits has been found, but the condition is compatible with normal intelligence (North *et al.* 1995). Epilepsy is relatively common. Sufferers from the condition nearly always have a number (usually more than five) of *café-au-lait* skin lesions. Lesser numbers of such spots are commonly found in unaffected individuals.

Treatment is symptomatic, and the outcome is variable depending on the spread of the lesions and the development of malignant changes.

Sturge–Weber syndrome

In Sturge–Weber syndrome there is an angiomatous malformation of the skin in an area corresponding to the distribution of one or more branches of the trigeminal nerve. A similar angioma is present on the interior of the skull, usually overlying the occipital lobe on the same side, but sometimes occupying a more widespread area. The cerebral ischaemia produced by the internal lesion may give rise to epilepsy and hemiplegia as well as other neurological symptoms. There may also be some degree of mental retardation. Anticonvulsant medication may be required for the epilepsy.

Management

These neurodermatoses may all sometimes be accompanied by severe psychiatric disturbances arising from brain dysfunction or as a psychological reaction to the condition. Involvement of the temporal lobes is particularly likely to result in behavioural and emotional disturbances. There are no characteristic psychiatric features, and aggressive behaviour as well as emotional disturbances are frequent. Frank psychotic states may also occur. Treatment is symptomatic and behavioural methods are likely to be especially useful. Emotional support for the families, with appropriate genetic counselling, should be a major part of management.

8.14 Immunodeficiency disorders

Bodily response to infection can be impaired by a deficiency in the immune system—the complex process involving especially immunoglobulins, proteins produced in plasma cells and circulating in body fluids (humoral immunity), and T-cells, lymphocytes produced in the thymus (cellular immunity). Deficiency in this system is sometimes responsible for an infant or young child being unusually susceptible to infection. The condition is occasionally inherited, but may be acquired as a complication of both infectious and non-infectious disease or its treatment. Some immunodeficiency is mild, transient, and of little significance to the child. Other forms, especially those produced by inherited conditions or drug therapy, may be very serious or even fatal. Treatment will depend on the nature and severity of the condition.

8.14.1 PSYCHOSOCIAL IMPLICATIONS

Children known to have unusually low resistance to infection often have to lead very protected lives. In mild and moderate forms of immunodeficiency it is often unclear even to the physicians involved how necessary this protection might be, so it is not surprising that parents are themselves confused and uncertain. This may result in unnecessary overprotection, or the child may be exposed to inappropriate hazards. If a child does contract or succumb to an overwhelming infection, parental guilt may be considerable.

The condition may, if mild, require no specific treatment, but in some circumstances prophylactic intramuscular injections of immunoglobulin are indicated.

Bone marrow transplantation is now highly successful in selected cases of immunodeficiency, as well as in severe aplastic anaemia, and is also used to treat some types of leukaemia. The marrow is usually transplanted from a parent or healthy sib of the affected child. Studies of the psychological effects of bone marrow transplantation on the patient, the sib, and the rest of the family have revealed the serious degree to which family members are under stress (Atkins and Patenaude 1987). A detailed study of the psychosocial impact of bone marrow transplantation is provided by Pot-Mees (1989). The best predictor of psychosocial outcome in terms of resilience and post-transplant adjustment is the amount of cohesion or conflict in the family beforehand (Phipps and Mulhern 1995). Any developmental delay or decline in children with leukaemia who have bone marrow transplantation is likely to be due to the cranial radiotherapy used as adjuvant therapy (Cool 1996).

The patient is likely to require transfer from a local hospital to a specialist centre. The family may feel rejected and abandoned by their local medical and nursing staff, and travelling difficulties may lead to a loss of contact between the child and family members.

The patients themselves may develop serious anxiety and depression related to the isolated circumstances in which they are nursed, and fear of death (a realistic but often unexpressed concern) is frequently present. The provision of age-appropriate direct emotional support for the child is of primary importance. The degree of pressure put on a sib to co-operate may present ethical problems. Although this is now an unusual outcome, sibs whose brother or sister subsequently dies may have fantasies that they have been responsible for the death.

These psychological problems can probably be reduced significantly if communication between local and specialist centre, between nursing and medical staff at the specialist centre, between family members, and between staff and family is open and honest, and if account is taken of the immature understanding and apparently irrational fears and fantasies of the patients and sibs so that appropriate explanations of procedures can be given. The relative unpredictability of complications such as graft versus host disease, and intense involvement of staff with patients and families, mean that psychological support for staff is particularly necessary. Such an approach may also improve compliance with post-transplant therapy (Phipps and DeCuir Whalley 1990).

In those conditions that are genetically determined, genetic counselling with the opportunity to discuss implications for future pregnancies is necessary.

8.15 Juvenile chronic arthritis

8.15.1 DEFINITION

Juvenile chronic arthritis is a condition in which a number of joints are involved in an inflammatory process, often resulting in chronic limitation of movement, deformity, and pain.

8.15.2 CLINICAL FEATURES

The illness commonly starts in the first 5 years of life, when fever, enlargement of the spleen, and lymph nodes are common. Arthritis is less prominent in this form of the condition, which is known as *Still disease*. In older children developing the condition, in whom prognosis is rather better, polyarthritis is a more salient feature. Although some children suffer only a single attack of acute arthritis and remain well subsequently, others go on to develop a chronic illness with remissions and relapses. It is these who suffer chronic disability and pain. Treatment is aimed at relieving pain, and increasing mobility, thus reducing social impairment.

8.15.3 PSYCHOSOCIAL FEATURES

It has been suggested that the onset of juvenile chronic arthritis can be precipitated by stressful events, but the evidence for this is poor, as the events taken into account might have been caused by the illness itself. Pathological immunological processes are certainly of causative importance, and it is possible that, in some children, stressful events can produce exacerbation by their effect on the immune system.

Despite earlier reports to the contrary, children with this condition do not appear to have higher than expected rates of behaviour and emotional problems (Wallander *et al.* 1988). However, in adolescence, sexual anxieties are common, and girls are particularly prone to depression (Wilkinson 1981). The use of steroids in treatment not uncommonly leads to stunting of growth with consequent adverse effects on self-image and self-esteem. There is no association between disease severity and psychosocial factors (Vandvik and Eckblad 1991; Baildam *et al.* 1995).

Young children with chronic arthritis appear to experience less pain than older children and adults with the same condition (Beales *et al.* 1983). It is suggested that this is because the young child, unlike older patients, does not attach such unpleasant meaning (disability, chronicity, etc.) to his pain every time he experiences it.

These studies confirm that clinicians should be aware of the special psychosocial problems relating to this condition (Ungerer *et al.* 1988). There is some evidence that social support provided by mentors (mothers of young adults with the condition), can be helpful in reducing mental health symptoms in families with a child with arthritis (Ireys *et al.* 1996). Great efforts should be made to ensure that immobility does not lead to social isolation. Counselling of adolescents may need to focus on sexual concerns, and teenagers need help to form realistic plans for future employment. Counselling directed towards what the adolescent will be able to do in later life may reduce the level of hopelessness and counter the tendency to experience pain as a reminder of chronic disability. On the other hand, the adolescent may also need to experience appropriate depression in relation to the reduction in quality of life.

9

Prevention and treatment

9.1 Preventive approaches

Preventive activity in the field of the psychosocial disorders of childhood can, like other forms of medical prevention, be classified as follows:

- *primary prevention*: action taken to prevent the development of the disorder in the first place, usually by removing the cause
- *secondary prevention*: action taken to identify the disorder at its onset, so as to prevent extension
- *tertiary prevention*: action taken to limit disability arising from an established condition.

Rational prevention is made easier if there is good understanding of the factors that may be related to the development of disorders (Graham 1995). The presence of a *risk factor* implies the individual has an increased likelihood of developing a disorder. *Protective factors* are those that reduce an individual's likelihood of developing the disorder, and *vulnerability factors* are those that increase that likelihood. Thus, for example, the presence of parental marital disharmony is a risk factor for conduct disorder. If a child at risk for this reason has a good relationship with an adult outside the family this can act as a protective factor, and if the child is educationally retarded, this may increase the child's vulnerability to develop such a disorder. Action to reduce risk and vulnerability factors, or to enhance protective factors, may therefore result in successful prevention.

Although perhaps the major responsibility for prevention lies in the social and educational policy areas, as far as health professionals are concerned the onus for prevention in this field lies largely, though not entirely, with those working in primary health care, such as general practitioners, community health doctors, and health visitors. Emphasis in this section will therefore be given to activities these professionals might undertake. Those involved in secondary care, such as paediatricians, psychologists, and psychiatrists, can, however, also undertake activities of major preventive significance, particularly if there is a focus on high-risk groups (Boyle and Offord 1990). Social policy measures of potential preventive significance will be discussed first.

9.1.1 PUBLIC POLICY ASPECTS OF PREVENTION

Alleviation of poverty

The presence of mild mental retardation is strongly linked to material disadvantage, and some conduct disorders also occur more frequently in disadvantaged groups. Although poverty in itself is only weakly linked to the presence of conduct disorders, its presence predisposes to a variety of family difficulties, such as family breakdown, that are much more strongly associated (Rutter and Madge 1976). Measures taken to reduce gross social inequality, and the sense of injustice that this evokes, may be expected to reduce rates of these problems.

Neighbourhood cohesiveness

The development of self-help groups, family centres, and other neighbourhood activities can provide helpful emotional support, especially for isolated mothers of young children (Haggerty 1980). The legal and social discouragement of racism can reduce tension in families belonging to ethnic minority groups. It should be remembered that many children in indigenous families also suffer psychologically as a result of racial tension.

Housing

Families with children need adequate space, both for everyday activities and for play. Avoidance of high-rise and other forms of cramped housing for families with young children could contribute to the prevention of behaviour disorders. Children living in accommodation for homeless families are at major risk for health, including behaviour problems (Bassuk and Rosenberg 1990). Adolescents also need a certain amount of personal space in their own homes.

Employment

There is a strong relationship between unemployment and criminality (Smith 1995). Availability of adequate work opportunities for parents, and good prospects of employment for teenagers, would almost certainly reduce the rate of maternal depression and minor affective disorders in teenagers (Banks and Jackson 1982). It would reduce anxiety, especially in teenagers with learning difficulties—a group that experiences most serious problems in obtaining employment.

Child protction

Legislation and social policy to prevent child abuse and neglect is described in Section 10.3. Although family support to parents who are in difficulties bringing up their children will always be the first duty of those working in social services departments, policies that encourage early adoption or long-term fostering in situations where parents are clearly not going to be able to took after their biological children are likely to reduce rates of antisocial disorder and mild mental retardation.

Social policy directed towards protecting children from exposure to illicit drugs and advertisements for cigarette smoking would reduce the numbers of children and teenagers whose health is affected by these substances. Protection of children from exposure to violence, and more especially perverted forms of violence shown on television and in videos, can also be seen as socially desirable and, at least possibly preventive in its effects (Strasburger 1995).

Accident prevention

Although mainly an issue concerning prevention of physical handicap, accident prevention is also relevant to psychosocial prevention, for disturbed, overactive children are most likely to be affected, and traumatic brain damage increases the risk of development of child psychiatric disorders. Health education, the development of safety devices in the home, and childproof tablet containers are all useful measures (see Section 8.4).

Education

Pre-school education plays a significant part in the prevention of mild mental retardation. Parent participation in the acquisition of reading can prevent reading disability. Promoting an academic ethos in secondary schools might reduce rates of truancy, as well as other forms of behavioural deviance.

Marital disharmony

Marital and family disharmony are major influences in the development of behaviour and emotional disorders. The ready availability of marital counselling from professionals who are sensitive to the needs of children might reduce rates of disturbance in youngsters inevitably affected by the marital problems of their parents (Stolberg and Garrison 1985).

Alcohol consumption

There is a strong relationship between alcohol consumption, violence in the home, and a range of child psychiatric disorders in both adolescents and parents (Royal College of Physicians 1995). Reducing levels of consumption through fiscal and social measures would reduce rates of psychosocial disorders.

9.1.2 SPECIFIC PREVENTIVE MEASURES BY HEALTH AND OTHER PROFESSIONALS

Preventive activity by professionals can be classified according to the stage in the life cycle in the individual towards whom it is directed.

Preparation for parenthood

Preparation begins in the childhood of the parent-to-be: an emotionally satisfying childhood is in many ways the best preparation for later parenthood. More specifically, sympathetic instruction and the opportunity for discussion in adolescence about the physical and emotional aspects of pregnancy, childbirth, and child-rearing will provide a basis for later learning from experience. Unfortunately, there are no satisfactory evaluations of parenting education programmes delivered in secondary schools. Better information about contraception, including emergency contraception, may well prevent unwanted pregnancies with their distressing sequelae. There is no evidence that the availability of such information increases promiscuity. Indeed, the reverse is the case (Mellanby *et al.* 1995).

Antenatal care

Pregnancy provides many opportunities for preventive activity (Newton 1988). Good antenatal care with regular check-ups reduces the rate of birth complications and subsequent brain damage and learning difficulties. Practical advice concerning avoidance of smoking and excessive alcohol intake should also produce a reduction in later learning difficulties in the offspring (Weinberg 1997). Providing parents-to-be with the opportunity for discussion of fears and fantasies about, for example, possible birth difficulties and congenital abnormalities will result in a more relaxed pregnancy and better outcome. Such discussion is particularly necessary when the pregnant woman suffers complications requiring complex technical investigation and treatment.

Birth and the neonatal period

Technically competent and sympathetic management with good communication between the mother and the birth attendant about the progress of the delivery will promote an initial positive attitude to the baby. The presence of other social supports during parturition has been shown to have a similarly positive effect (Klaus *et al.* 1986). Allowing the mother early contact with her child and the availability of rooming-in facilities provide a basis for later positive interaction. Early detection of maternal depression and abnormalities of mother–child interaction may require immediate intervention or follow-up that is more intensive than usual. Parents whose babies have to be admitted to special care baby units need extra support and as much opportunity as possible to continue to be involved in the care of their babies (Wolke 1997). Attention needs to be paid to the 'environment of care', avoiding inappropriate sensory input and providing an individualized approach, and there is some evidence this achieves a better developmental outcome. Early screening for phenylketonuria and hypothyroidism, with provision of appropriate treatment, reduces the rate of later mental retardation. A large number of studies carried out in the US have demonstrated that intensive home visiting programmes delivered by public health nurses to 'high risk' young mothers can produce measurable benefit to their children (Olds *et al.* 1986; Horacek *et al.* 1987).

Pre-school period

There are frequent opportunities for preventive activities during the pre-school period. A critical evaluation of surveillance procedures has suggested that regular examinations of young children should take place at 6 weeks, 3 months, 8 months, 21 months, 39 months, and around school entry (Polnay *et al.* 1996), but that the assessments carried out should be highly selective. These examinations allow checking of height and weight, a physical examination, identification of defects of hearing or vision, and an assessment of the child's developmental status. Further discussion of hearing, vision, language, and motor impairment is discussed in other sections of this book. The frequent attendance of young children at primary care consultations for minor infections and other health problems allows further opportunities for developmental surveillance, and discussion concerning child-rearing. Screening examinations of young children in primary care and attendance for health problems in primary or secondary care settings also provide an opportunity for prevention and early identification of emotional and behaviour problems. There is evidence that regular discussion of a child-centred approach to child-rearing reduces rates of later behavioural problems and enuresis (Cullen 1976; Gutelius *et al.* 1977). Such discussion can be provided by psychologists attached to health centres as well as by family practitioners and primary care paediatricians themselves (Kannoy and Schroeder 1985).

Observation of the parent–child interaction at clinic attendances may reveal causes for concern in a variety of ways. A mother may be noted to be slow and lethargic or unduly irritable in the way she handles her young child. Such behaviour may be symptomatic of maternal depression, perhaps secondary to difficulties she is having with her child or related to other life problems. A baby or young child may be noted to relate poorly to his mother, to be unduly active, to be markedly attention-seeking, or to show unusual behaviour in other ways.

When noting this type of behaviour in parent or child, or in the interaction between them, it is important not to jump to unwarranted conclusions. The observed behaviour may be highly situation-specific, the mother being under particular stress because of the clinic attendance, or the child showing behaviour that is atypical. Nevertheless, it is also important not to dismiss such observations as irrelevant, for they may be the first indicators of serious problems perhaps amenable to psychosocial intervention. Screening examinations should therefore include systematic questioning about the child concerning possible behavioural difficulties (eating, sleeping, compliance), relationships with other children (if age appropriate), and the presence of undue fearfulness. It may be useful to request the mother to complete a behaviour check-list before she is seen, so that this can be used as a basis for discussion, and Richman (1977) has provided such a check-list suitable for children aged $2\frac{1}{2}$–$4\frac{1}{2}$ years. There should also be routine questioning about the mother's physical and mental health, and the parental relationship. Questions can be framed in an unthreatening manner in relation to the child's needs:

- 'How are you feeling in yourself?'
- 'Do you feel you are able to cope with all the extra work X is giving you?'
- 'What about your husband/boyfriend? Do you find he is helping as much as he can?'

As with screening in other aspects of child care, identification of problems is pointless, and indeed potentially harmful, unless appropriate advice and intervention is available if problems are identified (Baird and Hall 1985). As indicated in other sections of this book, the limited but definite effectiveness, especially of some informal counselling procedures and behavioural intervention, does justify problem identification in a wide range of childhood behavioural and emotional disorders, provided that the practitioner can apply them himself or refer to an appropriate agency.

Pre-school programmes for disadvantaged children with a focus on promotion of development can result in an improved mental health outcome. Adjustment at age 19 years was found to be better in those young adults who had the experience of an educational programme at 3–4 years when compared with controls who had not had this experience (Berrueta-Clement *et al.* 1984).

The pre-school period also provides the best opportunities for the prevention of distress and subsequent psychiatric disorder in children who are hospitalized, although older children may also be affected. Preventive activity therefore needs to be age-appropriate. This issue is discussed in more detail in Section 7.6.

Middle childhood

At this age, preventive approaches naturally focus on prevention of learning failure. Parental involvement in teaching at the initial stages of reading, early identification by screening procedures of children failing to learn to read so that they can be given extra help before they become discouraged, and good parent–teacher communication are all likely to be effective preventive procedures.

In a significant number of children with health problems, it is of importance that teachers are aware of associated difficulties that may arise in school, either directly as a result of the physical condition or as a side-effect of treatment. Good family doctor or hospital communication with the child's teachers, either directly or through a school doctor or nurse, can prevent misunderstanding and unnecessary neglect or ignorance of the child's disabilities.

Various behavioural methods have been used in preventive programmes directed towards children of this age. The aims of such programmes have been, for example, to train children not to respond to the approaches of strangers in public places, to resist peer pressure to smoke and drink alcohol, to observe home safety rules, and to cope with stressful situations (Lee and Mash 1989). In addition, cognitive, problem-solving techniques have been used to help children relate to their peers and to adults in more satisfying ways (Spivack *et al.* 1976), but the benefit to emotional adjustment is uncertain. Parent training programmes directed towards parents of children of this age with mild to moderate conduct disorders have been demonstrated to be at least moderately effective (Bailey 1998).

Finally in this age group, school-based, multi-level preventive programmes directed towards parents, teachers, and children themselves have been shown to enhance academic achievement in disadvantaged children (Comer 1985) and to reduce rates of bullying in schools (Olweus 1989).

Adolescence

The life cycle of preventive activity is complete in the adolescent years, with the evident need for preparation for parenthood. Teenagers can benefit from the opportunity for group discussions of social (including sexual) relationships. Often such discussions appear to be most useful when they arise in relation to other subjects being studied, such as literature or human biology. The degree to which younger teenagers should be provided with information about sex and contraception is a controversial subject. However, there is good evidence that the provision of such information generally leads to a more, rather than a less, responsible attitude to sexual activity (Mellanby *et al.* 1995).

Counselling in schools or neighbourhood centres for teenagers, so that they can discuss life problems before these lead to adverse psychiatric reactions, can also have an important preventive role. Counsellors can also be helpful in advising youngsters at risk of becoming involved in drug-taking of techniques they can employ to resist encouragement from drug pushers.

In mid and late adolescence the prevalence of suicidal activity has stimulated interest in programmes directed towards reducing rates of self-destructive behaviour. A large number of school-based programmes exist in the US, but their effectiveness is uncertain, and their exclusive reliance on a stress-related explanation of suicidal activity may actually be counterproductive (Garland *et al.* 1989).

Finally in this age group, programmes directed towards the promotion of non-academic skills such as sports and manual crafts in less academically able youngsters have been shown to have modest but promising results in the reduction of antisocial behaviour (Offord 1987).

9.1.3 PREVENTIVE PRINCIPLES IN MANAGEMENT

Concern for the whole child and family

Especially in young children, any attempt to separate physical and mental health needs is doomed to failure. About a quarter of child consultations in general practice have a significant psychological component. Paediatricians estimate that about a third of their referrals are for 'psychosomatic' problems. Psychologists and psychiatrists need to be aware of physical conditions that may underlie the mental health problems with which they are dealing.

Knowledge about and respect for associated services

Professionals, however broad and comprehensive their own approach, need to be aware of what other groups of professionals have to offer, and how such help can be obtained. Thus general practitioners and clinical medical officers as well as psychiatrists need to have full awareness of the availability of special educational and social services in their locality.

Communication between professionals

Parents are sometimes confused by conflicting advice given to them by professionals who are unaware of previous opinions offered. The service provided, especially by the primary health care service (family doctors, health visitors, school nurses, etc.) can do much to prevent such confusion, but only if others who are in contact with families ensure that their participation is known to the primary health care-givers.

Availability of mental health consultation

Results of community surveys of disturbed children in the population make it clear that there will never be enough specialized psychologists and psychiatrists to deal with them. Even if there were, it is unlikely that it would be cost-effective to separate delivery of mental health services from other health services at primary care level. Further, many parents do not wish their children to be referred to psychiatrists and, although prejudice against mental health professionals is less prevalent than it used to be, it is improbable that community attitudes will ever change to a degree that makes referral universally acceptable. For all these reasons, non-mental health professionals will, for the foreseeable future, be involved in assessing and treating disturbed children and their families. The availability of advice from more highly trained professionals in this field would be one way of ensuring that problem children can be identified and treated early on. Many staff working in child and family psychiatric clinics now spend as much as a third of their time in such consultation services.

Consultation most appropriately takes the form of discussion of policy issues and of individual children who are causing concern. A comprehensive child mental health consultation service in a health district might involve:

- psychosocial meetings on the paediatric ward in the district general hospital
- consultation with social workers on difficult child care cases
- attendance at meeting of teachers in local special and ordinary schools
- discussion with residential child care workers concerning disturbed children in residential care
- ready availability for consultation to primary health care workers such as health visitors and general practitioners.

Only a well-staffed child mental health service is likely to be able to meet all the demands for consultation made upon it, but staff working in such services will themselves benefit from greater awareness of community needs and resources if they devote a significant amount of time to such consultation work. There is evidence (Mannino and Shore 1975) that those in receipt of consultation services do derive benefit from such activity.

Emphasis on parental involvement in decision-making

Although, when highly complex technical decisions need to be taken, parents will appropriately wish professionals to take full responsibility, in many other cases (the need for a special psychological assessment, treatment of a sleep disorder, etc.) greater success is likely to be achieved if decisions are taken *with* parents rather than *for* them. In particular, referrals for psychiatric consultation are only likely to be useful if parents are motivated. If they are not, and a serious problem exists, then it is those who still have to care for the child who will be in need of advice and counselling, and this too should be readily available.

Encouragement of voluntary activity

Professionals are sometimes wary of voluntary organizations and suspicious of the motives of those involved in their activities. Nevertheless, many parents of children with chronic physical or mental disorders have found great comfort and support in sharing their problems with others who have children with similar problems. The voluntary organizations dedicated to serve the needs of families where a child has a specific type of disability are often particularly helpful, both in providing information and in putting parents in touch with others in a similar predicament. In the UK, a useful booklet containing the names and addresses of relevant organizations is available (Contact-a-Family 1998), and a listing of all child mental health facilities in the UK is also available (Young Minds 1998). Other countries have similar publications.

Conclusions

If the mental health needs of children are met, there is at least a reasonable hope that the adults into which children grow will themselves be more caring and more sensitive to the needs of their own children. But the justification for a positive mental health approach to children does not just lie in making better adults. As Jack Tizard once wrote, 'Childhood is not just a preparation for life, it is a part of life'. Respect and concern for children who, because of immaturity, need special care and protection, is one of the criteria by which a society can judge its own worth.

9.2 Treatment

Treatment methods in child and family psychiatry are scientifically less well established than in most other branches of medicine. In particular, knowledge concerning the effectiveness of different types of treatment for particular disorders is often uncertain. Consequently, it is not surprising that treatment practice varies quite widely from centre to centre. Nevertheless, much useful knowledge is available (Kolvin *et al.* 1981). Further, although there is clearly a need for much more evaluation of treatment methods in this field, there is already a substantial amount of evidence available concerning the effectiveness of different techniques for specific disorders (Target and Fonagy 1996).

In the following section a number of methods of treatment are described, though it must be appreciated that many practitioners often use different forms of therapy in combination. In each case an attempt has been made to describe the form the treatment takes, the principles underlying it, indications and contra-indications for its use, and evidence for its effectiveness. Some examples are given of its application in different types of facility—primary care, paediatric, and psychiatric. For the sake of brevity, the case examples do not contain all relevant information. Names of children described, and some identifying data, have been altered to preserve anonymity.

Clearly, clinicians will vary greatly in their skills and opportunities to carry out these forms of treatment. The more highly specialized the clinician dealing with child psychiatric disorders, the more skilled he or she is likely to be in therapy, but there is no reason why all professionals concerned with children should not be capable of applying some of the principles described here. As with other forms of treatment, initial experience is likely to be more useful if it is supervised, and supervision by direct observation with the use of video and one-way screens, if such equipment is available, has many advantages.

One notable form of variation in treatment in specialist centres concerns the degree of co-therapy or joint therapy that is thought desirable. In some centres, virtually all treatment is carried out conjointly, whereas in others this way of working is unusual. One agreed principle of therapy in this field is that it is desirable for all doctors working with disturbed children to have ready access to colleagues with skills in psychology and social work as well as to have good contact with teachers when dealing with children of school age.

9.2.1 BEHAVIOURAL AND COGNITIVE PSYCHOTHERAPIES

Definition

Behavioural methods of treatment are those that are directed towards the development and encouragement of desirable behaviours, and the removal or at least reduction in frequency and severity of undesirable or challenging behaviours, by methods based on learning theory. The focus is on observable behaviour rather than underlying thoughts or feelings, though later developments of behaviour modification such as cognitive-behaviour therapy do deal with thought processes as well.

An essential and central feature of these methods is that they involve systematic analysis of the problem behaviour, objectively defined, as part of assessment. The treatment is accompanied by equally systematic monitoring of its effects with modification of the therapeutic programme if treatment is not producing the desired result. Features of behaviour modification in children are similar to those in adults, except that with children, parents and teachers and other involved individuals are usually used as agents ('co-therapists') of behavioural change.

The following account of treatment is necessarily limited in scope. A more detailed review of behavioural approaches is provided by Werry and Wollersheim (1989), a useful, highly practical account of the application of behavioural methods by Herbert (1981), and an account of cognitive methods by Graham (1998).

General principles of assessment for behaviour therapy

The form of assessment will depend on the time available, the nature and severity of the problem, and the skills and experience of the person making the assessment. Clearly a health visitor or family doctor using behaviour modification principles to deal with a sleep problem in a 2 year old child will not carry out as intensive an assessment as a psychologist referred a child with a severe and persistent obsessive–compulsive disorder. Nevertheless, the principles of assessment are likely to be similar.

Define a problem to be treated

Obtaining a description of the actual form of behaviour complained of by parents is an essential first step. Where, as is often the case, the child is showing more than one form of problem behaviour or deficit, it is necessary to establish which is to be the first target for change. Parents may have different views from professionals on this matter, and it is important to respect their views, as high parental motivation is required to achieve success. In-depth discussion may be needed to ascertain which behaviours are problematic to the child (e.g. social anxiety) and which are more troublesome for parents and teachers (e.g. disobedience, aggression). It is also necessary to prioritize the problem behaviours not only in terms of nuisance value but also regarding their likelihood of responding to intervention. It is often the case that the most troublesome behaviours are deeply entrenched and very resistant to change while more trivial behaviour problems may be relatively easily adapted and hence represent a good investment for initial efforts. As a general rule one should choose a behaviour likely to respond—not necessarily the most problematic.

Define the circumstances of the problem behaviour

Before treatment begins, it is necessary to obtain a clear idea, not only of the frequency and severity of the problem, but also of the circumstances that precede it (*antecedents*) and follow it (*consequences*) when it occurs. A basic assumption is that whether a form of behaviour changes will depend on whether there is a change in what happens before the behaviour or after it. Antecedents can be usefully split further into three groups:

- *predisposing factors*, which may be genetic (e.g. temperamental tendencies) or psychosocial (e.g. long-term sequelae of abuse and neglect experiences)
- *precipitating factors*, also known as 'triggers'—what cause the behaviour to happen when, where and with whom it does
- *perpetuating factors*, which maintain the behaviour.

Most of us demonstrate reasonably frequent challenging behaviours of varying types and degrees. However, these episodes are usually short-lived. The distinction from more serious problem behaviours is often their persistence and refractoriness to resolution as much as their severity.

Undertake a functional analysis of behaviour

Typically a diary or chart is kept over a period of time detailing the antecedents, behaviour, and consequences each time the problem in question arises. This is based on the learning theory model of causation and reinforcement of behaviour:

$$\text{antecedents} \rightarrow \text{behaviour} \rightarrow \text{consequences.}$$

A *functional analysis* is often necessary for the clinician and parents to understand fully what precipitates and maintains the problem behaviour—a necessary precursor to treatment. For example, if temper tantrums are the target behaviour, one needs to know how often they occur, who is present when they occur, in what setting and when they occur, what starts them off, how long they last, and what those present do when they occur (do nothing, give the child what he wants, smack the child, let the child off something unpleasant such as having to do his homework, etc.).

Baseline recording

Once it has been established which problem or problems are to be treated, it is necessary to obtain a baseline recording. This is usually achieved by the child, parent, and/or teacher keeping a chart of the frequency and maybe severity with which the problem occurs. If the clinician is especially interested in treating a particular condition such as bed-wetting, then he or she will probably develop a special chart for this purpose. It is useful, however, to have an all-purpose chart that can be used for a whole variety of problems. Figure 9.1 shows a chart that could be used to record a range of difficulties. Periods of time represented by each rectangle could involve a whole day (in which case the chart could be used for 5 weeks) or a segment of the day (e.g. morning, afternoon, or evening). What needs to be recorded on the chart will depend on the nature of the problem and the frequency of its occurrence. For example, if soiling occurring about three times a week is being treated, it will be necessary to chart all episodes that occur, or all periods during which the child is clean. If aggressive outbursts occurring several times a day are being treated, it may be more appropriate only to record what happens in one hour between 5 and 6 p.m. ('time sampling').

The process of keeping a baseline recording is sometimes, though not often, sufficient to achieve significant change in parental attitudes or child behaviour. Once parents see a graphic and precise illustration of the frequency and severity of the problem for the first time, they may decide that the problem is more trivial than they had thought and not worth troubling about. More often they may, through increased insight into the function of the behaviour, alter their own behaviour consequent on the child's behaviour, with the result that the child improves even before the clinician has brokered any more active intervention. Finally, problems parents have in keeping the chart may be useful diagnostically. Low motivation for change, sharp differences between parents over what constitutes a problem, and poor capacity for change may come to light as a result of chart-keeping.

Time	Nature of problem						
	Monday	Tuesday	Wednesday	Thursday	Friday	Saturday	Sunday

Fig. 9.1. Sample chart for recording occurrence of problems.

Table 9.1 Ways of increasing and decreasing behaviour

	Positive consequence	Negative consequence
Add	Reward—'positive reinforcement'	Punishment— 'aversion'
Subtract	Extinction	'Negative reinforcement'

Evolve a plan collaboratively

If record keeping proves insufficient and the resources and motivation are present, then a programme can be devised for counteracting the undesired behaviour and enhancing more appropriate ones. In this respect it is important to consider the principles of learning theory including classical and operant conditioning, and the means available for increasing and decreasing intensity and frequency of behaviour (Table 9.1).

Other general principles include the need to relate the above programme to each stage of the desired behaviour. Sometimes behaviour is an instantaneous event, for example wetting the bed. Often it consists of a chain of linked behaviours each of which needs to be developed, for example getting up, washed, and dressed in the morning, or mealtime or bedtime routines. In these instances it is often useful to reinforce the final behaviour in the chain until it is well developed and then to move back in stages ending with the earliest behaviour required ('reverse chaining'). All individuals involved with the programme must be crystal-clear about its nature and how they should behave towards the child, whether at home, school or elsewhere. A major difficulty in behavioural programmes is generalization—behaviour may improve at school but still be atrocious at home or vice versa. Also inconsistencies in how the programme is applied will drastically reduce the likelihood of success. Ratings are as necessary during the programme as in the baseline recording phase. An outline of the steps required in developing and instituting a programme, and general principles applicable to behavioural work with young people are listed in Figs 9.2 and 9.3.

Operant methods

Principles

The experimental work underlying the operant technique, pioneered especially by Skinner, indicated that the likelihood of a behaviour recurring depends on the significance of the event immediately following it to the person showing the behaviour. If the event following the behaviour is positively reinforcing or rewarding, then it will recur. If it is not reinforced or is punished, then it is less likely to recur and eventually will stop completely—a process known as *extinction*. An alternative, but related approach is *stimulus control*—changing the events preceding the behaviour, thus altering the likelihood that the same behaviour will recur. Figure 9.4 summarizes all this.

In childhood the most common form of positive reinforcement is social. Children are likely to repeat behaviour which gives pleasure to those of whom

1. Define objectively which behaviours are problematic:
   — to the child
   — to the family, teachers, etc.
2. Prioritize these behaviours.
3. Choose a behaviour likely to respond—**not** necessarily the most problematic.
4. Undertake a functional analysis with comprehensive description of behaviour (when, where, what, how, with whom), antecedents and consequences.
5. Evolve plan on the basis of above findings for counteracting maladaptive behaviour and enhancing appropriate behaviours. Consider methods of increasing and decreasing behaviours available.
6. Relate the above plan to each stage of the behavioural sequence in question.
7. Ensure plan is crystal clear to all involved. Ensure dissent can be voiced. Consider practicality of plan.
8. Rate response of behaviour to intervention.
9. React on basis of trends over time—not individual events.
10. Persist a reasonable time, considering possible reasons for success or failure.

Fig. 9.2. Step by step to a behavioural programme.

Consider:
— family
— friends
— teachers
Developmental level:
— understanding
— age appropriateness
— maintaining dignity and sense of control
Frequent readily obtainable rewards
Rewards that can be easily withdrawn
Personalize the programme
What is making the person do what (s)he does

Fig. 9.3. General principles of behaviour modification with young people.

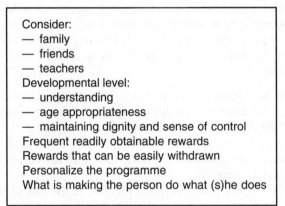

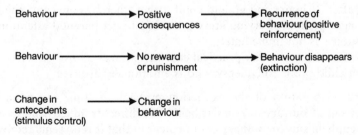

Fig. 9.4. Operant methods.

they are fond. Usually, but not necessarily, their parents and teachers are the most important positively reinforcing figures, but, as they get older, other children increasingly take on this role. If a teacher pays gratifying attention to bad behaviour (even if the attention takes the form of shouting at the child), then bad behaviour will recur, especially if attention is something of which the child is generally deprived. Material rewards, such as money, sweets, chocolates, other favourite foods, and watching television are usually positive material reinforcers. Further reward comes from the sense of satisfaction a child achieves at having succeeded in a task. Behaviour can also be reinforced 'vicariously'—that is, by observing another person benefiting from the behaviour in question, for example copying the bullying behaviour of a respected peer in the playground, or volunteering to help with cooking or shopping having seen a cartoon character receive praise and material rewards for having done these things.

Extinction generally occurs most rapidly following withdrawal of those things that are positive reinforcers. Thus, the withdrawal of love or attention from people of whom the child is fond is often the most powerful way of achieving extinction of the undesirable behaviour that children show. This works particularly effectively for sleeping and other night-time difficulties which are frequently reinforced by exhausted parents giving in and providing the child with the attention he or she wanted all along (Douglas and Richman 1984). In other children, the withdrawal of material goods, such as pocket money, special food or drink, and opportunity to watch television is more important.

Extinction, when it works, is an extremely elegant, swift, and enduring behavioural treatment. However, like any treatment it may be inappropriate for a number of reasons:

- Firstly, it may be impossible to prevent the contingent presentation of the reinforcer—e.g. no amount of exhortation stops the parents from rushing to their crying child the minute he starts up after lights out.
- Secondly, it may be undesirable to withhold the contingent reinforcer for practical reasons—the parents are willing to ignore the crying but the neighbours will complain bitterly.
- Thirdly, there is often a transient initial increase in the rate of the undesirable behaviour—the so-called *extinction burst*. This may make the programme inappropriate or dangerous (e.g. it is considered unsafe to risk a head-banging child increasing the behaviour, however temporarily).
- Fourthly, it may take too long—the parents give up ignoring their child's crying after $3\frac{1}{2}$ hours and go and comfort her, thereby conveying the message that longer periods of crying are worthwhile to get parental attention even if the response is not immediate!
- Fifthly, there may be other practical concerns such as a lowered seizure threshold in a child prone to epilepsy who is emotionally aroused.

A useful elaboration of the extinction principle is 'time out from positive reinforcement'. Contrary to popular belief this differs from exclusion, seclusion, or other euphemisms for solitary confinement in that it represents removal from a reinforcing environment, such as a playground or game with other children in a playroom, the return being conditional on a period of good behaviour. Time out should not normally consist of shutting a child in a room on his or her own—indeed some children may find this quite rewarding, particularly if there are fun activities such as television or computer games to hand. Being sat at a desk away from the other pupils in a classroom, or having to go and stand in the hall 'until you have calmed down for five minutes' is usually sufficient.

Punishment is a further technique which can be used to remove undesirable behaviour. Any unpleasant consequence of behaviour which makes that behaviour less likely to occur can be seen as punishing. Physical punishment by parents is the most frequently used, but many children do not respond to it by a reduction in their undesirable behaviour. Probably the extra attention they get when they are punished has a positive reinforcing or rewarding effect, and this result overrides negative experiences of physical pain. The experience of negative emotional states—anxiety, depression, and a sense of failure—is, by contrast, strongly punishing to many children. If, as a result of an unpleasant experience (for example being bullied by a group of boys on a particular corner of the street), a child experiences severe anxiety when he returns to that particular location, then he is less likely to return on a subsequent occasion. Of course, if he does return and the unpleasant experience is not repeated, then he will have less anxiety about making subsequent visits. Apart from the very real ethical concerns regarding punishment or 'aversion' programmes, there is evidence that any gains are more short lived than with reinforcement schedules, and that progressively increasing punishment may be needed to produce the same result. Thus there are scientific as well as moral objections to this approach although it is sometimes seen as a last resort, for example in children with learning disabilities who show life-threatening self-injury which has not responded to any other approach.

Nature of reinforcers
Whether something is positively reinforcing or punishing depends on the effect it has on behaviour. Virtually nothing is intrinsically reinforcing. What may be positively reinforcing to one child will not be so for another. For example, usually food will be positively reinforcing, but to an anorexic girl who hates the sight of food it may be punishing. Pain is usually punishing, but to a child preoccupied with guilt or with masochistic tendencies, it will be positively reinforcing or rewarding. Social interaction and lots of surprises are the spice of life for most of us but will be anathema to a child with an autistic spectrum disorder. Further, the strength and direction of reinforcement will depend to some degree on the child's relationship with the person administering or involved in it. A game of football is likely to be more positively reinforcing for a boy if it involves his father than his mother. A star chart for bed-wetting worked out in co-operation with a mother with whom a 6 year old has a good relationship is likely to be more effective than if the mother and child are in serious conflict.

A reinforcer can be defined as anything which increases the frequency or intensity of a behaviour. It therefore makes little sense to suggest that a reinforcer is not working. It would be more appropriate to say that a particular approach, or contingency, does not appear to be reinforcing for the behaviour in question. One then has to investigate why this is so and whether the programme needs to be adapted or indeed a different potential reinforcer found.

A reinforcement schedule may entail removal of an unpleasant stimulus in response to the desired behaviour (*negative reinforcement*) as well as the more often considered and applied positive reinforcement. Examples of negative reinforcement include a teacher's message to her pupils that the class will only be allowed to go out to play once the culprit who broke the window owns up. Owning-up behaviour is negatively reinforced by the prospect of not having to sit in a boring classroom during playtime. Peer pressure is also obviously of relevance here. Another example is the child stopping nagging and whinging in response to the parent giving sweets. Here, the parents sweet-giving behaviour is being negatively reinforced by the child's stopping the unpleasant behaviour. This example also illustrates the need for humility, and awareness of the reciprocal nature of behavioural programmes. It is rarely if ever the case that an adult has a child on a programme without the child having the adult on one as well.

Indications

Operant methods may be indicated with:

- *Conduct problems* such as aggressive behaviour, bullying, and stealing. Such behaviour may be reduced by stimulus control (e.g. by avoiding situations that produce conflict) or by systematic positive reinforcement (reward) for the non-occurrence of the antisocial behaviour. The differential reinforcement of other or incompatible behaviours (DRO or DRI), such as introducing rewards for alternative non-antisocial pastimes, is also a promising approach, especially when combined with problem-solving skills training and parent management training (Kazdin 1997; Webster-Stratton and Hammond 1997). DRO schedules have also been shown to be of use in eliminating inappropriate classroom behaviour (Ramasamy *et al.* 1996).
- *Problems related to anxiety* such as social withdrawal and difficulties in making friends. A combination of social skills training (see below) making it easier for the child to meet potential friends in a safe situation at home (stimulus control) and reward for even small steps in increasing social contacts may be effective.
- *Deficits of behaviour* such as mutism, aphasia, and language delay occurring in both otherwise normal and autistic children. Good results have been obtained using positive reinforcement methods, rewarding the child for utterances just a little in advance of those he is currently making.
- *Feeding difficulties* both in infants and in adolescents. In early feeding problems and failure to thrive (Section 4.2.3), removing the tension which may have built up around the feeding situation from the mother–child relationship by desensitization methods (see below) can be combined with social rewards, for example an increase in hugging and kissing if a child enjoys this, for more appropriate feeding behaviour. In the early treatment of anorexia nervosa,

enforced bed rest with the reward of increased physical activity for weight gain can be used as a form of positive reinforcement.

- *Hyperactivity*, where it is hoped to build up the child's ability to sit still and concentrate. Avoiding overstimulating situations (e.g. by ensuring that toys and games are produced one by one rather than all at once) is a form of stimulus control. Rewards can be instituted for longer and longer periods of concentration. Tasks requiring concentration can be broken down into separate steps, and the child rewarded for progress in each of them. Thus, when faced with a task, the child may be rewarded for learning to stop and consider what action he is going to take, but not for an immediate, thoughtless reaction. Treatment of hyperkinetic tendencies is a good example of multimodal approaches being of use. Combining the above stimulus control and reinforcement behavioural approaches with parent training, cognitive measures such as self-control techniques, and psychostimulant medication may be of particular benefit (Horn *et al.* 1991).
- *Habit disorders* such as enuresis and encopresis: providing an immediate reward on the morning after a dry bed (see Section 4.6.5 for this and other behavioural approaches to enuresis) is a form of positive reinforcement. The 'shaping' of appropriate behaviour involving the use of the toilet by positive reinforcement methods (see below) is often a useful adjunct in the treatment of encopresis (O'Brien *et al.* 1986). This can result in increased social competence and fewer behavioural problems—not just improved bowel habit (Young *et al.* 1995). Habits such as thumb sucking (Christensen and Sanders 1987) and hair pulling (Rothbaum 1992) may also be tackled in this way. Techniques such as response prevention and habit reversal may be used. The child is encouraged to identify the circumstances in which the habit occurs and then develop a competing response, for example enclosing the thumb inside the fingers in a closed fist for 20 seconds or so when these circumstances arise. Alternatively, such habits can be tackled by 'differential reinforcement'— rewarding with a token the absence of the behaviour for each 3 minute period over half an hour.

The indications, therefore, cover a very wide range of problems. Operant methods are particularly likely to be helpful where the problem is well circumscribed, and the family members (including the child) are motivated to achieve change. They are less likely to be effective when the problems are widespread, seem to emerge from deep-seated personality difficulties, or where motivation is low.

Practical applications

The mode of application will depend very much on the setting where the problem behaviour occurs, or where the deficit is most in evidence. Operant methods can be used effectively in the home (when applied by parents), at school, or in an in-patient or other residential setting. Probably its widest application for the health professional consists in its out-patient use with parents acting as 'co-therapists' with the clinician in attempting to alter or add to the child's behaviour, and it is this approach which will be described here.

Following assessment involving a functional analysis and baseline charting (see above), the parents and child then identify potential reinforcers or rewards. The child is then told that appropriate behaviour, i.e. not carrying out some undesirable activity such as a tantrum or carrying out a desirable activity such as helping with the dishes, will be followed by reward.

When choosing a behavioural target, change must be clearly within the child's capacity. Often it is necessary to 'shape' behaviour in the desired direction, and not attempt to produce a radical change very rapidly. Thus, for example, a child with encopresis might be reinforced first for sitting on the lavatory, then for attempting to pass a motion, and only finally for passing a motion into the lavatory pan. A child with a speech delay might be rewarded for making more and more appropriate sounds before he is rewarded for articulating words.

Reinforcers or rewards should, as far as possible, be social rather than material. A hug, kiss, or word of praise are more likely to produce lasting behavioural change than sweets or small-value coins, are financially less costly and, as far as sweets are concerned, less detrimental nutritionally. Nevertheless, for some children, material rewards are necessary, especially in the first stages of a behavioural programme. Whatever they may be, rewards should be given as soon as possible after the desired behaviour has occurred. Appropriate timing is essential. Promising a bicycle at Christmas if an encopretic boy is clean in September will probably have less effect than an immediate word of praise.

As well as positively reinforcing desirable behaviour, it is often useful to concentrate on removing rewards attached to undesirable activities (extinction). Parental attention to bad behaviour may be rewarding, and parents should be encouraged to ignore, rather than take notice of, undesirable behaviour. However, this is often easier said than done. It is often very difficult to help parents to work out ways of ignoring difficult behaviour, such as a child wrecking furniture or breaking crockery. Clearly in some circumstances, children do have to be given attention and stopped from doing things. Reinforcement can still be minimized in such circumstances, for example calm and quiet restraint rather loud remonstrations. Parents of children with such extreme behaviour are often best helped by devising techniques to help them avoid the development of such conflicts by the earlier application of positive reinforcement (working on the antecedents rather than the consequences). An additional technique involves the use of the time-out procedure, the parent removing the child from the place where the undesirable behaviour is gaining attention to a separate room or corner of the room where such behaviour can be quietly and calmly ignored until it stops. Assuming behavioural change is achieved in the desired direction, parents should be encouraged to 'fade' the rewards, so that the child is achieving well without them. This may need to be done slowly if the improvement is to be maintained. Initially the regular rewarding of desired behaviour can be changed to a regular intermittent schedule, with rewards only after every second, third, fourth, etc. demonstration of the desired behaviour. Later the schedule can be changed to an irregular intermittent schedule with rewards all the less predictable because of uncertainty as to when they will be received. Intermittent irregular reinforcement schedules are probably amongst the most difficult to establish but at the same time the most resistant to extinction.

Desensitization

Principles

The development of normal and abnormal fear and anxiety reactions is described in Section 4.4.1. Thinking of fear and avoidance as emotional and behavioural responses that can be both learned and unlearned has proved a useful concept in treatment. Normal coping mechanisms for dealing with a feared situation include a cautious but sustained approach towards the source of fear until the situation has been mastered and the fear conquered. At each stage the person involved must feel confident and assured before proceeding further. Desensitization involves a systematic application of this principle of a graded approach to overcoming anxiety.

Indications

Phobias, especially those confined to one or two feared objects or situations, are the main indications for this form of treatment. In particular, fear of the dark, of insects, dogs and other animals, and of separation from familiar figures may be treated in this way, but any reasonably well-defined phobia is likely to respond.

Practical application

- *Establishing a hierarchy of feared situations.* The first step in treatment is to develop a 'fear hierarchy' of situations, linked to the phobia. In a dog phobia, the least-feared situation might involve seeing a small dog on television or in a picture book while in the company of the father, and the most-feared might be meeting a large dog coming towards the child on the same side of the road while the child is unaccompanied. In severe separation anxiety, the least-feared situation might involve mother going into another room while the child is in the company of the father, and the most-feared might involve both mother and father going away for the weekend, leaving the child in the company of a relative. In each case, there might well be as many as a dozen intermediate feared situations.
- *Graded exposure.* Parents should be encouraged to expose the child to the least-feared situation until this has been mastered before proceeding to the next stage. At each stage anxiety can be reduced by reassuring and praising the child, thus achieving greater relaxation and reinforcement for the desired behaviour. The procedure is usually best carried out in the home by parents, but occasionally the nature of the fear may mean that treatment needs to be carried out in school or a clinic. In children, exposure to the feared situation in reality is usually necessary, but in adolescents and adults, phobias may be treated in this way by getting the individual to imagine feared situations while gradually achieving greater relaxation and freedom from anxiety (*covert desensitization*).

- *Relaxation*. In adolescents and sometimes in younger children with phobias and anxiety states, teaching relaxation may also be of value. This often involves a combination of deep breathing exercises, imagining a calm and relaxing scene (*imagery*) and conscious attempts to achieve reduction of muscular tension by concentrating on one muscle group after another, tensing and then relaxing them. The subject may first be encouraged to concentrate on ensuring his respiratory movements are easy and relaxed, then his stomach muscles, neck muscles, limbs, etc., until he has the impression that his entire body is in a pleasant relaxed state. The child or adolescent may be encouraged to practise relaxation on his own two or three times a day maybe with the aid of a pre-recorded cassette. Relaxation may be used on its own, or in association with desensitization techniques described above.

Parents of young children may be able to grasp the principles and apply desensitization methods so sensitively that very little help beyond an initial explanatory session is required. On the other hand, in the unusual case where the phobia is severe or parents have difficulties in applying the method, a great deal of regular supervision may be necessary. Work with adults suggests that a hierarchy and relaxation exercises are not necessary for therapeutic change, exposure being the single important principle. This may be the case but in clinical practice, especially with young people, compliance stands the best chance of being maximized if all three components are applied.

Other behavioural techniques
A number of other behavioural techniques have been described as useful in children, but appear to have more limited application.

Classical conditioning
The conditioning method derives originally from the model of classical conditioning developed by Pavlov. Working with dogs, he paired an unconditioned stimulus (food) with another stimulus (a bell) until the latter itself became effective and 'conditioned' to trigger the response of salivary secretion. Classical conditioning methods are little used in child psychiatry today, although the bell and pad treatment of enuresis (Section 4.6.5) can be seen as one example of its use. One explanation of the effectiveness of the bell and pad lies in the view that the bell becomes a conditioned stimulus, paired with the unconditioned stimulus (bladder distension) and produces sphincter contraction. However, the treatment can also be considered as a form of operant conditioning, or as a combination of operant and classical conditioning. Either way it remains an exceptionally successful example of behavioural treatments (Evans and Meadow 1990).

Flooding
The flooding method has been used in phobias, and involves sudden massive exposure to the object of which the child is afraid. It is not more effective than desensitization, but might have a place where desensitization has failed or where

a particularly rapid response is needed. Parents and child must agree that it is worth undergoing an extremely unpleasant, albeit transient, experience so that the phobia can be relieved. One naturally occurring example of flooding occurs when a child with no previous experience of hospital and with a fear of hospitals and doctors has to be admitted as an emergency. Such an experience may produce a sharp increase in anxiety, from which it may take the child months to recover. However, the flooding of the feared situation can also result in the child losing his original fear providing the anxiety subsides before the child leaves hospital. Failure in this respect will result in the child associating hospitals even more with anxiety and fear, and being away from hospitals as calming. Rapid return to school in a child with school phobia is another example of flooding.

Aversion therapy

Aversion therapy involves the use of the same principle as the operant methods described above. Although, of course, many parents do use physical punishment to reduce the likelihood of repetition of undesirable behaviour as a routine, the technique has very little application for professional use. It has, however, been employed on an in-patient basis in children with severe learning disabilities who show very severe self-destructive behaviour. Mild electric shocks, spraying of water 'mists' in the face, and lemon juice on the tongue have all been used as aversive stimuli. Even in these cases, very careful consideration to ethical issues must be given. More humane approaches are usually possible if sufficient thought is given and sufficient resources available.

Response prevention

The response prevention technique is used in children and, more commonly, adolescents who are compelled to carry out rituals as part of obsessive–compulsive disorders (Shafran 1998). An analogous technique of *thought blocking* is used for ruminative thoughts. The conduct of the rituals relieves anxiety, and the cycle of behaviour is therefore self-reinforcing. By encouraging the patient to desist from the rituals for longer and longer periods, the cycle can be broken (Wolff and Wolff 1991). Response prevention is often linked with exposure exercises—the individual being encouraged to place himself deliberately in settings increasingly likely to trigger the obsessive–compulsive tendencies while practising restraint. This treatment may need to be carried out on an in-patient basis with the assistance of nursing staff (Bolton *et al.* 1983), if the problems are resistant to out-patient treatment.

Social skills training

This technique, either in group or in individual sessions, may be used in children who have difficulty in their relationships with adults or others of their own age (Spence and Donovan 1998). There may be difficulties in making or keeping friends, or the child may be a constant target of bullying. Such difficulties may have arisen because of constitutional factors, because children have been exposed to inappropriate models, or because the child has, for other reasons, not acquired the skills needed to develop relationships successfully. In any event, a series of social skills training techniques, especially those involving role-playing, have been devised to counter such problems. Parents may, for example, be encouraged to practise with their children the problematic situation that they have in relating to peers, so as to improve their skills in this direction. Alternatively the professional involved can undertake such role play with the child himself. Such techniques can be used to help children with obesity or physical deformities to practise how they are going to behave when they are teased or asked embarrassing questions by other children.

Social skills training may also incorporate cognitive methods described below in a form of treatment known as *interpersonal cognitive problem-solving* (Pellegrini and Urbain 1985). Children may, for example, be asked to reflect systematically on conflicts in which they have been involved, and then work out alternative strategies they could adopt in the future when similar situations arise, in order to avoid such conflicts while still being appropriately assertive (Thompson *et al.* 1995).

Evidence for effectiveness
There is now a large literature involving single case studies and studies of small groups of patients demonstrating that behavioural methods can be effective in a wide range of childhood disorders (Herbert 1994). However, there is a lack of information on the degree to which these methods are generally applicable, on long-term outcome, and on the degree of expertise required to apply them. Beliefs that removing one symptom would merely result in the development of others (symptom substitution) have not been confirmed, and behavioural approaches remain a scientifically proven, cost-effective, and patient-friendly therapeutic approach for childhood psychopathology. It is of note that, as with other forms of psychological treatment, the principles of behavioural psychotherapies can be applied by relatively untrained professionals, and in mild problems one would often expect a successful outcome. Resistant and severe problems will need referral to more highly skilled professionals, who will often apply rather similar methods, but more systematically, and with more attention to detail.

Cognitive psychotherapy

Cognitive therapy refers to a group of techniques which have developed from the basic notion that psychological change can be brought about by attention to, and attempts to alter, the thought processes (cognitions) of the individual (Spence 1994; Graham 1998a). It is assumed that underlying psychological problems relate to a deficiency or distortion of cognitive techniques which individuals use to appraise themselves and events occurring around them, and to generate expectations regarding future occurrences. These misinterpretations, or *maladaptive cognitions*, result in the development of both inappropriate states of mind and detrimental behavioural patterns. Cognitive principles aimed at altering these maladaptive cognitions are usually combined with behavioural techniques and referred to as *cognitive–behavioural therapy* (CBT). CBT deals with the present (the 'here and now') and is problem-orientated. As with traditional behavioural approaches goals are clearly defined, and active exchanges are undertaken between therapist and client, in collaboration, as a means of working towards a consensus on what constitutes appropriate appraisals of situations and occurrences. Practical homework tasks may then be undertaken to test out the validity of these beliefs, which can be further adapted in the light of experience. The techniques developed from a growing awareness that therapeutic attempts aimed exclusively at the emotions or behaviour tended to be ineffective in producing change, and were highly vulnerable to relapse, or prone to a high prevalence of residual symptoms. A major factor appeared to be the individual's thought processes, which often remained unaltered despite at least temporary behavioural or emotional improvement. More traditional analytic approaches, while sometimes improving the individual's sense of well-being, often did little to change thought processes. In contrast, by altering the young person's cognitions through a problem-orientated process of 'collaborative empiricism' therapists found themselves able to achieve genuine and enduring improvements not only in cognitive functioning but also in behaviour and emotional state. The central assumption in cognitive approaches is that dysfunctional behaviours and emotions derive from distorted thinking. These cognitions should therefore be the primary focus for therapeutic intervention. Earlier beliefs by professionals that such sophisticated thinking only develops just prior to adolescence has been superseded by awareness of just how young a child can be and still benefit from these techniques. Thus age and intellectual level are not exclusion criteria *per se*. Of more importance is the ability to entertain alternative possible explanations to those held, and to be prepared to test out alternative hypotheses through practical exercises.

Just as a functional behavioural analysis can be undertaken examining antecedents, behaviour and consequences, so too can an analysis of cognitions be performed as illustrated by the path:

antecedent event → belief → emotional and behavioural consequence.

Documenting of multiple examples, both in the therapy session, and as part of a homework exercise, helps in gaining understanding of how particular beliefs are triggered and reinforced, and how these beliefs in turn can encourage either useful or maladaptive mood states and behaviours. Recognition of the significance of choice of words can be a crucial turning point. The therapist can encourage the rephrasing of sentences to cut out absolutes, e.g. **must, should, can't**. Substituting **won't** may begin to re-establish a person's control over his or her own behaviour. Also of use is encouraging the patient to view a situation through someone else's eyes in order to see that the distorted beliefs are not supported by real evidence. Depersonalizing the discussion can reduce anxiety and allow for rational thought (e.g. 'If a friend of yours were to be making himself very unwell but seemed to be unaware of what he was doing to himself, how might you feel? What would you want other people to do for your friend?'). Overall, therefore, the therapist does not act to persuade the child or family that their views are illogical or inconsistent with reality. The skill is to assist the child and family in discovering this for themselves.

Maladaptive beliefs can be grouped into three areas—the so-called *cognitive triad* which comprises beliefs about oneself, the future and one's surrounding environment. Thus low self-esteem is a common finding in association with a negative view of the future in adolescents with depression ('I shall always be a failure, nothing can help') along with a negative view of people and happenings around one ('Everybody is well meaning but they just don't understand') (Harrington 1993). Maladaptive cognitions are often self-defeating and extreme as in the case of anorexia nervosa ('I have absolutely no self-control over food intake once I've started eating ... mustn't eat another crumb if I'm going to stay this weight') (Turk 1993). Certain logical errors and inappropriate thought processes are particularly common:

- *Magnification* or *catastrophizing*: exaggerating the intensity, stressfulness or significance of events; embellishing situations with surplus meaning that is not supported by objective evidence. 'I left home without checking the door three times yesterday. That's it, I can't control myself at all.'
- *Personalization* or *self-reference*: relating external events to oneself. 'Two people laughed and whispered something to each other when I walked by—they were probably commenting on my appearance.'
- *Superstitious thinking*: believing in cause–effect relationships between non-contingent events. 'If I eat sugar it will be converted instantly into stomach fat.'
- *Self-fulfilling prophecy*: making predictions about outcomes of events, and then acting in ways that ensure that prediction will occur. 'This is my last chance—if I don't succeed this time, it's hopeless.'
- *Dichotomous* or *all-or-nothing thinking*: thinking in extreme, absolute 'black and white' terms. 'Either you're a success or a failure. There's no half way. You can't sit on the fence.'
- *Arbitrary inference*: the tendency to draw a negative conclusion on the basis of subjective impressions, even in the absence of concrete evidence to support these views. 'People are only happy when their parents live together—I shall never be happy.'
- *Selective abstraction*: repeatedly judging a situation on the basis of a fragment of the information available, focusing only on certain negative aspects and ignoring contradictory factors. 'You say there are so many good reasons to gain weight. Well, if it weren't for my dieting I'd never have got that gymnastics medal. There you are, I'm right!'
- *Overgeneralization*: a general conclusion is drawn on the basis of a single incident, so that an isolated setback is interpreted as evidence of global lack of ability. 'I gained a pound in weight two weeks ago. I can never control my weight. I need to diet more vigorously.'

In addition there are some issues of particular relevance to work with children:

- *Cognitive distortions* versus *cognitive deficiencies*. Many of the techniques described above relate to distorted thought processes and inappropriate logical inferences. For children, however, the difficulty is often more one of a simple deficiency in cognitive skills. To an extent this is a developmental trait which often rectifies over time. Nonetheless, steps can be taken to compensate for the child's lack of cognitive sophistication and facilitate more advanced thinking. Thus, educational approaches and prompts to consider a situation from different perspectives and to concentrate on learning from experience, take priority over cognitive restructuring exercises. The problem solving approach becomes particularly applicable here.

- *Need for self-control.* In anorexia nervosa the child can be perceived as needing to impose unrealistically strict limits on eating behaviour for fear of catastrophic 'letting go'. A gentler, more appropriate self-control technique can be taught. If necessary this can commence with spoken instructions from parents under the therapist's supervision. The child can then progress to using his or her own overt speech and ultimately private internal commands to modulate and control desirable and undesirable behaviours. The use of a graded hierarchy breaks down an apparently insurmountable task into smaller, more manageable, ones. It also helps the transfer of control over the child's behavioural problems from therapist through parents to the child himself, thereby enhancing independence and self-esteem.

- *Use of games.* The child's co-operation, and application to important therapeutic tasks, is enhanced by presenting activities in the form of enjoyable games rather than arduous endeavours. Examples include the 'I wonder what would happen if ...' game, which conveniently precedes the 'Let's see what actually happens when ...' game. Using analogies from every day life help as in the 'Stop and think' approach developed from road crossing instructions every child is exposed to early in life (Kendall 1989). The only limiting variable in this technique is the therapist's ingenuity in creating enjoyable games which also serve important therapeutic functions.

These approaches have considerable potential for therapy with children with a wide range of psychopathology (Graham 1998a). For example, the self-denigrating thoughts of a depressed adolescent can be seen as resulting from distortions of the incoming information from other people and there is now evidence that cognitive approaches are useful for depressed youngsters (Reinecke *et al.* 1998), in particular those who are younger and less severely impaired (Jayson *et al.* 1998). Post-traumatic stress and other associated emotional difficulties in sexually abused children can be reduced by cognitive–behavioural means particularly when parental interventions are included (Cohen and Mannarino 1998). Cognitive self-management strategies can enhance outcome when combined with behavioural programmes for enuresis (Ronen *et al.* 1995) and childhood obesity (Duffy and Spence 1993). Useful cognitive approaches for young people with obsessive–compulsive disorder have also been described (March 1995).

Case examples

Informal behaviour modification—general practitioner
Tracy was a 2 year old girl brought to her general practitioner by her mother because of her sleep problem. Her mother requested sleep medicine for Tracy,

or for herself. Tracy would not settle in her bed. She kept coming downstairs crying if her mother left her in her bedroom. Eventually she would settle by about 11.00 p.m. but then she would wake around 2.00–3.00 a.m., and come into her parents' bedroom. They would take her back to her room, give her sweet drinks, and play with her a little to try to settle her, but she would continue to cry and scream. Eventually after much coming and going they would take her into their bed. This was happening virtually every night. Tracy's young parents, who did not have a particularly good relationship between themselves, argued about how to overcome the problem, father thinking Tracy should be left at night to 'cry it out', while mother took a softer line. Mother was mildly depressed, tearful, and irritable. She said that she was at the end of her tether.

The general practitioner suggested that mother keep a chart to record what actually happened each night for a fortnight—what time Tracy went to bed, what she did, the times she woke in the night, and what the parents did when she woke. He arranged to see Tracy again in 10 days and said that it was important that father also came on that occasion. He said that if mother felt she might lose control of her temper with Tracy, she was to contact him immediately. When the family returned, it was clear from the chart mother had kept that Tracy was not waking each night but only about three times a week. However, on one to two nights a week she seemed to be up a good deal of the night. The general practitioner asked the parents which behaviour they would most like to change and the parents chose her night waking as the most stressful. The general practitioner discussed with the parents how they would feel about just letting Tracy 'cry it out' when she woke in the night, but mother was not happy about this, and even father admitted the neighbours would probably complain. The parents agreed a programme with the general practitioner whereby when Tracy woke and came into their bedroom in the night, father would take her back into her own room. Tracy preferred her mother to look after her in the night, and it would be less rewarding for her if father did it. She would not be given a drink and on no account would her father play with her. Father was asked if this would not be too exhausting for him, but he said he was having a quiet time at his work and could cope. Mother was asked to continue to keep a chart. Tracy was extremely difficult for the first few nights, even a little worse than she usually was, and the parents, especially father, were on the verge of giving in to her and taking her into their bed. However, on the fifth night she appeared to accept the inevitable—woke up only once at about 3.00 a.m., whimpered but did not call out and went back to sleep. Subsequently her bad nights decreased to about once a fortnight. The parents were still having a problem getting her to stay in her bedroom when she was put to bed in the evening, but decided they did not want any more help because they could cope with this problem themselves.

Behaviour modification—paediatrician (with advice from psychologist)
Jason was a 7 year old boy who presented in the paediatric out-patient department with encopresis. He had been clean and dry by 3 years, but had started soiling when he began school just before 5 years. He had found his reception

class teacher unsympathetic and had been frightened of her. The soiling occurred every day—weekends and holidays as well as schooldays. He said he did not know when he was passing a motion. The motions were said to be normal in colour and consistency. There were no other significant behaviour problems and, although his parents seemed rather irritable with each other, there were no obvious family or other stresses. Physical examination was negative, and it was decided no physical investigations were indicated. The paediatrician decided to institute a behaviour modification programme along the lines he had tried previously in consultation with a psychologist. He explained the nature of the problem to the parents and to Jason in terms of a habit that had become established. He asked the mother to chart the times each day when the soiling occurred, together with what happened before and after this event. The results of this behavioural analysis made it clear that the soiling did indeed occur at any time of the day, and that after the soiling mother would become irritable with Jason and behave in an inconsistent way. Sometimes she would make him wash his pants, sometimes not. Sometimes she would try to make him go to the toilet after he had passed a motion, though she was not clear why she did this. After discussion concerning Jason's particular likes and dislikes, a behavioural programme was instituted in which Jason was given a book in which to stick stars—one star for sitting on the toilet and two if he tried to pass a motion. At this stage no reward was given for passing a motion into the toilet, but only for trying. He was collecting football stickers, and six stars earned him one of these. His mother was encouraged not to comment on his soiling, but just to change his pants when she noticed he had messed himself. It was suggested that Jason, with his mother's help, rang the paediatrician's secretary (to whom he was introduced) to report progress each week, and a further appointment was given in 3 weeks' time. At this appointment mother reported that he had been to the toilet regularly for a few days, but then lost interest in the stickers and had started to refuse to go when she reminded him. A further discussion revealed that Jason would very much like to go to a football match with his father, and it was agreed that 25 stars, earned as previously, would win him this outing. He became dramatically co-operative and the paediatrician wondered whether his original formulation was accurate, or whether the boy was low in self-esteem partly because he had previously been rather ignored by his father.

Jason was in fact rather scared by the crowd at the football match he went to, so rewards were changed to small sums of money with which he bought sweets or football stickers. His father was encouraged to take him out more regularly. Jason began to pass motions into the toilet and his soiling improved though he continued to mess himself about once a week, mainly at home.

Behaviour modification and medication—psychiatrist
Victor was a 12 year old boy with a history of multiple tics going back 4 years. The tics were unusually severe and involved his head, neck, trunk, and arms. Over the previous 9 months he had started to make involuntary screeching noises. He had never shown any other serious behaviour or learning problems, though he was occasionally in trouble at school for disruptive activities and was

somewhat below average in his educational attainments. He was the youngest of three boys. His oldest brother had been in quite serious trouble for various offences, but appeared now, at 20 years, to have settled down to a regular job. The parents were warm and caring, but they had great difficulty in accepting that the movements were beyond Victor's control.

Victor's Tourette syndrome (Section 3.1.4) was initially treated with a combination of counselling and medication. He was put on haloperidol in doses up to 0.5 mg three times a day. On this dose he had a severe dystonic reaction. The drugs were stopped for three days, and it was found that he could tolerate 0.5 mg twice a day. On this dose his tics were definitely reduced, but still present. It was therefore decided to embark on a behaviour modification programme. A behavioural analysis, carried out by getting the parents to chart the tics (with Victor's knowledge and co-operation) showed that the tics were worst in the evenings when both parents were present. They were especially marked when his parents told him to stop the movements and also appeared worse on evenings when he had physical education the following day (because of his movements he found this very embarrassing). With a knowledge of the current frequency of tics, Victor was encouraged to try the effect of massed practice—deliberately and repeatedly indulging in his tics as a means of ultimately reducing the frequency and intensity. He practised making his noise as often and as loudly as he could for 10 minutes each day, morning and evening. This programme had no effect on the frequency of tics at other times, and Victor complained it gave him a sore throat. A further contact was made with the school, which agreed he could be excused PE.

Victor's parents then agreed that Victor should chart their behaviour in telling him to stop making his noise. The mere fact that Victor was charting their behaviour produced a dramatic effect, and they almost completely stopped telling him off overnight. This also produced a further slight improvement in tic frequency.

Over the next 3 years, Victor was maintained on haloperidol. Every 3–4 months an attempt was made to stop the medication, but it was clear each time that he was benefiting from it. At about the time he left school, at the age of 16 years, he was able to stop the drug and his tics gradually improved, though they did not cease completely.

9.2.2 INDIVIDUAL PSYCHOTHERAPY

Definition

In contrast to behavioural methods of treatment, where the focus is on observable behaviour, psychotherapeutic techniques involve the use of understanding the internal world of the child or adolescent in order to help resolve internal conflicts and master developmental tasks. This can be done for example by making a child or adolescent become aware of the meaning of symptoms to himself and to other people so that he can, if he wishes, change his behaviour. Most individual psychotherapeutic approaches have evolved from psychoanalytic theory and psychoanalytic practice.

Psychotherapy can be formal or informal. If formal, it involves the practitioner setting aside a particular time (usually for 45–50 minutes once or more times a week) during which no interruptions are permitted. Formal psychotherapy is usually carried out by practitioners who have had training in a particular school of psychotherapy, and who would usually expect to see their patients or 'clients' at a regular time at least over several weeks, and sometimes over several months. The therapist's goal is to help the child or adolescent express feelings and thoughts, understand causes of behaviour, and form a relationship with the therapist. With younger children, play usually is the major tool. Depending on the frequency and duration of treatment, the goals of individual psychotherapy differ. Classical psychoanalysis with five sessions a week, extended over several months to years, aims at achieving major structural changes in the child's personality. Short-term individual psychotherapy has more immediate goals, and tends to be focused on a limited number of issues such as helping the child cope with a physical illness, or with death in the family.

Informal psychotherapy is, as its name implies, less highly structured. Appointments may be made on a more *ad hoc* basis, though an agreement for a predetermined number of sessions might be made at the outset. The child might be seen for varying periods of time. Interruptions, though unwelcome, might be tolerated, if urgent. The practitioner is likely to be less highly trained in psychotherapy, but will nevertheless apply many of the same principles. Indeed, some highly trained psychotherapists practise informal as well as formal psychotherapy. Informal psychotherapy is practised by many general practitioners, social workers, psychologists, psychiatrists, and paediatricians. Elements of psychotherapy enter into many encounters between children, parents, and professionals. For example, a doctor working out with a teenager why he keeps on forgetting to take his anticonvulsant medication might well use his knowledge of the unconscious mechanism of denial during a medical consultation. Further, elements of psychotherapy are often involved in the application of other methods of treatment, both psychological (such as behaviour modification) and non-psychological (e.g. medication). But psychotherapy, formal or informal, can really only be said to take place when time is set aside specifically for the purpose of achieving greater understanding of feelings and behaviour.

Principles of individual psychotherapy

There are a number of fundamental notions which need to be accepted with some conviction in order to practice individual psychotherapy (Shapiro 1989). These are:

- that there is unconscious mental functioning
- that observable symptoms may be driven by internalized conflicts (parts of which are out of awareness), or by developmental deviance based on deprivation
- that symptoms have meaning and significance to the child or adolescent and affect his or her adaptation to the environment by how they are construed in the larger social community

- that there is a critical role for displacing (transferring) internalized conflicts and maladaptive relationships on to the therapist, so that the patient–therapist relationship can be interpreted and understood so as to lead to success in the wider task of removing repetitive maladaptive behaviour and symptoms.

Although there are many schools of psychotherapy, those who practise it share a number of principles (Reisman 1973) that can be summarized as follows:

- The child should be allowed the time he needs to express his feelings and thoughts.
- Practitioner and child should, early on in their meetings, try and focus on some particular goals. These goals might involve the eradication of particular symptoms, but they are more likely to involve the achievement of understanding in some area of the patient's life, for example why he feels so angry with his parents, or why he has so much difficulty making friends. Sometimes, before this goal can be reached, the child may need to attain a preliminary goal—the ability to recognize his own real feelings and put a name to them.
- The practitioner communicates his respect for the child's own feelings and thoughts, no matter how unacceptable these might be to the family, teachers, and others around. This does not mean that the practitioner communicates approval, only his acceptance, emotional empathy, and wish to help the child understand himself, so that he can change if he wants to.
- While the practitioner expresses his willingness to help the child recognize and understand his feelings, he communicates at the same time that responsibility for trying to change rests with the child.

Mechanisms of change in individual psychotherapy

Russ (1998) summarizes a number of factors that may be involved in how change occurs in psychotherapy:

- *Catharsis and labelling of feelings.* An important factor in individual psychotherapy helping the child to make his or her feelings less overwhelming and more understandable is the labelling of affect, with the therapist verbalizing the child's feelings. Also, the mere fact that the individual can express feelings and release emotions is traditionally regarded as an important therapeutic element.
- *Corrective emotional experience.* The therapist's non-punitive, empathic, and accepting attitude towards the child's feelings and thoughts may serve as a normalizing experience. For instance, the child may fear punishment as a result of his or her hostile feelings, whereas the therapist's attitude means that the child can accept his or feelings without anxiety.
- *Insight and working through.* The therapist helps the child to re-experience earlier conflicts. This will aid the child in gaining insight into the origins of conflicts and feelings. However, often cognitive insight is not enough, and emotional re-experiencing, with working through earlier conflicts is necessary to obtain mastery and symptom reduction.

- *Learning alternative problem-solving techniques and coping strategies.* Therapists vary in the way they actively introduce better problem-solving and coping strategies for the child.
- *Development of internal structure.* Children with structural deficits such as disturbed social relationships are thought to be helped by using the relationship with the therapist to develop more healthy internal psychological structures.

Techniques

The following techniques have been found helpful in applying the above principles.

Voluntary attendance

At the initial interview it is important to establish with the child that he does indeed wish to come. Most therapists are experienced in dealing with initial reluctance of a child or adolescent to come to treatment. In the majority of cases this initial resistance is overcome when the child or adolescent learns that the therapist is genuinely interested and non-judgemental, and that he can be expected to give support. Some children attend only because they are virtually forced to by parents or teachers. This may be acceptable as far as assessment is concerned, but is not compatible with ongoing psychotherapy, formal or informal. Therefore, if a child or adolescent does not wish to attend, this should usually be respected, though in some highly specialist units dealing with, for example, very severely disturbed mute or anorexic children, it is sometimes thought desirable for attendance to be insisted upon by parents and professionals acting together. Ambivalence can be dealt with by suggesting that the child might like to begin therapy and see how it goes. In accepting a refusal of therapy, one can make clear that the child is welcome to attend in the future if he changes his mind. Initial resistance to treatment should be separated from resistance during the process of treatment. It may be that the re-experiencing of conflict evokes so much anxiety that the child or adolescent no longer wishes to come. In those cases it is important that both patient and parents are persuaded to continue.

Establishing the pattern of attendance

At the beginning of the sessions, it is as well to make clear how many there are likely to be, and how they are going to be arranged, formally or informally. The practitioner should make clear how he is going to deal with possible interruptions.

Clarifying the reason for attendance

The practitioner should also make explicit at the beginning the purpose and nature of the sessions. This might be put along the following lines:

You told me that you get angry with your parents/often feel very worried/get panicky about going to school/can't make friends/find yourself messing about with your insulin, etc. We are going to meet to try and work out why this happens so that you can change if you want to. If you tell me about yourself, your feelings, about what's happening in your life and how you feel about things, together we may be able to make more sense of what's going on.

Defence mechanisms
In trying to make sense of the child's world, the practitioner will probably make particular use of the concept of unconscious defence mechanisms—means by which the child protects himself against emotionally unbearable thoughts (Freud 1966). These are described, in relation to ways in which parents deal with the unacceptable sides of having a child with a chronic physical handicap, in Section 7.3.3. If these defence mechanisms (denial, projection, repression, regression, etc.) are very strong, it is less likely they will be altered by psychotherapy, and indeed, in some circumstances, it may be unwise to attempt to do so. However, some children are able to become aware of their unacceptable aggressive, sexual, or other feelings, and, if the practitioner conveys his acceptance of these feelings, the child may have a reduced need to defend himself against them in a maladaptive way. For example, a child who is in trouble for fighting, and who blames other children for all the episodes that occur, may be using projection as a defence mechanism: 'I feel very angry with other people.' = 'Other people feel angry with me.' If he can be helped by the therapist to understand his aggressive feelings and then to accept them in himself, his need to use the defence of projection may be reduced and his behaviour may change.

Making connections
Another technique for helping the child make sense of himself is to point out possible connections of which the child may previously have been unaware. Connections may be made, for example, between:

- the child's behaviour in one current situation and another, for example in everyday life and in the session with the therapist
- the child's behaviour in the past and in the present, for example the first time the child was separated from his parents and a more recent event
- feelings and particular situations, for example the child may feel angry whenever he thinks he is going to be forced to do something
- a symptom and a particular situation, for example a row with mother and suicidal thoughts.

Making clarifying suggestions
In making suggestions that might help the child to make sense of himself, it is preferable to put ideas forward tentatively. The child is the only arbiter of the helpfulness of a suggestion. However, sometimes it is fairly obvious that a child is rejecting an idea that would make some sense of his predicament. In these circumstances it may be worth going on to question how upset the child would be if the suggestion were valid.

Observing the child in therapy
In the therapeutic session, the practitioner should constantly be aware of clues the child is providing to the way he is thinking or feeling. The way the child reports events of the previous week is likely to be at least as important as

what actually happened. In this way, the practitioner will be in a better position to pick up inconsistencies in the child's behaviour that it may be helpful for the child to be aware of, for example, if a child describes in positive tones a time when he played a game with his sister when he has previously only described arguments with her. The meaning of non-verbal messages should also be considered.

Respect for the child

The therapist should attempt to enhance the self-esteem of the child by taking him seriously, and approving of his coping behaviour. The child's self-esteem will not be enhanced by the therapist pretending to approve of undesirable behaviour, but attempting to examine why undesirable behaviour occurs without condemning it is likely to have a more positive effect.

Use of play and drawing

Many children, especially younger children, find it hard to talk about their feelings. They may require play and drawings to express feelings which have not yet been given a verbal form in their minds. The practitioner should have available a supply of toys (especially families of dolls), coloured pencils, and felt-tip pens or paints for this purpose. Obviously, for the therapist, the technical quality of what is produced is irrelevant—the drawings, etc. are useful in so far as they provide a starting point to understand and talk about feelings, etc. Some children will not play, draw, or talk, yet they continue to attend in mute silence. The practitioner can probably best help the child by tolerating and accepting the silences for minutes at a time, but occasionally making suggestions why it is so hard for the child to communicate. A child's drawings or play can also provide clues to thoughts and feelings in a way that can be used in therapy. A drawing with a violent theme can be employed to discuss a child's fears of being harmed. Play with a family of dolls or the drawing of a family can help the clinician (and thus the child) understand the child's wishes concerning his or her own family.

Stopping treatment

If, at the beginning of therapy, the practitioner and child have agreed on a particular number of sessions, there will be no problem about deciding when to stop. In other circumstances, termination should ideally occur when the problem is resolved, but may well be necessary when no further progress is being made or when the child no longer wants to come. If termination occurs in a planned way, then there should be an opportunity at the end for the child to discuss how he feels about stopping. Children may well go through a sequence of feelings about treatment terminating (particularly if it has been prolonged). Denial may be followed by bargaining, anger, sadness, and only finally acceptance. At the very end there should be a firm arrangement whereby the child should either be seen at a follow-up appointment or know he can contact the therapist again if the need arises.

Indications for individual psychotherapy with children

- *Emotional disorders*: although the rather rarely occurring specific phobias are better helped by behaviour modification techniques, and behavioural management advice is also helpful in a wide range of conditions in which anxiety is prominent, psychotherapy is probably the treatment of choice when anxiety and depression are diffuse and chronic.
- *Physical conditions* in which psychological factors are prominent in aetiology: usually as a supplement to family therapy, individual treatment can be helpful for children in this category with, for example, abdominal pain, chronic headaches, and asthma.
- Criteria that are less well established include situations in which a child with a physical condition is *failing to comply* with treatment, *social disorders* in which the most prominent features are withdrawal and inability to relate to other children, and some special symptoms such as *encopresis*. In many of these conditions, psychotherapy can be supplementary to other forms of treatment, such as family therapy.

If these conditions are present, positive indications for psychotherapy would include situations in which the child and family are well motivated for psychotherapy, the condition is not obviously entirely reactive to factors within the family, and the child has already shown some capacity for making connections, i.e. has some degree of psychological mindedness for his symptoms. In specialist settings, it is often helpful for the parents to receive counselling at the same time as the child is undergoing therapy.

The age of the child is relevant. Children under the age of 6–7 years will find it difficult to communicate verbally about their problems. Although in theory, and to some degree in practice, children under this age can communicate their feelings through play, there is little systematic evidence that connections made in therapy in this way generalize to everyday life. Other methods, including family therapy and behaviour modification, are more likely to be applicable. In contrast, the older the child the more likely he is to benefit from psychotherapy. It should, however, be added that some highly trained analytic child therapists do claim effectiveness for this form of treatment with very young children.

Contraindications

There is no evidence that the type of therapy described above, or indeed intensive psychotherapy, is helpful for children with autism (pervasive developmental disorder) or attention deficit disorder, or for conduct disorders unless symptoms of emotional disturbance (anxiety or depression) are prominent. Psychotherapy is contraindicated in these conditions because the child is likely to show poor capacity for symbolic thought, short attention span, and difficulties in forming interpersonal relationships—all of which make interpretive forms of psychotherapy difficult or impossible to apply.

Evidence for effectiveness

Although individual psychotherapy with children and adolescents is often said to be more of an art than a science and remains untested (Russ 1998), there is evidence for the effectiveness of child psychotherapy (Eisenberg *et al.* 1965; Fonaghy and Moran 1990; Rosenthal and Levine 1971; Gurman and Kniskern 1979) in some circumstances. Although the size of the effect of psychotherapy with children is similar to that found with adults, in general behavioural approaches have been found to be superior to non-behavioural approaches (Weisz and Weiss 1993). From work examining therapist effectiveness in student counselling (Truax and Carkhuff 1967) one can reasonably assume that improvement is related not only to the nature of the child's condition, but also to therapist qualities, especially capacity for warmth, accurate empathy, and genuineness. Also by generalizing from work with adults (Reid and Shyne 1969) one may assume that brief, focused therapy, with a finite number of sessions arranged at the outset is, in general, more effective than therapy conducted without clear goals.

Case examples

Informal individual psychotherapy—general practitioner

An overweight 11 year old girl, Jennifer, was brought by her very slim and attractive mother to the general practitioner. There were no complaints about her, apart from her obesity and tendency to overeat. She was indeed over the 97th percentile in weight, but only of average height. The general practitioner knew there were considerable problems in the family. Father was now living at home, but had previously left home on three or four occasions for months at a time—unable to make up his mind whether to live with another younger woman or with his family. Jennifer was the second of four children and the oldest girl. The general practitioner suspected that the mother was having an affair herself because he noted she came for birth control checks when her husband was away. Previous attempts by the general practitioner to treat the obesity with a restricted diet had been unsuccessful.

He tried to talk to the girl and found her unresponsive. With her mother present she looked at him stonily, chewed gum, answered his questions monosyllabically. Yes, she would like to be thinner. No, there was nothing she was worried about. He asked to see the girl by herself and made little further progress. She denied she was worried her father might leave home again—they did not need their father. If he wanted to go, that was his business. They had managed without him before.

The general practitioner said he would like to see mother and daughter again in a fortnight's time and put aside a further 25 minutes to talk to the girl. Ideally, he would also like to have seen the father, but it was clear he would not attend. On this second occasion the girl was initially somewhat more forthcoming, then began to cry. Her father was threatening to leave home again. She hated the idea, not because she missed her father, but because when he left, her mother was irritable with all the children, made her do more housework, so that she could not go out with friends. They were much more hard up. Her younger sister was taken into her mother's bed and Jennifer admitted she was a bit jealous. Her younger sister was always messing up her games with her friends. The general practitioner said he really understood why she had to eat so much. She must be very unhappy. He said he did not think she could go on a diet in the circumstances. The girl said, on the contrary, she thought she could. He asked if she could talk to her friends about her problems and she said she could not—she was too ashamed. The general practitioner suggested there might be other girls in the same boat. He said at least she should not feel a failure if she found she could not stop eating. He suggested her way of responding to feeling sad was to eat more, while her mother just got cross and irritable when she was sad. The girl agreed and added that she thought it would be better for the family if her mother ate more rather than being cross and irritable when she was sad. The general practitioner offered further appointments, but the girl said she would come and see him if she wanted another talk. She did not lose weight, but at least managed to avoid putting on any more. The next time she came was for birth control advice when she was 15 years old. She was slimmer and more forthcoming. The general practitioner was able to talk with her about her need for affection in a way she obviously found helpful in deciding whether to sleep with her boyfriend.

Informal individual psychotherapy—paediatrician
Paul was a 14 year old boy with cystic fibrosis that had been diagnosed in infancy. An older brother had died of the same condition 2 years previously, aged 16 years. There was an unaffected 20 year old sister. The family members had always had difficulty in expressing their feelings to each other, and to the social worker who had known them for the previous 5 years. The paediatrician had been responsible for Paul's hospital care since just after the diagnosis had been made, but he also found difficulty in knowing what was going on in the family. Paul had been rather little affected by his condition until about the age of 10 years, since then he had had three hospital admissions with infections that had been difficult to treat.

Over the last 6 months, Paul had changed from being a rather cheerful, active boy, keen on games and with many friends, to being morose, sullen, and isolated. He was rather unco-operative when undergoing physiotherapy both at home and during the present admission. The nurses on the ward were worried about him, and the social worker was away.

The paediatrician assumed he was depressed because of increasing awareness of his prognosis. He decided to see the boy on his own and in fact saw him three times before his discharge. He and Paul talked about Paul's interests, how the football team Paul supported was doing. He then asked what sort of things Paul was worried might happen over the next few months. Paul said he supposed he would just go 'jogging along'. There was nothing more. The paediatrician asked if he was worried about his mother, and immediately Paul's eyes filled with tears. He said he thought his mother was going to crack up. She had been very upset by the death of Gerald (the older brother), but no one else but he, Paul knew about this. The paediatrician asked how Paul remembered his brother, and Paul immediately said that it had not been too bad for Gerald because his mother was always with him. It was obvious that Paul was angry with Gerald, and also that he was frightened of being left alone when he was very ill. The paediatrician commented that it was very natural for Paul to feel angry with Gerald, but he knew sometimes people felt bad about being angry with someone who had died.

He asked Paul later on what worries he had about himself and Paul again denied having any. However, as the paediatrician was about to leave the cubicle on one occasion, Paul asked him if the thought they might discover a cure for cystic fibrosis. The paediatrician said that was not impossible—there was research going on all the time, but he did not want to raise Paul's hopes.

After he left Paul, the nurses noticed the boy crying, and there was a certain amount of anger amongst the junior nurses towards the paediatrician who, it was felt, had upset Paul unnecessarily. This led to a useful discussion at the next ward psychosocial meeting about whether it was, in fact, better for teenagers to be encouraged to deny the implications of their condition, or to encourage the expression of sad feelings. No conclusion was reached, but both medical and nursing staff were left with a better idea of the complexity of the issue, and the need to treat each individual case on its merits. The paediatrician continued to see Paul in out-patients after his discharge, and felt he was now much more open in expressing his feelings.

Individual psychotherapy—psychiatrist
Sally was a 10 year old girl with widespread fears and anxieties. Her parents both complained that she took hours to settle in her bedroom because she kept coming downstairs. She frequently woke in the night with nightmares. She was too fearful to stay in another's girl's home if she went out to play, so either girls came to her to play or she was unable to see her friends. She would not go to the shops by herself. School attendance was reasonably regular, but she often tried to get out of school by complaining of physical symptoms.

The family background was disturbed and provided some but probably not a full explanation why Sally was so anxious. Two family interviews were held, but it became clear that, for various reasons, father was not prepared to attend any more. The widespread nature of the fears made it improbable that behavioural methods would be effective, and it was decided to embark on a brief course of 8–10 sessions of psychotherapy. The focus was to be on the understanding of the source of Sally's anxieties, so that she could obtain better control over them.

The first session was largely taken up with setting Sally at ease and discussing why she felt so anxious with the psychiatrist away from her mother. She was clearly uncomfortable in the situation, but managed to stay for 45 minutes. In the second and third sessions she started to draw rather stereotyped pictures of a house and garden. One house had three girls and their mother living in it (Sally was an only child). Why no boys? No, boys were rough. There were a lot of naughty boys at school. If they had any sense, girls did not want boys around. The psychiatrist wondered how far aggression was a problem for Sally. On the fourth session the psychiatrist was unavoidably 20 minutes late, and Sally was obviously fed up. The psychiatrist commented on this, but Sally denied it, saying she did not mind. She had been quite happy in the waiting room. The psychiatrist suggested that it was hard for Sally to admit she was angry. He suggested it might be hard for her to admit she was angry at home too. The next session was taken up with a similar theme. Prior to the sixth session the social worker, who was seeing the mother, told the psychiatrist that Sally appeared slightly less anxious, that her mother was finding her more disobedient and aggressive to her. The final three sessions were taken up with the psychiatrist preparing Sally for termination of the sessions, while Sally tested the psychiatrist out. She tried to mark the table and then the wall with felt pens, swore at the psychiatrist when he firmly prevented behaviour he had told her would not be allowed, and then sulked. The psychiatrist made connections concerning her mixed feelings about him and her feelings about her parents and teachers. He suggested it was very hard for her to be a little girl who had to do what adults told her to—both with him and with her mother. Sally agreed with this, and said this was because grown-ups were stupid. Towards the end of the final session she became tearful. The psychiatrist wondered about offering further sessions, but decided against this, partly as a result of pressure on his own time.

The girl's anxieties outside the session decreased during and after the therapy. Over the next 3 years, during which she was seen for review appointments, her general anxiety also decreased, perhaps partly as a result of the natural history of the condition and partly as a result of the therapy. She became a rather isolated, shy teenager, but her sleep problems completely waned and she was able to stay the night with friends without difficulty.

9.2.3 FAMILY THERAPY

Definition

Family therapy involves an attempt to understand a presenting problem as arising from the nature of the family relationships rather than locating its source in any one individual. When a child's behaviour is presented as problematic, it would normally involve seeing together, for at least part of the time, the child and both parents (if there are two parents still in the household), as well as any brothers and sisters, if this is acceptable to them and the other members of the family. There are many different types and schools of family therapy, well described in Gorell-Barnes (1995). The essential ingredients of all forms of family therapy involve an attempt to enable family members to see presenting problems as arising from their interactions and to improve communication between family members, thus indirectly reducing individual symptomatology.

Principles

Most family therapy is at least partly rooted in systems theory. This assumes that family functioning can usefully be viewed as a single self-controlling entity. If one part of the system changes, this will have an impact on other parts, until a new homeostasis is reached. The family system can be seen to have boundaries, and there may be sub-systems (such as mother–daughter or sib–sib relationships) within the family that have their own boundaries.

Within this framework numerous different schools of family therapy have been developed. In particular, the *structural* family therapists rely on strongly interventionist approaches within the family sessions. For example, in the session, they may insist the family changes its seating arrangements, speak for other members, or embrace each other when this does not normally occur. *Strategic* family therapists place emphasis on identifying the different meanings arrived at by different family members of the same interactions and thus improve patterns of communication. The *Milan school* involves to a much greater degree the reactions of the therapy team to the family, and the way the therapists themselves interact with the family.

Further, family therapists are likely to be influenced in their family work by their theoretical orientation in work with individuals. Thus, those with a basic *behavioural* approach will tend to use techniques such as reinforcement, contracting, and systematic recording of events between sessions. Those with a *psychoanalytic* framework will look for the way unconscious processes affect family interactions. For example, a therapist may characterize a whole family as prone to the use of denial or projection as a means of dealing with anxiety.

Assessment

When a child is referred for a behaviour or emotional problem, or is seen for a physical complaint which turns out to have a strong functional component, assessment of family relationships with a view to family therapy may be informal or formal. Formal family therapy will generally involve trained professionals in the child mental health services, some of whom specialize in family therapy. Informal therapy will be provided by the less highly trained who will nevertheless find it helpful to use concepts and techniques derived from specialist workers.

A formal family assessment involves seeing together as many family members living under the same roof as possible, to observe their characteristics, mode of communication, and interaction. A specific period of time, normally 1–2 hours, is set aside for this purpose, and towards the end of this time, the therapist will usually feed back to the family the observations he is making and assess the impact this has.

Informal family therapy or family counselling

Paediatricians and general practitioners are often involved in counselling small groups of family members. Usually this involves listening and talking to mothers or both parents and a child identified as having a problem.

For example, a general practitioner may note that the mother of a boy with asthma is unnecessarily overprotective. He may see the parents together with the child on a couple of occasions, and facilitate the father's feelings that his son could be allowed more independence. The family doctor might sympathize with the mother's predicament but support the father in his wish to help mother and son to separate. A paediatrician faced with a teenage diabetic girl failing to comply with treatment might arrange to see parents and child together to discuss the situation. He might discover that the girl's refusal was part of a wider rebellion. He might give the parents, on the one hand, and the girl, on the other, the opportunity to discuss their feelings about independence and autonomy. Then he might sympathize with the parents in their worries about their daughter's behaviour, but support the daughter's wish to achieve her identity in her own way. He might succeed in persuading the girl in this way to fight her battles in areas that do not involve her health.

The distinction between this form of family counselling and formal family therapy is not clear-cut. The following account of family assessment and treatment is probably most likely to be used by those working in a psychiatric department, but many of the principles and techniques can be applied in other settings and with less time available than is usually the case in the child and family psychiatric clinic.

Formal family therapy

The whole family (i.e. all those living in the same physical household) is invited to attend. It is particularly important for both parents and the identified child to be present, but the effectiveness of the family approach is enhanced by the attendance of brothers and sisters.

To assess family functioning it is important to elicit family interaction. This can usually be successfully achieved by asking the family to focus on various topics. One can begin with the nature of the problem behaviour of the identified child, the way in which the referral came about, and the attitude of all the family members to the attendances. While discussing this particular topic, it is especially important to elicit the feelings of the identified child, and to ascertain whether or not he thinks there are other, perhaps bigger problems in the family. If the sibs do not speak spontaneously, they should also be asked their views. Members of the family can be asked to talk directly to each other.

Other topics which can be used to elicit family interaction include finding out about the way in which family tasks, such as shopping, keeping the house clean, and looking after the children, are shared; the out-of-home activities undertaken by family members, separately and together; the development of the family, including the way the parents met, the circumstances of the children's births, the times when the family moved house, children started school, etc.; and the impact on the different family members of recent stressful events.

Family assessments can and normally should be combined with individual assessment of the child to explore the mental state or feelings in more detail. It is often also sensible to offer parents separate sessions without the children. During family assessment the therapist will find it helpful to use certain techniques. He should be aware of the ways in which the more silent family members show their feelings and make a particular effort to comment on their form of non-verbal expressions and to get them to talk. He should refrain from taking sides, but make sure that everyone's opinions and feelings are as fully expressed as possible. He should make tentative observations of the family's functioning during the sessions and check out with family members whether they perceive these observations to be accurate. Such observations can be considered under the following headings:

- *Family structure*
  - Who sits next to whom, speaks for whom?
  - Are there any special alliances or coalitions in the family?
  - Are family members overinvolved ('enmeshed') or too detached from each other?
  - Are the intergenerational barriers respected, or do the parents behave like children?
  - Are the children taking on parental roles?
- *Communication*
  - Are feelings about important family matters readily expressed?
  - Are messages about what the parents and children would like of each other clearly communicated?
  - Do the children understand and accept the sanctions imposed by the parents?
- *Family atmosphere*
  - Is this tense or relaxed, depressed or cheerful?
  - Do the family use humour to release tension or heighten it?
  - Does the atmosphere change, for example, when the child identified as a problem is being discussed or the parents start to talk about problems they have together?
- *Potential for change*
  - How rigid and inflexible does the family seem when family members discuss and argue among themselves?
  - Can they tolerate differences between themselves?
  - How well do family members take up the tentative suggestions made by the therapist?

Treatment

After the preliminary assessment has been completed, usually in one but perhaps in two sessions, the therapist should decide whether treatment is indicated and if it is, draw up a treatment plan with the family.

Format

Treatment might involve family sessions alone, or family sessions combined with marital or individual sessions. The main advantage of not having separate individual or marital sessions is that inevitably those not present at such sessions develop fantasies about what is being said about them behind their backs. On the other hand it is inappropriate to discuss parental sexual problems with children present, and other family matters may also be regarded as secret from the children. When a member of the family requests a separate session, it is reasonable to check out with the family present whether this concerns something all family members do not already know about. If the therapist accedes to the request for a separate session and it turns out to concern a matter it is reasonable for the rest of the family to know about, then it should be suggested that the whole family be involved in further discussions. The length and frequency of treatment should be discussed with the family. It would be reasonable, for example, to suggest that there be 6–10 sessions held at fortnightly or three-weekly intervals over 3–6 months.

Techniques

It is useful to develop a focus for the sessions with the family fairly early on. This might involve achieving improvement in communication, helping the family to understand why a particular behaviour problem in a child is occurring and how they might cope with it better, how a family member, for example the father, might be more integrated with family life, etc.

The therapist should comment on positive as well as negative aspects of family functioning. When examples of good coping behaviour, clear expressions of feelings, etc. come up, then this should be positively commented upon by the therapist. The therapist should also positively comment on the adaptive functions of behavioural problems. Thus, he can say of a child who is having temper tantrums that he is really very good at getting his own way. The question is whether he could not succeed in getting his own way in another more acceptable fashion. A child soiling his pants could be congratulated on finding such an effective way of showing how angry he is with his parents, etc. Of course, the therapist should make clear he does not approve of this behaviour, but establish that he sees its function and is intent on helping a child find other modes of expression. The therapist should facilitate communication of feelings as well as information. He can ask how one family member thinks another feels about a particular problem and then ask them to check this out in the session. He should promote the establishment of appropriate boundaries between the generations, communicating, for example, how confusing it must be for the children if parents behave like them at one point in time, and then expect to be obeyed at another.

The more experienced therapist will use a variety of other techniques (Street and Dryden 1988) to promote more adaptive family functioning. An example of a more advanced technique is the paradoxical challenge (Cade 1984). The therapist may suggest that it would be better for the family if a particular form of maladaptive behaviour did not change, Thus, for example, in a child not attending school the therapist might suggest that, if the child did attend school, the mother, unable to cope with the separation, would have a breakdown, and that the father would have to stay at home to look after her. Perhaps it would be better for the child to remain off school. Some families respond to such a challenge when they have failed to respond to more conventional therapy by taking positive moves to achieve better functioning, but clearly this is not the sort of technique to be used lightly by a less experienced therapist.

Indications

Most child and adolescent psychiatric disorders (emotional and conduct problems, management difficulties in the pre-school period, anorexia nervosa, tics, psychosomatic disorders, etc.) may respond to family therapy. It should, however, be applied only when the presenting symptom can be seen on initial assessment to be maintained by mechanisms involving other members of the family. If, after assessment, the therapist strongly suspects that the presenting problem is not centred in the child but within the family relationships more generally, then, if there are no contraindications (see below) family therapy is indicated.

Contraindications

There are some cases where family therapy should not be applied, for example:

- The problem is mainly centred not in the family but in the child, for example in cases of childhood autism, severe personality problems, or where a child has clearly responded to a specific physical or psychological trauma unrelated to family life. Occasional family sessions may be helpful in such cases to help family members cope better together, but family therapy should not be the main mode of treatment.
- One member of the family has a serious mental illness such as paranoid schizophrenia or a marked personality disorder which prevents a realistic perception of family relationships. (Psychoeducational methods to reduce expressed emotion in families where a family has schizophrenia, will involve parents—see Section 5.6.2—but this would not fall into the usual definition of family therapy given above.)
- Effective resolution of the problem can be achieved by a cheaper form of treatment not involving the father or mother taking time off work or the other children time off school.

Relative but not absolute contraindications for using family therapy as an exclusive approach include a family on the point of breakdown, the presence of a serious marital problem, the presence of 'legitimate' family secrets, and apparently unmodifiable scapegoating of one particular family member. When a family approach is used in these cases, family sessions may be combined with individual or marital therapy.

Evidence for effectiveness

There is evidence that family therapy is helpful in a variety of cases in which the child is the presenting problem (Diamond *et al.* 1997). Controlled studies, discussed in the relevant sections, have demonstrated slight but definite improvement in children with a range of behavioural and emotional disorders as well as psychosomatic conditions such as asthma. In a review of 19 controlled studies of variable quality of the effectiveness of family therapy, 15 of which involved children, about three-quarters of the patients treated did better than they would have done if the subjects had received no treatment or an alternative treatment (Markus *et al.* 1990).

Family therapy is more likely to be effective where the therapist is sufficiently flexible to integrate family approaches with other forms of therapy, including, where indicated, individual sessions and medication. Therapists will also need to adapt their techniques to take account of differences in family functioning in ethnic minority groups, and in families with different structures, e.g. those with single parents, foster and adoptive parents, and separated and divorced parents. There is increasing acceptance that it is helpful for family therapists to acknowledge that the causes of presenting problems lie in factors such as temperamental differences and individual experiences, as well as in past and present family interactions. Indications of positive outcome include the family's success in 're-framing' individual problems in terms of family interactions where this is appropriate, and the replacement of cross-generational with inter-generational coalitions (Diamond *et al.* 1997).

Case examples

Informal family therapy—family practitioner

Jonathan was a 3 year old brought to his general practitioner for an opinion on a mole on his back, which turned out to be a pigmented naevus of no particular significance. However, examination of the mole turned out to be a traumatic experience, as Jonathan first would not allow his shirt to be taken off, then screamed, shouted, and wriggled while the doctor tried to examine him, and finally finished with a monumental temper tantrum when his mother tried to put his shirt back on again.

When calm was eventually restored, the family doctor enquired if this sort of thing happened often, and his young mother was soon in tears saying she could not manage the boy at all, her husband was little help, she felt she was going to lose control of herself with him, and she was on the verge of a 'breakdown'. The family doctor asked if she and her husband would bring Jonathan back in 10 days' time for a further talk.

At this next appointment Jonathan was once again very difficult and started to play with the doctor's telephone and open his desk drawers while the parents were trying to talk to him. Neither parent seemed to make much attempt to stop Jonathan, though each looked at the other expectantly, obviously with this in mind. The family doctor asked who normally controlled him in this situation, and the father said he thought it was his wife's job. The mother said she had Jonathan all day and her view was that when father was home, he ought to take this responsibility. The doctor said he wondered if really the parents wanted to stay together because they were obviously making life impossible for each other. Both parents were very angry at this suggestion and jointly rounded on the doctor for making it. The doctor said in that case they looked as though they wanted the family to stay together but Jonathan to run it. Was he not a little young to take this responsibility?

The parents then both described their own childhoods of which the doctor knew something, as he had looked after them before they married. They had each had a very strict upbringing. They admitted they both hated the idea of bringing Jonathan up not to have what he wanted. The doctor did not comment on this, and the parents saw themselves that they would have to set firmer controls. No further appointments were made, and there was no systematic follow-up, but the doctor noted that when, 3 months later, he had to listen to Jonathan's chest, his shirt came off without demur.

Informal family therapy—paediatric out-patients

An 8 year old girl, Amanda, was referred by her general practitioner to paediatric out-patients with recurrent abdominal pain. The pain had begun a year previously—it was intermittent in frequency, occurring for a few hours every 8–9 days. It was not accompanied by vomiting or alteration of bowel habit. The pain was severe, and made Amanda cry. It never woke her at night. The pain stopped her going to school when it occurred, but she also had it at weekends and during school holidays.

She was an only child who lived with her parents in a residential area of the city. There did not seem to be any obvious stresses at home or at school. Physical examination was negative and, in particular, she had no abdominal tenderness.

The child was accompanied only by her mother. The paediatrician noted that the girl kept darting anxious glances at her mother. He also observed that Amanda was very neatly and smartly dressed and kept brushing imaginary flecks of dust from her skirt. The mother seemed rather obsessional in the way in which she seemed to have to get every detail of the occurrence of the pain precisely accurate.

In answer to questions it became clear that the mother thought the pain might be due to ulcerative colitis from which a maternal aunt had suffered. The paediatrician was reassuring, but ordered a blood count, urine examination, and straight radiography of the abdomen. He asked to see the girl again in a fortnight and requested that her father should come as well on that occasion.

Investigations were negative. The paediatrician diagnosed non-organic recurrent abdominal pain and saw the family on three further occasions for about 20 minutes each time to monitor progress before referring back to the family practitioner. He discussed possible links between tension and pain with the family (of which they were already aware) and the family members talked about how Amanda could be helped to be less tense and anxious. When Amanda was asked to draw a picture, using felt pens, it was clear that she was unduly worried both about getting her hands dirty and about producing a perfect picture. The parents obviously disagreed about how relevant this behaviour might be to her pain, but could not express their disagreement to each other. Amanda looked more uncomfortable at this point. The paediatrician suggested that possibly parental disagreements might make Amanda less anxious if they were able to express them more clearly. Over the next few weeks Amanda's pains virtually ceased, although the family relationships appeared unchanged. The paediatrician was uncertain whether the interviews had resulted in pain alleviation or whether this was due to the natural history of the condition. A further possibility was that in fact the pains were persisting, but the parents denied them so that they need no longer attend interviews they themselves found painful.

Family therapy—psychiatrist

Helen, aged 12 years, was referred to a child psychiatrist with an established diagnosis of anorexia nervosa. At about the age of $10\frac{1}{2}$ years, she had been a rather plump girl and a chance remark about her appearance by a PE teacher

had humiliated her. She began to diet and became preoccupied with her appearance. She exercised excessively and lost a stone in weight. Her parents eventually
took her to the family practitioner who was alarmed at her appearance and
referred her immediately. The paediatrician who saw her treated her on an
out-patient basis over several months, but eventually referred her to a child
psychiatrist. By now mealtimes were a nightmare, with the parents and Helen's
16 year old sister Jasmine all shouting at her in order to get her to eat and then
at each other when they failed to do so.

There was no significant family history. Helen was a very good girl who
worked conscientiously at school. The parents said of their own relationship that
they got on extremely well with each other until Helen's problems had begun.
They said Jasmine presented no problems.

Helen was admitted to an in-patient unit and put on a behavioural regime to
encourage her to gain weight. She was allowed increased activity for each 2 kg
increase in weight. This programme was initially successful, but her weight
began to plateau out before she reached the target at which she could go home
for a weekend. Family interviews were arranged, although the father, in particular, set up obstacles to such sessions. The interviews were immediately illuminating. Father, who was a senior civil servant, sat slightly apart from his wife and
two daughters. He was clearly excluded from much family life. It transpired that
he worked very long hours and often did not know what had been going on at
mealtimes. He undercut his wife's remarks at every opportunity. Mother was
closely identified with her daughters and included herself when referring to their
activities. For example she said to Jasmine, 'We are very good at maths, aren't
we dear?' When the psychiatrist pointed out that she had repeated this phrasing
in another connection, father, with heavy sarcasm, said 'Did you hear what the
doctor said, dear, or are you totally deaf?' After three sessions of this nature a
family meal was arranged in which it became clear that the parents could not
agree on how to get Helen to eat and undercut each other's efforts constantly.
The psychiatrist pointed this out, and was able to help them at the second meal
to agree a strategy to encourage their daughter to eat. When her parents joined
forces, Helen began to take notice of this and eat distinctly more than she had
previously.

Marital sessions were arranged, and revealed that the parents had had an
appalling relationship for years. No sexual relationships had occurred for over
2 years. The parents began to discuss separation without any apparent self-
consciousness that their attitude now totally negated all they had said about
their relationship when first seen. Further family interviews were held when the
parents were encouraged to express some, though not all, of this problem to their
children. Helen, who had previously said little in family interviews without
looking at her mother for approval, began to speak more for herself. She reached
a satisfactory weight and managed to maintain it, though she continued to have
some personality problems. The parents refused further interviews once she was
home from hospital. One year follow-up revealed that the girl had not relapsed
and the parents were still together, with some improvement in the quality of their
own relationship.

Children of divorced or separating parents

The assessment and management of children with psychiatric disorders, developmental delay, or physical conditions, when the parents are divorced or separated, present special problems.

In assessing the child's difficulties, a decision has to be made whether to see the parents together or separately. The wishes of the parent who has control and custody should be respected and taken into account. Every effort, however, should be made to see the parent living apart, if he or she still has contact with the child, even if such contact is rather tenuous. Further, even though a divorced parent may not have a legal right to be involved in decision-making concerning a child's future, it is usually helpful to ascertain this parent's views, without in any way undermining the legal parent's position.

Children of parents living together face particular difficulties in their lives. They may be used as pawns in a continuing marital dispute by parents who, although physically separated, are still emotionally joined together by their dislike of each other. They may be used as message-bearers by parents who cannot bring themselves to communicate directly. They may be at risk of emotional upset arising because the separated parent does not keep to access times in a regular and predictable way. They may have to listen to their parents denigrating each other when they are fond of both of them. They often have to be flexible enough to make relationships with new partners their parents may find, and be able to cope with the ambivalent feelings these new parental figures elicit in them.

The rate of psychiatric disorders in the children of divorced parents is distinctly higher than that in the general population (Hetherington *et al.* 1982). Nevertheless, perhaps surprisingly, most children in this situation do not develop emotional disturbances, though of course their lives are always profoundly affected. It is clinically relevant that children whose parents have a disharmonious marriage are less likely to show disturbance if they have a good relationship with an adult outside the family, take part in an activity for which they receive positive recognition, and enjoy good relationships with their sibs (Jenkins and Smith 1990).

In the management of children whose parents have divorced or are in the process of separating or divorcing, it is likely to be particularly important to arrange separate interviews for the child, so that he can express his feelings and views about the situation privately. Counselling of parents can be undertaken separately or together, depending on the wishes of the parents, with priority being given to the legal parent. The role of the counsellor involved in providing advice concerning children during the process of divorce and separation is beyond the scope of this book, but is well discussed elsewhere (e.g. Levy 1985).

9.2.4 GROUP THERAPY

Definition

The treatment of children and parents in groups can, like individual, family, and behavioural therapy, be both formal and informal. In formal therapy, groups are set up with a particular therapeutic purpose in mind. But group therapy can also be informal, and this occurs especially when, because individuals are already in group settings, such as schools, children's homes, or in-patient units, the opportunity can readily be taken to use group dynamics in a positive, therapeutic manner. Obviously, group processes also occur between staff working in different professional settings such as children's wards and special schools.

Principles

Group therapists can use a number of different underlying theories to underpin their practices:

- *Psychodynamic:* in groups run along psychoanalytic or psychodynamic lines, the emphasis is on the interpretation of unconscious aspects of group interaction. Thus a child who encouraged another in the group to get into trouble might be helped to see that it was he who had the wish to be disruptive himself.
- *Behavioural:* group settings can be used to apply behavioural therapies, taking advantage of the group in different ways. Thus an operant conditioning approach in a classroom might be more effective when applied to a particular child in that setting than when applied individually because reward or reinforcement could involve the whole class of children. A group setting may be particularly appropriate for the use of cognitive behavioural methods: group members assisting each other to check the validity of their self-cognitions.

  In the application of social skills training, a group provides a real-life opportunity to apply such skills with the therapist present and able to monitor the outcome. In a broad sense, social skills training forms part of all group treatments. The way in which limits are set and observed, the laying down of rules, the way in which aggressive behaviour and social isolation are dealt with—all provide possible opportunities for learning social relationships (Sands and Golub 1974).
- *Nurturant:* especially in young children, but also in older, deprived children, application of group treatments may allow children to receive care and attention, as well as experience in sharing, in ways they would otherwise have missed.

Therapeutic groups can also involve groups of parents and groups of families. Parent groups have been set up antenatally (to discuss and interact about issues relating to prospects of parenthood), and postnatally (to consider early experiences and problems in bringing up children). Parent groups have also been established for those whose children have similar behavioural or emotional problems. Thus behaviour modification principles and practice can be effectively and perhaps more economically imparted to groups of parents whose children show, for example, aggressive behaviour. Parent groups run on behavioural lines have also been effective for those with severely developmentally retarded young children. Finally, groups for parents whose children suffer from the same physical condition such as leukaemia or cystic fibrosis have also been found helpful (e.g. Bywater 1984). These provide a combination of support, practical self-help, and information.

Informal group therapy for children themselves has been described in nursery schools and other pre-school educational intervention units, ordinary schools for older children, special schools for maladjusted children, children's homes, and in-patient and day psychiatric units for children and adolescents. More formal group therapy usually takes place in child and family psychiatry departments, but also in special schools and units.

Voluntary self-help groups have been set up for many purposes, either entirely by parents themselves or with initial professional stimulus. Paediatricians and paediatric nurses can play a helpful role here. Examples are groups for parents of very young children run by the National Childbirth Trust, and the very large numbers of parent organizations set up to provide support for parents with children suffering from particular physical conditions. Organizations now exist in the majority of economically developed countries for parents of children with most chronic physical conditions. Many such organizations have now achieved national or even international status, and also have active local branches. In the child mental health field in the UK, Young Minds, MENCAP, and the National Society for Autistic Children are particularly active, and similar organizations exist in other countries.

Practical issues

The setting up of formal groups in a clinical child psychiatric setting presents a number of practical problems, especially difficulties in finding a room of sufficient size and a suitable time when group participants can all attend. For this reason, most formal groups involving children and adolescents take place on in-patient or day units. The age range of the children to be admitted to a group needs attention. It is helpful to think in terms of three main age groups whose needs will differ sufficiently to require age-separation: 4–7 year olds, 8–12 year olds, and adolescents (Lask 1989). Groups generally work better if they are composed of children with similar problems, and, in early and mid-adolescence, if they are single sex. Decisions have to be made about whether the group should be open (allowing newcomers to enter after the group has started) or closed. If inexperienced, group leaders or therapists need the opportunity for supervision. It is helpful to specify to participants the aims of the group, the nature of the limits to be set, the degree of confidentiality, and the likely number of sessions (usually 10–20) to be held. If group therapy is to be combined with individual sessions administered by the same therapist, the possibility of confusion needs to be considered.

Indications and contraindications

Children most likely to benefit from formal group therapy are those with difficulties in their social relationships, especially undue shyness, social isolation, and other forms of anxiety in social situations. Antisocial children may benefit from behavioural techniques applied in a group setting. Children and adolescents who have suffered similar traumatic experiences (e.g. those who have suffered sexual abuse) may benefit from the opportunity to share their experiences and feelings in a group.

Those less likely or unlikely to benefit, at least from formal methods, include those who, like autistic children, do not have the necessary cognitive skills to form social relationships, For other children, such as those where, for example, faulty family communication or intrapsychic problems are predominant, group therapy will not be the preferred mode of treatment.

Evidence for effectiveness

Most evaluative studies of group therapy suffer from serious methodological problems (Abramowitz 1976). However, Kolvin *et al.* (1981) in a careful con-trolled study were able to show that group therapy carried out in schools with groups of 7 year olds and 12 year olds resulted in improvement of neurotic problems (in the younger group) and antisocial as well as neurotic problems in the older age group. Follow-up confirmed that improvement was still detectable 3 years after the children were first assessed, and this form of therapy was more effective than others with which it was compared, such as parent counselling and teacher consultation regimes. Fine *et al.* (1991) demonstrated in a group of adolescents with depressive disorders that, compared to social skills groups, short-term therapeutic support groups were more effective initially, but less so in the longer term.

9.2.5 DRUG THERAPY

Introduction

Medication has a limited but increasing role in the treatment of the psychiatric disorders of childhood and adolescence. Nevertheless, occasionally, appropriate use of medication for the right individual with the right problem can produce highly beneficial effects, especially when used in combination with other forms of psychological, educational, familial, and social intervention. In general, drugs should be given in dosages appropriate to the child's body weight and, where facilities are available, it is desirable to check plasma levels. However, therapeutic dosages can vary substantially from person to person. Unusual or idiosyncratic adverse effects are relatively common, particularly in young people with abnormal central nervous system development, and plasma drug levels may not correlate with clinical response. Hence, paediatric psychopharmacology remains a compli-cated area and highly specialist advice is best sought sooner rather than later.

A number of general principles apply irrespective of medication being considered:

- Medication should never be the initial intervention. Consider psychological, educational, family, and social approaches first. If these are insufficient then consider the cautious addition of medication while maintaining the other approaches.
- Thorough multidisciplinary assessment must be undertaken as a preliminary to any prescription.

- Other interventions should have been tried.
- If problems still persist, consider adding medication as an adjunct to the above approaches and as a means to an end—not an end in itself.
- Treat symptoms (e.g. aggression, overactivity, self-injury) not a syndrome (e.g. autism) or an underlying condition (e.g. fragile X syndrome).
- Undertake a clinical trial of medication. Does it work or not? Are there side-effects?
- Consider the cost–benefit ratio. What is the likelihood of improvement? How important is this? What is the likelihood of side-effects? How serious might they be?
- Beware of the increased risk of side-effects in people with learning disabilities and neurodevelopmental disorders.
- If medication is ineffective, stop it!
- If medication does work, give it for the minimum time possible with frequent monitoring and reviews regarding continuing need and possible side-effects.
- Do not ask whether medication works for people with a particular condition. Ask whether a specific medication may work for a specific behavioural problem.

Most parents are naturally anxious about the use of drugs to treat their children's disorders. Even if the clinician is convinced that a trial of medication would benefit a child, he will wish to take parental anxieties into account when recommending medication. A period of delay to try the effects of other forms of treatment is not usually harmful. Parents are most likely to be persuaded of the need for medication if the clinician explains that his use of drugs is very sparing, that a close eye will be kept for side-effects, that the child will be taken off the drugs as soon as possible, and that the drugs he is prescribing are not, as far as is known, addictive. It is useful to explain to parents that as a rule drugs are not prescribed for emotional or behavioural problems in young people, but as with all good rules there are a few exceptions and this may be one of them.

Because drugs have such a limited place in this age group, only a small number of them will be described here. Fuller information may be found elsewhere (Green 1995; Kaplan and Hussain 1995). Because recommended dosages change, all dosages provided here should be checked before use with a recent edition of an authoritative guide such as the *British National Formulary* (British Medical Association and Pharmaceutical Society of Great Britain 1998).

Hypnotics

Monosymptomatic sleep disorders should wherever possible be treated with advice and behavioural management (see Section 4.3.2). As a short-term measure it is reasonable to use trimeprazine.

Trimeprazine tartrate syrup (Vallergan forte)
Dosage   Approximate dose for 3–6 year old, 3 mg/kg in one dose, i.e. 30–60 mg (1–2 teaspoons).

Side-effects Some children are made less sleepy and more irritable. Headaches, dry mouth.

Comment Use only for periods up to 2 weeks because of habituation.

Benzodiazepines (e.g. diazepam, nitrazepam) and barbiturates are usually contra-indicated because of their addiction potential, rapid habituation necessitating increased dosage and the risk of paradoxical excitation. Other possible hypnotics include *chloral hydrate* (in younger children), *dichloralphenazone*, and *promethazine* (in older children and adolescents). Antidepressant medication given at night (especially *imipramine hydrochloride* and *amitriptyline hydrochloride*—see below) will often improve insomnia in children suffering from depression and may even be beneficial in the absence of depressive symptoms.

There is increasing interest in the endogenous neuropeptide *melatonin* which is produced by the pineal gland and released in response to visually experienced falling light levels. Oral supplements have been shown to facilitate sleep onset and to reduce night-time waking in children with developmental disabilities who have failed to respond to psychological interventions (Jan *et al.* 1994). Melatonin is currently unlicensed and is available only on a named patient basis from the manufacturers. The only major contra-indication seems to be possible aggravation of seizures in children with already-existing epilepsy. Dosage depends on the strength of preparation available but is usually 2–3 mg 30–60 minutes before bedtime increasing to 6–9 mg as required. Single dosage is required. Multiple dosing on each occasion the child wakes is not of benefit. It is important to ensure that the preparation used is a synthetic one, rather than one which has been derived from human or animal tissue, because of the theoretical risk of slow virus transmission.

Minor tranquillizers (anxiolytic agents)

Anxiolytics are little used in child and adolescent psychiatric practice, partly because attacks of anxiety tend to be more episodic, are usually attributable to a specific cause and are less often 'free-floating' than in adulthood. However, short courses (1–3 weeks) of long-acting benzodiazepine medication (*diazepam* or *chlordiazepoxide*) may be indicated for subacute anxiety states in combination with counselling, psychotherapy, behaviour modification, or other therapeutic methods. Longer courses should not be prescribed because of the risk of dependency. Diazepam may also be indicated in sleep disorders such as night terrors and sleep walking when persistent, severe and unresponsive to psychological approaches, and as a pre-anaesthetic for induction of sleep. Rectal diazepam may be indicated in status epilepticus, and has the advantage that parents can be instructed in its use.

Diazepam syrup or tablets

Mechanism Potentiates γ-aminobutyric acid (GABA) activity.

Dosage 2–10 mg daily in two divided doses for children aged 6–12 years; can be increased to 6–15 mg in three divided doses for 13–16 year olds.

Side-effects   Drowsiness, irritability, dizziness, dry mouth, paradoxical excitation.
Comment   Dependency occurs with prolonged usage. For short-term effects, such as to reduce morning anxiety in school-refusing children, it is advisable to use a benzodiazepine with more rapid effects (e.g. lorazepam), but not for more than a few days because of the dependency risk.

Major tranquillizers (neuroleptic agents)

Major tranquillizers are usually reserved for use in psychotic states, for multiple, complex tics, and for the treatment of very severe aggressive outbursts especially in children who have severe learning disabilities. The relief of acute psychotic symptomatology is often dramatic. Maintenance treatment is also of value in the prevention of relapses of schizophrenic states. Drugs to be mentioned here are phenothiazines (*chlorpromazine*) a butyrophenone (*haloperidol*), a diphenylbutylpiperidine (*pimozide*), a substituted benzamide (*sulpiride*), and a benzisoxazole derivative (*risperidone*).

Chlorpromazine syrup, tablets, or intramuscular injection
Mechanism   Blocks activity of dopamine receptors in limbic system.
Dosage   50 mg increasing to 150 mg in 2 or 3 divided doses (approximate maintenance dose for average-sized 13–16 year old with a psychotic state). Higher doses may be necessary in acute states.
Side-effects   Dry mouth, postural hypotension, Parkinsonian symptoms (slowness, rigidity, tremor, salivation), restlessness, acute dystonia. Tardive dyskinesia (a syndrome characterized by delayed onset of stereotyped facial and tongue movements with choreoathetosis) may occur after usage for variable periods of time, and is sometimes irreversible. Withdrawal emergent symptoms consisting of a range of movement disorders may occur when dosage reduction is attempted. Neuroleptic malignant syndrome is a rare but potentially fatal complication consisting of pyrexia, muscle rigidity and the potential for multi-system failure (see Turk and Lask 1991 for review).
Comment   In childhood and adolescence, for use only in diagnosed schizophrenia and acute hypomanic psychotic states because of the potential for serious adverse effects.

Haloperidol syrup, tablets, or intramuscular injection
Mechanism   Blocks dopamine receptors in limbic system.
Dosage   Initially 0.025 mg/kg body weight per day in divided doses, increasing to 0.05 mg/kg per day in divided doses. Higher doses may be prescribed in older adolescents with acute hypomanic or schizophrenic states.
Side-effects   Less drowsiness than chlorpromazine but more likely to cause extrapyramidal side-effects, especially acute dystonic reactions, sometimes with relatively low dosage. Apathy, depression, dry

mouth and nasal congestion are also possible. Orphenadrine 50 mg three times a day or procyclidine 5 mg three times a day can be used to prevent recurrences of extrapyramidal symptoms if they occur, but should not be prescribed routinely.

Comment Main usage of this drug in child and adolescent psychiatry is in treatment of multiple, complex tics, especially Tourette syndrome, in which symptomatic improvement, though not usually complete relief, can often be achieved. It can be used in similar dosage to treat severe outbursts of agitation or aggressive behaviour, especially in young people with severe learning disabilities or autism but care must be taken to minimize treatment duration.

Pimozide
Mechanism Used in tablet form, it acts by similar mechanisms to the phenothiazines and butyrophenones and tends to have a similar side-effect profile, although it may be tolerated better by individuals who have experienced unacceptable side-effects from the above medications.

Dosage Can be administered in a once daily dose of 2–12 mg, or can be taken in divided doses.

Comment As well as having reasonable antipsychotic properties it has been used successfully in the treatment of Tourette syndrome and other severe tic disorders.

Sulpiride
Mechanism A specific antagonist at postsynaptic D_2 dopamine receptors. It also blocks presynaptic dopamine autoinhibitory receptors thereby increasing the concentration of transmitter presented to the postsynaptic receptors. The long half-life (about 10 hours) allows for twice daily dosage (usually 100–800 mg twice daily). It has been said to be particularly useful for 'negative' symptoms of schizophrenia such as apathy, inertia, social withdrawal, and loss of affect, and also has some antidepressant activity.

Side-effects Typical of dopamine antagonists and include dystonic reactions, parkinsonism, akathisia (persistent motor restlessness), tardive dyskinesia and galactorrhoea. However they are less frequent than with other neuroleptic agents. Sedation is rare.

Comment Increasingly being prescribed for Tourette syndrome in young people.

Risperidone (a benzisoxazole derivative)
Mechanism Blocks dopamine 2 and α_1 and α_2 adrenoceptors as well as $5HT_2$ receptors and histamine H_1 receptors. Has a therapeutic effect on both positive and negative symptoms of schizophrenia.

Dosage Should commence with 1 mg twice daily, increasing cautiously with maintenance on the lowest dose possible which should not usually exceed 4 mg twice daily.

Side effects With lower doses extrapyramidal side-effects are not common. Agitation, anxiety and insomnia are less common than with haloperidol. Other possible side-effects include postural hypotension, anxiety, insomnia, headache, fatigue, impaired concentration, dizziness, blurred vision, gastrointestinal symptoms and weight gain.

Comment Of particular benefit for individuals with predominantly negative symptoms, those who have not responded to conventional neuroleptics, and those who have experienced unacceptable extrapyramidal side-effects from them. However, case reports suggest that side-effects may be more common in young people, in particular extrapyramidal symptoms, low mood, weight gain and galactorrhoea (Mandoki 1995).

Other neuroleptic agents sometimes used in psychotic states include the piperidine derivative *thioridazine* which has few extrapyramidal adverse effects but can be quite sedating, and the piperazine derivatives *trifluoperazine* and *fluphenazine* which are less sedating and which have anti-emetic properties as well. In maintenance treatment of schizophrenia, 'depot' injections of fluphenazine decanoate, haloperidol decanoate, or the thioxanthine *flupenthixol decanoate* may be used at intervals of 2–4 weeks.

Stimulant medication

Stimulant medication is of value in pervasive, severe forms of the hyperkinetic syndrome (attention deficit hyperactivity disorder). It is also effective in narcolepsy. In hyperkinetic disorders it should be used in combination with counselling, behaviour modification, special educational measures, and occasionally dietary exclusions.

Methylphenidate tablets (10 mg)

Mechanism Activates inhibitory neuronal pathways. Children with the hyperkinetic syndrome may show underarousal, although findings are inconsistent. This explanation of mechanism is therefore inadequate, and the effects of stimulants remain largely unexplained.

Dosage Initial dose 0.15 mg/kg in one dose before breakfast, increasing to 0.3–0.6 mg/kg in two divided doses, before breakfast and at lunch time. Approximate initial dose in 4–8 year olds is 5 mg at breakfast. Increase stepwise by 5 mg increments mornings and lunch times every 3–4 days up to a maximum of 20 mg breakfast and lunch time.

Side-effects Lack of response in one third, and worsening of target behaviours in a few individuals, especially those with abnormal CNS development. Reduction in appetite with concomitant weight loss. Temporary growth retardation may occur but rectifies when medication is stopped. Excitement, muscular twitching, nervous tics. Dizziness, light-headedness, headaches, tummy aches, insomnia. Very small possibility of small pulse and blood pressure rises.

Comment   There is a substantial literature testifying to the benefits of methylphenidate in disorders of overactivity and attention. There are few
arguments for delaying prescription if the diagnosis is not in doubt.
Response can be rapid and dramatic but only rarely produces
complete symptom resolution. Because of the short half-life, benefits rarely extend beyond 4 hours from time of dosage. Hence
dosage regime must be adjusted carefully to cover important phases
of the day, for example classwork.

Dexamphetamine sulphate tablets
Mechanism   Similar to methylphenidate.
Dosage   Similar to methylphenidate. Tablets are available as 5 mg enabling
finer adjustments of drug regime at lower doses than with methylphenidate.
Side-effects   Similar to methylphenidate. Worth trying where unacceptable
adverse reactions preclude the use of methylphenidate—some
individuals do not show cross-sensitivity.
Comments   Can be used as an alternative to methylphenidate. Adverse reactions with stimulants may be reduced by using medication only on
schooldays, i.e. not at weekends or in school holidays. Addiction
has not been recorded with use of this medication in childhood. To
avoid abuse, it is particularly important not to prescribe large
quantities, and to monitor usage regularly. This medication should
not be used for overactive children with tics or twitching which
may be worsened. Height, weight, pulse, and blood pressure must
be monitored regularly.

   Pemoline sulphate has also been used successfully for the treatment of overactivity and attentional deficits. The longer half-life allows for once daily dosing
and a more consistent and sustained effect. However, recent concerns regarding
possible liver toxicity have lead to its withdrawal from the UK market.

   α_2 *Adrenergic agonists* are also of use in hyperkinetic (attention deficit hyperactivity) disorders.

Clonidine tablets
Mechanism   Uncertain
Dosage   25–50 µg before bedtime or earlier if afternoon and evening excitation is a problem.
Side-effects   Sedation, cognitive blunting, hypotension.
Comment   Of particular use where evening and bedtime settling is a problem
or where attentional deficits and overactivity co-exist with Tourette
syndrome or other tic disorders. Can be prescribed in conjunction
with methylphenidate or dexamphetamine for this purpose. Main
effects are on behaviour. Less useful in enhancing concentration.

   Guanfacine is an alternative α_2 adrenergic agonist which is gaining popularity in North America. It is said to have fewer hypotensive and sedative effects than clonidine. Open study using 1.5 mg/day showed enhanced vigilance and concentration and diminished impulsiveness, distractibility, and tics (Chappell *et al*. 1995).

Antidepressant medication

Antidepressant medication should only be used in children and adolescents in combination with counselling and psychotherapy. It should be reserved for those depressive disorders where there is severe and persistent depression of mood with biological symptoms (appetite and sleep disturbance, diurnal mood variation) and with either reduction in energy or agitation. In these circumstances, until the late 1990s, the tricyclic drugs (*imipramine* and *amitriptyline hydrochloride*) were regarded as the medication of choice. However, meta-analysis of controlled trials of tricyclic drugs in childhood depression have revealed largely negative results (Hazell *et al*. 1995). In general, their use for this purpose in children under the age of 10 years is now not advised, and the selective serotonin reuptake inhibitors may be more effective in the adolescent age group. Because the tricyclics are still quite widely prescribed, details of their mechanism of action, etc. are provided here.

Imipramine hydrochloride (syrup, tablets)

Mechanism	Affects action of neurotransmitters, especially serotonin and noradrenaline, probably by blockage of pre- and postsynaptic receptors. However, this is now regarded as only a partial explanation of their mechanism, which remains largely undetermined.
Dosage	2–3.5 mg/kg per day in two or three divided doses. Approximate initial dose in 10–15 year olds is 25 mg twice daily, increasing by 25 mg increments to 50 mg three times daily in adolescents.
Side-effects	Dry mouth and drowsiness are common. Blurred vision, constipation, nausea, postural hypotension, sweating, rashes. In high doses cardiotoxic effects occur.
Comment	Use in depressive disorders marked by apathy and anergia. ECG monitoring is required if doses of 3.5 mg/kg daily or higher are applied. Therapeutic effects occur only after 7–14 days' medication. Doses of 25–50 mg last thing at night may be used for symptomatic relief of bed-wetting over periods of 1–2 weeks in children aged 7 years or more. Also of use in treating persistent enuresis which is unresponsive to behavioural measures (Rushton 1989) and in hyperkinetic disorders(attention deficit hyperactivity) unresponsive to psychostimulants. Although less effective generally than methylphenidate it can still help reduce hyperactive and impulsive behaviour (Popper 1997).

Amitriptyline hydrochloride

Mechanism, dosage, side-effects	As for imipramine hydrochloride. Prescribing main dosage at night before sleep reduces the risk of drowsiness in the day.

Comment Use in depressive disorders marked by agitation and restlessness. Therapeutic effects only occur after 7–14 days' medication
although sedation which may benefit sleep develops earlier. Dosage
of 25–50 mg at night may be used for symptomatic relief of bed-
wetting over periods of 1–2 weeks in children aged 7 years or older.
Relapse usually occurs when the drug is discontinued.

Enuresis can also be treated pharmacologically with the vasopressin analogue
desmopressin (DDAVP). This can be taken by nasal insufflation (Evans and
Meadow 1992) or as tablets (Matthieson *et al.* 1994) and is a convenient and
safe means of inducing dry nights for short durations such as sleepovers with
friends or relatives, or holiday breaks.

The *selective serotonin reuptake inhibitors* (SSRIs) are a recently developed
family of drugs which inhibit the removal (reuptake) of the monoamine neurotransmitter serotonin (5-hydroxytryptamine) from synapses in the brain and so
prolong their effect on the receptors. Their main indication is for depression
where they produce fewer side-effects, especially sedation and anticholinergic
effects, than the older tricyclic antidepressants while being of at least equal
clinical benefit. However they have also been found to have marked antiobses-
sional qualities making them extremely useful in highly ruminative forms of
depression and in obsessive–compulsive disorder. They all have similar untoward
effects including nausea, diarrhoea, sedation, insomnia, anxiety, agitation, dry
mouth, and blurred vision. Control of pre-existing diabetes mellitus may be
impaired.

Fluoxetine tablets or syrup
Dosage 4–20 mg depending on age and response in one daily dose.
Comment Double-blind, randomized, placebo-controlled evaluation has confirmed the benefits of fluoxetine for children and adolescents (7–17
years old) in the acute phase of a nonpsychotic major depressive
disorder although complete remission of symptoms was rare (Emslie
et al. 1997). Double-blind cross-over placebo-controlled trial has
similarly confirmed the benefits of fluoxetine for obsessive–compulsive disorder in children and adolescents (Riddle *et al.* 1992). There
is, however, some concern that fluoxetine may cause or aggravate
self-injurious ideation or behaviour in some individuals, emphasizing the need for particularly vigilant monitoring of mental state in
patients on this medication (King *et al.* 1991).

Clomipramine is another antidepressant found to be of especial value in
obsessive-compulsive disorders in childhood (Flament *et al.* 1985) as well as in
the treatment of narcolepsy. Controlled comparisons of fluoxetine and clomipramine in the treatment of obsessive–compulsive disorder suggest they are of
similar therapeutic benefit but fluoxetine may cause fewer side-effects (Pigott
et al. 1990). A further SSRI, *fluvoxamine*, has also been reported to be of benefit
in adolescents with obsessive–compulsive disorder or major depressive disorder
at doses of 100–300 mg daily (Apter *et al.* 1994).

Other drugs used in depressive disorders of childhood and adolescence include the monoamine oxidase inhibitors, especially *phenelzine*. Because of the risk of serious side-effects due to dietary non-compliance, regular use of these drugs is not advised in this age group.

In the rarely occurring bipolar affective disorders in older children and adolescents, *lithium carbonate* can be effective in the prevention of relapses (Delong and Aldersdorf 1987). However, the therapeutic window allowing benefits without adverse effects is narrow and side-effects are frequent and potentially serious. These include sedation, tremor, muscle jerking, and precipitation of epilepsy. Nausea, vomiting, diarrhoea, and abdominal pain are dose related. Long-term complications include increased appetite, nephrogenic diabetes insipidus and hypothyroidism. Careful and regular monitoring to avoid overdosage and side-effects is therefore essential yet complex, and should be carried out by those experienced in its use in adult patients.

Anticonvulsant medication

A description of the range of anticonvulsant medication is outside the scope of this book. The general use of anticonvulsants in episodic psychiatric disorders in childhood without clinical evidence of seizure activity is not advised. The presence of EEG abnormalities alone is not thought to be sufficient ground for use of such medication for behavioural purposes.

All types of anticonvulsant medication may have adverse as well as occasionally beneficial effects on behaviour, emotional development, and learning in children with epilepsy (Section 3.8.2). Their use should be closely monitored with this in mind, and difficult behaviour or learning difficulties should indicate the possible need for a change in medication.

Carbamazepine is now prescribed for recurrent mood disorders in adults. Some child psychiatrists are starting to use it in children and adolescents as a safer alternative to lithium for bipolar affective disorders. It can also sometimes be useful for intermittent unpredictable outbursts of aggression or other challenging behaviour in young people with learning disabilities. However, it is not without side-effects which include dizziness, drowsiness, double-vision, nausea and vomiting, and rashes. It should never be combined with lithium therapy because of increased neurotoxicity. Similar therapeutic claims have been made anecdotally for *sodium valproate*. Other newer anticonvulsants (*lamotrigine*, *vigabatrin*, *gabapentin*) can all aggravate or precipitate behaviour problems even if epilepsy is improved.

Monitoring of medication

All forms of medication require careful monitoring, especially in the initial stages of their use. Where appropriate, plasma levels should be measured. These usually tell the clinician more about compliance than whether therapeutic dosage has been reached because of the highly variable plasma levels often associated with improvement. Observations by parents, teachers, and children themselves are a most valuable source of information. The clinician should, however, also make use of his own observations, as parents may, for one reason or another, be biased in favour of or against the use of medication, and this may affect their perception of its effects. There are an increasing number of standardized rating scales which are of use in monitoring behavioural response to medication and these can form a useful objective record. Drugs are, however, unlikely to be effective if parents or children themselves are opposed to their use. When it is reported that children are refusing medication, this may indicate that parents are ambivalent about its use. Conversely, overenthusiasm for medication may be an indication of a risk of neglecting other equally important interventions whether they be psychological, educational or social.

If the child is at school, teachers should always be informed that a child is on medication, and told of its mode of action and likely benefits and possible side-effects. Their observations of the effect of drugs on the child's learning and school behaviour will always be invaluable in monitoring dosage, and should be regularly obtained.

Medication should not be continued unless it is producing clear benefit. This will usually be within 3–4 days with antipsychotic agents, and 2–4 weeks with stimulants and antidepressants. Even if a particular drug has had an initial beneficial effect, an attempt should be made to see how the child copes without the drug from time to time. The point in time at which discontinuation should be attempted will vary with the medication (e.g. after about 3 months with antidepressants, after about 6 months with stimulants, after 2–3 years fit-free with anticonvulsants) and will also vary considerably from child to child. Children will sometimes stay on long-term medication for many years quite unnecessarily if periodic monitoring of this type does not occur.

9.2.6 MISCELLANEOUS THERAPIES

Hypnotherapy

Hypnosis produces a special state of awareness in which an individual is particularly likely to accept from another person, or from himself, suggestions resulting in alterations of sensation or behaviour. Such alterations may then be generalized and experienced in ordinary awareness. There is some debate over whether hypnosis produces an altered state distinct from that produced by other relaxation therapies.

Although the popular view of hypnosis is that it involves one individual, the hypnotist, imposing his will on a subject, perhaps against the subject's will, the therapeutic use of hypnosis for children consists of a very different process. The therapist instead acts as a coach to teach the subject self-hypnosis in order to achieve for himself alterations in sensation or behaviour. The technique used usually involves relaxation-imagery and biofeedback as part of self-hypnosis (Olness 1989).

After an assessment procedure in which an indication for hypnosis is established, the procedure that is to be undertaken is explained to the child:

I am going to help you to relax and then to imagine things that will (help your pain, improve your skin rash, make your headache less painful or less frequent, etc.).

The child is then taught how to achieve muscle relaxation and encouraged to concentrate on images that will result in symptom relief. Imagery that might be effective is arrived at by a discussion between the child and the therapist. Thus the therapist might suggest the child imagines he has a lever inside his head that can control pain, and the child might indicate the lever could work better if, when he thought of it, he also imagined he was lying on a beach in the sun. The child is encouraged to practise self-hypnotic techniques by himself when symptoms occur in everyday life outside the consulting room.

Children of 5 years and even younger can be taught self-hypnosis and indeed, because imaginative skills peak at around the age of 9 years, children are particularly suitable subjects for this form of treatment. The techniques have been used either as the main form of treatment or as an adjunct to therapy in a wide range of common and less common disorders in childhood, including enuresis, headaches, fear of injections, and organically determined as well as psychogenic pain.

There is limited but clear-cut evidence for its effectiveness in a range of situations including pain control. More detailed information on the use of hypnosis in childhood (not to be undertaken without a period of training) is available in Olness and Gardner (1988). The establishment of a hypnotherapy service based in a psychiatric department in a children's hospital has been described by Sokel *et al.* (1990).

Dietary treatment

Dietary measures are used in a wide variety of childhood disorders, and their use often has implications for psychosocial development. Thus, in metabolic disorders such as phenylketonuria and galactosaemia, diets low in phenylalanine and galactose are preventive against the development of mental retardation. In contrast, calorie restriction in obesity and calorie control in anorexia nervosa are examples of dietary treatment in conditions with a significant psychological component in aetiology.

The value of a few-food diet, with gradual introduction of new foods or additives, one at a time, to identify those associated with a worsening of symptoms, has now been confirmed in a number of placebo controlled trials (Carter *et al.* 1993; Schmidt *et al.* 1997) in treatment of the hyperkinetic syndrome (Section 3.4.2). However, it is clear that avoidance of foods, such as sugar, without previous identification of their adverse effects, is most unlikely to result in benefit. Few-food diets have also sometimes been found helpful in the treatment of other stress-related disorders, such as migraine and asthma, but their value in these conditions remains uncertain.

Electroconvulsive therapy (ECT)

The use of ECT is very rarely indicated indeed in children and adolescents. However, it may be beneficial in youngsters with severe depressive illnesses, producing major social impairment, where these have failed to respond to two adequate courses of different forms of antidepressant medication. It is also effective in catatonic states occurring as manifestations of schizophrenia.

ECT should be administered to adolescents only by staff working in centres with experience of this form of treatment. Although the use of ECT in teenagers appropriately produces ethical concerns, there is no reason to withhold the treatment, merely because of age considerations, in those patients likely to benefit symptomatically from it. For a fuller discussion of the use of ECT in adolescents, see Walter and Rey (1997), and guidelines provided by Freeman (1995).

10

Services

Children with mental health problems and their families are served by general health, specialist mental health, education, social, and voluntary services. In this chapter, a description based on UK services is provided, but this will be of relevance to those working in other countries. The relatively unusual features of the health care system in the UK are the comprehensive nature of the primary care service, with family doctors and health visitors (public health nurses) covering the entire population—a service that is free at the point of delivery—and an integration of the preventive and curative services. However, these features are shared by Scandinavian and other western European countries and there are similarities with other health care systems.

10.1 The estimation of service needs

Service needs can be estimated by knowledge of the prevalence of disorders, the efficacy of preventive and curative methods, and the motivation of the population to receive services (Health Advisory Service 1995). Estimates of the prevalence of disorders are provided in the relevant sections elsewhere in this book. A comprehensive epidemiologically based needs assessment for services for child mental health disorders has been provided by Wallace *et al.* (1995), and an estimate of costs by Light and Bailey (1993).

There are several important principles in developing models of care (Wallace *et al.* 1995):

- The majority of child and adolescent mental health problems can be dealt with in primary care.
- Specialists should provide assessment and treatment for other groups.
- The service should be patient centred and there should be patient choice.
- Specialist services should accommodate the spectrum of need.
- Services should be concentrated in areas of greatest need. Professional isolation should be avoided, and there should be good inter-agency collaboration.
- In addition, services should deliver the most cost-effective methods of assessment and treatment and, as far as possible, the choice of methods should be based on the best available scientific evidence.

10.2 Health services for children with mental health problems

The structure of health services for children with behaviour and emotional problems is illustrated in Fig. 10.1.

Tier one: Primary level with interventions by

- Family doctors
- Health visitors
- School nurses
- Social services
- Voluntary agencies
- Teachers
- Residential social workers

Tier two: Professional groups working as individuals

- Clinical child psychologists
- Paediatricians, especially community
- Educational psychologists
- Psychotherapists
- Child and adolescent psychiatrists
- Child psychiatric nurses (community)
- Social workers
- Occupational therapists

Tier three: A specialist multidisciplinary team

- Child and adolescent psychiatrists
- Social workers
- Clinical psychologists
- Community psychiatric nurses
- Child psychotherapists
- Occupational therapists
- Art, music and drama therapists

Tier four: Highly specialist tertiary level services

- In-patient units
- Specialist teams for sexual abuse
- Secure forensic adolescent units
- Eating disorder units
- Specialist teams for neuro-psychiatric problems

Fig. 10.1. Health services for disturbed children and their families.

Mental health services can be considered in four tiers (Health Advisory Service 1995):

- *Tier 1* includes all those agencies that offer first-line services to the public and with whom they make direct contact. Family doctors and health visitors, teachers, school nurses, school medical officers, social workers in child care teams, family aides, carers, and support workers from the statutory and voluntary sectors comprise this tier.

  Although this is often little appreciated, this tier of services is already deeply involved in assessing and providing first line treatment for children with mental health problems and their families. For example, psychosocial problems and physical problems with an important psychosocial component form a large part of family practice consultations with children (Bailey *et al.* 1978), and about a quarter of child attenders at family practitioners show psychiatric disorders (Garralda and Bailey 1986).
- *Tier 2* consists of mental health professionals working as individuals, though they also form part of multidisciplinary teams. They include psychiatrists, psychologists, social workers, psychotherapists, community psychiatric nurses, and occupational therapists. Again they provide assessment and treatment as

well as advice to those working in Tier 1, as well as to more specialist professionals in other fields such as paediatricians. Finally, they act as gatekeepers for Tiers 3 and 4.

- *Tier 3* provides multidisciplinary team assessment for more complex problems by those working as individuals in Tier 2. The teams may be generic, dealing with a range of problems, or specialist, for example in substance abuse or family therapy.
- *Tier 4* consists of very specialized services such as those provided in psychiatric in-patient units or by day units specialising in the assessment and treatment of rare disorders such as autism or psychiatric problems in children with severe hearing impairment.

General and paediatric health services will be considered first, and an account will then be given of specialist child mental health services.

10.2.1 PRIMARY GENERAL AND PAEDIATRIC HEALTH SERVICES

Family doctor services

Psychosocial problems and physical problems with an important psychosocial component form a large part of general practice consultations with children. One study (Bailey *et al.* 1978), found that 'pure' psychological problems accounted for 4% of such consultations, physical symptoms with definite psychological problems for 7%, and physical symptoms with possibly important psychological factors for a further 16%. A further 9% of consultations were for 'undifferentiated' disorders in which psychological factors were probably relevant. In all, including overlap, 32% of child referrals to general practitioners were for one of these four reasons. As about 90% of 0–4 year olds and 60% of 5–14 year olds attend their general practitioners at least once a year, this means that family doctors regularly see a high proportion of their child patients for psychosocial reasons. Independent assessment of child attenders at family practitioners suggests that about a quarter show psychiatric disorder (Garralda and Bailey 1989) and, not surprisingly, disturbed children are more likely to present with complaints such as anxiety and bed-wetting. Parents of disturbed children are particularly likely to be socially stressed at the time of consultation.

There are a number of special characteristics of these primary care consultations. The child is usually accompanied only by the mother, there is usually a physical presenting symptom, and the consultation is usually relatively brief (in the UK lasting an average of about 10–12 minutes). The disorders that present are often difficult to classify using a formal psychiatric classification.

Facilities

The frequency of primary care consultation for psychosocial reasons means that the facilities available to conduct these should be adequate. There should be a good supply of toys and books suitable to divert the child, and learn about his developmental level as well as something of his fantasy life. Such toys and books need to be as carefully looked after as the sphygmomanometer and tendon hammer, and put away when not in use. There should be sufficient privacy for confidential material to be communicated without being overheard.

The consultation

The principles of assessment for a psychosocial problem are described elsewhere (Section 1.5). In primary care, evaluation inevitably has to be rapid, though it is helpful if, when the need arises, the practitioner can put aside time for a longer consultation. Concentration on the reason for attendance at the present time, on the onset, nature, and severity of the presenting symptom, and on the presence or absence of other family problems, is usually profitable. The nature of treatment suggested will depend on the type of problem presented. Encouragement to return if the problem persists will enable the practitioner to identify those chronic disorders that require referral. Many family practitioners and primary care paediatricians have difficulty in identifying appropriate children for referral (Dulcan *et al.* 1990), and there is an important need for the training of doctors in primary care for psychosocial aspects of their work.

Experienced health visitors and family practitioners will, for example, be alert to the fact that a mother who brings a child with an apparently trivial physical complaint may be using this symptom as an 'admission ticket' for a discussion of a problem that is more important to her (e.g. a behaviour problem in the child, or a marital difficulty) which she would be reluctant to raise without some prompting.

Child health clinics

These are run both by the community health services and increasingly by health visitors (child health nurses) and family practitioners for surveillance and preventive activities. The preventive service offered includes vaccination and immunization, weighing and measuring, physical (especially sensory) examination, and developmental checks. In the UK over 90% of babies are brought to these clinics in the first year of life but subsequently, in most areas, attendance drops off fairly sharply. Although most work in these clinics is directed towards pre-school children, some authorities also run special clinics on the same premises for school-aged children. Special clinics for children with enuresis and obesity are those most commonly arranged.

Although it is generally agreed that regular surveillance of a child population for checks on hearing, vision, etc. is desirable, there is less agreement about the value of identifying behaviour and emotional problems (Hall 1989). However, check-lists suitable for this purpose in young children have been developed (Richman *et al.* 1982), and found of value especially by health visitors. It is important for health visitors and doctors conducting surveillance examinations to enquire routinely about the presence of behaviour and emotional disorders, bearing in mind their frequency, significance, and impact on family life.

There are significant psychosocial aspects to the delivery of a comprehensive, preventive programme. Children living in disorganized families, of low socio-economic status, and from minority ethnic groups are most likely to be missed. An outreach system with careful record-keeping can, nevertheless, achieve good results even in deprived areas. There is evidence that child-centred counselling of mothers of infants and toddlers based in family practice can reduce rates of behaviour and emotional problems occurring subsequently.

There is in any event a large psychosocial component to work in child health clinics. Mild and moderate developmental delays are often produced by understimulation and poor social circumstances. Early feeding problems of psychosocial origin and failure to thrive are commonly identified as causes for concern in children seen in clinics. They offer an opportunity for counselling of mothers in child-rearing practices. In toddlers, behaviour problems such as sleep difficulties and other adjustment problems are often mentioned to doctors or health visitors by mothers in need of advice and counselling.

Such clinics should contain attractive and well-kept play material as well as adequate equipment for weighing and measuring, developmental assessment, sensory testing, and physical examination. There should be a room available that can be used for discussion of confidential matters. Good communication between community health doctors and nurses and general practitioners will ensure that if conditions requiring treatment are identified, therapy can be readily arranged.

Links with other agencies

Primary medical care involving psychosocial problems is likely to be much more effective if there are opportunities for close working with other professionals and agencies. The health visitor (district community nurse) working as part of a primary health care team will, in fact, often be able to take responsibility for a major component of this work. Attachment of social workers to general practice is becoming more frequent. Regular outreach visits from child psychiatric agency staff to primary care facilities have occasionally been described. Especially in small communities, the general practitioner will be able to make useful contacts with local schools and social workers.

10.2.2 SECONDARY GENERAL PAEDIATRIC HEALTH SERVICES

Community paediatric team

The community paediatric team consists of a community paediatrician, community nurse, educational psychologist, social worker, speech therapist, and physiotherapist (Polnay *et al.* 1996). Other specialists, such as a hospital paediatrician, audiologist, orthopaedic surgeon, occupational therapist, and child psychiatrist may also attend as required, and sometimes do so regularly. Children suspected of developmental disorders, physical or mental handicap, and sensory deficits, are often referred to such teams for further assessment and advice, especially concerning future schooling. Such teams are often sited in a hospital- or community-based child development centre, where children are assessed and may attend subsequently on a daily, weekly, or less frequent basis, for further assessment and treatment. Mental handicap and learning disorders, epilepsy, and behaviour problems are the diagnoses most frequently made in children attending child development centres (Bax *et al.* 1988), so the contribution of mental health professionals is clearly essential.

As already indicated, children suffering from neurological conditions and mental handicap have high rates of emotional and behavioural disorders. Parents of children with disabilities are also in need of counselling. There is therefore a strong case for those working in such units to have well-developed skills in the assessment of psychiatric disorders and in parent counselling. Close links with the child psychiatric service are desirable, and there are considerable advantages in a regularly occurring psychiatric liaison consultation service (Evered *et al.* 1989).

School medical service

The school medical service is staffed largely by school nurses and doctors, speech therapists, and physiotherapists. In most authorities, all children are medically screened on school entry (Whitmore and Bax 1986) but, subsequently, screening examinations are usually selective. In some authorities even the school entry medical examination is selective, based on a screening procedure carried out by the school nurse (O'Callaghan and Colver 1987). Regular examinations are more likely to be held for children attending special schools, such as schools for the physically or mentally handicapped.

As well as the medical examination of children with learning problems and behavioural difficulties so as to identify underlying physical causes (e.g. sensory defects), staff of the school health service may also be asked to ensure that teachers understand the nature of physical disorders suffered by children they are teaching. Children may be referred to them because of suspicion of ill-treatment or neglect. Although the school psychologist is likely to be the main source of advice, school doctors and nurses may be asked about children with emotional and behaviour problems, especially if the child has an associated physical condition. They may also be asked to provide information to teachers to help them run classes on health education, sex education, birth control, and preparation for parenthood. Teachers may also require help in identifying and dealing with drug abusers. Members of the school health service are required to assess and produce medical reports on children thought to be in need of special education.

For most of these tasks, school doctors and nurses require training in the psychosocial aspects of their work. Good communication with general practitioners, hospital paediatric services, social workers, educational psychologists, and other staff working in child psychiatric units is essential.

Hospital care

In about 5–10% of children attending general paediatric clinics a mental health problem is the main reason for attendance (Garralda and Bailey 1989), though psychosocial factors are prominent in a much higher proportion. About a quarter of such children are showing concomitant psychiatric disorder at the time of referral, and the families of disturbed children are particularly likely to be under stress. Vomiting and feeding difficulties, failure to thrive, abdominal pain, constipation, and chronic headache all very frequently have strong psychosocial implications and are common reasons for referral.

There are many advantages to the provision of separate out-patient facilities for children and, in developed countries, these are increasingly available. The availability of trained paediatric nursing staff, and the provision of appropriate decoration, toys, and books are more likely to occur if there are separate out-patient facilities for children. As psychosocial problems are so common, it is important that privacy is available so that parents can feel comfortable when communicating confidential information.

The distress of anticipating painful procedures in child out-patients can be reduced in a number of ways. A satisfactory appointment system geared to the needs of families has been achieved in some out-patient departments. Obviously, medical staff may sometimes be required to attend to emergencies, but planning ahead can sometimes reduce this occurrence. The provision of play staff in the out-patient department can do much to reduce unnecessary anxiety, especially if there are unexpected delays. Preparation for procedures is as important in out-patient as in in-patient care. Children with chronic disorders should, if at all possible, be seen for review appointments by the same member of staff whenever they attend. The continuing attendance of children merely because they have 'interesting' conditions should be discouraged. There should be clear aims for every out-patient attendance and, if junior staff are involved, these aims should be made explicit to them. If satisfactory care can be carried out by the general practitioner or health visitor, with a referral back to hospital as necessary, this should always be preferred to continuing hospital or out-patient appointments.

Ready availability of a paediatric medical social worker and member of a child psychiatric team for appropriate referrals will also improve the quality of care available for children seen in out-patients who have psychosocial components to their problems. Psychosocial aspects of the care of hospitalized children are discussed in Section 7.6.

The considerable psychosocial component in paediatric practice means that there is a real need for paediatricians to receive training in psychosocial aspects of their work (Graham and Jenkins 1985).

10.2.3 SPECIALIST CHILD MENTAL HEALTH SERVICES

A comprehensive mental health service for children and adolescents may be expected to include the following.

Child and family psychiatric clinic or out-patient departments

The out-patient facility may be situated either in the community, usually in a health centre or education authority premises, or form part of the local hospital service. The department is usually staffed by a child psychiatrist, psychologist (educational and/or clinical), and social worker. In some parts of the UK, especially around London, child psychotherapists may also be members of clinic staff. The clinics generally take referrals from a range of other professionals—especially general practitioners, paediatricians, teachers, and social workers (including probation officers). Clinics situated in education authority premises usually have a high proportion of school referrals with behaviour problems and learning difficulties. Services based in health centres see a high proportion of young children and children with physical complaints thought to be of psychological origin.

Assessment and treatment are usually provided by all the professionals working in the clinic, with a variable degree of specialization (see below). In some clinics, most families are seen by more than one professional (working conjointly); in others this is unusual. Most children and families are seen in the clinic, but home visiting is a prominent feature of the work of some clinics. A relatively new development in the UK is the establishment in some districts of a community child psychiatric nursing service. In most clinics a good deal of emphasis is placed on outreach consultation with other agencies, so that often as much as one-third of a child mental health professional's time is spent discussing problems with other professionals, especially teachers and social workers (Black *et al.* 1974).

Psychiatric day centres

Children are admitted for whom continuing home care is practicable and desirable, but who, it is thought, will benefit from a full daily programme of care. In the younger, pre-school age group, these are often children with severe developmental disorders and management problems. In older children, school refusal and behavioural disorders in the school setting are common reasons for admission (Kiser *et al.* 1995).

Most day centres cater for a fairly narrow age range: pre-school (2–5 years), middle childhood (6–12 years), or teenage (13 years or older). Centres dealing with the pre-school group usually involve the parents very actively in the treatment programme, and some will accept the child only if one or both parents attend at the same time. Treatment usually consists of both group and individual therapy, with the type of therapy depending on the orientation of the clinic. There is an increasing tendency to use focused behavioural methods.

The staffing pattern is very variable. Some are staffed mainly by social workers and others by nurses and nursing aides. There is also variable input from mental health professionals, but in many cases there is committed input from one or two psychiatrists or psychologists. There is a variable amount of contact with paediatric facilities, special schools, and day nurseries depending on where the centre is sited and the ages of the children admitted. Evidence is lacking for the effectiveness of such centres (Richman *et al.* 1983) in terms of symptom improvement, but they have an important and valuable assessment function, and delayed development may be accelerated (Cohen *et al.* 1987). Further, children and families are helped and supported over crises and escalations in chronic conditions by attendance at such centres.

Walk-in centres

There is a variety of other types of assessment and treatment facilities for disturbed children and adolescents. Walk-in centres for adolescents, who might not be prepared to accept conventional patterns of referral through general practitioners, etc., are becoming more common. These are most commonly staffed by social workers and volunteer counselling staff, sometimes with a mental health professional available for consultation. A small number of such facilities staffed mainly by psychologists, psychiatrists and psychotherapists have been described.

In-patient units

The need for specialized psychiatric residential assessment and treatment facilities for children and adolescents will depend on the availability of other residential facilities. Thus, a high level of special residential educational provision for children with emotional and behavioural disorders, and ready availability of substitute care by social service departments for children whose parental care has broken down, will reduce the need for in-patient facilities. Nevertheless, a proportion of severely disturbed children will require such specialized psychiatric facilities. These include:

- children with complex paedo-psychiatric disorders (e.g. non-organic seizures, anorexia nervosa, encopresis) which have failed to respond to out-patient treatment or paediatric management
- children where home care has broken down or threatened to break down and who are, for example, too aggressive or too anxious to be placed in social service or educational facilities
- children with severe psychiatric disorders, for example psychotic depression and schizophrenia, who, it is thought, would benefit from the special skills available in an in-patient unit.

The age range of children admitted to psychiatric in-patient units usually ranges from 5–6 years up to puberty, and in adolescent units from puberty up to 17–18 years. There is, however, much variation. The main assessment and therapeutic input is usually provided by skilled nurses with psychiatric and/or paediatric training as well as the other mental health disciplines. Schooling is usually available on the premises of the unit, and other professionals, for example occupational therapists and speech therapists, may play a very active part.

The assessment and treatment philosophy of in-patient units varies considerably. Some admit only a highly selected group of disturbed children; others are much less selective. Some base their treatment mainly on psychoanalytic principles, others on behavioural principles. Most are eclectic, and put a good deal of emphasis on working with the family and trying to ensure that gains made in the unit are maintained at home. On discharge, a significant proportion of children are transferred to other residential units, especially residential schools for children with emotional and behaviour problems.

Mental health professionals

The following description is applicable in the UK, although a similar pattern of professional work and training exists in other developed countries.

Child and adolescent psychiatrists

Consultants have had specialized training in child psychiatry in this field for $3\frac{1}{2}-4\frac{1}{2}$ years, following a medical education, general medical and surgical experience, preferably some paediatric experience, and experience in general (adult) psychiatry. In the field of child mental health, although his work will cover the whole range of child psychiatric disorders, the psychiatrist has a special contribution to make where the presenting complaints are somatic, there is a possibility of psychosis, autism, or other serious mental disorder in the child, one or other parent is suffering from a mental illness, or there is a possibility that medication might be helpful to the child.

Child psychologists

There are two types of child psychologist in the UK, educational and clinical.

- Normally the *educational psychologist* will have initially obtained a teaching qualification and then taught in ordinary or special school for some time. He or she will then have taken a 1 year postgraduate course in educational psychology. He/she will spend a good deal of time working in schools, and will have special skills in the evaluation of learning and behavioural problems and in the development of remedial programmes.
- Following a first degree in psychology, and (usually) some practical experience in a health service or social service setting, *clinical psychologists* have taken a 2–3 year postgraduate course in clinical psychology. The special skills of the clinical psychologist lie in systematic assessment of behavioural deviance, and the development and evaluation of behavioural programmes, but many have also developed skills in counselling and psychotherapy. Some clinical psychologists work in the field of mental handicap, where their work particularly involves devising individualized and group programmes for the promotion of social and cognitive development.

Social workers

Social workers have usually taken a first degree and had some practical experience before embarking on the certificate of qualification in social work (CQSW). Their special skills lie in the evaluation of family situations in which the child is at risk, and there is a need for family support, with concern that the child may not be receiving adequate care and protection. They have statutory responsibilities where a child is seriously at risk. Their counselling skills are likely to be highly developed.

Child psychotherapists

Child psychotherapists are normally expected to have a first degree, followed by some practical experience in working with children in a field such as teaching, before embarking on a course lasting at least 4 years that includes a personal psychoanalysis. Their special skills are in individual psychotherapy with children, and assessment of the role psychodynamic factors are playing in psychological or psychosomatic problems, but increasingly they are using their skills in consultation and liaison services.

Common skills

All child mental health professionals (except for child psychotherapists, who are usually more specialized) have shared skills in the systematic assessment of behavioural and emotional disorders of children. They are all skilled in the counselling of both individual parents and children. Most are likely to be able to apply both psychodynamic and behavioural methods in the treatment of mental health problems in children and families. They are able to provide consultation with professionals working in other agencies. In many child and family psychiatric clinics and departments, a substantial proportion of the work is carried out interchangeably by members of all the disciplines represented.

Organization of child mental health services

Organization varies considerably from country to country, and the following description applies only to the UK.

The child and adolescent psychiatric service is staffed by child psychiatrists (employed by the health authority), social workers (employed by the local authority's social services department), and educational psychologists (employed by the local authority education department). Clinical psychologists and psychotherapists are employed by the health authority. These professionals all work together, usually in premises maintained by the health authority (hospital or health centre), or local education authority. Each health district and local authority determines its own pattern of service to ensure that, as far as possible, a full range of residential and community facilities is available, if not within the area at least reasonably close by. Disturbed children and adolescents may be placed outside the health district in a regional in-patient unit. A local education authority may arrange for disturbed pupils to attend a special school run by its own or another authority.

Each clinical department determines its own pattern of work within a contract negotiated with a purchasing authority. Thus the way of dealing with referrals, sharing of work, exercise of individual clinical responsibility, supervision, etc. is locally arranged. In most clinics, a substantial amount of work is 'extramural' and involves consultation with a number of different agencies outside the clinic, including ordinary and special schools, paediatric services, and the juvenile courts. In many areas, the demands made on the child mental health service mean that it is overstretched and priorities have to be established. This usually involves an emphasis on care for the most severely disturbed, on the use of short-term focused treatment procedures, and on consultation with other non-mental health professionals to enable them to work more successfully with disturbed children and their families.

10.3 Social services and child protection

The majority of parents are able to provide conditions for their children that are adequate or more than adequate to enable them to thrive physically, emotionally, and intellectually. A significant minority are, however, unable to provide this level of care. Indications that children are not receiving adequate care include evidence of physical neglect, failure to thrive, or slow intellectual development, as well as non-accidental injury and emotional and sexual abuse. Some of these problems may, of course, be due to factors other than inadequate parental care. Certain types of behaviour, such as primary attachment disorders, may also indicate emotional deprivation.

As well as these signs in the child of inadequate parental care, there are also a number of risk factors in the family and environment that should alert the professional to the possibility that care might be inadequate. Professionals should, however, be wary of jumping to conclusions concerning inadequacy of care on the basis of the presence of one or more of these risk factors. Many children brought up in unusual circumstances do in fact receive excellent care. There are, for example, many one-parent families in which the quality of child care is better than in some two-parent families. The following is a brief summary of family and environmental factors that suggest a child may be at risk of inadequate care.

- *Parental marital disharmony.* About 1 in 5 children are brought up in families where the parental relationship is characterized by constant disagreements, quarrelling and interpersonal tension, and more severe forms of domestic violence.
- *Marital breakdown and divorce.* About 1 in 4 children will have experienced the breakdown of the parental relationship by the age of 16 years. In many cases there will have been a prolonged period of parental disharmony, sometimes with parental separation, before the breakdown occurs.
- *Lone parent families.* About 1 child in 5 is, in the late 1990s, brought up by one parent; in about 1 in 10 cases of lone parenthood, the lone parent is the father (Office of National Statistics 1997). Single parents vary greatly in the amount of social support they receive from the other parent, from family members, friends, neighbours, and professional agencies.
- *Parental mental illness.* The impact of parental mental health problems, such as depression, disturbed personality functioning, alcoholism, and psychosis is discussed in Section 1.3
- *Poverty.* It has been estimated that about 1 in 8 children in the UK are living at or below the poverty line, calculated on the basis of their parents' entitlement to income support.
- *Poor housing.* Many children live in unsatisfactory, cramped accommodation with inadequate indoor or outdoor space to play. About 1% of children in the UK are living in accommodation made available to homeless families by local authorities, and these are at considerable psychosocial risk (Vostanis *et al.* 1997).

- *Racism*. Children of ethnic minorities readily identifiable by their colour are frequently subject to harassment by other children and adults . The widespread extent of racial abuse has been well documented.

It is a central task of the social worker, usually employed in the local authority's social services department, to monitor and seek to improve the lives of those children whose care appears inadequate or who are at risk. The Children Act 1989 states that when a court determines any question with regard to the upbringing of a child, the child's welfare shall be the court's paramount consideration. The Act goes on to describe parental inadequacy in terms of lack of 'reasonable parental care' resulting in the child suffering significant harm or being likely to suffer significant harm. However, all other professionals in contact with children and families have a duty to identify situations of unsatisfactory child care, to provide what help they can, and, in situations of serious risk and inadequacy, to refer the child to the local social services department. Various means of informal and formal protection for the child are possible.

10.3.1 FAMILY SUPPORT

The family unit is the main source of protection for children. Consequently, the main aim of those involved in ensuring the care and protection of children is to support the cohesiveness of the family unit and prevent family breakdown.

Part III of the Children Act (mentioned above) states that it shall be the general duty of every local authority to safeguard the welfare of the children within their area who are in need, by providing a range of appropriate services. Children 'in need' are defined as those in whom health or development are likely to be significantly impaired or who are disabled. Health includes both physical and mental health, and development includes emotional, social, and behavioural as well as physical development.

Various approaches to family support are possible. In all cases voluntary action is regarded as preferable to compulsory, legal measures, but in certain circumstances, the law has to be invoked for the protection of the child.

Anticipatory action

The anticipation of crises in family life can diminish adverse effects on children. Thus if, for example, a woman with schizophrenia becomes pregnant, careful assessment of her capacity to care for her child will become necessary. Family centres can frequently provide monitoring and support. The social services department is responsible for co-ordinating a range of services such as domiciliary support, respite care or, if necessary, removal of the child either by voluntary agreement or legal intervention. In all instances, arrangements for contact by the parent and other appropriate family members will be promoted as long as this is considered consistent with the welfare of the child. Similar action will be indicated in many other circumstances, for example on the release of a violent partner from prison or when a lone parent has to go into hospital.

Social work with families in crisis or under chronic stress

Partnership with service users
In all instances, social workers try to work *with* parents, but in those situations where the parent is unable or unwilling to provide adequate care, social workers, by virtue of their prime responsibility to support and protect the child, may well be in conflict with the parent. Social work practice is frequently informed by psychodynamic and attachment theories, but, generally speaking, has more supportive and fewer interpretative features than formal psychotherapy. In more recent times, social workers have tended to focus more on achievement of behavioural change and with empowering their clients, especially those who are vulnerable because of discrimination against them on grounds of race, gender, religion, or culture.

Financial provision
Professionals can ensure that families are in receipt of those statutory benefits to which they are entitled. Social workers are also able to assess financial need in families and, if appropriate, arrange for payment of discretionary benefits. Health professionals should be aware of benefits to which parents of handicapped children are entitled. For example, in the UK, disability living allowance is payable to parents of children aged 2–16 years who are severely disabled and require a great deal of extra attention.

Other practical assistance
Professionals can also assist children of families under stress by checking that they are receiving appropriate health care and education, or in other ways, for example by arranging placements for pre-school children in day nurseries or school-age children in holiday play schemes. Children in problem families or with chronic disabilities may be considerably helped by the availability of family centres or the provision of a family aide who may visit the family daily and provide practical assistance as well as counselling.

Brief respite care
Families can also be supported in times of stress by temporary arrangements whereby a child spends a short period in a children's home, in day or short-term foster care, or, in the case of children with unusual nursing needs, in hospital. Such care may be particularly helpful for handicapped children who may place extra strain on a family's resources.

Child-minding

Most child-minding is provided by other family members, but a substantial proportion is carried out for a daily charge by women who look after a small number of children in their own homes. The quality of such day care varies considerably, from the highly satisfactory to the very inadequate. Some children receive care that is a considerable improvement on the care they receive in their own home, while others may be looked after in a crowded, poorly illuminated room with no toys and little contact with adults. Child-minding is regulated in the UK by the Children Act 1989. Local authorities have a duty to keep a register of people who use their homes to look after children aged under 8 years for payment. Inspection of the premises and of the circumstances in which children are being looked after must be carried out at least once a year. Children whose mothers go out to work and arrange adequate substitute care with child-minders do not appear to be significantly emotionally or intellectually advantaged or disadvantaged by the experience (Graham 1990), although clearly their opportunities for making a wider range of relationships with both adults and other children are likely to be increased.

Day nurseries, nursery schools, playgroups

- *Day nurseries*, run by social services departments and staffed mainly by nursery nurses, provide care especially for children whose mothers are in special need, through social disadvantage or illness. They may take children of any age up to school entry.
- *Nursery schools*, run by local authority education departments, provide more formal learning experiences for children aged 3–5 years.
- *Playgroups*, usually run by voluntary agencies, provide less formal experience often for a limited number of half days per week, for children usually aged between $2\frac{1}{2}$ and 5 years.

The quality of care in all these types of establishment varies considerably, and consequently it has not been possible to draw general conclusions concerning the value of attendance.

10.3.2 SUBSTITUTE CARE FOR CHILDREN

Children may be placed in substitute care on residential basis either voluntarily or following court proceedings.

Children's homes

Substitute care for children in children's homes is now generally seen as an unsatisfactory form of care, except on a short-term basis. Nevertheless, there remain a number of children for whom other forms of care are unavailable. In contrast to former times, children's homes now usually contain relatively small numbers of children (usually 6–12) and provide much more personalized care. Some do achieve a high level of care, but the quality is uneven (Berridge and Brodie 1997). Unsatisfactory features of some children's homes in the UK include rapid turnover of staff and a high proportion of relatively inexperienced, untrained staff (Utting 1997).

Outcome

Early descriptions of the cognitive and personality outcome of children reared in children's homes painted a gloomy picture. The mortality of infants admitted into such homes was high. A high proportion of older children were seriously disturbed and had poor educational attainments. In adulthood, the rate of personality disorder was also raised. These findings related to children who had been brought up in large and often impersonal homes in the pre-war years.

Following the Second World War, the quality of care in children's homes improved. Staffing ratios were increased, and staff showed increased awareness and sensitivity to psychological problems shown by the children themselves. Nevertheless, staff turnover usually remained high, so that children still often did not have the opportunity of a continuous relationship with one or two adults. Rates of behaviour and emotional problems in children in children's homes remained elevated (Wolkind and Rutter 1973). Early cognitive development, including language development (Tizard *et al.* 1972), was usually normal, though in later childhood educational retardation was common.

Follow-up studies of girls reared in children's homes in the 1960s into adulthood suggest that they have high rates of psychiatric problems (Wolkind and Kruk 1985) and show more inadequacy in caring for their own children than do controls (Quinton and Rutter 1985). Nevertheless, a high proportion have a reasonably favourable personality development; their capacity to look after their own children is much enhanced if they meet a supportive partner.

These findings point to the need to provide family care and, if appropriate, adoption for children whose biological parents are unable to look after them. Inevitably, because of problems such as difficulty in obtaining parental consent, or severe behavioural difficulties in the child or young person, family care will not be feasible in some circumstances. The training and continuity of staff working in such homes remain a matter of concern.

Permanency planning

The consequences of the provision of inadequate substitute care and delays in decision-making by social workers, courts, and indeed parents themselves, have led to a realization that there is always a need to make a long-term plan for children whose parents cannot take full responsibility for them. The concept of 'permanency planning' has been introduced with this in mind. Those concerned with the welfare of such children, including mental health professionals, need to ensure that children do not drift from one set of unsatisfactory temporary placements to another.

Foster care

Fostering involves the care and maintenance of a child by a person who is not a relative, guardian, or custodian. Long-term fostering is the usual arrangement when care is no longer possible for the child in his biological family, but arrangements for adoption cannot be made. Although, in some circumstances, the consent to adoption by biological parents who cannot themselves look after a child is no longer necessary, there are still a number of situations in which adoption is not feasible. Local authorities have statutory duties concerning the selection of foster carers and supervision of foster care. Although most fostering arrangements are dictated by impending or actual family breakdown, fostering has also been employed positively as a means of rehabilitating adolescents with antisocial problems (Hazel 1977). In the US, treatment fostering schemes with built-in mental health service provision deal with children with a wide range of psychiatric disorders. This is a promising development, and a review of 40 published studies showed many positive results (Reddy and Pfeiffer 1997).

Outcome

Some children spend the whole of their childhood and adolescence in a single long-term fostering placement. Others have multiple foster placements over a long period of time, and, for yet others, a brief period of foster care may be a single interruption in a childhood otherwise spent with the biological family. It is not surprising therefore that follow-up studies of children who have been fostered are few and that outcome is very mixed. It seems likely that children who have multiple foster placements have a high likelihood of developing disturbance, but it is improbable that this can be attributed entirely to fostering. Such children usually experience, in addition, numerous separations, deprivation, and inconsistency of care (Berridge and Cleaver 1987).

Nevertheless, certain special problems concerned with fostering have emerged. Children undergoing this experience are particularly likely to be confused about their relationship to their original family as well as to the foster family. Their uncertain and temporary status often creates particular insecurity. They may be sensitive to rejection and respond to threats of further change with angry or anxious reactions.

There are various implications of these findings. The selection and support of foster parents needs careful appraisal, though in some communities, identification of sufficient, suitable families to foster children presents difficulties. While children are in foster care, it is desirable for children to remain in contact with their biological parents providing this is what the child wants, it is considered consistent with the child's welfare, and it is not seriously disruptive to the foster placement. To avoid confusion and distress, such contact may need to be facilitated and supervised. As far as possible, where repeated foster placements are necessary for a child, they should be arranged with the same family. Foster parents who are temporarily fostering children with chronic physical disorders or mental handicap need to know as much about the management of the disorder as do the biological parents. If, as is often the case, the fostered children show signs of psychiatric disorder, their foster carers need to have easy access to appropriate mental health professional advice.

Adoption

For children whose natural parents have no prospect of providing adequate care for them in the future, it is generally agreed that adoption into another family with permanent and legally binding transfer of parental rights is the most satisfactory procedure. Adoption proceedings can be taken by a local authority social services department, a registered adoption agency, or a parent or guardian direct.

Once parents have adopted a child, they have the same rights and duties as biological parents.

Applications to adopt a child are considered by an Adoption Panel. The panel considers social work reports and medical assessments of the child, the biological parents and the prospective adopters. When a decision has been reached that adoption is in the best interests of the child, that the prospective adopters are suitable, and the match between the needs of the child and the parenting offered by the prospective adopters is appropriate, then the child can be placed. The prospective adopters can apply for an Adoption Order 3 months after placement. The court will then appoint a guardian ad litem, that is a social worker or probation officer appointed by the court to ensure the child's interests are fully represented in the decision it will make. The consent of the biological parent to the adoption is normally required, though in certain special circumstances, for example mental illness, mental handicap, or prolonged parenting incapacity, consent may be dispensed with.

The easier availability of contraception and more permissive legislation for abortion has meant that there is a smaller number of babies available for adoption to infertile couples. Consequently, a much higher proportion of adoptions now involve more 'difficult to place' children. These include older, often disturbed children, those of mixed race or black parentage, and children with mental and/or physical handicaps. There are specialist adoption agencies to facilitate arrangements for adoption of these children with special needs.

Outcome

The educational and behavioural outcome of children adopted in the first few months of life and reared throughout childhood in the same adoptive family is very similar to that of a biological child brought up in the same circumstances. If the family is able to provide reasonably warm, consistent care and the child is not exposed to unusual stress, the chances of problematic behaviour are low. Nevertheless, there may be some differences. A great majority of adopted children have normal intelligence, but the correlation between the IQ of adopted children and their adoptive parents is lower than that between non-adopted children and their biological parents. Adopted children, especially adopted boys, have slightly higher rates of behavioural disturbance than non-adopted children, and these differences increase towards adolescence (Lambert and Streather 1980). However, rates in adoptive children are still distinctly lower than those in children brought up in homes broken by divorce or separation, or in lone parent families. As adopted children reach adolescence, they do experience more uncertainty and confusion about their identity than children reared in biological families, and this can, on occasion, lead to serious problems.

Children adopted later in childhood do not have such a favourable outcome. Nevertheless, such children are capable of making warm, positive attachments to adoptive parents, and late-adopted children who have previously been mainly reared in children's homes do better behaviourally than if they are returned to their biological families or stay in children's homes (Tizard 1977). At one point, it was not thought possible or desirable for physically and mentally handicapped children to be adopted, but this practice has now become much more common, and follow-up suggests that the great majority of such adoptions are highly successful, at least if they are carefully planned (Wolkind and Kozaruk 1983). Adoption does not, of course, affect the likelihood of children inheriting strongly genetically determined conditions such as schizophrenia and certain metabolic disorders from their biological parents.

The implications of these studies of adopted children are reasonably clear-cut. Adoption is, in general, a successful practice for children for whom it is obvious early on that care by biological parents is not feasible. Later adoption has a less good outcome, but is preferable to other alternatives. There is no reason why children with disabilities should not be adopted, provided suitable parents can be identified, prepared to take the responsibility with knowledge of the problems they will face. Though this is a controversial area, it is better for black children to be adopted into suitable black families if they are available, but, if they are not, adoption into white families is much preferable to alternatives with less expectation of permanency. There is good evidence that school, social class, and peer group influence adolescent identity to a greater degree than skin colour (Tizard and Phoenix 1995).

Changes in legislation and social work practice in the 1980s mean that a number of biological parents are retaining contact with their children after they have been adopted. Adopted individuals now have the right, once they reach adulthood, to obtain information about their biological parents. These changes require careful monitoring to ensure that the generally positive results of adoption are not prejudiced by them.

Finally, there has been considerable interest in the increased scale of international adoptions. Such children do have an increased risk for the development of psychiatric disorders (Versluis-den Bieman and Verhulst 1995).

10.3.3 LEGISLATION

The system of legislation concerning the welfare of children in England and Wales (the Scottish system is somewhat different) is mainly regulated by the 1989 Children Act. The following legal procedures can be invoked for the protection and welfare of children.

Emergency Protection Order (EPO)

An EPO is a short-term order (for 8 days, with the possibility of extension for up to a further 7 days), that can be applied for if urgent action is required to protect a child. Anyone can make an application for an EPO but, in fact, application will usually be made to a magistrate by a local authority or National Society for the Prevention of Cruelty to Children (NSPCC) social worker, though it may also be made to a judge. The court must be satisfied that the child is likely to suffer significant harm unless he is removed from where he is to another place, or he is kept where he is (Department of Health 1989). Following the granting of an EPO, the applicant must allow reasonable contact with parents unless the court attaches extra provisions to the order relating to access.

Child Assessment Order

A Child Assessment Order can be made for up to 7 days by a magistrate after receiving an application from a local authority or NSPCC social worker. The court must be satisfied that the applicant has reasonable cause to believe that the child is suffering, or is likely to suffer harm, that an assessment is required to enable the applicant to determine whether this is indeed the case, and that it is unlikely that a satisfactory assessment can be made unless an order is obtained. In practice, such an order is rarely made.

Care, interim care, and supervision orders

Care and supervision orders can be made for a longer period following application by a local authority or NSPCC social worker. The child must be suffering, or be likely to suffer, significant harm because of a lack of reasonable parental care, or because he is beyond parental control. The question what is 'reasonable' parental control is likely to give rise to considerable legal debate, but it is the intention that parents who are handicapped in their parenting by mental ill-health or low intelligence to such a significant degree that they require help with their children will be expected to show that they are prepared to accept such help (Department of Health 1989). The philosophy of the Children Act is to expect parents to be responsible and, before parental rights can be removed to any degree, it has to be shown that significant harm is attributable to lack of parental care.

A *Care Order* gives the local authority parental responsibility for the child, but the authority must determine to what extent the parent can continue to exercise responsibility. Parents are expected to retain their duty to care for the child and raise him to moral, physical, and emotional health in all ways that are compatible with the Care Order. Even though a child may be 'in care' and removed from the family, social workers will make every attempt to work in partnership with the family, respect their wishes, etc. Children in care may live at home under supervision of the social services department.

A form of legal protection less extreme than a Care Order is a *Supervision Order*, which a magistrate may also grant to a social services department. This order, often made in relation to adolescents in trouble, provides a social worker such as a probation officer with the legal right to advise and assist the child and family while the child lives at home.

Local authority accommodation

Local authorities have a duty under Section 20 of the Children Act 1989 to provide accommodation for children whose parents are unable, for one reason or another, to look after them, or who have no one taking parental responsibility for them. The parents of children who are looked after voluntarily in local authority accommodation in this way do not lose their parental rights or responsibility and, except in certain unusual circumstances (for example if the child is over 16 and objects to removal), may remove their children from such accommodation.

Wardship

In cases where an individual has good reason to believe that a child's welfare is at risk, then an application can be made to the High Court for a child to be made a *ward of court*. Wardship proceedings are now unusual as the provisions of the 1989 Children Act cover most of the situations where they might previously have been considered.

Separation and divorce

Children whose parents are separating or intending to divorce are entitled to the same legal protection as other children and indeed must be regarded as requiring special attention as far as their care is concerned. Parents engaged in divorce proceedings are encouraged to make a joint statement of the arrangements they propose for their children. These statements are considered by the district judge, who, perhaps assisted by a court welfare officer, decides whether it would be in the child's interests for a specific order under Section 8 of the 1989 Children Act to be made, or whether the parental arrangements proposed are satisfactory and can be agreed without further legal action.

Section 8 orders may specify various conditions on behalf of the child's welfare:

- A *Residence Order* states with whom the child is to live.
- A *Contact Order* requires the person with whom the child lives to allow the child to visit or stay with the person named in the order—usually, but not always, this will be the other parent.

Normally both parents will be expected to retain their parental responsibility to care for the child and raise him to physical, moral, and emotional health, in so far as this is compatible with any specific agreed arrangements or orders that are made.

Disputes regarding residence, contact, or other matters may be settled informally or by recourse to the courts. Professionals may be asked to provide expert advice in cases of conflict, and some principles on which advice can be given are provided below.

Consent to and refusal of treatment

Normally, with children under the age of 16 (minors), parental consent is legally necessary to carry out any medical procedures such as prescribing medication, admitting the child to hospital, or performing an operation. It is also, in the great majority of cases, good practice for parents to be fully involved in such decisions concerning their children. In the UK, it was ruled in 1984 that, for certain procedures, i.e. the prescription of contraceptives to girls under the age of 16 years, practitioners could, in unusual circumstances, where this seemed in the best interests of the girl, act without the knowledge and consent of parents. Further, when a parent withholds consent to treatment in such a manner that a child's health or welfare are clearly endangered, then an application can be made for a Care Order as described above. If the delay involved in obtaining such an order would put the child's health at serious risk (e.g. when parental religious beliefs preclude a life-saving blood transfusion), then, in the UK, emergency treatment may be undertaken.

Normally, if doctors and parents are agreed on a course of action for a child involving the giving or withholding of treatment, it can be assumed that the agreed decision is in the child's best interests. In certain cases, however, such as those involving decisions to withhold life-saving treatment from babies with conditions that would result in later severe handicap, or very poor quality of life, it is legally open to social services departments to take action, under the 1989 Children Act, such as application for an Emergency Protection Order. Most authorities believe that, at least in the great majority of cases, decisions concerning the treatment of young children should be left to parents and their professional advisers.

The position regarding consent to and refusal of treatment in older children is more complex. It is good practice to obtain both the permission of parents and the assent of children to all procedures. When a child thought to be capable of forming a sufficiently mature judgement refuses treatment, despite understanding all the implications of this decision, then parents cannot now override the wishes of the child. In these circumstances, the provisions of the 1983 Mental Health Act, which allows for compulsory admission and/or treatment, if the child's safety is at risk, may need to be invoked. This Act requires an application by the nearest relative or an approved social worker, as well as medical recommendations for compulsory admission or treatment.

10.3.4 ROLE OF PROFESSIONALS IN CHILD WELFARE

Social workers

Social work in relation to children and families has many aims. In the community, the social worker will see it as her or his duty to provide both practical and emotional support to families where the child is at risk of neglect or other forms of harm. She or he will invoke legal procedures for the protection of the child when this seems necessary, and will often act as the 'key worker' when a number of professionals whose activities need to be co-ordinated, are concerned with caring for a family.

Specialism in social work was much reduced in the UK after the publication of the Seebohm Report in 1968, but in most local authority social services departments, a significant amount of specialism continues. Hospital social workers attached to paediatric units from social service departments apply social work skills to families with children with physical and psychosocial problems. Most social service departments have specialist units concerned with family placement (adoption, fostering, etc.) and residential care. Child and family psychiatric departments usually have social workers attached full-time to their multidisciplinary teams.

Although the majority of social workers are employed by the local authority social services department, voluntary agencies such as the NSPCC also provide a significant number. Some are employed by voluntary bodies with a specific interest in a particular health problem, such as visual impairment or epilepsy.

Health professionals

It is the responsibility of all health professionals to inform a social worker if they are seriously concerned for the future safety of a child, or have reason to believe that a child has been neglected, injured, or otherwise abused. Doctors and nurses are sometimes understandably reluctant to make referrals to social workers because they fear, often realistically, that their positive relationship with the parents will be threatened if they do. Clearly, there will be situations—where there is only insubstantial suspicion of neglect, for example—when a health professional may feel prepared to accept the heavy responsibility for not informing a social worker about his concerns.

General practitioners and paediatricians undertake responsibility for the medical examination of infants and children who are to be placed for adoption. It is important that prospective adoptive parents are aware of any special health risks of the child they are preparing to adopt and, if the child has a physical or mental condition, its likely course. In providing this information, the paediatrician will need to have access to all available data on the health of the parents, any other family history, and details of the pregnancy, birth, and any postnatal complications or illnesses. In past days, in questionable cases, the adoption of babies was often considerably delayed to see whether an infant's early development proceeded normally. It is now realized this is misguided, because of the benefits of early adoption (see above). Prospective parents should obviously be told if there are realistic doubts about a child's development, so that they can make as informed a decision as possible.

Paediatricians or general practitioners examine children admitted into the care of local authorities to determine whether the child needs medical treatment, has any transmissible disease or injuries, or shows evidence of neglect (Bamford 1979). Nude weight and height (or length) should also be carefully obtained as a baseline for future assessment.

Psychiatrists may be requested to advise concerning what type of placement for a child will provide the best conditions for personality development and least risk of behavioural or emotional disorder. They may also be asked to assess the relevance of a possible mental disorder, either in terms of the risk of such disorder in the child, or in relation to the fitness of a mentally ill adult to parent. Criteria that can be used in making these judgements are described below.

The psychiatrist may also be involved in consultation concerning procedures for assessing the suitability of substitute parents, especially prospective foster and adoptive parents. Finally, he may be asked to provide an opinion for children following separation and divorce arrangements, especially where there is dispute between parents concerning custody or access.

Conflicts concerning child care

Although social workers have prime responsibility for decision-making concerning appropriate placement for children and for assisting the courts where legal procedures are taken, health professionals, such as paediatricians and psych-iatrists, may also be asked for advice. In considering what advice to give, major considerations must be the identification of the environment which will be most favourable to personality development and reduce the risk of behavioural and emotional disorders (Wolkind 1984). The following considerations will be relevant:

- The *quality of the existing placement* in terms of the health and personality of the main people caring for the child, the strength of attachment of the child to them, and the quality of health care and social stimulation they are provid-ing. The assessment of the fitness of a parent suffering from mental illness to parent a child requires the special knowledge of a psychiatrist knowledgeable in the likely outcome of different disorders (Oates 1984).
- The *quality of the proposed alternative placement* using the same criteria. This is often more difficult to appraise because of the hypothetical nature of the judgements involved. Nevertheless, it is usually possible to make some in-formed judgement of the quality of care likely to be available.
- The *age of the child* and the *length of time* he has been in his existing placement. Children aged from 6 months to about 3–4 years are especially likely to show prolonged adverse reactions to a change in placement, unless this is very carefully arranged with the new parental figures only gradually taking over care.
- The *temperament of the child* and the presence of already existing *behavioural and emotional disorders*. Children with adverse temperamental characteristics, especially those who are volatile, easily upset, and irregular in their eating and sleeping habits are more in need of continuous, warm care than other children, with perhaps more phlegmatic temperaments.
- The presence of a *physical disorder*. Children with physical conditions, espe-cially those involving brain dysfunction, are particularly liable to develop behavioural and emotional disorders when under stress.
- The degree to which prospective 'parents' can *accept their own limitations*, and are motivated to turn to outside help if the child-care situation becomes intolerable is relevant. The availability of such help if it is required is also of relevance.

A fuller description of the factors that mental health professionals will wish to take into account in giving an opinion in cases of disputed adoption, Residence and Contact Orders, etc. is provided by Black *et al.* (1998).

Preparation of reports to the court

Increasingly, when courts are dealing with cases of abuse or suspected abuse, or where there is conflict between parents over contact or the residence of a child, health professionals including psychiatrists and paediatricians are requested for their views. In these circumstances, as far as is possible, the professional should see his main duty as promoting the welfare of the child.

Useful guidelines on the writing of court reports are provided by Black *et al.* (1998). The report should open with the name and date of birth of the child, and with a statement of the professional position of the person writing the report and how he became involved in the case. The introduction should continue by stating the questions the person writing the report was asked to address, and the way the assessment was carried out. Usually this would involve interviews with the various members of the family and professionals concerned, but a report may be prepared entirely on the basis of an examination of documentation if this is agreed beforehand.

An account should be given of the events in the child's life before the assessment, the major problems that have occurred, and the measures previously taken to deal with them. The assessment interviews should be reported with particularly detailed accounts of the relevant sections of the interviews, making it clear whether remarks made were spontaneous or in response to specific questioning. An account of the results of any investigations, psychological or physical, that have been carried out should be added.

There should be a summary of the information, a conclusion, and a list of recommendations. The feasibility of any recommendations concerning therapy should be checked out before they are made. The report should always be signed and a list of relevant documents that have been consulted appended.

10.4 School influences and special education

10.4.1 SCHOOL INFLUENCES

Formal school attendance begins in the UK at the age of 5 years or even earlier; in most other countries schooling begins a year or two later. The value of attendance at pre-school facilities such as playgroups, nursery schools, and kindergartens for the prevention and treatment of behaviour and emotional problems in young children has been the subject of considerable research.

For children relatively deprived of stimulation and care at home, focused pre-school educational programmes have been shown to have short and long-lasting benefit for behavioural and educational outcomes, providing they are of high quality (Graham 1995). Requirements for a successful outcome include a developmentally appropriate curriculum, adequate adult–child ratios (e.g. a group of no more than 20 3–5 year olds with 2 adults), sensitivity to the child's non-educational needs, developmentally appropriate evaluation procedures, high-quality caregiver–child verbal interactions and an experienced leader of the programme.

Benefits for deprived children attending less adequate facilities are much less certain, as they are for children already receiving good stimulation at home. However, attendance at a well-run playgroup or nursery school is likely to improve social skills in children and prepare them for later formal schooling as well as to allow parents, especially mothers who wish it, the opportunity to work at least part-time, or to enjoy some time on their own. In contrast, attendance at chaotic or repressive facilities will clearly have a negative effect on the child. It is unwise therefore to generalize about the effects of pre-school attendance.

In older children, the characteristics of the schools they attend have been shown to have an important effect (Rutter *et al.* 1979). Some schools obtain consistently better academic results, as well as lower rates of delinquency and behaviour problems, and higher attendance rates than do other schools. The reasons lie partly in the type of pupil intake, but schools themselves also make a difference. The internal organization of schools is more important than physical features such as the size of the school and the age of the school buildings (Maughan 1988).

School characteristics that make a positive difference include (Rutter *et al.* 1979):

- placing emphasis on rewards and praise for good work and behaviour
- providing a comfortable environment for all children in which they feel free to approach staff for help
- ensuring that responsibility is shared out between different children and that all feel they are participating in an important aspect of school life
- an academic life placing emphasis on the importance of academic work with teachers preparing lessons conscientiously, turning up punctually for lessons, marking homework promptly
- ensuring teachers act as good models for behaviour
- effective management of children in groups, rather than concentrating on them as individuals
- a strong school organization with effective behaviour policies
- early identification of behaviour problems with interventions by well-trained staff.

The level of physical resources, the age and structure of the buildings, size of class, and the degree of emphasis on punishment are of rather little importance.

The processes whereby certain school characteristics lead to better outcomes are unknown, but the impact they have on child self-esteem and sense of self-efficacy may well be relevant (Rutter 1979).

10.4.2 SPECIAL EDUCATION

The first attempts to provide special schooling were made in the late nineteenth century when facilities were set up for children with physical and mental handicaps. From that time until the 1960s, in most developed countries an increasing amount of separate, special educational provision was created. Children were largely allocated to facilities on the basis of their medical diagnosis—deafness, blindness, etc. At this point it became clear that this approach was unsatisfactory (Department of Education and Science 1978) because:

- medical diagnosis was often a poor guide to educational need
- many children had multiple handicaps, and their needs were poorly met in schools set up for one disability alone
- many children in ordinary schools were discovered to have special needs that were not being met at all

• separate education seemed to have many disadvantages for children; the main dangers were seen to be stigmatization, lack of opportunity to mix with non-handicapped children, and unnecessarily low expectations for educational performance.

As a result, there has been a move towards integrating handicapped children into ordinary schools, though it is recognized that some children with very special needs will still need to be educated separately. Placement is now based on educational need rather than medical diagnosis. This trend is exemplified by the passing of the Disabilities Act PL 102–109 in the US, and the Education Act (1993) in the UK.

Types of special educational need

As many as 1 child in 5 will have some sort of special educational need at some stage in their school careers. Types of help needed may include:

• a more favourable staff ratio to provide extra time to give to the child
• teachers with special training to deal with children with particular handicaps
• the ready availability of other professionals, for example speech therapists, psychologists
• special equipment, for example to assist children with sensory disorders
• a special classroom regime; for example, some children may benefit from a highly structured, and others from a particularly permissive atmosphere
• special building features; for example the building may need to have ramps to be suitable for a child in a wheelchair.

Special educational provision

It is agreed that ideally there should be a 'continuum of special educational provision' to match the continuum of special educational needs that children show (Anderson 1976). A useful review of types of educational interventions for children with learning disabilities in the US is provided by Lerner (1989). Currently, in the UK such provision consists, or should consist of:

• Extra help provided in the ordinary classroom. This might involve, for example, the employment of a teaching aide to work part-time, or the application of a behaviour modification programme in the classroom, by the teacher in consultation with a psychologist.
• Part-time withdrawal of the child to a small remedial group held within the school. Extra help for children behindhand with reading is often provided in this way.
• Part-time withdrawal to a class held in a separate unit or school. Units of this type exist for children with more serious learning or behavioural problems as well as for those with hearing problems.
• Full-time special education in a separate day school or unit. Special schools are available in most education authorities for the following types of problem:
  — *mild mental retardation:* schools for children with moderate learning difficulties.

— *moderate and severe mental retardation*: schools for children with severe learning difficulties.

— *psychiatric disorders*: schools for children with emotional and behaviour difficulties.

— *physical disability*: schools for the physically handicapped, and for specific sensory disabilities.

— *autism and communication disorders*: schools for autistic and aphasic children.

It should be noted that American terminology in this field differs from British. In the US, the term 'learning difficulty' is reserved for specific learning difficulties, such as dyslexia. Some ordinary schools and schools for children with learning difficulties have 'assessment units' where young pre-school children with handicaps can be placed, assessed, and educated before moving on to ordinary or special schools.

• Full-time special education in a separate residential school. These exist for the same categories as day schools. Residence may be on a weekly or termly boarding basis.

Assessment for special education

As part of their work, teachers assess children's progress and identify those with learning and behavioural problems. In England and Wales guidance on the steps teachers should take when they identify a problem is provided in a Code of Practice (Department for Education and Employment 1994). If they need outside help, they first call on help that is available from within the school, for example from a specialist teacher, a year head, head teacher, or the school nurse. If a child requires further assessment, then outside professionals—the school doctor, an outside advisory teacher, psychologist, or psychiatrist—may be invoked. These professionals are, however, likely to be involved with only a minority of children with problems, though in the US in particular there is increasing demand for psychologists and psychiatrists to work in a consultation role in schools (Jellinek 1990). The type of involvement will obviously depend on the nature of the problem, but it may include a personal assessment of the child, or merely a discussion between the outside professional and members of the school staff. Consultation with teachers can be carried out along similar lines to those followed with other professionals. Involvement of parents in the assessment process, and in the production of an educational plan, is not only highly desirable, but is a statutory requirement.

Most children with educational problems will be educated with relatively minor special arrangements in ordinary schools, though in a number of such children, behavioural problems of some significance are not identified and an opportunity for mental health consultation is lost (Mattison *et al.* 1986). In a small minority (perhaps about 2%), it becomes clear that this is insufficient. If children have a need for special education or provision, then a full assessment must be carried out leading to a 'statement' of the child's special educational needs (under the terms of the Education Act 1993). The aim of the assessment should be to make clear what the child needs and how this can be provided, while retaining as far as possible components of normal education and contact with ordinary children without special needs.

There are two main pathways to a full assessment:

- In some children, mainly those with severe learning difficulties and physical disabilities, it is clear well before they go to school that they will need special education.
- In others, especially those with mild and moderate learning difficulties, the need becomes apparent only when the child has been at school for some time. Health professionals have obligations especially involving the first group (Polnay *et al.* 1996). If a doctor thinks a child he is seeing is likely to require special education, then he should:
  — discuss the matter with the parents
  — in the case of children over the age of 2 years, inform the education authority of his view of the child's needs
  — if appropriate, suggest the part a voluntary organization might play in helping.

In children under 2 years, the education authority should only be contacted with parental agreement. With a child over the age of 2 years, parental agreement is highly desirable, but not mandatory.

The outcome of the full assessment should consist of five main components. There should be:

- *reports* from
  — the *child's teacher*
  — an *educational psychologist*
  — *health professionals*
- a *statement from the parents* about what they consider to be the child's special needs
- a *statement from the education authority* summarizing the child's needs and what special provision is thought necessary to be made available.

Parents are expected to see the final statement as well as the reports on which it is based. If they do not agree with the statement they have the right to appeal.

Health professionals should provide relevant information that will both assist in the preparation of the statement of the child's educational needs and be useful to the teachers responsible for the child's further education. Their main task is to summarize the child's physical and psychological needs, particularly for any special professional help (e.g. speech therapy, psychotherapy), medication, diet, and aids to daily living. If the child needs any special classroom regime such as a highly structured or permissive setting, this should be stated.

Those receiving the statement of educational needs must be aware of family problems that might be affecting the child's learning. For example, continuing social work support may need to be arranged. It is often difficult to phrase an account of the situation in a way that is acceptable to parents who, of course, will read the report. However, it is usually possible to frame statements in a way that makes it clear that, though the parents are finding it difficult to be, for example, as tolerant and appropriately protective to their children as they should be, they are nevertheless doing the best they can for their children. Communication of potentially shameful or embarrassing information may pose problems. Such information can only be disclosed with parental consent, and indeed it is always helpful to tell parents roughly what one is intending to put into a report before one writes it. It is usually possible to phrase statements in such a way that teachers receiving the information can know that there are serious domestic problems in a child's background, without going into details of desertion, alcoholism, marital infidelity, or other sensitive matters.

Health professionals should not attempt to make educational recommendations themselves: that is the responsibility of the education authority. They may, however, sometimes wish to engage in behind-the-scenes advocacy on behalf of a child to ensure that delay in placement is not too long, or that an apparently very appropriate placement is brought to the attention of the education authority. Mental health professionals should be involved in the assessment of disruptive children at risk of exclusion from school. Advice on placement is often problematic because what may be best for the child in question may not be best for other children or the teacher. This raises ethical issues best dealt with by open discussion (Graham 1998b).

Contributions to assessment are only a small part of the role played by health professionals—paediatricians, nurses, psychiatrists, etc.—in educational medicine. In particular, such professionals are important in helping teachers and others in ordinary and special schools to understand and cope with the physical and psychiatric problems of children in their care. With parental permission, information relevant to teacher's concerns needs to be transmitted to school doctors via the school health service following in-patient admissions and out-patient attendances. Visits to schools by health professionals working in hospitals can be especially helpful when a child's physical or psychiatric problems are causing unusual concern.

The value of special education for disturbed children

A discussion of the teaching methods used with children with emotional and behavioural problems is outside the scope of this book (but see Laslett 1977). A wide diversity of methods is used, often strongly influenced by psychodynamic or behavioural theories. The personal warmth and concern of the teacher are major influences. Other important factors are thought to include

- firm discipline not based on punishment
- a well-thought-out academic programme
- the opportunity of continuity of relationships provided by staff stability
- the availability of personal counselling for the student.

Though there are many studies of interventions for specific problems in the ordinary and special school setting, there are few studies investigating the type of school experience that produces the best outcomes. However, Wrate *et al.*

(1985) studied the effects of different types of education on a sizeable group of children with neurotic and conduct disorders. They found that children treated in ordinary schools did better than those placed in special schools for slow learning children and schools for the maladjusted, though children with conduct disorders did not fare well in any setting. This study needs replication, for obviously, if confirmed, the findings have major implications for the organization of special education. Rutter and Bartak (1973) were able to show that autistic children in schools with a structured, goal-setting approach to education made more cognitive gains than those in schools with a more permissive relationship-fostering approach. The capacity of the children to make relationships did not differ between the two types of school. There is a need for further evaluative studies—perhaps a fitting expression to end this book because it applies to so many aspects of child psychiatry.

References

Abbeduto, L. and Hagerman, R. J. (1997) Language and communication in fragile X syndrome. *Mental Retardation and Developmental Disabilities Research Reviews* 3, 313–22.

Abramowicz, H. K. and Richardson, S. A. (1975) Epidemiology of severe mental retardation in children: community studies. *American Journal of Mental Retardation* 80, 18–39.

Abramowitz, C. V. (1976) The effectiveness of group therapy with children. *Archives of General Psychiatry* 33, 320–6.

Achenbach, T., Howell, C., Quay, H., and Conners, C. (1991) National survey of problems and competencies among four-to-sixteen year-olds: parent's reports for normative and clinical samples. *Monographs of the Society for Research in Child Development, serial no 225*, 56.

Achenbach, T. M. (1991a) *Manual for the child behavior checklist/4–18 and 1991 profile.* Department of Psychiatry, University of Vermont, Burlington, VT.

Achenbach, T. M. (1991b) *Manual for the teacher's report form and 1991 profiles.* Department of Psychiatry, University of Vermont, Burlington, VT.

Achenbach, T. M. (1991c) *Manual for the youth self-report and 1991 profiles.* Department of Psychiatry, University of Vermont, Burlington, VT.

Achenbach, T. M. and McConaughy, S. H. (1997) *Empirically based assessment of child and adolescent psychopathology. Practical applications.* Sage, London.

Agnarsson, U. and Clayden, G. (1990) Constipation in childhood. *Maternal and Child Health* 15, 252–6.

Ainsworth, M., Blehar, M. C., Waters, E., and Wall, S. (1978) *Patterns of attachment: a psychological study of the strange situation.* Lawrence Erlbaum, Hillsdale, NJ.

Alberts-Corush, J., Firestone, P., and Goodman, J. T. (1986).Attention and impulsivity characteristics of the biological and adoptive parents of hyperactive and normal control children. *American Journal of Orthopsychiatry* 56, 413–23.

Allen, A., Leonard, H., and Swedo, S. (1995a) Case study: a new infection-triggered, auto-immune subtype of pediatric OCD and Tourette's syndrome. *Journal of the American Academy of Child and Adolescent Psychiatry* 34, 307–11.

Allen, A., Leonard, H., and Swedo, S. (1995b) Current knowledge of medication for the treatment of childhood anxiety disorders. *Journal of the American Academy of Child and Adolescent Psychiatry* 34, 976–86.

Alsaker, F. (1995) Timing of puberty and reactions to pubertal changes. In *Psychosocial disturbances in young people*, ed. M. Rutter, and D. Smith, Wiley, Chichester, pp. 37–82.

American Academy of Child and Adolescent Psychiatry (1997) Practice parameters for the forensic evaluation of children and adolescents who may have been physically or sexually abused. *Journal of the American Academy of Child and Adolescent Psychiatry* 36, 423–4.

American Academy of Pediatrics (1996) Timing of elective surgery on the genitalia of male children with particular reference to the risks, benefits and psychological effects of surgery and anesthesia. *Pediatrics* 97, 590–4.

American Psychiatric Association (1994) *Diagnostic and statistical manual of mental disorders*, 4th edn. American Psychiatric Association, Washington, DC.

Anders, T. and Eiben, L. (1997) Pediatric sleep disorders: a review of the past ten years. *Journal of the American Academy of Child and Adolescent Psychiatry* 36, 9–20.

Anderson, E. (1976) Special schools or special schooling for the handicapped: the debate in perspective. *Journal of Child Psychology and Psychiatry* 17, 151–5.

Anderson, E., Clarke, L., and Spain, B. (1982) *Disability in adolescence*. Methuen, London.

Apley, J. and Hale, B. (1973) Children with recurrent abdominal pain: how do they grow up? *British Medical Journal* 3, 7–9.

Apley, J. and MacKeith, R. (1968) *The child and his symptoms*. Blackwell Scientific, Oxford.

Appleton, R. E. (1996) The new antiepileptic drugs. *Archives of Disease in Childhood* 75, 256–62.

Apter, A., Ratzoni, G., King, R. A. *et al.* (1994) Fluvoxamine open-label treatment of adolescent inpatients with obsessive–compulsive disorder or depression. *Journal of the American Academy of Child and Adolescent Psychiatry* 33, 342–8.

Aries, P. (1973) *Centuries of childhood*. Penguin, Harmondsworth.

Asarnow, J. R. (1994) Childhood onset schizophrenia. *Journal of Child Psychology and Psychiatry* 35, 1345–71.

Asarnow, R., Brown, W. and Strandburg, R. (1995) Children with a schizophrenic disorder: neurobehavioural studies. *European Archives of Psychiatry and Clinical Neurosciences* 245, 70–9.

Assessment of Performance Unit (1978) *Assessing the performance of children*. DES Report on Education No. 93. Department of Education and Science, London.

Atkins, D. M. and Patenaude, A. F. (1987) Psychosocial preparation and follow-up for pediatric bone marrow transplant patients. *American Journal of Orthopsychiatry* 57, 246–52.

Attwood, T. (1988) *Asperger's syndrome*. Jessica Kingsley, London.

Aydin, B., Yaprak, L., Akarsus, D., Okten, N. and Ulgen, M. (1997) Psychosocial aspects of psychiatric disorders in children with thalassaemia major. *Acta Paediatrica Japonica* 39, 354–7.

Ayres, A. J. (1979) *Sensory integration and the child*. Western Psychological Services, Los Angeles.

Azima, F. and Dies, K. (1989) Clinical research in adolescent group psychotherapy: status, guidelines and directions. In *Adolescent group psychotherapy*, ed. F. Azima and L. Richmond, International Universities Press, Madison, CT, pp. 193–223.

Badian, N. A. (1996) Dyslexia: a validation of the concept at two age levels. *Journal of Learning Disabilities* 29, 102–12.

Baildam, E. M., Holt, P. J., Conway, S. C., and Morton, M. J. (1995) The association between physical function and psychological problems in children with juvenile chronic arthritis. *British Journal of Rheumatology* 34, 470–7.

Bailey, A., Bolton, P., Butler, L. *et al.* (1993) Prevalence of the fragile X anomaly amongst autistic twins and singletons. *Journal of Child Psychology and Psychiatry* 34, 673–88.

Bailey, A., Phillips, W. and Rutter, M. (1996) Autism: towards an integration of clinical, genetic, neuropsychological, and neurobiological perspectives. *Journal of Child Psychology and Psychiatry* 37, 89–126.

Bailey, V. F. (1998) Conduct disorders in young children. In *Cognitive behaviour therapy for children and families*, ed. P Graham, Cambridge University Press, Cambridge, pp. 99–114.

Bailey, V., Graham, P., and Boniface, D. (1978) How much child psychiatry does a general practitioner do? *Journal of the Royal College of General Practitioners* 28, 621–6.

Baird, G. and Hall, D. M. B. (1985) Developmental paediatrics in primary care. What should we teach? *British Medical Journal* **291**, 583–6.

Baker, A. W. and Duncan, S. P. (1985) Child sexual abuse: a study of prevalence in Great Britain. *Child Abuse and Neglect* **9**, 457–68.

Baker, R. C., Kummer, A. W., Schultz, J. R., and Gonzalez-Del-Rey, J. (1996) Neuro-developmental outcome of infants with viral meningitis in the first three months of life. *Clinical Pediatrics* **35**, 295–301.

Baldwin, J. A. and Oliver, J. E. (1975) Epidemiology and family characteristics of severely abused children. *Journal of Preventive and Social Medicine* **29**, 205–21.

Bamford, F. N. (1979) Medical examinations of children admitted to care. In *Medical aspects of adoption and foster care*, ed. S. N. Wolkind, Heinemann, London, pp. 16–21.

Banks, M. and Jackson, P. (1982) Unemployment and risk of minor psychiatric disorder in young people: cross-sectional and longitudinal evidence. *Psychological Medicine* **12**, 786–98.

Barkley, R. A. (1989) Hyperactive girls and boys: stimulant drug effects on mother–child interactions. *Journal of Child Psychology and Psychiatry* **30**, 379–90.

Barkley, R. A., Anastopoulos, A. D., Guevremont, D. C., and Fletcher, K. E. (1991) Adolescents with ADHD: patterns of behavioral adjustment, academic functioning, and treatment utilization. *Journal of the American Academy of Child and Adolescent Psychiatry* **30**, 752–61.

Baron-Cohen, S. (1989) The autistic child's theory of mind: a case of specific developmental delay. *Journal of Child Psychology and Psychiatry* **30**, 285–97.

Baron-Cohen, S. (1991) Do people with autism understand what causes emotion? *Child Development* **62**, 385–95.

Baron-Cohen, S., Cox, A., Baird, G. *et al.* (1996) Psychological markers in the detection of autism in infancy in a large population. *British Journal of Psychiatry* **168**, 158–63.

Barr, R., Boyce, W. T., and Zeltzer, L. K. (1996) The stress–illness association in children: a perspective from the biobehavioural interface. In *Stress, Risk and Resilience in Children and Adolescents*, ed. R. J. Haggerty, L. R. Sherrod, N. Garmezy and M. Rutter, Cambridge University Press, Cambridge, pp. 182–224.

Bassuk, E. K. and Rosenberg, L. (1990) Psychosocial characteristics of homeless children and children with homes. Pediatrics **85**, 257–61.

Baumer, J. H., David, T. J., Valentine, S. J., Roberts, S. J., and Hughes, R. (1981) Many parents think their child is dying when having a first febrile convulsion. *Developmental Medicine and Child Neurology* **23**, 462–4.

Baumrind, D. (1967) Child care practices anteceding three patterns of preschool behaviour. *Genetic Psychology Monographs* **75**, 43–88.

Bax, M. C. O. and Colville, G. A. (1995) Behaviour in mucopolysaccharide disorders. *Archives of Disease in Childhood* **73**, 77–81.

Bax, M., Hart, H., and Jenkins, S. M. (1990) *Child development and child health: the pre-school years*. Blackwell Scientific, Oxford.

Bax, M. C. O., Robinson, R. J., and Gath, A. (1988) The reality of handicap. In *Child health in a changing society*, ed. J. A. Forfar, Oxford University Press, Oxford, p. 116.

Baxter, L. R. and Guze, G. H. (1993) Neuroimaging. In *Handbook of Tourette's syndrome and related tic disorders*, ed. R. Kurlan, Marcel Dekker, New York, p. 289.

Bayley, N. (1993) *Bayley scales of infant development: birth to two years*. Psychological Corporation, New York, 2nd Edition.

Beales, J. G., Keen, J. H., and Holt, P. J. (1983) The child's perception of the disease and the experience of pain in juvenile chronic arthritis. *Journal of Rheumatology* **10**, 61–5.

Beasley, M., Costello, P., and Smith, I. (1994) Outcome of treatment in young adults with phenylketonuria detected by routine neonatal screening between 1964 and 1991. *Quarterly Journal of Medicine* 87, 155–60.

Beck, A. T. (1967) *Depression: clinical, theoretical and experimental aspects.* Harper and Row, New York.

Beck, A. T. (1976) *Cognitive therapy and the emotional disorders. International Universities Press,* New York.

Beck, A. T., Rush, A. J., Shaw, B. F., and Emery, G. (1979) *Cognitive therapy of depression.* Wiley, New York.

Beitchman, J. H., Nair, R., Clegg, M., Ferguson, B., and Patel, P. G. (1986) Prevalence of psychiatric disorders in children with speech and language disorders. *Journal of the American Academy of Child and Adolescent Psychiatry* 25, 528–35.

Bellman, M. (1966) Studies in encopresis. *Acta Paediatrica Scandinavica,* Suppl. 170.

Belson, W. (1975) *Juvenile theft: the causal factors.* Harper and Row, London.

Bender, B. G., Belleau, L., Fukuhara, J. T., Mrazek, D., and Strunk, R. C. (1987) Psychomotor adaptation in children with chronic severe asthma. *Pediatrics* 79, 723–7.

Bender, B. G., Harmon, R. J., Linden, M. G., and Robinson, A. (1995) Psychosocial adaptation of 39 adolescents with sex chromosome abnormalities. *Pediatrics* 96, 302–8.

Bengi-Arslan, L., Verhulst, F., Van der Ende, J., and Erol, N. (1997) Understanding childhood (problem) behaviors from a cultural perspective: comparison of problem behaviors and competencies in Turkish immigrant, Turkish and Dutch children. *Social Psychiatry and Psychiatric Epidemiology,* in press.

Bentovim, A. (1988) Understanding the phenomenon of sexual abuse: a family systems view of causation. In *Child sexual abuse within the family,* ed. A. Bentovim, A. Elton, J. Hildebrand, M. Tranter, and E. Vizard, Wright, London, pp. 40–58.

Bentovim, A. and Gray, J. (In Press) Illness induction syndrome. *Child Abuse and Neglect.*

Berg, I. (1970) A follow-up study of school phobic adolescents admitted to an in-patient unit. *Journal of Child Psychology and Psychiatry* 11, 37–47.

Berg, I., Butler, D., and Hall, G. (1976) The outcome of adolescent school phobia. *British Journal of Psychiatry* 128, 80–5.

Berg, I., Consterdine, M., Hullin, R., McGuire, R., and Tyrer, S. (1978) A randomly controlled trial of two court procedures in truancy. *British Journal of Criminology* 18, 232–44.

Berg, R., Svensson, J., and Astrom, G. (1981) Social and sexual adjustment of men operated for hypospadias during childhood: a controlled study. *Journal of Urology* 125, 313–17.

Berger, M., Yule, W., and Rutter, M. (1975) Attainment and adjustment in two geographic areas. II. The prevalence of specific reading retardation. *British Journal of Psychiatry* 126, 510–19.

Berridge, D. and Brodie, I. (1998) *Children's homes revisited.* Jessica Kingsley, London.

Berridge, D. and Cleaver, H. (1987) *Fostering breakdown.* Basil Blackwell, London.

Berrueta-Clement, J. R., Schweinhart, L. J., Barnett, W. S., Epstein, A. S., and Weikart, D. P. (1984) *Changed lives: the effects of the Perry pre-school program on youth through age 19.* High Scope Press, Ypsilanti, MI.

Bertagnoli, M. W. and Borchardt, C. M. (1990) A review of ECT for children and adolescents. *Journal of the American Academy of Child and Adolescent Psychiatry* 29, 302–7.

Berwick, D. M., Levy, J. C., and Kleinerman, R. (1982) Failure to thrive: diagnostic yield of hospitalisation. *Archives of Disease in Childhood* 57, 347–51.

Bewley, B. R. (1979) Teachers smoking. *British Journal of Preventive and Social Medicine* 33, 219–22.

Biederman, J. (1987) Clonazepam in the treatment of prepubertal children with panic-like symptoms. *Journal of Clinical Psychiatry* **48**, 38–41.

Biederman, J., Munir, K., Knee, D. *et al.*(1986) A family study of patients with attention deficit disorder and normal controls. *Journal of Psychiatric Research* **20**, 263–74.

Biederman, J., Faraone, S., Milberger, S. *et al.* (1996) Is childhood oppositional defiant disorder a precursor to adolescent conduct disorder? Findings from a four year follow-up study of children with ADHD. *Journal of the American Academy of Child and Adolescent Psychiatry* **35**, 1193–2004.

Bijur, P. E., Golding, J., and Haslum, M. (1988) Persistence of occurrence of injury: can injuries of pre-school children predict injuries of school-aged children? *Pediatrics* **82**, 707–12.

Billard, C., Gillet, P., Signoret, J. *et al.* (1992) Cognitive functions in Duchenne muscular dystrophy: a reappraisal and comparison with spinal muscular atrophy. *Neuromuscular Disorders* **2**, 371–8.

Bingley, L., Leonard, J., Hensman, S., and Lask, B. (1980) Comprehensive management of children on a paediatric ward. *Archives of Disease in Childhood* **55**, 555–61.

Bird, H., Canino, G., Gould, M. *et al.* (1988) Estimates of the prevalence of childhood maladjustment in a community survey in Puerto Rico: the use of combined measures. *Archives of General Psychiatry* **45**, 1120–6.

Bird, H., Gould, M., Yager, T. *et al.* (1989) Risk factors of maladjustment in Puerto Rican children. *Journal of the American Academy of Child and Adolescent Psychiatry* **28**, 847–50.

Bird, H. and Kestenbaum, C. (1988) A semi-structured approach to clinical assessment. In C. J. Kestenbaum and D. T. Williams (eds) *Handbook of clinical assessment of children and adolescents*, pp. 19–30. New York, New York University Press.

Birley, J. and Brown, G. (1970) Crises and life change preceding the onset or relapse of acute schizophrenia: clinical aspects. *British Journal of Psychiatry* **116**, 327–33.

Bishop, D. (1993) Autism, executive functions and theory of mind: a neuropsychological perspective. *Journal of Child Psychology and Psychiatry* **34**, 279–93.

Bishop, D. V. M. (1983). *Test for reception of grammar*. National Foundation for Educational Research, Slough.

Bishop, D. V. M. (1992) The underlying nature of specific language impairment. *Journal of Child Psychology and Psychiatry* **33**, 3–66.

Black, D. and Urbanowicz, M. (1987) Family intervention with bereaved children. *Journal of Child Psychology and Psychiatry* **28**, 467–76.

Black, D., Black, M., and Martin, F. (1974) A pilot study of the use of consultant time in psychiatry. *British Journal of Psychiatry*, Supplement. News and Notes, September, pp. 3–5.

Black, D., Harris Hendriks, J., and Wolkind, S. (1998) *Child Psychiatry and the law*. Royal College of Psychiatrists, Gaskell Press, London, 3rd Edition.

Blagg, N. R. and Yule, W. (1984) The behavioural treatment of school refusal: a comparative study. *Behaviour, Research and Therapy* **22**, 119–27.

Blair, A. (1992) Working with people with learning difficulties who self-injure: a review of the literature. *Behavioural Psychotherapy* **20**, 1–23.

Blair, H. (1977) Natural history of childhood asthma. *Archives of Disease in Childhood* **52**, 613–19.

Blurton-Jones, N., Rossetti Ferreira, N. C., Farquhar Brown, M., and Macdonald, L. (1978) The association between perinatal factors and later night waking. *Developmental Medicine and Child Neurology* **20**, 427–34.

Bohman, M. (1978) Some genetic aspects of alcoholism and criminality. *Archives of General Psychiatry* **35**, 269–76.

Bolton, D. (1996) Developmental issues in obsessive compulsive disorder. *Journal of Child Psychology and Psychiatry* **37**, 131–7.

Bolton, D., Collins, S., and Steinberg, D. (1983) The treatment of obsessive–compulsive disorder in adolescence. *British Journal of Psychiatry* **142**, 456–64.

Bolton, P. F., Murphy, M., MacDonald, H., Whitlock, B., Pickles, A., and Rutter, M. (1997) Obstetric complications in autism: consequences or causes of the condition? *Journal of the American Academy of Child and Adolescent Psychiatry* **36**, 272–81.

Bolton, P. and Griffiths, P. (1997) Association of tuberous sclerosis of the temporal lobes with autism and atypical autism. *Lancet* **349**, 392–5.

Bools, M. (1996) Factitious illness by proxy. Munchausen syndrome by proxy. *British Journal of Psychiatry* **169**, 268–75.

Botvin, G. J., Erg, A., and Williams, C. L. (1980) Preventing the onset of cigarette smoking through life-skills training. *Preventive Medicine* **9**, 135–43.

Bowlby, J. (1971) *Attachment and loss. Volume 1. Attachment*. Penguin, Harmondsworth.

Bowlby, J. (1975) *Attachment and loss. Volume 2. Separation, anxiety and anger*. Penguin, Harmondsworth.

Bowlby, J. (1980) *Attachment and loss. Volume 3. Loss*. Penguin, Harmondsworth.

Bowman, E. S. (1993) Etiology and clinical course of pseudoseizures. Relationship to traumas, depression and disorientation. *Psychosomatics* **34**, 333–42.

Boyle, M. H. and Offord, D. R. (1990) Primary prevention of conduct disorder. *Journal of the American Academy of Child and Adolescent Psychiatry* **29**, 227–33.

Bradbury, M. and Meadow, S. R. (1995) Combined treatment with enuresis alarm and desmopressin for nocturnal enuresis. *Acta Paediatrica* **84**, 1014–8.

Bradley, S. and Zucker, K. (1997) Gender identity disorder: a review of the past ten years. *Journal of the American Academy of Child and Adolescent Psychiatry* **36**, 872–80.

Brandhagen, D., Feldt, R., and Williams, D. (1981) Long-term psychologic implications of congenital heart disease: a 24 year follow-up. *Mayo Clinic Proceedings* **66**, 474–9.

Brazelton, T. B. (1962) A child-oriented approach to toilet training. *Pediatrics* **29**, 121–8.

Brazelton, T. B., Koslowski, O., and Main, M. (1974) The origin of reciprocity: the early mother–infant interaction. In *The effect of the infant on its caregiver*, ed. M. Lewis and L. A. Rosenblum, Wiley, New York, pp. 49–76.

Bregman, J. D. (1991) Current developments in the understanding of mental retardation part 2: psychopathology. *Journal of the American Academy of Child and Adolescent Psychiatry* **30**, 861–72.

Bregman, J. D. and Hodapp, R. M. (1991) Current developments in the understanding of mental retardation Part 1: biological and phenomenological perspectives. *Journal of the American Academy of Child and Adolescent Psychiatry* **30**, 707–19.

Brent, D. A., Perper, J., and Goldstein, C. (1988) Risk factors for adolescent suicide. *Archives of General Psychiatry* **45**, 581–8.

Brenton, D. and Lilburn, M. (1996) Maternal phenylketonuria: a study from the United Kingdom. *European Journal of Paediatrics* **155** Suppl. 1, S177–180.

Breslau, N. (1985) Psychiatric disorder in children with physical disabilities. *Journal of the American Academy of Child Psychiatry* **24**, 87–94.

Breslau, N. (1990) Does brain dysfunction increase children's vulnerability to environmental stress? *Archives of General Psychiatry* **47**, 15–20.

Breslau, N. and Prabucki, K. (1987) Siblings of disabled children. *Archives of General Psychiatry* **44**, 1040–6.

Breslau, N., Weitzman, M., and Messenger, K. (1981) Psychosocial functioning of siblings of disabled children. *Pediatrics* **67**, 344–53.

Brett, E. (1997) *Paediatric neurology*. Churchill Livingstone, Edinburgh, 3rd Edition.

Brewster, A. B. (1982) Chronically ill children's concepts of their illness. *Pediatrics* 69, 355–62.

Brinch, M., Isager, T., and Tolstrup, K. (1988) Anorexia nervosa and motherhood: reproduction and mothering behaviour of 50 woman. *Acta Psychiatrica Scandinavica* 77, 611–17.

British Medical Association and Pharmaceutical Society of Great Britain (1998) *British National Formulary*. British Medical Association, London.

Brooke, O. G., Anderson, H. R., Bland, J. M., Peacock, J. L., and Stewart, C. M. (1985) Effects on birthweight of smoking, alcohol, caffeine, socio-economic factors and psycho-social stress. *British Medical Journal* 298, 795–801.

Brown, B. (1979) Beyond separation: some new evidence on the impact of brief hospital-ization in young children. In *Medicine, illness and society. Beyond separation: further studies of children in hospital*, ed. D. Hall and M. Stacey, Routledge and Kegan Paul, London.

Brown, D. G. (1972) Stress as a precipitant factor of eczema. *Journal of Psychosomatic Research* 16, 321–7.

Brown, G. W. and Davidson, S. (1978) Social class, psychiatric disorder of mother and accidents to children. *Lancet* i, 378–80.

Brown, G. W. and Harris, T. (1978) *Social origins of depression*. Tavistock, London.

Brown, J. B. and Lloyd, H. (1975) A controlled study of children not speaking at school. *Journal of the Association of Workers with Maladjusted Children* 10, 49–63.

Brown, W. T. (1996) The molecular biology of the fragile X mutation. In *Fragile X syndrome: diagnosis, treatment and research*, ed. R. J. Hagerman, and A. Silverman, Johns Hopkins University Press, Baltimore.

Bruininks, R. H. (1978) *Bruininks–Oseretsky test of motor proficiency*. American Guidance Service, Circle Pines, MN.

Bryant-Waugh, R. and Lask, B. (1995) Eating disorders in children. *Journal of Child Psychology and Psychiatry* 36, 191–202.

Bryant-Waugh, R., Knibbs, J., Fosson, A., Kaminski, Z., and Lask, B. (1988) Long-term follow-up of patients with early onset anorexia nervosa. *Archives of Disease in Child-hood* 63, 5–9.

Budd, K. and Chugh, C. (1998) Common feeding problems in young children. *Advances in Clinical Child Psychology* 20, 138–212.

Burke, P., Meyer, V., Kocoshis, S., Orenstein, D., Chandra, R., and Sauer, J. (1989) Obsessive–compulsive symptoms in childhood inflammatory disease and cystic fibrosis. *Journal of the American Academy of Child and Adolescent Psychiatry* 28, 525–7.

Burton, L. (1974) *Care of the child facing death*. Routledge and Kegan Paul, London.

Burton, L. (1975) *The family life of sick children*. Routledge and Kegan Paul, London.

Button, E. J., Sonuga-Barke, E., Davies, J., and Thompson, M. (1996) A prospective study of self-esteem in the prediction of eating problems in adolescent schoolgirls: question-naire findings. *British Journal of Clinical Psychology* 35, 193–203.

Byrne, E. A. and Cunningham, C. C. (1985) The effect of mentally handicapped child-ren on families: a conceptual review. *Journal of Child Psychology and Psychiatry* 26, 847–64.

Bywater, M. (1981) Adolescents with cystic fibrosis: psychosocial adjustment. *Archives of Disease in Childhood* 56, 538–43.

Bywater, M. (1984) Coping with a life-threatening illness: an experiment in parents' groups. *British Journal of Social Work* 14, 117–27.

Cade, B. (1984) Paradoxical techniques in therapy. *Journal of Child Psychology and Psychiatry* 25, 509–16.

Cadman, D., Boyle, M., Szatmari, P., and Offord, D. R. (1987) Chronic illness, disability, and mental and social well-being: findings of the Ontario Child Health Study. *Pediatrics* **79**, 805–13.

Cadoret, R. J., Cain, C., and Crowe, R. R. (1983) Evidence for gene-environment interaction in the development of adolescent antisocial behaviour. *Behavioral Genetics* **13**, 301–10.

Cadoret, R., Yates, W., Troughton, E. *et al.* (1995) Genetic environmental interaction in the genesis of aggressivity and conduct disorders. *Archives of General Psychiatry* **52**, 916–24.

Cairns, S. N. and Lansky, S. B. (1980) MMPI indicators of stress and marital discord among parents of children with chronic illness. *Death Education* **4**, 29–42.

Calnan, M. W., Dale, J. W., and Fonseka, C. P. de (1976) Suspected poisoning in children. Study of the incidence of true poisoning and poisoning scare in a defined population. *Archives of Disease in Childhood* **51**, 180–5.

Cameron, M. and Hill, P. (1996) Hyperkinetic disorder: assessment and treatment. *Advances in Psychiatric Treatment* **2**, 94–102.

Cameron, R. J. (1990) Curriculum-related assessment. In *Educational assessment in the primary school*, ed. J. Beech and L. Harding, NFER-Nelson, Windsor.

Campbell, A. (1984) Failure to thrive. In J. Forfar and G. Arneil (eds) *Textbook of Pediatrics* 475–9, Churchill Livingstone, Edinburgh.

Campbell, L., Kirkpatrick, S., Berry, C., and Lamberti, J. (1995) Preparing children with congenital heart disease for cardiac surgery. *Journal of Pediatric Psychology* **20**, 313–328.

Campbell, S. B. (1986) Developmental issues in childhood anxiety. In *Anxiety disorders of childhood*, ed. R. Gittelman, Guilford, New York, pp. 24–57.

Campbell, S. (1995) Behaviour problems in pre-school children: a review of recent research. *Journal of Child Psychology and Psychiatry* **36**, 113–149.

Caplan, H. (1970) Hysterical 'conversion' symptoms in childhood. M.Phil Dissertation, University of London.

Caplan, M. G. and Douglas, V. I. (1969) Incidence of parental loss in children with depressed mood. *Journal of Child Psychology and Psychiatry* **10**, 225–36.

Capute, A. J., Shapiro, B. K., Palmer, F. B., Ross, A., and Wachtel, R. C. (1985) Normal gross motor development: the influence of race, sex and socioeconomic status. *Developmental Medicine and Child Neurology* **27**, 635–43.

Carlin, M. E. (1990) The improved prognosis in cri-du-chat (5p–) syndrome. In *Key Issues in Mental Retardation Research*, ed. W. I. Fraser, Routledge, London, pp. 64–73.

Carlson, G. A. and Cantwell, D. P. (1980) Unmasking masked depression in children and adolescents. *American Journal of Psychiatry* **137**, 445–9.

Carr, J. (1970) Mental and motor development in young mongol children. *Journal of Mental Deficiency Research* **14**, 205–20.

Carr, J. (1985) The effect on the family of a severely mentally handicapped child. In *Mental Deficiency: The Changing Outlook*, 4th edn, ed. A. M. Clarke, A. D. B. Clarke, and J. M. Berg, Methuen, London.

Carr, J. (1988) Six weeks to twenty-one years old: a longitudinal study of children with Down's syndrome and their families. *Journal of Child Psychology and Psychiatry* **29**, 407–32.

Carter, C., Urbanowicz, M., Hemsley, R., Mantilla, L., Strobel, S., Graham, P., and Taylor, E. (1993) Effects of a few foods diet in attention deficit disorder. *Archives of Disease in Childhood* **69**, 564–8.

Caspi, A., Moffitt, T., Newman, D., and Silva, P. (1996) Behavioral observations at 3 years predict adult psychiatric disorders. *Archives of General Psychiatry* **53**, 1033–9.

Cassell, S. and Paul, M. (1967) The role of puppet therapy on the emotional responses of children hospitalised for cardiac catheterisation. *Journal of Pediatrics* **71**, 233–9.

Caveness, W. F., Merritt, H. F., and Gallup, G. H. (1974) A survey of public attitudes towards epilepsy in 1974 with an indication of trends over the past twenty-five years. *Epilepsia* **15**, 523–6.

Cederblad, M. (1968) A child psychiatric study on Sudanese Arab children. *Acta Psychiatrica Scandinavica* **200** Suppl.

Cederblad, M. and Rahmin, S. (1986) Effects of rapid urbanisation on child behaviour and health in a part of Khartoum, Sudan; I Socio-economic changes 1965–1980. *Social Science Medicine* **22**, 713–21.

Central Statistical Office (1995) *Social trends, 1995.* HMSO, London.

Cepeda, M. L., Yang, Y. M., Price, C. C., and Shah, A. (1997) Mental disorders in children and adolescents with sickle-cell disease. *Southern Medical Journal* **90**, 284–7.

Cerreto, M. C. and Travis, L. B. (1984) Implications of psychological and family factors in the treatment of diabetes. *Pediatric Clinics of North America* **31**, 689–710.

Chamberlain, R. N., Christie, P. N., Holt, K. J., Huntley, R. M., Pollard, R., and Roche, M. C. (1983) A study of schoolchildren who had identified virus infection during infancy. *Child: Care, Health and Development* **9**, 29–47.

Chaplais, J. du Z. and Macfarlane, J.A. (1984) A review of 404 'late walkers'. *Archives of Disease in Childhood* **59**, 512–16.

Chappell, P. B., Riddle, M. A., Scahill, L. *et al.* (1995) Guanfacine treatment of comorbid attention-deficit hyperactivity disorder and Tourette's syndrome: preliminary clinical experience. *Journal of the American Academy of Child and Adolescent Psychiatry* **34**, 1140–6.

Charlton, A., Larcombe, I., Meller, S. *et al.* (1991) Absence from school related to carers and other chronic conditions. *Archives of Diseases in Childhood* **66**, 1217–22.

Chasnoff, I. (1988) Drug use in pregnancy: parameters of risk. *Pediatric Clinics of North America* **35**, 1403–12.

Cheasty, M., Clare, A. W., and Collins, C. (1998) Relations between sexual abuse in childhood and adult depression: case control study. *British Medical Journal,* **316**, 198–201.

Chess, S. and Fernandez, P. (1980) Neurologic damage and behavior disorders in rubella children. *American Annals of the Deaf* **125**, 998–1001.

Child Accident Prevention Trust (1989) *Basic principles of child accident prevention: a guide to action.* Child Accident Prevention Trust, London.

Child Growth Foundation (1994) *Standardised Growth Charts.* Child Growth Foundation, London.

Christensen, A. P. and Sanders, M. R. (1987) Habit reversal and differential reinforcement of other behaviour in the treatment of thumb-sucking: an analysis of generalisation and side-effects. *Journal of Child Psychology and Psychiatry* **28**, 281–95.

Christensen, M. F. and Mortensen, O. (1975) Long term prognosis in children with recurrent abdominal pain. *Archives of Disease in Childhood* **50**, 110–14.

Christodoulou, G. N., Gargoulas, A., Papalouvkasa, A., Marinopoulou, A., and Sideris, E. (1977) Primary peptic ulcer in childhood. Psychosocial, psychological and psychiatric aspects. *Acta Psychiatrica Scandinavica* **56**, 215–22.

Chu, C. E. and Connor, J. M. (1995) Molecular biology of Turner's syndrome. *Archives of Disease in Childhood* **72**, 285–6.

Chu, C. E., Donaldson, M. D., Kelnar, C. J. *et al.* (1994) Possible role of imprinting in the Turner syndrome. *Journal of Medical Genetics* **31**, 840–2.

Ciaranello, A. L. and Ciaranello, R. D. (1995) The neurobiology of autism. *Annual Review of Neurosciences* **18**, 101–28.

Clausen, J. A. (1975) The social meaning of differential physical and sexual maturation. In *Adolescence in the life cycle: psychological change and social content*, ed. S. E. Dragastin and G. H. Elder, Halsted, London, pp. 25–48.

Clay, M. (1985) *The early detection of reading difficulties*, 3rd edn. Heinemann, Tadworth, Surrey.

Clayden, G. S. (1988) Reflex anal dilatation associated with severe chronic constipation in children. *Archives of Disease in Childhood* 63, 832–6.

Clayton-Smith, J. (1993) Clinical research on Angelman syndrome in the United Kingdom: observations on 82 affected individuals. *American Journal of Medical Genetics* 46, 12–15.

Clements, S. (1966) Minimal brain dysfunction in children. *NINDS Monograph No. 3*, US Public Health Services, Washington, DC.

Cohen, J. A. and Mannarino, A. P. (1998) Factors that mediate treatment outcome of sexually abused preschool children: six and 12-month follow-up. *Journal of the American Academy of Child and Adolescent Psychiatry* 37, 44–51.

Cohen, N. J., Bradley, S., and Kolers, N. (1987) Outcome evaluation of a therapeutic day treatment program for delayed and disturbed pre-schoolers. *Journal of the American Academy of Child Psychiatry* 26, 687–93.

Cohn, A. H. (1983) *An approach to preventing child abuse*. National Committee for the Prevention of Child Abuse, Chicago.

Cohn, J. F. and Tronick, E. (1989) Specificity of infants' response to mothers affective behaviour. *Journal of the American Academy of Child and Adolescent Psychiatry* 28, 242–8.

Cohn, S. (1988) Assessing the gifted child and adolescent. In *Handbook of clinical assessment of children and adolescents, Vol. 1*, ed. C. J. Kestenbaum and D. T. Williams, New York University Press, New York, pp. 355–76.

Collacott, R. A., Cooper, S.-A., Branford, D., and McGrother, C. (1998) Behaviour phenotype for Down's syndrome. *British Journal of Psychiatry* 172, 85–9.

Colland, V. (1993) Learning to cope with asthma: a behavioral self-management program for children. *Patient Educational and Counselling* 22, 141–52.

Colley, A. F., Leversha, M. A., Voullaire, L. E., and Rogers, J. G. (1990) Five cases demonstrating the distinctive behavioural features of chromosome deletion 17(p11.2 p11.2) (Smith–Magenis syndrome). *Journal of Paediatrics and Child Health* 26, 17–21.

Colley, J. R. T. and Reid, D. D. (1970) Urban and social class origins of childhood bronchitis in England and Wales. *British Medical Journal* 2, 213.

Comer, J. P. (1985) The Yale–New Haven Primary Prevention Project: a follow up study. *Journal of the American Academy of Child Psychiatry* 24, 154–60.

Condon, J. T. (1987) Psychological and physical symptoms during pregnancy: a comparison of male and female expectant parents. *Journal of Reproductive and Infant Psychology* 5, 207–19.

Connell, H. M. and McConnel, T. S. (1981) Hydrocephalus in infancy: psychiatric sequelae. *Developmental Medicine and Child Neurology* 23, 505–17.

Conners, C. K. (1973) Rating scales for use in drug studies with children. *Psychopharmacology Bulletin (Special Issue, Pharmacotherapy of Children)*, 24–84.

Contact-A-Family (1998) *Parents Support Organisations Register*. Contact-A-Family, London.

Cool, V. A. (1996) Long-term neuropsychological risks in pediatric bone marrow transplant: what do we know? *Bone Marrow Transplant* 18, 545–9.

Cooper, P. J. and Goodyer, I. (1993) A community study of depression in adolescent girls. I: Estimates of syndrome and syndrome prevalence. *British Journal of Psychiatry* 163, 369–74.

Cooper, P. J., Campbell, A. E., Day, A., Kennerly, H., and Bond, A. (1988) Non-psychotic psychiatric disorder after childbirth. *British Journal of Psychiatry* 152, 799–806.

Cooper, S. (1987) The fetal alcohol syndrome. *Journal of Child Psychology and Psychiatry* 28, 223–8.

Corbett, J. (1981) Epilepsy and mental retardation. In *Epilepsy and Psychiatry*, ed. E. H. Reynolds and M. R. Trimble, Churchill Livingstone, Edinburgh, pp. 138–46.

Corbett, J. A., Harris, R., Taylor, E., and Trimble, M. (1977) Progressive disintegrative psychosis of childhood. *Journal of Child Psychology and Psychiatry* 18, 211–19.

Corbett, J. A., Trimble, M. R., and Nicol, T. C. (1985) Behavioral and cognitive impairment in children with epilepsy: the long-term effects of anti-convulsant therapy. *Journal of the American Academy of Child Psychiatry* 24, 17–23.

Cornish, K. M. and Munir, F. (1998) Receptive and expressive language skills in children with cri-du-chat syndrome. *Journal of Communication Disorders* 31, 73–82.

Cornish, K. M. and Pigram, J. (1996) Developmental and behavioural characteristics of cri du chat syndrome. *Archives of Disease in Childhood* 75, 448–50.

Costello, A. M. de L., Hamilton, P., Baudin, J. *et al.* (1989) Prediction of neurodevelopmental impairment at four years from brain ultrasound appearances of very pre-term infants. *Developmental Medicine and Child Neurology* 30, 711–22.

Cowen, L., Mok, J., Corey, M., MacMillan, H., Simmons, R., and Levison, H. (1986) Psychologic adjustment of the family with a member who has cystic fibrosis. *Pediatrics* 77, 745–53.

Cox, A., Hopkinson, K., and Rutter, M. (1981) Psychiatric interviewing techniques. II. Naturalistic study: eliciting factual information. *British Journal of Psychiatry* 138, 283–91.

Cox, J. L., Connor, Y., and Kendell, R. E . (1982) Prospective study of the psychiatric disorders of childbirth by personal interview. *British Journal of Psychiatry* 140, 111–19.

Crijnen, A., Achenbach, T., and Verhulst, F. (1997) Comparisons of problems reported by parents of children in 12 cultures: total problems, externalizing and internalizing. *Journal of the American Academy of Child and Adolescent Psychiatry* 36, 1269–77.

Crowell, J., Keener, M., Ginsburg, N., and Anders, T. (1987) Sleep habits in toddlers 18 to 36 months old. *Journal of the American Academy of Child and Adolescent Psychiatry* 26, 510–15.

Cullen, K. J. (1976) A six year controlled trial of prevention of children with behavioural disorders. *Journal of Pediatrics* 88, 662–6.

Cunningham, C. C., Morgan, P. A., and McGucken, R. B. (1984) Down's syndrome: is dissatisfaction with disclosure of diagnosis inevitable? *Developmental Medicine and Child Neurology* 26, 33–9.

Cytryn, L., Cytryn, E., and Rieger, E. (1967) Psychological implications of cryptorchidism. *Journal of the American Academy of Child Psychiatry* 6, 131–42.

Dahl, J. A., Melin, L., and Leissner, P. (1988) Effects of a behavioural intervention on epileptic seizure behaviour and paroxysmal activity: a systematic replication of three cases of children with intractable epilepsy. *Epilepsia* 29, 172–83.

Dahl, R., Holttum, J., and Trubnick, L. (1994) A clinical picture of child and adolescent narcolepsy. *Journal of the American Academy of Child and Adolescent Psychiatry* 33, 834–41.

Daud, L, Garralda, M. E., and David T. (1993) Psychosocial adjustment in pre-school children with atopic eczema. *Archives of Disease in Childhood* 69, 670–6.

Davie, R., Butler, N., and Goldstein, H. (1972) *From birth to seven: report of the National Child Development Study*. Longmans, London.

de Groot, C. M., Bornstein, R. A., Spetie, L., and Burriss, B. (1994) The course of tics in Tourette syndrome: a 5-year follow-up study. *Annals of Clinical Psychiatry* 6, 227–33.

De Jonge, G. A. (1973) Epidemiology of enuresis: a survey of the literature. In *Bladder Control and Enuresis. Clinics in Developmental Medicine Nos. 48/49*, ed. I. Kolvin, R. MacKeith, and S. R. Meadow, Heinemann/Spastics International Medical Publications, London, pp. 109–17.

Deale, A., Chalder, T., Marks, I., and Wessely, S. (1997) Cognitive behavior therapy for chronic fatigue syndrome: a randomized controlled trial. *American Journal of Psychiatry* 154, 408–14.

Di Gallo, A., Barton, J., and Parry-Jones, W. (1997) Road traffic accidents: early psychological consequences in children and adolescents. *British Journal of Psychiatry* 170, 358–62.

Delong, G. R. and Aldersdorf, A. L. (1987) Long-term experience with lithium treatment in childhood: correlation with clinical diagnosis. *Journal of the American Academy of Child and Adolescent Psychiatry* 26, 389–94.

DeMaso, D., Campis, L., Wypij, D., Bertram, S., Lipschitz, M., and Freed, M. (1991) The impact of maternal perceptions and medical severity on the adjustment of children with congenital heart disease. *Journal of Pediatric Psychology* 16, 137–49.

DeMaso, D., Twente, A., Spratt, E., and O'Brien, P. (1995) Impact of psychologic functioning, medical severity and family functioning in pediatric heart transplantation. *Journal of Heart-Lung Transplantation* 14, 1102–8.

Department for Education and Employment (1994) *Code of Practice.* Department for Education, London.

Department of Education and Science (1978) *Special educational needs.* HMSO, London.

Department of Health (1989) *Working together.* HMSO, London.

DeVaugh-Geiss, J., Maroz, G., Biederman, J. *et al.* (1992) Clomipramine hydrochloride in childhood and adolescent obsessive–compulsive disorder—a multi-center trial. *Journal of the American Academy of Child and Adolescent Psychiatry 31*, 45–9.

Diamond, G. S., Serrano, A. C., Dickey, M., and Sonis, W. A. (1997) Current status of family-based outcome and process research. *Journal of the American Academy of Child and Adolescent Psychiatry* 35, 6–16.

Diamond, L. J. and Jaudes, P. K. (1983) Child abuse in a cerebral-palsied population. *Developmental Medicine and Child Neurology* 25, 169–74.

Dische, S., Yule, W., Corbett, J., and Hand, D. (1983) Childhood nocturnal enuresis: factors associated with outcome of treatment with an enuretic alarm. *Developmental Medicine and Child Neurology* 25, 67–80.

Dodge, J. A. (1972) Psychosomatic aspects of infantile pyloric stenosis. *Journal of Psychosomatic Research* 16, 1–5.

Dorman, C., Hurley, A. D., and D'Avignon, J. (1988) Language and learning disorders of older boys with Duchenne muscular dystrophy. *Developmental Medicine and Child Neurology* 28, 316–27.

Dorner, S. (1976) Adolescents with spina bifida: how they see their situation. *Archives of Diseases in Childhood* 51, 439–44.

Douglas, J. (1998) Therapy for parents of difficult pre-school children. In *Cognitive behavioural therapy for children and families,* ed. P. J. Graham, Cambridge University Press, Cambridge.

Douglas, J. and Richman, N. (1984) *My Child Won't Sleep.* Penguin, London.

Douglas, J. W. B., Ross, J. M., and Simpson, H. R. (1968) *All our future: a longitudinal study of secondary education.* Peter Davies, London.

Dow, S. P., Sonies, B. C., Scheib, D., Moss, S. E., and Leonard, H. L. (1995) Practical guidelines for the assessment and treatment of selective mutism. *Journal of the American Academy of Child and Adolescent Psychiatry* 34, 836–46.

Downey, J., Ehrhardt, A. A., Morishima, A., Bell, J. J., and Gruen, R. (1987) Gender role development in two clinical syndromes. Turner syndrome versus constitutional short stature. *Journal of the American Academy of Child and Adolescent Psychiatry* 26, 566–73.

Drotar, D., Baskiewicz, A., Irvin, N., Kennell, J., and Klaus, M. (1975) The birth of an infant with a congenital malformation: a hypothetical model. *Pediatrics* 56, 710–17.

Drotar, D., Doershuk, C., Stern, R., Boat, T., Boyer, W., and Matthews, L. (1981) Psychological functioning of children with cystic fibrosis. *Pediatrics* 67, 338–43.

Dubowitz, V. and Hersov, L. (1976) Management of children with non-organic (hysterical) disorders of motor function. *Developmental Medicine and Child Neurology* 18, 358–68.

Duffy, G. and Spence, S. (1993) The effectiveness of cognitive self-management as an adjunct to a behavioural intervention for childhood obesity: a research note. *Journal of Child Psychology and Psychiatry* 34, 1043–50.

Dulcan, M. K., Costello, E. J., Costello, A. J., Edelbrock, C., Brent, D., and Janiszewski, S. (1990) The pediatrician as gatekeeper to mental health care for children: do parents' concerns open the gate? *Journal of the American Academy of Child and Adolescent Psychiatry* 29, 453–8.

Dummit, E. S., Klein, R. G., Tancer, N. K., Asche, B., and Martin, J. (1996) Fluoxetine treatment of children with selective mutism: an open trial. *Journal of the American Academy of Child and Adolescent Psychiatry* 35, 615–21.

Dummit, E. S., Klein, R. G., Tancer, N. K., Asche, B., Martin, J., and Fairbanks, J. A. (1997) Systematic assessment of 50 children with selective mutism. *Journal of the American Academy of Child and Adolescent Psychiatry* 36, 653–60.

Dunn, J. (1988) Sibling influence and child development. *Journal of Child Psychology and Psychiatry* 29, 119–28.

Dutton, P. V., Furnell, J. R. G., and Speirs, A. L. (1985) Environmental stress factors associated with toddler diarrhoea. *Journal of Psychosomatic Research* 29, 85–8.

Dykens, E. M. (1995) Measuring behavioral phenotypes: provocations from the 'new genetics'. *American Journal on Mental Retardation* 99, 522–32.

Dykens, E. M. and Cassidy, B. C. (1995) Correlates of maladaptive behavior in children and adults with Prader–Willi syndrome. *American Journal of Medical Genetics (Neuropsychiatric Genetics)* 60, 546–9.

Dykens, E. M. and Clarke, D. J. (1997) Correlates of maladaptive behaviour in individuals with 5p- (cri du chat) syndrome. *Developmental Medicine and Child Neurology* 39, 752–6.

Dykens, E. M., Hodapp, R. M., Ort, S., Finucane, B., Shapiro, L. R., and Leckman, J. F. (1989) The trajectory of cognitive development in males with fragile X syndrome. *Journal of the American Academy of Child and Adolescent Psychiatry* 28, 422–6.

Dykens, E. M., Hodapp, R. M., Walsh, K., and Nash, L. J. (1992) Adaptive and maladaptive behavior in Prader–Willi syndrome. *Journal of the American Academy of Child and Adolescent Psychiatry* 31, 1131–6.

Earls, F. and Richman, N. (1980) The prevalence of behaviour problems in three year old children of West Indian born parents. *Journal of Child Psychology and Psychiatry* 21, 99–106.

Eaton-Evans, J. and Dugdale, A. E. (1988) Sleep patterns of infants in the first year of life. *Archives of Diseases in Childhood* 63, 647–9.

Eaves, L., Silberg, J., Meyer, J. *et al.* (1997) Genetics and developmental psychopathology: 2. The main effects of genes and environment on behavioural problems in the Virginia twin study of adolescent behavioural development. *Journal of Child Psychology and Psychiatry* 38, 965–80.

Egger, J., Carter, C., Graham, P., Gumley, D., and Soothill, J. (1985) A controlled trial of oligoantigenic treatment in the hyperkinetic syndrome. *Lancet* i, 540–5.

Ehlers, S. and Gillberg, C. (1993) The epidemiology of Asperger syndrome: a total population study. *Journal of Child Psychology and Psychiatry* 34, 1327–50.

Eisenberg, L., Conners, K., and Sharpe, L. (1965) A controlled study of the differential application of out-patient psychiatric treatment for children. *Japanese Journal of Child Psychiatry* 6, 125–32

Eiser, C. (1989) Childrens' concepts of illness: towards an alternative to the stage approach. *Psychology and Health* 3, 93–101.

Eiser, C. (1993) *Growing up with a chronic disease.* Jessica Kingsley, London.

Eiser, C. and Town, C. (1987) Teacher's concerns about chronically sick children: implications for paediatricians. *Developmental Medicine and Child Neurology* 29, 56–63.

Eiser, C., Havermass, T., and Casas, R. (1993) Healthy children's understanding of their blood: implications for explaining leukaemia to children. *British Journal of Educational Psychology* 63, 528–537.

El Abd, S., Turk, J., and Hill, P. (1995) Annotation: psychological characteristics of Turner syndrome. *Journal of Child Psychology and Psychiatry* 36, 1109–25.

El Abd, S., Wilson, L., Howlin, P., Patton, M.A., Wintgens, A.M., and Wilson, R. (1997) Agenesis of the corpus callosum in Turner syndrome with ring X. *Developmental Medicine and Child Neurology* 39, 119–24.

Elliott, C., Murray, D., and Pearson, L. (1996) *British Ability Scales.* Manuals 1–4. NFER, Nelson, Windsor.

Ellis, A. (1962) *Reason and emotion in psychotherapy.* Lyle Stewart, New York.

Emery, A. E. H. (1985) Infanticide, filicide and cot death. *Archives of Disease in Childhood* 66, 505–7.

Emslie, G. J., Rush, A. J., Weiberg, W. A., Kowatch, R. A., Hughes, C. W., Carmody, T., and Rintelmann, J. (1997) A double-blind randomized, placebo-controlled trial of fluoxetine in children and adolescents with depression. *Archives of General Psychiatry* 54, 1031–7.

Engstrom, I. and Lindquist, B. (1991) Inflammatory bowel disease in children and adolescents: a somatic and psychiatric investigation. Acta Paediatrica Scandinavica 80, 640–7.

Epstein, L., Valonski, A., Wine, R., and McCurley, J. (1994) Ten year outcomes of behavioural family-based treatment for childhood obesity. *Health Psychology* 13, 373–83.

Epstein, L. H., Myers, M. D., and Anderson, K. (1996) The association of maternal psychopathology and family socio-economic status with psychological problems in obese children. *Obesity Research* 4, 65–74.

Eth, S. R. and Pynoos, R. S. (1985) *Post-traumatic stress disorder in children.* American Psychiatric Association, Washington, DC.

Evans, J. H. and Meadow, S. R. (1992) Desmopressin for bed wetting: length of treatment, vasopressin secretion, and response. *Archives of Disease in Childhood* 67, 184–8.

Evans, J. H. C. and Meadow, S. R. (1990) What's new in enuresis? *Maternal and Child Health* 15, 178–82.

Evered, C. J., Hill, P. D., Hall, D. M., and Hollins, S. C. (1989) Liaison psychiatry in a child development clinic. *Archives of Disease in Childhood* 64, 754–8.

Eysenck, M. and Keane, M. T. (1990) *Cognitive psychology.* Lawrence Erlbaum, Hove, Sussex.

Farrington, D. (1995) The development of offending and antisocial behaviour from childhood: key findings from the Cambridge study in delinquent development. *Journal of Child Psychology and Psychiatry* **36**, 929–64.

Farrington, D. P. (1977) The effects of public labelling. *British Journal of Criminology* **17**, 112–25.

Feingold, B. F. (1975) Hyperkinesis and learning difficulties linked to artificial food and colors. *American Journal of Nursing* **75**, 797–803.

Feldman, F., Cantor, D., Soll, S., and Bachrach, W. (1967) Psychiatric study of a consecutive series of thirty-four patients with ulcerative colitis. *British Medical Journal* **3**, 14–17.

Ferdinand, R. and Verhulst, F. (1995) Psychopathology from adolescence into young adulthood: an 8 year follow-up study. *American Journal of Psychiatry* **152**, 1586–94.

Fergusson, D. M., Lynskey, M. T., and Horwood, L. J. (1997) Childhood sexual abuse and psychiatric disorder in young adulthood. I: Prevalence of sexual abuse and factors associated with sexual abuse. *Journal of the American Academy of Child and Adolescent Psychiatry* **35**, 1355–64.

Ferrari, M., Matthews, S., and Barabas, G. (1983) The family and child with epilepsy. *Family Process* **22**, 53–60.

Ferrier, L. J., Bashir, A. S., Meryash, D. L., Johnston, J., and Wolff, P. (1991) Conversational skills of individuals with fragile-X syndrome: a comparison with autism and Down syndrome. *Developmental Medicine and Child Neurology* **33**, 776–788.

Fine, S. (1979) Incidence of visual handicap in childhood. In *Visual handicap in children* (ed V. Smith and J. Keen). Spastic International Medical Publications, Heinemann, London.

Fine, S., Forth, A., Gilbert, M., and Haley, G. (1991) Group therapy for adolescent depressive disorder: a comparison of social skills and therapeutic support. *Journal of the American Academy of Child and Adolescent Psychiatry* **30**, 79–85.

Finkelhor, D. (1979) *Sexually victimised children*. Free Press, New York.

Firth, M., Gardner-Medwin, D., Hosking, G., and Wilkinson, E. (1983) Interviews with parents of boys suffering from muscular dystrophy. *Developmental Medicine and Child Neurology* **25**, 466–71.

Fish, D., Smith, S., Quesney, L., Andermann, F., and Rasmussen, T. (1993) Surgical treatment of children with medically intractable frontal or temporal lobe epilepsy: results and highlights of 40 years experience. *Epilepsia* **34**, 244–247.

Fishler, K., Koch, R., Donnell, G., and Graliker, B. V. (1966) Psychological correlates in galactosemia. *American Journal of Mental Deficiency* **71**, 116–25.

Fishman, M. and Palkes, H. (1974) The validity of psychometric testing in children with congenital malformations of the central nervous system. *Developmental Medicine and Child Neurology* **16**, 180–5.

Fitzpatrick, C., Barry, C., and Garvey, C. (1986) Psychiatric disorder among boys with Duchenne Muscular Dystrophy. *Developmental Medicine and Child Neurology* **28**, 589–95.

Flament, M. F., Rapoport, J. L., Berg, C. J., and Kilts, C. (1985) A controlled trial of clomipramine in childhood obsessive compulsive disorder. *Psychopharmacology Bulletin* **21**, 150–152.

Flament, M. F. *et al.* (1990). Childhood obsessive-compulsive disorder. *Journal of Child Psychology and Psychiatry* **31**, 363–80.

Fogelman, D., Tibbenham, A., and Lambert, L. (1980) Absence from school: findings from the National Child Development Study. *In Out of school* (ed. L. Hersov and I. Berg), pp. 25–48. John Wiley, Chichester.

Fombonne, E. (1995) Eating disorders: time trends and possible explanatory mechanisms. In: M. Rutter and D. Smith (ed.). *Psychosocial disorders in young people*. Chichester: Wiley, pp. 616–685.

Fombonne, E., Du Mazaubrun, C., Cans, C., and Grandjean, H. (1997) Autism and associated medical disorders in a French epidemiological survey. *Journal of the American Academy of Child and Adolescent Psychiatry* 36, 1561–9.

Fonagy, P., and Moran, G. S. (1990) Studies on the efficacy of child psychoanalysis. *Journal of Consulting and Clinical Psychology* 58, 684–695.

Fonagy, P., Moran, G. S., Lindsay, M. K. M., Kurtz, A. B., and Brown, R. (1987) Psychological adjustment and diabetic control. *Archives of Disease in Childhood* 62, 1009–13.

Fonagy, P., Streele, H., and Steel, M. (1991) Maternal representativeness of attachment during pregnancy predicts the organisation of infant-mother attachment at one year. Child Development 62, 891–905.

Fonagy, P., Target, M., Steele, M., and Gerber, A. (1995) Psychoanalytic perspectives on developmental psychopathology. In: D. Cicchetti and D. J. Cohen (ed.). *Developmental psychopathology. Vol. 1: Theories and methods.* Chichester: Wiley, pp 504–54.

Fordham, K. E. and Meadow, S. R. (1988) Controlled trial of standard pad and bell alarm against mini-alarm for nocturnal enuresis. *Archives of Disease in Childhood* 64, 651–6.

Forrest, G. C., Claridge, R. S., and Baum, J. D. (1981) Practical management of perinatal death. *British Medical Journal* 282, 31–2.

Forrest, G. C., Standish, E., and Baum, D. (1982) Support after perinatal death: a study of support and counselling after perinatal bereavement. *British Medical Journal* 285, 1475–8.

Forssman, H. and Thuwe, I. (1966) One hundred and twenty children born after application for therapeutic abortion refused. *Acta Psychiatrica Scandinavica* 42, 71–88.

Fosson, A., Knibbs, J., Bryant-Waugh, R., and Lask, B. (1987) Early onset anorexia nervosa. *Archives of Disease in Childhood* 62, 114–18.

Fournier, J.-P., Garfinkel, B. D., Bond, A., Beauchesne, H., and Shapiro, S. K. (1987) Pharmacological and behavioral management of enuresis. *Journal of the American Academy of Child and Adolescent Psychiatry* 26, 845–53.

Fraiberg, S. (1977) *Insights from the blind*. Basic Books, New York.

Frank, D. A. and Zeisel, S. H. (1988) Failure to thrive. *Pediatric Clinics of North America* 35, 1187–206.

Frankenburg, W. K., Dodds, J. B., Fandal, A. W., Kazuk, E., and Cohrs, M. (1975) *Denver Developmental Screening Test*. Ladoca Project and Publishing Foundation, Denver.

Freeman, C. (1995) ECT in those under 18 years old. In *ECT handbook*, ed. C. Freeman, Royal College of Psychiatrists, London, pp. 18–21.

Freeman, J. (1983) Emotional problems of the gifted child. *Journal of Child Psychology and Psychiatry* 24, 481–5.

Freeman, R. D. (1970) Psychiatric problems in adolescents with cerebral palsy. *Developmental Medicine and Child Neurology* 12, 64–70.

Freeman, R. D. (1977) Psychiatric aspects of sensory disorders and intervention. In *Epidemiological approaches in child psychiatry*, ed. P. J. Graham, Academic Press, London, pp. 275–304.

Freeman, R. D. (1989) Blind children's early emotional development: do we know enough to help? *Child: Care, Health and Development* 15, 3–28.

Freud, A. (1966) *Normality and pathology in childhood*. Hogarth, London.

Fritz, G. K., Fritsch, S., and Hagino, O. (1997) Somatoform disorders in children and adolescents. A review of the past ten years. *Journal of the American Academy of Child and Adolescent Psychiatry* 36, 1329–38.

Frydman, M. (1981) Social support, life-events and psychiatric symptoms: a study of direct, conditional and interaction effects. *Social Psychiatry* 16, 69–78.

Fuggle, P., Shand, G. A., Gill, L. J., and Davies, S. C. (1996) Pain, quality of life and coping in sickle-cell disease. *Archives of Disease in Childhood* 75, 199–203.

Fulcher, K. Y. and White, P. D. (1997) Randomised controlled trial of graded exercise in patients with chronic fatigue syndrome. *British Medical Journal* 314, 1647–52.

Fundudis, T., Kolvin, I., and Garside, R. (eds) (1979) *Speech retarded and deaf children: their psychological development.* Academic Press, London.

Furniss, T., Bingley-Miller, L., and Bentovim, A. (1984) Therapeutic approach to sexual abuse. *Archives of Disease in Childhood* 59, 865–70.

Galante, R. and Foa, D. (1986) An epidemiological study of psychic trauma and treatment effectiveness for children after a natural disaster. *Journal of the American Academy of Child Psychiatry* 25, 357–63.

Galatzer, A., Nofar, E., Beit Halachmi, N. *et al.* (1981) Intellectual and psychosocial functions of children, adolescents and young adults before and after operations for craniopharyngioma. *Child: Care, Health and Development* 7, 307–16.

Gambrill, E. (1983) Behavioral intervention with child abuse and neglect. *Progress in Behaviour Modification* 15, 1–56.

Garber, H. J., McGonigle, J. J., Slomka, G. T., and Monteverde, E. (1992) Clomipramine treatment of stereotypic behaviors and self-injury in patients with developmental disabilities. *Journal of the American Academy of Child and Adolescent Psychiatry* 31, 1157–60.

Garber, J., Zeman, J., and Walker, L. S. (1990) Recurrent abdominal pain in children: psychiatric diagnoses and parental psychopathology. Journal of the American Academy of Child and Adolescent Psychiatry 29, 648–56.

Gardner, R. J. M., and Sutherland, G. R. (1996) Prenatal diagnostic procedures. In *Chromosome abnormalities and genetic counselling*, Oxford University Press, Oxford, pp. 336–44.

Garland, A., Shaffer, D., and Whittle, B. (1989) A national survey of school based, adolescent suicide prevention programs. *Journal of the American Academy of Child and Adolescent Psychiatry* 28, 931–4.

Garralda, M. E. (1984) Hallucinations in children with conduct and emotional disorders. *Psychological Medicine* 14, 589–96.

Garralda, M. E. and Bailey, D. (1986) Children with psychiatric disorders in primary care. *Journal of Child Psychology and Psychiatry* 27, 611–24.

Garralda, M. and Bailey, D. (1989) Psychiatric disorders in general practice referrals. *Archives of Disease in Childhood* 64, 1727–33.

Garralda, M. E., Jameson, R. A., Reynolds, J. M., and Postlethwaite, R. J. (1988). Psychiatric adjustment in children with chronic renal failure. *Journal of Child Psychology and Psychiatry* 29, 79–91.

Garrison, C. Z., Waller, J. L., Cuffer, S. P., McKeown, R. E., Addy, C., and Jackson, K. (1997) Incidence of major depressive disorder and dysthymia in young adolescents. *Journal of the American Academy of Child and Adolescent Psychiatry* 36, 458–65.

Garson, A., Benson, R. S., Ivler, L., and Patton, C. (1978) Parental reactions to children with congenital heart disease. *Child Psychiatry and Human Development* 9, 86–94.

Gath, A. (1989) Living with a mentally handicapped brother or sister. *Archives of Disease in Childhood* 64, 513–16.

Gath, A. and Gumley, D. (1984) Down's syndrome and the family: follow-up of children first seen in infancy. *Developmental Medicine and Child Neurology* 26, 500–8.

Gath, A. and Gumley, D. (1987) Retarded children and their siblings. *Journal of Child Psychology and Psychiatry* 28, 715–30.

Gatherer, A., Parfitt, J., Porter, E., and Vessey, M. (1979) *Is health education effective?* Health Education Council, London.

Gayton, W. F., Friedman, S. B., Tavormina, J. F., and Tucker, F. (1977) Children with cystic fibrosis: psychological test findings of patients, siblings and parents. *Pediatrics* **59**, 888–94.

Geller, B. and Luby, J. (1997) Child and adolescent bipolar disorder: a review of the past ten years. *Journal of the American Academy of Child and Adolescent Psychiatry* **36**, 1168–76.

Gergen, P. J., Mullaly, P. I., and Evans, R. (1988) National survey of prevalence of asthma among children in the United States, 1976–1980. *Pediatrics* **81**, 1–7.

Ghaziuddin, M. and Gerstein, L. (1996) Pedantic speaking style differentiates Asperger syndrome from high-functioning autism. *Journal of Autism and Developmental Disorders* **26**, 585–95.

Gibb, C. (1992) The most common cause of learning difficulties: a profile of fragile-X syndrome and its implications for education. *Educational Research* **34**, 221–8.

Gibbens, T. C. N. (1974) Preparing psychiatric case reports. *British Journal of Hospital Medicine* **11**, 278–84.

Gibbs, M. V. and Thorpe, J. G. (1983) Personality stereotype of noninstitutionalised Down syndrome children. *American Journal of Mental Deficiency* **87**, 601–5.

Gilbert, R. (1994) The changing epidemiology of SIDS. *Archives of Diseases in Childhood* **70**, 445–9.

Gill, M., Daly, G., Heron, S., Hawi, Z., and Fitzgerald, M. (1997) Confirmation of association between attention deficit hyperactivity disorder and a dopamine transporter polymorphism. *Molecular Psychiatry* **2**, 311–13.

Gill, O. and Jackson, B. (1984) *Adoption and race.* Batsford, London.

Gillberg, C. (1991) Outcome in autism and autistic-like conditions. *Journal of the American Academy of Child and Adolescent Psychiatry* **30**, 375–82.

Gillberg, C. (1992) Subgroups in autism: are there behavioural phenotypes typical of underlying medical conditions? *Journal of Intellectual Disability Research* **36**, 201–14.

Gillberg, C. and Schaumann, H. (1989) Autism: specific problems of adolescence. In *Diagnosis and Treatment of Autism*, ed: C. Gillberg, Plenum: New York, pp. 375–82.

Gillberg, C., Persson, U., Grufman, M., and Temner, U. (1986) Psychiatric disorders in mildly and severely mentally retarded urban children and adolescents. Epidemiological aspects. *British Journal of Psychiatry* **149**, 69–74.

Gillberg, I. C., Gillberg, C., and Ahlsen, G. (1994) Autistic behaviour and attention deficits in tuberous sclerosis: a population-based study. *Developmental Medicine and Child Neurology* **36**, 50–6.

Gillies, D., Sills, M., and Forsythe, I. (1986) Pizotifen (Sanomigran) in childhood migraine. *European Neurology* **25**, 32–5.

Gilman, J. T. and Tuchman, R. F. (1995) Autism and associated behavioral disorders: pharmacotherapeutic intervention. *Annals of Pharmacotherapy* **29**, 47–56.

Giovannoni, J. M. and Becerra, R. M. (1979) *Defining child abuse.* Free Press, New York.

Gittelman-Klein, R. and Mannuzza, S. (1989) The long-term outcome of the attention deficit disorder/hyperkinetic syndrome. In *Attention deficit disorder: clinical and basic research*, ed. T. Sagvolden and T. Archer, Lawrence Erlbaum, Hillsdale, NJ, pp. 71–91.

Glaser, D. and Bentovim, A. (1987) Psychological aspects of congenital heart disease. In *Paediatric cardiology*, ed. R. H. Anderson, F. J. Macartney, E. A. Shinebourne, and M. Tynan, Churchill Livingstone, Edinburgh.

Goldenberg, J. N., Brown, S. B., and Weiner, W. J. (1994) Coprolalia in younger patients with Gilles de la Tourette Syndrome. *Movement Disorders* **9**, 622–5.

Golombok, S., Spencer, A., and Rutter, M. (1983) Children in lesbian and single-parent households: psychosexual and psychiatric appraisal. *Journal of Child Psychology and Psychiatry* 24, 551–72.

Goodman, R. (1997a) Child mental health: an over-extended remit. *British Medical Journal* 314, 813–14.

Goodman, R. (1997b) Psychological aspects of hemiplegia. *Archives of Disease in Childhood* 76, 177–8.

Goodman, R. and Graham P. (1996) Psychiatric problems in children with hemiplegia. *British Medical Journal* 312, 1065–9.

Goodman, R. and Stevenson, J. (1989) A twin study of hyperactivity. II. The aetiological role of genes, family relationships and perinatal adversity. *Journal of Child Psychology and Psychiatry* 30, 691–709.

Goodyer, I. M. (1990) *Life, experiences, development and childhood psychopathology.* Wiley, Chichester.

Goodyer, I. (1992) Stressful life events and childhood illnesses. *Archives of Diseases in Childhood* 67, 673–674.

Goodyer, I. and Taylor, D. C. (1985) Hysteria. *Archives of Disease in Childhood* 60, 680–1.

Goodyer, I. M., Wright, C., and Altham, P. M. E. (1987) The impact of recent life events in psychiatric disorders of childhood and adolescence. *British Journal of Psychiatry* 151, 179–85.

Goodyer, I., Herbert, J., Altham, P., Pearson, J., Secher, S., and Shiers, H. (1996) Adrenal secretion during major depression in 8–16 year olds. I: Altered diurnal rhythms in salivary cortisol and dehydroepiandrosterone (DHEA) at presentation. *Psychological Medicine* 26, 245–56.

Goodyer, I., Herbert, J., Secher, S., and Pearson, J. (1997a) Short-term outcome of major depression: I Co-morbidity and severity at presentation as predictors of persistent disorder. *Journal of the American Academy of Child and Adolescent Psychiatry* 36, 179–87.

Goodyer, I., Herbert, J., Tamplin, A., Secher, S., and Pearson, J. (1997b) Short-term outcome of major depression. II: Life events, family function and friendship difficulties as predictors of persistent disorder. *Journal of the American Academy of Child and Adolescent Psychiatry* 36, 474–80.

Gorrell-Barnes, J. (1995) Family therapy. In *Child and adolescent psychiatry: modern approaches*, ed. M. Rutter, E. Taylor and L. Hersov, Blackwell Scientific, Oxford, pp. 946–67.

Gortmaker, S., Must, A., Sobol, A., Peterson, K., Colditz, G., and Dietz, W. (1996) Television viewing as a cause of increasing obesity among children in the United States. *Archives of Pediatric and Adolescent Medicine* 150, 356–62.

Graham. P. (1982) Child psychiatry in relation to primary health care. *Social Psychiatry* 17, 109–16.

Graham, P. (1984) Paediatric referral to a child psychiatrist. *Archives of Disease in Childhood* 59, 1103–5.

Graham, P. (1990) Maternal employment. *Archives of Disease in Childhood* 65, 565–6.

Graham, P. (1995) Prevention. In *Child and adolescent psychiatry: modern approaches*, ed. M. Rutter, E. Taylor and L. Hersov, Blackwell Scientific, Oxford, pp. 815–28.

Graham, P. (ed). (1998a) *Cognitive behaviour therapy for children and families.* Cambridge University Press, Cambridge.

Graham, P. (1998b) Ethics in child psychiatry. In *Psychiatric ethics*, ed. S. Bloch and J. Chodoff, Oxford University Press, Oxford.

Graham, P. and Jenkins, S. (1985) Training of paediatricians for psychosocial aspects of their work. *Archives of Disease in Childhood* 60, 777–80.

Graham, P., Wolkind, S., and Dingwall, R. (1985) Research issues in child abuse. *Social Science and Medicine* 21, 1217–28.

Grattan-Smith, P., Fairly, M., and Procopis, P. (1988) Clinical features of conversion disorder. *Archives of Diseases in Childhood* 63, 408–14.

Green, J. (1990) Is Asperger's a syndrome? *Developmental Medicine and Child Neurology* 32, 743–7.

Green, J. M., Dennis, J., and Bennets, L. A. (1989) Attention disorder in a group of young Down's syndrome children. *Journal of Mental Deficiency Research* 33, 105–22.

Green, M. and Solnit, A. J. (1964) Reactions to the threatened loss of a child: a vulnerable child syndrome. *Pediatrics* 34, 58–66.

Green, W. H. (1995) *Child and Adolescent Clinical Psychopharmacology*. Williams and Wilkins, Baltimore.

Green, W. H., Padron-Gayol, M., Hardesty, A., and Bassiri, M. (1992) Schizophrenia and childhood onset: a phenomenological study of 38 cases. *Journal of the American Academy of Child and Adolescent Psychiatry* 31, 968–76.

Grey, M. J., Genel, M., and Tamborlane, W. V. (1980) Psychosocial adjustment of latency aged diabetics: determinants and relationship to control. *Pediatrics* 65, 69–73.

Griffiths, R. (1954) *The abilities of babies*. McGraw-Hill, New York.

Grubman, S., Gross, E. Lerner-Weiss, E. *et al.* (1995) Older children and adolescents living with perinatally acquired human immunodeficiency virus infection. *Pediatrics* 95, 657–63.

Guilleminault, C., Carskadon, M., and Dement, W. C. (1974) On the treatment of rapid eye movement narcolepsy. *Archives of Neurology* 30, 90–3.

Gurman, A. and Kniskern, D. P. (1979) Research on marital and family therapy. In *Handbook of psychotherapy and behavior change*, ed. S. Garfield and A. Berger, Brunner Mazel, New York.

Gustafsson, P. A., Kjellman, N. -I. M., Ludvigsson, J., and Cederblad, M. (1987) Asthma and family interaction. *Archives of Disease in Childhood* 62, 258–63.

Gutelius, M. F., Kirsch, A. D., MacDonald, S., Brooks, M. R., and McErlean, T. (1977) Controlled study of child health supervision: behavioral results. *Pediatrics* 60, 294–304.

Gyulay, J. E. (1978) *The dying child*. McGraw-Hill, New York.

Hagberg, B. (1993) *Rett Syndrome—Clinical and Biological Aspects. Clinics in Developmental Medicine No. 127*. MacKeith Press, London.

Hagberg, B. and Hagberg, G. (1984) Prenatal and perinatal risk factors in a survey of 681 Swedish cases. In *The Epidemiology of the Cerebral Palsies*, ed. F. Stanley and E. Alberman, Blackwell Scientific, Oxford.

Hagberg, B., Hagberg, G., Lewerth, A., and Lindberg, V. (1981) Mild mental retardation in Swedish school children. II. Etiological and pathogenetic aspects. *Acta Paediatrica Scandinavica* 70, 445–52.

Hagerman, R. J. (1996) Physical and Behavioral Phenotype. In R. J. Hagerman and C. Cronister (ed.): *Fragile X Syndrome: Diagnosis, Treatment and Research*. Johns Hopkins University Press, Baltimore, pp. 3–87.

Hagerman, R. J., and Cronister, A. C. (1996) *Fragile X Syndrome: Diagnosis, Research and Treatment*. Johns Hopkins University Press, Baltimore,

Haggard, M. and Hughes, E. (1991) *Screening children's hearing*. HMSO, London.

Haggerty, R. J. (1980) Life stress, illness and social support. *Developmental Medicine and Child Neurology* 22, 391–400.

Hall, D. M. B. (ed.) (1989) *Health for all children*. Oxford Medical Publications, Oxford.

Hamblin, T. J., Hussain, J., Akbar, A. N., Tang, Y. C., Smith, J. L., and Jones, D. B. (1983) Immunological reason for chronic ill health after infectious mononucleosis. *British Medical Journal* **287**, 85–9.

Hamburg, D. and Hamburg, B. (1980) A life-span perspective on adaptation and health. In *Family and health: epidemiological approaches*, ed. B. Kaplan and M. Ibrahim, University of South Carolina Press, Chapel Hill.

Hammer, L. (1992) The development of eating behaviour in childhood. *Pediatric Clinics of North America.* **39**, 379–94.

Happé, F. and Frith, U. (1996) The neuropsychology of autism. *Brain* 119, 1377–400.

Harbord, M. G. and Manson, J. I. (1987) Temporal lobe epilepsy in childhood: re-appraisal of etiology and outcome. *Pediatric Neurology* 3, 263–8.

Haring, N. G., Lovitt, T. C., Eaton, M. D., and Hanson, C. L. (1978) *The 4th R: research in the classroom.* Charles Merrill, Columbus, OH.

Harrington, R. (1993) Psychological treatments. In *Depressive disorder in childhood and adolescence*, Wiley, Chichester, pp. 151–67.

Harrington, R., Fudge, H., and Rutter, M. (1990) Adult outcomes of child and adolescent depression. I: Psychiatric status. *Archives of General Psychiatry* 47, 465–73.

Harrington, R., Wood, A., and Verduyn, C. (1998) Principles and practice of cognitive behaviour therapy with clinically depressed adolescents. In: *Cognitive behaviour therapy for children and families*, ed. P. Graham, Cambridge University Press, Cambridge, pp. 156–93.

Harris, B. H., Schwaitzberg, S. D., Seman, T. M., and Herrmann, C. (1989) The hidden morbidity of pediatric trauma. *Journal of Pediatric Surgery* 24, 103–5.

Harris, D. B. (1963) *Children's drawings as measures of intellectual maturity: a revision and extension of the Goodenough Draw-A-Man Test.* Harcourt, Brace and World, New York.

Harris, J. C. (1995) Mental Retardation. In *Developmental Neuropsychiatry*, Volume 2, ed. J. Harris, Oxford University Press, Oxford, pp. 91–126.

Harrison, J. E. and Bolton, P. F. (1997) Annotation: tuberous sclerosis. *Journal of Child Psychology and Psychiatry* 38, 603–14.

Hattie, J. and Edwards, H. (1987) A review of the Bruininks–Oseretsky test of motor proficiency. *British Journal of Educational Psychology* 57, 104–13.

Hawton, K. (1982) Attempted suicide in children and adolescents. *Journal of Child Psychology and Psychiatry* 23, 497–503.

Hawton, K., Fagg, J., Simkin, S., Bale, E., and Bond, A. (1997) Trends in deliberate self-harm in Oxford, 1985–95. Implications for clinical services and the prevention of suicide. *British Journal of Psychiatry* 171, 556–60.

Hazell, P., O'Connell, D., Heathcote, D., Robertson, J., and Henry, D. (1995) Efficacy of tricyclic drugs in treating child and adolescent depression: a meta-analysis. *British Medical Journal* 310, 897–901.

Health Advisory Service (1995) *Child and adolescent mental health services: together we stand.* HMSO, London.

Hellings, J. A. and Warnock, J. K. (1994) Self-injurious behavior and serotonin in Prader–Willi syndrome. *Psychopharmacology Bulletin* 30, 245–50.

Henderson, S. E. and Hall, D. (1982) Concomitants of clumsiness in young schoolchildren. *Developmental Medicine and Child Neurology* 24, 448–60.

Hendren, R., Hodde-Vargas, J., Yeo, R., Vargas, L., Brooks, W., and Ford, S. (1995) Neuropsychophysiological study of children at risk for schizophrenia: a preliminary report. *Journal of the American Academy of Child and Adolescent Psychiatry* 34, 1284–91.

Henggeler, S. (1999) Multisystemic therapy: an overview of clinical procedures, outcomes and policy implication. *Child Psyhology and Psychiatry Reveiw* 4, 2–10.

Hensey, O. J., Williams, J. K., and Rosenbloom, L. (1983) Intervention in child abuse: experience in Liverpool. *Developmental Medicine and Child Neurology* 25, 606–11.

Herbert, M. (1981) *Behavioural treatment of problem children: a practice manual.* Academic Press, London.

Herbert, M. (1994) Behavioural methods. In *Child and adolescent psychiatry, modern approaches*, ed.. M. Rutter, E. Taylor and L. Hersov, Blackwell Scientific, Oxford, pp. 858–79.

Hersov, L. A. (1960) Persistent non-attendance at school. *Journal of Child Psychology and Psychiatry* 1, 130–6.

Herzog, D. B. and Copeland, P. M. (1985) Eating disorders. *New England Journal of Medicine* 313, 294–303.

Heston, L. (1966) Psychiatric disorder in foster and home-reared children of schizophrenic mothers. *British Journal of Psychiatry* 113, 819–25.

Hetherington, E. M., Cox, M., and Cox, R. (1982) Effects of divorce on parents and children. In *Non-traditional families*, ed. M. E. Lamb, Lawrence Erlbaum, Hillsdale, NJ, pp. 233–88.

Hewison, J, and Tizard, J. (1980) Parental involvement and reading attainment. *British Journal of Educational Psychology* 50, 209–15.

Hill, R. A., Standen, P. J., and Tattersfield, A. E. (1989) Asthma, wheezing and school absence in primary schools. *Archives of Disease in Childhood* 64, 246–51.

Hindley, P. (1997) Psychiatric aspects of hearing impairment. *Journal of Child Psychology and Psychiatry* 38, 101–17.

Hindley, P. and Brown, R. M. A. (1994) Psychiatric aspects of specific sensory impairments. In *Child and adolescent psychiatry, modern approaches*, ed.. M. Rutter, E. Taylor and L. Hersov, Blackwell Scientific, Oxford, pp. 720–36.

Hindley, P., Hill, P., and Bond, D. (1993) Interviewing deaf children, the interviewer effect: a research note. *Journal of Child Psychology and Psychiatry* 34, 1461–7.

Hindley, P. A., Hill, P. D., McGuigan, S., and Kitson, N. (1994) Psychiatric disorder in deaf and hearing impaired children and young people: a prevalence study. *Journal of Child Psychology and Psychiatry* 35, 917–34.

Hoare, P. (1984a) The development of psychiatric disorder among schoolchildren with epilepsy. *Developmental Medicine and Child Neurology* 26, 3–13.

Hoare, P. (1984b) Psychiatric disturbance in the families of epileptic children. *Developmental Medicine and Child Neurology* 26, 14–19.

Hoare, P. and Kerley, S. (1991) Psychosocial adjustment of children with chronic epilepsy and their families. *Developmental Medicine and Child Neurology* 33, 201–15.

Hobson, R. F. (1986) The autistic child's appraisal of expressions of emotion. *Journal of Child Psychology and Psychiatry* 27, 321–42.

Hochberg, Z., Gardos, M., and Benderly, A. (1987) Psychosexual outcome of assigned females and males with 46XX virilising congenital adrenal hyperplasia. *European Journal of Paediatrics* 146, 497–9.

Hodapp, R. M., Dykens, E. M., Ort, S. I., Selinsky, D. G., and Leckman, J. F. (1991) Changing patterns of intellectual strengths and weaknesses in males with fragile X syndrome. *Journal of Autism and Developmental Disorders* 21, 503–16.

Hodges, J. and Tizard, B. (1989) Social and family relationships of ex-institutional adolescents. *Journal of Child Psychology and Psychiatry* 30, 77–97.

Holland, A., Sicotte, N., and Treasure, J. (1988) Anorexia nervosa: evidence for a genetic basis. *Journal of Psychosomatic Research* 32, 561–71.

Hollingworth, C. E., Tanguay, P. E., Grossman, G., and Pabst, P. (1980) Long-term outcome of obsessive-compulsive disorders in childhood. Journal of the *American Academy of Child Psychiatry* 19, 134–44.

Hollis, C. (1995) Child and adolescent (juvenile onset) schizophrenia. A case-controlled study of premorbid developmental impairments. *British Journal of Psychiatry* **166**, 489–95.

Holtzman, N. A., Kronmal, R. A., Doorninck, W., Azen, C., and Koch, R. (1986) Effect of age at loss of dietary control on intellectual performance and behavior of children with phenylketonuria. *New England Journal of Medicine* **314**, 593–8.

Horacek, H. J., Ramey, C. T., Campbell, F. A., Hoffmanuk, K. P., and Fletcher, R. H. (1987) Predicting school failure and assessing early intervention with high-risk children. *Journal of the American Academy of Child and Adolescent Psychiatry* **26**, 758–63.

Horn, W. F., Ialongo, N. S., Pascoe, J. M. *et al.* (1991) Additive effects of psycho-stimulants, parent training, and self-control therapy with ADHD children. *Journal of the American Academy of Child and Adolescent Psychiatry* **30**, 233–40.

Howe, G., Feinstein, C. Reiss, D., Molock, S., and Berger, K. (1993) Adolescent adjustment to chronic physical disorders. I: Comparing neurological and non-neurological conditions. *Journal of Child Psychology and Psychiatry* **34**, 1153–71.

Howlin, P. (1988) Living with impairment: the effects on children of having an autistic sibling. *Child: care, health and development* **14**, 395–408.

Howlin, P. and Rutter, M. (1987) *Treatment of autistic children*. Wiley, New York.

Howlin, P., Wing, L., and Gould, J. (1995) The recognition of autism in children with Down syndrome: implications for intervention and some speculations about pathology. *Developmental Medicine and Child Neurology* **37**, 406–14.

Hsu, L. K. G., Crisp, A. H., and Harding, B. (1979) Outcome of anorexia nervosa. *Lancet* **i**, 61–5.

Huesmann L. R. (1986) Psychological processes promoting the relation between exposure to media violence and aggressive behavior by the viewer. *Journal of Social Issues* **42**, 125–39.

Hunt, G. M. and Holmes, A. E. (1976) Factors related to intelligence in treated cases of spina bifida. *American Journal of Diseases in Childhood* **130**, 823–7.

Hunt, H. and Wills, D. M. (1983) The family and the young visually handicapped child. In *Pediatric ophthalmology: current aspects*, ed. K. Wybar and D. Taylor, Marcel Dekker, New York, pp. 95–105.

Hutchings, B. and Mednick, S. A. (1974) Registered criminology in the adoptive and biological parents of registered male adoptees. In *Genetics, environment and psycho-pathology*, ed. S. A. Mednick, F. Schulsinger, F. Higgins, and B. Bell, North-Holland, Amsterdam, pp. 215–27.

Hutton, C. and Bradley, B. (1994) Effects of sudden infant death on bereaved siblings: a comparative study. *Journal of Child Psychology and Psychiatry* **35**, 723–32.

Illingworth, R. S. (1991) *The normal child*. Churchill Livingston, London.

Ireys, H. T., Sills, E. M., Kolodner, K. B., and Walsh, B. B. (1996) A social support intervention for parents of children with juvenile rheumatioid arthritis: results of a ran-domized trial. *Journal of Pediatric Psychology* **21**, 633–641.

Iwaniec, D., Herbert, M., and McNeish, A. J. (1985) Social work intervention with failure to thrive children and their families. II. Behavioural social work intervention. *British Journal of Social Work* **15**, 357–89.

Jamieson, C. R., van der Burgt, I., Brady, A. F. *et al.* (1994) Mapping a gene for Noonan syndrome to the long arm of chromosome 12. *Nature Genetics* **8**, 354–60.

Jan, J. E., Freeman, R. D., and Scott, E. P. (1977) *Visual impairment in children and adolescents*. Grune and Stratton, New York.

Jan, J. E., Groenveld, M., Sykanda, A. M., and Hoyt, C. S. (1987) Behavioural charac-teristics of children with permanent cortical visual impairment. *Developmental Medi-cine and Child Neurology* **29**, 571–6.

Jan, J. E., Espezel, H., and Appleton, R. E. (1994) The treatment of sleep disorders with melatonin. *Developmental Medicine and Child Neurology* **36**, 97–107.

Jarvelin, M. R., Moilanen, I., Vikevainen-Tervonen, L., and Huttunen, N. -P. (1990) Life changes and protective capacities in enuretic and non-enuretic children. *Journal of Child Psychology and Psychiatry* **31**, 763–74.

Jastak, J. F. and Jastak, S. (1978) *The Wide Range Achievement Test*, revised edn. Jastak Associates, Wilmington, DE.

Jay, B. (1979) Genetic causes of visual handicap: prevalence and prevention. In *Visual handicap in children* (ed. V. Smith and J. Keen) Heinemann/Spastic International Medical Publications, London, pp. 94–101.

Jayson, D., Wood, A., Kroll, L., Fraser, J., and Harrington, R. (1998) Which depressed patients respond to cognitive-behavioral treatment? *Journal of the American Academy of Child and Adolescent Psychiatry* **37**, 35–9.

Jellinek, M. S. (1990) School consultation: evolving issues. *Journal of the American Academy of Child and Adolescent Pyschiatry* **29**, 311–14.

Jenkins, J. M. and Smith, M. A. (1990) Factors protecting children living in disharmonious homes: maternal reports. *Journal of the American Academy of Child and Adolescent Psychiatry* **29**, 60–9.

Jenkins, S., Bax, M., and Hart, H. (1980) Behaviour problems in preschool children. *Journal of Child Psychology and Psychiatry* **21**, 5–17.

Johnson, D., McCabe, M., Nicholson, H. *et al.* (1994) Quality of long-term survival in children with medulloblastoma. *Journal of Neurosurgery* **80**, 1004–10.

Johnson, H. G., Ekman, P., Friesen, W., Nyhan, W. L., and Shear, C. (1976) A behavioral phenotype in the de Lange syndrome. *Pediatric Research* **10**, 843–50.

Johnson, S. B. (1988) Psychosocial aspects of juvenile diabetes. *Journal of Child Psychology and Psychiatry* **29**, 729–38.

Johnstone, F. D. and Forfar, J. O. (1984) Pre-natal paediatrics. In *Textbook of Paediatrics*, 3rd edn, ed. J. O. Forfar and G. C. Arneil, Churchill Livingston, London, p. 104.

Joleff, N. and Ryan, M. M. (1993) Communication development in Angelman's syndrome. *Archives of Disease in Childhood* **69**, 148–50.

Jones, D. (1992) *Interviewing children who have been sexually abused*, 4th edn. Royal College of Psychiatrists, Gaskell Press, London.

Jordan, R. and Powell, S. (1995) *Understanding and Teaching Children with Autism.* Wiley, Chichester.

Jorde, L. B., Mason-Brothers, A., Waldmann, R. *et al.* (1990) The UCLA–University of Utah epidemiological survey of autism: genealogical analysis of familial aggregation. *American Journal of Medical Genetics* **36**, 85–8.

Kafantaris, V. (1995) Treatment of bipolar disorders in children and adolescents. *Journal of the American Academy of Child and Adolescent Psychiatry* **34**, 732–41.

Kahn, A., Sottiaux, B. P., Appelboom-Fondu, J., Blum D., Rebuffat, E., and Levitt, J. (1989) Long-term development of children monitored as infants for an apparent life-threatening event during sleep: a ten year follow-up study. *Pediatrics* **83**, 668–73.

Kales, A., Soldatos, C. R., Bixler, E. O. *et al.* (1980) Hereditary factors in sleepwalking and night terrors. *British Journal of Psychiatry* **137**, 111–18.

Kallarackal, A. and Herbert, M. (1976) The happiness of Indian immigrant children. *New Society* **34**, 422–4.

Kaminer, R. K., Jedrysek, E., and Soles, B. (1984) Behavior problems of young retarded children. In *Perspectives and progress in mental retardation, vol. II—biomedical aspects*, ed. J. M. Berg and J. M. de Jong, Johns Hopkins University Press, Baltimore.

Kandel, D. B., Davies, M., Karuis, D., and Yamaguchi, K. (1986) The consequences in young adulthood of adolescent drug involvement. *Archives of General Psychiatry* 43, 746–54.

Kannoy, K. W. and Schroeder, C. S. (1985) Suggestions to parents about common behavior problems in a paediatric primary care office: 5 years of follow-up. *Journal of Pediatric Psychology* 10, 15–30.

Kaplan, C. A. and Hussain, S. (1995) Use of drugs in child and adolescent psychiatry. *British Journal of Psychiatry* 166, 291–8.

Kashani, J. H., Konig, P., Shepperd, J. A., Wilfley, D., and Morris, D. A. (1988) Psychopathology and self-concept in asthmatic children. *Journal of Pediatric Psychology* 13, 509–20.

Kasius, M. C., Ferdinand, R. F., Van de Berg, H., and Verhulst, F. C. (1997) Associations between different assessment approaches of child and adolescent psychopathology. *Journal of Child Psychology and Psychiatry* 38, 625–32.

Kazak, A. E., Reber, M., and Snitzer, L. (1988) Childhood chronic disease and family functioning: a study of phenylketonuria. *Pediatrics* 81, 224–30.

Kazdin, A. (1997) Psychosocial treatments for conduct disorder in children. *Journal of Child Psychology and Psychiatry* 38, 161–78.

Kazdin, A. E. (1987) *Conduct disorders in childhood and adolescence.* Sage, Newbury Park.

Kemmer, F. W., Bisping, R., Steingruber, H. J. *et al.* (1986) Psychological stress and metabolic control in patients with type 1 diabetes mellitus. *New England Journal of Medicine* 314, 1078–84.

Kendall, P. C. (1989) *Stop and Think Workbook.* Temple University Department of Psychology, Philadelphia, PA.

Kendell, R. E., Rennie, D., Clark, J. A., and Dean, C. (1981) The social and obstetric correlates of psychiatric admission in the puerperium. *Psychological Medicine* 11, 341–50.

Kennedy, W. A. (1965) School phobia: rapid treatment of fifty cases. *Journal of Abnormal Psychology* 70, 285–9.

Kessler, R., Davis, C., and Kendler, K. (1997) Childhood adversity and adult psychiatric disorder. *Psychological Medicine* 27, 1101–19.

Keuzenkamp-Jansen, C. W., Fijnvandraat, C., Kneepens, C., and Douwes, A. (1996) Diagnostic dilemmas and results of treatment for chronic constipation. *Archives of Disease in Childhood* 75, 36–41.

King, M. D., Day, R. E., Oliver, J. S., Lush, M., and Watson, J. M. (1981) Solvent encephalopathy. *British Medical Journal* 283, 663–5.

King, N. J., Mulhall, J., and Gullone, E. (1989) Fears in hearing-impaired and normally hearing children and adolescents. *Behaviour Research and Therapy* 27, 577–80.

King, R. A., Riddle, M. A., Chappell, P. B. *et al.* (1991) Emergence of self-destructive phenomena in children and adolescents during fluoxetine treatment. *Journal of the American Academy of Child and Adolescent Psychiatry* 30, 179–86.

Kingsbury, S. (1996) Pathos: a screening instrument for adolescent overdose: a research note. *Journal of Child Psychology and Psychiatry* 37, 609–11.

Kirk, S. A., McCarthy, J. J., and Kirk, W. D. (1968) *The Illinois Test of Psycholinguistic Abilities (Revised).* University of Illinois Press, Urbana.

Kiser, L., Culhane, D., and Hadley, T. (1995) The current practices of child and adolescent partial hospitalisation: results of a national survey. *Journal of the American Academy of Child and Adolescent Psychiatry* 34, 1336–42.

Klaus, M. and Kennell, J. (1976) *Maternal-infant bonding. The impact of early separation or loss on family development.* Mosby, St. Louis.

Klaus, M. H., Kennell, J. H., Robertson, S. S., and Sosa, R. (1986) Effects of social support during parturition on maternal and infant morbidity. *British Medical Journal* **293**, 585–7.

Klein, R. G. and Mannuzza, S. (1991) Long-term outcome of hyperactive children: a review. *Journal of the American Academy of Child and Adolescent Psychiatry* **30**, 383–7.

Klein, S. D., Simmons, R. G., and Anderson, C. R. (1984) Chronic kidney disease and transplantation in childhood and adolescents. In *Chronic illness and disabilities in childhood and adolescence*, ed. R. Blum, Grune and Stratton, London, pp. 1429–557.

Klin, A. and Volkmar, F. R. (1993) Elective mutism and mental retardation. *Journal of the American Academy of Child and Adolescent Psychiatry* **32**, 860–4.

Klin, A., Volkmar, F. R., Sparrow, S. S., Cicchetti, D. V., and Rourke, B. P. (1995) Validity and neuropsychological characterization of Asperger syndrome: convergence with nonverbal learning disabilities syndrome. *Journal of Child Psychology and Psychiatry* **36**, 1127–40.

Klonoff, H., Low, M. D., and Clark, C. (1977) Head injuries in children: a prospective five year follow-up. *Journal of Neurology, Neurosurgery and Psychiatry* **40**, 1211–19.

Koblenzer, C. S. and Koblenzer, P. J. (1988) Chronic intractable atopic eczema. Its occurrence as a sign of impaired parent–child relationship and psychologic developmental arrest: improvement through parent insight and education. *Archives of Dermatology* **124**, 1673–7.

Koegel, R., Schreibman, L., O'Neil, R. E., and Burke, J. C. (1983) The personality and family-interaction characteristics of parents of autistic children. *Journal of Consulting and Clinical Psychology* **51**, 683–92.

Kolvin, I. (1971) Psychoses in childhood—a comparative study. In *Infantile autism: concepts, characteristics and treatment*, ed. M. Rutter, Churchill Livingstone, London, pp. 7–26.

Kolvin, I. and Fundudis, T. (1981) Elective mute children: psychological development and background factors. *Journal of Child Psychology and Psychiatry* **22**, 219–232.

Kolvin, I., Garside, R. F., Nicol, A. R., MacMillan, A., Wolstenholme, F., and Leitch, I.M. (1981) *Help starts here: the maladjusted child in the ordinary school*. Tavistock, London.

Kolvin, I., Miller, F. J. W., Scott, D., Gatzanis, M., and Fleeting, M. (1988) *Adversity and destiny: explorations in the transmission of deprivation—Newcastle thousand families study*. Gower, Aldershot.

Kovacs, M. and Gatsonis, C. (1989) Stability and change in childhood-onset depressive disorders: longitudinal course as a diagnostic validator. In *The validity of psychiatric diagnosis*, ed. L. N. Robins and J. E. Barrett, Raven Press, New York, pp. 57–75.

Kovacs, M. and Pollock, M. (1995) Bipolar disorder and comorbid conduct disorder in childhood and adolescence. *Journal of the American Academy of Child and Adolescent Psychiatry* **34**, 715–23.

Kramer, H. H., Awiszus, D., Sterzel, U., Van Halteren, A., and Classen, R. (1989) Development of personality and intelligence in children with congenital heart disease. *Journal of Child Psychology and Psychiatry* **30**, 299–308.

Kreitman, N. (1977) *Parasuicide*. Wiley, Chichester.

Krener, P. (1996) Neurological and psychosocial aspects of HIV infection in children and adolescents. In *Child and Adolescent Psychiatry: A Comprehensive Textbook*, ed. M. Lewis, Williams and Wilkins, Baltimore, pp. 1006–15.

Kroll, L. and Shaw, M. (1994) Inpatient psychiatric treatment for diabetic teenagers. *Archives of Disease in Childhood* **71**, 470–4.

Kumar, R. and Robson, K. (1978) Previous induced abortion and ante-natal depression in primiparae: preliminary report of a survey of mental health in pregnancy. *Psychological Medicine* **8**, 711–15.

Kun, L. E., Mulhern, R. K., and Crisco, J. J. (1983) Quality of life in children treated for brain tumours: intellectual, emotional and academic function. *Journal of Neurosurgery* **58**, 1–6.

Kupst, M. J. and Schulman, J. L. (1988) Long-term coping with pediatric leukemia: a 6 year follow-up study. *Journal of Pediatric Psychology* **13**, 7–22.

Kupst, M. J., Schulman, J. L., Davis, A. T., and Richardson, C. C. (1983) The psychological impact of pediatric bacterial meningitis on the family. *Pediatric Infectious Diseases* **2**, 12–17.

Labropoulos, S. and Beratis, S. (1995) Psychosocial adjustment of thalassaemic children's siblings. *Journal of Psychosomatic Research* **39**, 911–19.

Lambert, L. and Streather, J. (1980) *Children in changing families: a study of adoption and illegitimacy.* Macmillan, London.

Lamont, M. A. and Dennis, N. R. (1988) Aetiology of mild mental retardation. *Archives of Disease in Childhood* **63**, 1032–8.

Lannering, B., Markey, I., Lundberg, A., and Olsson, E. (1990) Long-term sequelae after pediatric brain tumors: their effect on disability and quality of life. *Medical Pediatric Oncology* **18**, 304–10.

Lansdown, R. (1981) Cleft lip and palate: a prediction of psychological disfigurement? *British Journal of Orthodontics* **8**, 83–8.

Lansdown, R. and Benjamin, G. (1985) The development of the concept of death in children aged five to nine years. *Child: Care, Health and Development* **11**, 13–20.

Lansdown, R. and Polak, L. (1975) A study of the psychosocial effects of facial deformity in children. *Child: Care, Health and Development* **1**, 885–91.

Lask, B. (1988*a*) Novel and non-toxic treatment for night terrors. *British Medical Journal* **297**, 592.

Lask, B. (1988*b*) Psychological aspects of gastrointestinal disorders. In *Essentials of paediatric gastroenterology*, ed. P. Milla and D. Muller, Churchill Livingstone, Edinburgh.

Lask, B. (1989) Family therapy and group therapy. In *Studies on child psychiatry*, ed. B.J. Tonge, G. D. Burrows, and J. S. Werry, Elsevier, Amsterdam, pp. 431–42.

Lask, B. (1995) Psychosocial aspects of cystic fibrosis. In *Cystic fibrosis*, ed. M. E. Hodson and D. M. Gehdes, Chapman and Hall, London, pp. 315–27.

Lask, B. and Matthew, D. (1979) Childhood asthma—a controlled trial of family psychotherapy. *Archives of Diseases in Childhood* **54**, 116–19.

Lask, B. and Bryant-Waugh, R. (1993) *Childhood onset anorexia and related eating disorders.* Hove, Lawrence Erlbaum.

Laslett, R. (1977) *Educating maladjusted children.* Crosby Lockwood Staples, London.

Lassman, L. and Arjona, V. E. (1967) Pontine gliomas of childhood. *Lancet* **i**, 913–15.

Last, C., Hansen, C., and Franco, N. (1997) Anxious children in adulthood: a prospective study of adjustment. *Journal of the American Academy of Child and Adolescent Psychiatry* **36**, 645–52.

Last, C. G. and Francis, G. (1988) School phobia. In *Advances in clinical child psychology, Vol. 11*, ed. B. Lahey and A. Kazdin, Plenum, New York.

Lawson, D., Metcalfe, M., and Pampiglione, G. (1965) Meningitis in childhood. *British Medical Journal* **1**, 557–62.

Lazarus, R. S. and Folkman, S. (1984) *Stress, appraisal and coping.* Springer-Verlag, New York.

Le Couteur, A., Bailey, A., Goode, S., Pickles, A. *et al.* (1996) A broader phenotype of autism: the clinical spectrum in twins. *Journal of Child Psychology and Psychiatry* 37, 785–802.

Leach, D. (1980) Assessing children with learning difficulties: an alternative model for psychologists and teachers. *Journal of the Association of Educational Psychologists* 5, 16–23.

Lee, C. M. and Mash, E. J. (1989) Behaviour therapy. In *Studies on child psychiatry*, ed. B. J. Tonge, G. D. Burrows, and J. Werry, Elsevier, Amsterdam, p. 424.

Leff, J. (1978) Social and psychological causes of the acute attack. In *Schizophrenia: towards a new synthesis*, ed. J. K. Wing. Academic Press, London.

Leicester, J. (1982) Temper tantrums, epilepsy and episodic dyscontrol. *British Journal of Psychiatry* 141, 262–6.

Lenke, R. R. and Levy, H. L. (1980) Maternal phenylketonuria and hyperphenyla-lanaemia. An international survey of the outcome of treated and untreated pregnancies. *New England Journal of Medicine* 303, 1202–8.

Lerner, J. W. (1989) Educational interventions in learning disabilities. *Journal of the American Academy of Child and Adolescent Psychiatry* 28, 326–33.

Leslie, S. (1988) Diagnosis and treatment of hysterical conversion reactions. *Archives of Diseases in Childhood* 63, 506–11.

Leung, P. W. L. and Connolly, K. J. (1996) Distractibility in hyperactive and conduct-disordered children. *Journal of Child Psychology and Psychiatry* 37, 305–12.

Leventhal, J. M. (1988) Can child maltreatment be predicted during the peri-natal period: evidence from longitudinal cohort studies. *Journal of Reproductive Infant Psychology* 6, 139–61.

Levine, M. D. and Bakow, H. (1976) Children with encopresis: a study of treatment outcome. *Pediatrics* 58, 845–52.

Levy, A. M. (1985) The divorcing family: its evaluation and treatment. In *The clinical guide to child psychiatry*, ed. D. Shaffer, A. E. Ehrhardt, and L. L. Greenhill, Free Press, New York, pp. 353–70.

Levy, F., Hay, D. A., McStephen, M., Wood, C., and Waldman, I. (1997) Attention deficit hyperactivity disorder: a category or a continuum? Genetic analysis of a large-scale twin study. *Journal of the American Academy of Child and Adolescent Psychiatry* 36, 737–44.

Lewis, C., Hitch, G. J., and Walker, P. (1994) The prevalence of specific arithmetic difficulties and specific reading difficulties in 9- to 10-year-old boys and girls. *Journal of Child Psychology and Psychiatry* 35, 283–92.

Light, D. and Bailey, V. (1993) Pound foolish. *Health Services Journal* II, 6–18.

Lilford, R., Stratton, P., Godsil, S., and Pravad, A. (1994) A randomised trial of routine versus selective counselling in perinatal bereavement from congenital disease. *British Journal of Obstetrics and Gynaecology* 101, 291–6.

Lishman, W. A. (1978) *Organic psychiatry*, Blackwell Scientific, Oxford, p. 244.

Lloyd, J. K. and Wolff, O. H. (1976) Obesity. In *Recent advances in paediatrics*, ed. D. Hull, pp. 306–31. Churchill Livingstone, Edinburgh.

Logan, F. A., Gibson, B., Hann, I. M., and Parry-Jones, W. (1993) Children with hemophilia: same or different. *Child: Care, Health and Development* 19, 261–73.

Lombroso, P. J., Scahill, L., King, R. A., Lynch, K. A. *et al.* (1995) Risperidone treatment of children and adolescents with chronic tic disorders: a preliminary report. *Journal of the American Academy of Child and Adolescent Psychiatry* 34, 1147–52.

Lotter, V. (1978) Follow-up studies. In *Autism: a reappraisal of concepts and treatments*, ed. M. Rutter and E. Schopler, Plenum Press, New York, pp. 475–95.

Lou, H. C., Henriksen, L., and Bruhn, P. (1984) Focal cerebral hypoperfusion in children with dysphasia and/or attention deficit disorder. *Archives of Neurology* 41, 825–9.

Lou, H. C., Henriksen, L., Bruhn, P., Borner, H., and Nielsen, J. B. (1989) Striatal dysfunction in attention deficit and hyperkinetic disorder. *Archives of Neurology* 46, 48–52.

Lowe, M. and Costello, A. J. (1976) *Symbolic play test*. NFER, Windsor.

Lucas, A., Morley, R., Cole, T. J. *et al.* (1992) Breast milk and subsequent intelligence quotient in children born pre-term. *Lancet* 339, 261–4.

Ludman, L., Spitz, L., and Lansdown, R. (1990) Developmental progress of newborns following neonatal surgery. *Journal of Pediatric Surgery* 25, 469–71.

Lynch, M. A. and Roberts, J. (1982) *Consequences of child abuse*. Academic Press, London.

Maccoby, E. E. and Jacklin, L. N. (1980) Psychological sex differences. In *Scientific foundations of developmental psychiatry*, ed. M. Rutter. Heinemann Medical, London.

MacGregor, R., Pullar, A., and Cundall, D. (1994) Silent at school—elective mutism and abuse. *Archives of Disease in Childhood* 70, 540–1.

Macy, C. (1986) Psychological factors in nausea and vomiting in pregnancy: a review. *Journal of Reproductive and Infant Psychology* 4, 23–55.

Maguin, E. and Loeber, R. (1996) Academic performance and delinquency. *Crime and Justice* 20, 145–264.

Maguire, P. (1983) The psychological sequelae of childhood leukaemia. *Recent Results in Cancer Research* 88, 47–56.

Maino, D. M., Wesson, M., Schlange, D., Cibis, G., and Maino, J. H. (1991) Optometric findings in the fragile X syndrome. *Optometry and Vision Science* 68, 634–40.

Mandoki, M. W. (1995) Risperidone treatment of children and adolescents: increased risk of extrapyramidal side effects? *Journal of Child and Adolescent Psychopharmacology* 5, 49–67.

Mandoki, M. W., Sumner, G. S., Hoffman, R. P., and Riconda, D. L. (1991) A review of Klinefelter's syndrome in children and adolescents. *Journal of the American Academy of Child and Adolescent Psychiatry* 30, 167–72.

Mannino, F. V. and Shore, M. F. (1975) The effects of consultation: a review of empirical studies. *American Journal of Community Psychology* 3, 1–21.

March, J. (1995) Cognitive behavioral therapy for children and adolescents with OCD: a review and recommendations for treatment. *Journal of the American Academy of Child and Adolescent Psychiatry* 34, 7–18.

Marchi, M. and Cohen, P. (1990) Early childhood eating behaviors and adolescent eating disorders. *Journal of the American Academy of Child and Adolescent Psychiatry* 29, 112–17.

Marcovitch, H. (1997) Managing chronic fatigue in children. *British Medical Journal* 314, 1635–36.

Markova, I., Macdonald, K., and Forbes, C. (1980a) Impact of haemophilia on child-rearing practices and parental cooperation. *Journal of Child Psychology and Psychiatry* 21, 153–62.

Markova, L., Macdonald, K., and Forbes, C. (1980b) Integration of haemophiliac boys into normal schools. *Child: Care, Health and Development* 6, 101–9.

Markova, L., Phillips, J. S., and Forbes, C. D. (1984) The use of tools by children with haemophilia. *Journal of Child Psychology and Psychiatry* 25, 261–71.

Marks, I. (1987) The development of normal fear: a review. *Journal of Child Psychology and Psychiatry* 28, 667–98.

Markus, E., Lange, A., and Pettigrew, T. F. (1990) Effectiveness of family therapy—a meta analysis. *Journal of Family Therapy* 12, 205–22.

Marlow, N., Roberts, B., and Cooke, R. (1988) Motor skills in extremely low birthweight children at the age of six years. *Archives of Disease in Childhood* **64**, 839–47.

Marteau, T. M., Bloch, S., and Baum, D. (1987) Family life and diabetic control. *Journal of Child Psychology and Psychiatry* **28**, 823–34.

Mason, S. and Hillier, V. F. (1993) Young scarred children and their mothers—a short-term investigation into the practical, social and psychological implications of thermal injury to the pre-school child. *Burns* **19**, 507–10.

Matheny, A. P. (1986) Injuries among toddlers: contributions from child, mother and family. *Journal of Pediatric Psychology* **11**, 163–76.

Matthew, H. S., Solan, A., and Barabas, G. (1995) Cognitive functioning in Lesch–Nyhan syndrome. *Developmental Medicine and Child Neurology* **37**, 715–22.

Matthiesen, T. B., Rittig, S., Djurhuus, J. C., and Norgaard, J. P. (1994) A dose titration, and an open end 6-week efficacy and safety study of desmopressin tablets in the management of nocturnal enuresis. *Journal of Urology* **151**, 460–3.

Mattison, R. E., Humphrey, F. J., Kales, S. N., Handford, H. A., Finkenbinder, R. L., and Hernit, R. C. (1986) Psychiatric background and diagnosis of children. Evaluation for special class placement. *Journal of the American Academy of Child Psychiatry* **25**, 514–20.

Mattson, A. and Gross, S. (1966) Social and behavioral studies on hemophiliac children and their families. *Journal of Pediatrics* **68**, 952–64.

Matus, I. (1981) Assessing the nature and clinical significance of psychological contributions to childhood asthma. *American Journal of Orthopsychiatry* **51**, 327–41.

Maughan, B. (1988) School experiences as risk/protective factors. In *Studies of psychosocial risk*, ed. M. Rutter, Cambridge University Press, Cambridge.

Maughan, B. (1995) Annotation: long-term outcomes of developmental reading problems. *Journal of Child Psychology and Psychiatry* **36**, 357–71.

Maughan, B. and Rutter, M. (1998) Continuities and discontinuities in antisocial behaviour from childhood to adult life. *Advances in Clinical Child Psychology* **20**, 1–47.

Maughan, B. and Yule, W. (1994) Reading and other learning disabilities. In *Child and adolescent psychiatry: modern approaches*, ed. M. Rutter, E. Taylor and L.Hersov, Blackwell Scientific, Oxford, pp. 647–65.

Maughan, B., Gray, G., and Rutter, M. (1985) Reading retardation and antisocial behaviour: a follow-up into employment. *Journal of Child Psychology and Psychiatry* **26**, 741–58.

McBurney, A. K. and Eaves, L. C. (1986) Evolution of developmental and psychological test scores. In *Sequelae of low birthweight: the Vancouver Study*, Clinics in Developmental Medicine Nos. 95/96 (ed. H. G. Dunn), pp. 54–67. MacKeith Press, London.

McCauley, E., Ito, J., and Kay, T. (1986) Psychosocial functioning in girls with Turner's syndrome and short stature: social skills, behavior problems and self-concept. *Journal of the American Academy of Child Psychiatry* **25**, 105–12.

McClure, G. M. (1994) Suicide in children and adolescents in England and Wales. *British Journal of Psychiatry* **165**, 510–14.

McCubbin, H. I., McCubbin, M. A., Patterson, J. M., Cauble, A. E., Wilson, L. R., and Warwick, W. (1983) CHIP—Coping Health Inventory for Parents: an assessment of parental coping patterns in the care of the chronically ill child. *Journal of Marriage and the Family* **45**, 359–70.

McDermott, J. and Finch, S. (1967) Ulcerative colitis in children: reassessment of a dilemma. *Journal of the American Academy of Child Psychiatry* **6**, 512–25.

McFarlane, A. C. (1988) Recent life events and psychiatric disorder in children: the interaction with preceding extreme adversity. *Journal of Child Psychology and Psychiatry* **29**, 677–90.

McGrath, P. and Goodman, J. (1998) Cognitive behavioural approaches for pain in childhood. In *Cognitive behaviour therapy for children and families,*. ed. P. J. Graham, Cambridge University Press, Cambridge, pp. 143–55.

McGreevy, P. and Arthur, M. (1987) Effective behavioural treatment of self-biting by a child with Lesch–Nyhan syndrome. *Developmental Medicine and Child Neurology* 29, 536–40.

McGuffin, P. (1987) The new genetics and child psychiatric disorder. *Journal of Child Psychology and Psychiatry* 28, 215–22.

McNichol, K. N., Williams, H. C., Allan, J., and McAndrews, I. (1973) Spectrum of asthma in children III: Psychological and social components. *British Medical Journal* 4, 16–20.

Meadow, R. (1982) Munchausen syndrome by proxy. *Archives of Disease in Childhood* 57, 92–8.

Meadow, R. (1985) Management of Munchausen syndrome by proxy. *Archives of Disease in Childhood* 60, 385–93.

Meadow, R. (1998) Munchausen Syndrome by Proxy perpetrated by men. *Archives of Disease in Childhood* 78, 210–16.

Mechanic, D. (1978) *Medical sociology*, 2nd edn. Free Press, Glencoe, IL.

Mellanby, A., Phelps, F., Crichton, N. J., and Tripp, J. (1995) School sex-education: an experimental programme with educational and medical benefit. *British Medical Journal* 31, 414–17.

Meyer, R. J. and Haggerty, R. J. (1962) Streptococcal infection in families. *Pediatrics* 29, 539–49.

Miller, McC. and Plant, M. (1996) Drinking, smoking and illicit drug use among 15 and 16 year olds in the United Kingdom. *British Medical Journal* 313, 394–7.

Mills, M., Puckering, C., Pound, A., and Cox, A. (1984) What is it about depressed mothers that influences their children's functioning? In *Recent research in developmental psychopathology*, ed. J. Stevenson, pp. 11–17. Pergamon, Oxford.

Milner, J., Bungay, C., Jellinek, D., and Hall, D. (1996) Needs of disabled children and their families. *Archives of Diseases in Childhood* 76, 399–404.

Minchom, P., Ellis, N., Appleton, P. *et al.* (1995) Impact of functional severity on self-concept in young people with spina bifida. *Archives of Disease in Childhood* 73, 48–52.

Minde, K. K. (1978) Coping styles of twenty-four adolescents with cerebral palsy. *American Journal of Psychiatry* 135, 1344–9.

Minde, K. K., Whitelaw, A., Brown, J., and Fitzhardinge, P. (1983) Effect of neonatal complications in premature infants on early parent-infant interactions. *Developmental Medicine and Child Neurology* 25, 763–77.

Minde, K., Faucon, A., and Falkner, S. (1994) Sleep problems in toddlers: Effects of treatment on their daytime behavior. *Journal of the American Academy of Child and Adolescent Psychiatry* 33, 1114–21.

Minuchin, S. (1974) *Families and family therapy*. Tavistock, London.

Mitchell, W. G., Gorrell, R. W., and Greenberg, R. A. (1980) Failure to thrive in primary care. *Pediatrics* 65, 971–7.

Monck, E. and Graham, P. (1988) Suicide ideation in a total population of 15–19-year-old girls. In *Tentatives de Suicide à l'Adolescence*, Centre Internationale de l'Enfance, Paris, pp. 167–76.

Money, J. (1975) Psychologic counselling: hermaphroditism. In *Endocrine and genetic diseases of childhood and adolescence*, 2nd edn. W. B. Saunders, Philadelphia.

Money, J. and Ehrhardt, A. (1972) *Man and woman: boy and girl. The differentiation and dimorphism of gender identity from conception to maturity*. Johns Hopkins University Press, Baltimore.

Money, J., Schwartz, J., and Lewis, V. J. (1984) Adult herotosexual status and fetal hormonal masculinization and demasculinization: 46 XX congenital virilizing adrenal hyperplasia and 46 XY androgen insensitivity syndrome compared. *Psychoneuroendocrinology* 9, 405–14.

Moran, G., Fonagy, P., Kurtz, A., Bolton, A., and Brook, C. (1991) A controlled study of the psychoanalytic treatment of brittle diabetes. *Journal of the American Academy of Child and Adolescent Psychiatry* 30, 926–35.

Morton, R. E., Ali Khan, M., Murray-Leslie, C., and Elliott, S. (1995) Atlantoaxial instability in Down's syndrome: a five year follow-up study. *Archives of Disease in Childhood* 72, 115–19.

Mouridsen, S. E. (1995) The Landau-Kleffner syndrome: a review. *European Child and Adolescent Psychiatry* 4, 223–28.

Mrazek, D. (1992) Psychiatric complications of pediatric asthma. *Annals of Allergy* 69, 285–90.

Mrazek, D. A., Casey, B., and Anderson, I. (1987) Insecure attachment in severely asthmatic pre-school children: is it a risk factor? *Journal of the American Academy of Child and Adolescent Psychiatry* 26, 516–20.

Mrazek, D., Klinnert, M., Mrazek, P., and Macey, T. (1991) Early asthma onset: consideration of parenting issues. *Journal of the American Academy of Child and Adolescent Psychiatry* 30, 277–82.

Mullen, P., Martin, J., Anderson, J., Romans, S., and Herbison, G. (1994) The effect of child sexual abuse on social, interpersonal and sexual function in adult life. *British Journal of Psychiatry* 165, 35–47.

Mullen, P., Martin, J., Anderson, J. *et al.* (1996) The long-term impact of the physical, emotional and sexual abuse of children: a community study. *Child Abuse and Neglect* 20, 7–22.

Mureau, M., Slijper, F., van der Meulen, J., Verhulst, F., and Slob, A. (1995) Psychosexual adjustment of men who underwent hypospadias repair: a norm-related study. *Journal of Urology* 154, 1351–5.

Mureau, M., Slijper, F., Slob, A., and Verhulst, F. (1997) Psychosocial functioning of children, adolescents and adults following hypospadias surgery: a comparative study. *Journal of Paediatric Psychology* 22, 371–87.

Murphy, G., Hulse, J.A., Jackson, D. *et al.* (1986) Early treated hypothyroidism: development at 3 years. *Archives of Disease in Childhood* 61, 761–5.

Murphy, M. S. (1993) Management of recurrent abdominal pain. *Archives of Diseases in Childhood* 69, 409–19.

Murray, D. and Cox, J. (1990) Screening for depression with the Edinburgh Depression Scale. *Journal of Reproductive and Infant Psychology* 8, 99–107.

Murray, R. M. (1994) Neurodevelopmental schizophrenia: the rediscovery of dementia praecox. *British Journal of Psychiatry Supplement*, 6–12.

Naditch, M. P. (1974) Acute adverse reactions to psychoactive drugs. *Journal of Abnormal Psychology* 83, 394–403.

National Center for Clinical Infant Programs (1994) *Diagnostic Classification of Mental Health and Developmental Disorders of Infancy and Early Childhood*. National Center for Clinical Infant Programs, Arlington, VA.

Neale, M. D. (1988) *Neale analysis of reading ability manual*, revised British edn. Macmillan, London.

Needleman, H., Gunnoe, C., Leviton, A. *et al.* (1979) Deficits in psychologic and classroom performances of children with elevated dentine lead levels. *New England Journal of Medicine* 300, 689–95.

Neligan, G. A., Kolvin, I., Scott, D. McI., and Garside, R. F. (1976) Born too soon or too small. *Clinics in Developmental Medicine*, No. 61. Heinemann, London.

Neuchterlein, K. H. (1986) Childhood precursors of adult schizophrenia. *Journal of Child Psychology and Psychiatry* 27, 133–44.

Neuman, R. J., Geller, B., Rice, J., and Todd, R. (1997) Increased prevalence and earlier onset of mood disorders among relatives of prepubertal versus adult probands. *Journal of the American Academy of Child and Adolescent Psychiatry* 36, 466–73.

Newacheck, P. W., Budetti, P. P., and Halfon, N. (1986) Trends in activity-limiting chronic conditions among children. *American Journal of Public Health* 76, 178–84.

Newberger, C. S. and White, K. M. (1989) Cognitive foundations for parental care. In *Child maltreatment*, ed. D. Cicchetti and V. Carlson, Cambridge University Press, Cambridge, pp. 302–16.

Newson, J. and Newson, E. (1963) *Patterns of infant care in an urban community*. Penguin, Harrnondsworth.

Newton, R. W. (1988) Psychosocial aspects of pregnancy: the scope for intervention. *Journal of Reproductive and Infant Psychology* 6, 23–39.

NHS Centre for Reviews and Dissemination (1997) Effective health care: preventing and reducing the adverse effects of unintended teenage pregnancies. University of York, York.

Njiokiktjien, C. (1994) Dyslexia: a neuropsychiatric puzzle. *Acta Paedopsychiatrica* 56, 157–67.

Nobes, G. and Smith, M. (1997) Physical punishment of children in two-parent families. *Clinical Child Psychology and Psychiatry* 2, 271–81.

Nolan, T., Debelle, G., Oberklaid, F., and Coffey, C. (1991) Randomized trial of laxatives in treatment of childhood encopresis. *Lancet* 338, 523–7.

North, K., Joy, P., Yuille, D., Cocks, N., and Hutchins, P. (1995) Cognitive function and academic performance in children with neurofibromatosis type 1. *Developmental Medicine and Child Neurology* 37, 427–36.

Northam, E., Anderson, P., Adler, R., Werther, G., and Warne, G. (1996) Psychosocial and family functioning in children with insulin-dependent diabetes at diagnosis and one year later. *Journal of Pediatric Psychology* 21, 699–717.

Nunn, K. (1986).The episodic dyscontrol syndrome in childhood. *Journal of Child Psychology and Psychiatry* 27, 439–46.

Nurcombe, B., Seifer, R., Scioli, A., Tramontana, M. G., Grapentine, W. L., and Beauchesne, H. C. (1989) Is major depressive disorder in adolescence a distinct diagnostic entity? *Journal of the American Academy of Child and Adolescent Psychiatry* 28, 333–42.

Nyhan, W. L. (1972) Behavioral phenotypes in organic genetic disease. *Pediatric Research* 6, 1–9.

Nyhan, W. L. (1976) Behaviour in the Lesch-Nyhan syndrome. *Journal of Autism and Childhood Schizophrenia* 6, 235–42.

O'Brien, G. and Yule, W. (1995) *Behavioural phenotypes*. MacKeith, London.

O'Brien, S., Ross, L. V., and Christopherson, E. R. (1986) Primary encopresis: evaluation and treatment. *Journal of Applied Behavioral Analysis* 19, 137–45.

O'Callaghan, E. M. and Colver, A. F. (1987) Selective medical examinations on starting school. *Archives of Disease in Childhood* 62, 1041–3.

O'Connor, N. and Hermelin, B. (1984) Idiot savant calendrical calculations. *Psychological Medicine* 14, 801–6.

Oakley, A. (1988) Is social support good for the health of mothers and babies? *Journal of Reproductive and Infant Psychology* 6, 3–21.

Oakley, A., Hickey, D., Rajan, L., and Rigby, A. V. (1996) Social support in pregnancy: does it have long-term effects? *Journal of Reproductive and Infant Psychology* 14, 7–22.

Oates, M. (1984) Assessing fitness to parent. In *Taking a stand*, British Agencies for Adoption and Fostering, London, pp. 29–41.

Oates, M. (1988) The development of an integrated community orientated service for severe post-natal mental illness. In *Motherhood and mental illness. 2. Causes and consequences*, ed. I. F. Brockington. Wright, London.

Oddy, M. (1984) Head injury during childhood: the psychological implications. In *Closed head injury: psychological, social, and family consequences*, ed. N. Brooks, Oxford University Press, Oxford, pp. 179–94.

Offer, D. and Schonert-Reichl, K. (1992) Debunking the myths of adolescence: findings from recent research. *Journal of the American Academy of Child and Adolescent Psychiatry* **31**, 1003–14.

Office of National Statistics (1996) *Birth statistics. FMI no. 23.* HMSO, London.

Office of National Statistics (1997) *Social Trends 27.* HMSO, London.

Office of Population Censuses and Surveys (1989) The prevalence of disability among children. *OPCS Surveys of Disability in Great Britain, Report No. 3.* HMSO, London.

Offord, D. R. (1987) Prevention of behavioural and emotional disorders in children. *Journal of Child Psychology and Psychiatry* **28**, 9–20.

Offord, D., Boyle, M., Szatmari, P. *et al.* (1987) Ontario Child Health Study: II Six month prevalence of disorder and rates of service utilization. *Archives of General Psychiatry* **44**, 832–6.

Offord, D., Boyle, M. H., and Racine, Y. (1989) Ontario Child Health Study: correlates of disorder. *Journal of the American Academy of Child and Adolescent Psychiatry* **28**, 856–60.

Oke, S. and Mayer, R. (1991) Referrals to child psychiatry—a survey of staff attenders. *Archives of Diseases in Childhood* **66**, 862–865.

Olds, D., Henderson, C. R., Tatelbaum, R., and Chamberlin R. (1986) Improving the delivery of pre-natal care and outcomes of pregnancy: a randomized trial of nurse home visitation. *Pediatrics* **77**, 16–28.

Oliver, C. (1995) Annotation: self-injurious behaviour in children with learning disabilities: recent advances in assessment and intervention. *Journal of Child Psychology and Psychiatry* **30**, 909–27.

Oliver, C. and Holland, A. J. (1986) Down's syndrome and Alzheimer's disease: a review. *Psychological Medicine* **16**, 307–22.

Olness, K. (1989) Hypnotherapy: a cyberphysiologic strategy in pain management. *Pediatric Clinics of North America* **36**, 873–84.

Olness, K. and Gardner, G. G. (1988) *Hypnosis and hypnotherapy with children.* Grune and Stratton, Philadelphia.

Olson, H. C., Strei, S. S., Guth, A. P. *et al.* (1997) Association of prenatal alcohol exposure with behavioral and learning problems in early adolescence. *Journal of the American Academy of Child and Adolescent Psychiatry* **36**, 1187–94.

Olsson, B. and Rett, A. (1987) Autism and Rett syndrome: behavioural investigation and differential diagnosis. *Developmental Medicine and Child Neurology* **29**, 429–41.

Olweus, D. (1989) Bully/victim problems among schoolchildren: basic facts and effects of a school based intervention program. In *The development and treatment of childhood aggression*, Erlbaum, Hillsdale, NJ.

Oostra, B. A., Jacky, P. B., Brown, W. T., and Rousseau, F. (1993) Guidelines for the diagnosis of fragile X syndrome. *Journal of Medical Genetics* **30**, 410–13.

Orvaschel, H. (1988) Structured and semi-structured psychiatric interviews for children. In *Handbook of clinical assessment of children and adolescents*, ed. C. J. Kestenbaum and D.T. Williams, New York University Press. New York, pp. 31–42.

Ottinger, D. and Simmons, J. (1964) Behaviour of human neonates and prenatal maternal anxiety. *Psychological Reports* 14, 391–4.

Palmai, G., Storey, P. B., and Briscoe, O. (1967) Social class and the young offender. *British Journal of Psychiatry* 113, 1073–82.

Panitch, H. S. and Berg, B. O. (1970) Brain stem tumors of childhood and adolescence. *American Journal of Diseases in Childhood* 119, 465–72.

Parmelee, A. H. (1986) Children's illnesses: their beneficial effects on behavioral development. *Child Development* 57, 1–10.

Parsons, T. (1951) *The social system*. Free Press, Glencoe, IL.

Parush, S., Sohmer, H., Steinberg, A., and Kaitz, M. (1997) Somatosensory functioning in children with attention deficit hyperactivity disorder. *Developmental Medicine and Child Neurology* 39, 464–8.

Patterson, G. R. (1982) *Coercive family process*. Castalia, Eugene, OR.

Patterson, G. R., Reid, J. B., and Dishion, T. (1992) *Antisocial boys*. Castalia, Eugene, OR.

Payton, J. B., Burkhart, J. E., Hersen, M., and Helsel, W. J. (1989*a*) Treatment of ADDH in mentally retarded children: a preliminary study. *Journal of the American Academy of Child and Adolescent Psychiatry* 28, 761–7.

Payton, J. B., Steele, M. W., Wenger, S. L., and Minshew, N. J. (1989*b*) The fragile X marker and autism in perspective. *Journal of the American Academy of Child and Adolescent Psychiatry* 28, 417–21.

Pearman, D. A., Pumariega, A., and Seilheimer, D. (1991) The development of psychiatric symptomatology in patients with cystic fibrosis. *Journal of the American Academy of Child and Adolescent Psychiatry* 30, 290–7.

Pelligrini, D. S. and Urbain, E. S. (1985) An evaluation of inter-personal cognitive problem-solving training with children. *Journal of Child Psychology and Psychiatry* 26, 17–41.

Penner, K. A., Johnstom, J., Faircloth, B. H., Irish, P., and Williams, C. A. (1993) Communication, cognition, and social interaction in the Angelman syndrome. *American Journal of Medical Genetics* 46, 34–9.

Peterson, A. L., Campise, R. L., and Azrin, N. H. (1994) Behavioral and pharmacological treatments for tic and habit disorders: a review. *Journal of Developmental and Behavioral Pediatrics* 15, 430–41.

Peterson, L. (1989) Coping by children undergoing stressful medical procedures: some conceptual, methodological and therapeutic issues. *Journal of Consulting and Clinical Psychology* 57, 380–7.

Petty, L. K., Ornitz, E. M., Michelman, J. D., and Zimmerman, E. G. (1984) Autistic children who become schizophrenic. *Archives of General Psychiatry* 41, 129–35.

Phipps, S. and De Cuir-Whalley, S. (1990) Adherence issues in pediatric bone-marrow transplantation. *Journal of Pediatric Psychology* 15, 459–75.

Phipps, S. and Mulhern, R. K. (1995) Family cohension and expressiveness promote resilience to the stress of pediatric bone marrow transplant: a preliminary report. *Journal of Developmental and Behavioral Pediatrics* 16, 257–63.

Pigott, T. A., Pato, M. T., Bernstein, S. E. *et al.* (1990) Controlled comparisons of clomipramine and fluoxetine in the treatment of obsessive–compulsive disorder. *Archives of General Psychiatry* 47, 926–32.

Pike, M. and Stores, G. (1994) Klein–Levin syndrome: a cause of diagnostic confusion. *Archives of Disease in Childhood* 71, 355–7.

Piven, J. and Palmer, P. (1997) Cognitive deficits in parents from multiple-incidence autism families. *Journal of Child Psychology and Psychiatry* 38, 1011–21.

Piven, J., Palmer, P., Landa, R., Santangelo, S., Jacobi, D., and Childress, D. (1997) Personality and language characteristics in parents from multiple-incidence autism families. *American Journal of Medical Genetics (Neuropsychiatric Genetics)* **74**, 398–411.

Platt, M. J. and Pharaoh, P. (1996) Child Health Statistical Review, 1996. *Archives of Diseases in Childhood* 75, 527–33.

Pless, I. B., Cripps, H. A., Davies, J. M. C., and Wadsworth, M. (1989) Chronic physical illness in childhood: psychological and social effects in adolescence and adult life. *Developmental Medicine and Child Neurology* 31, 747–55.

Plomin, R. (1991) A behavioral genetic approach to learning disabilities and their subtypes. In *Subtypes of learning disabilities*, ed.: L. V. Feagans, E. J. Short, and L. J. Meltzer, Lawrence Erlbaum, Hillsdale, NJ, pp. 83–111.

Plomin, R. and Daniels, R. (1987) Why are children in the same family as different from one another? *Behavioral and Brain Sciences* 10, 1–60.

Polnay, L., Blair, M., Horn, N., and Nathan, D. (1996) *Manual of community paediatrics*. Churchill Livingstone, Edinburgh.

Popper, C. W. (1997) Antidepressants in the treatment of attention-deficit/hyperactivity disorder. *Journal of Clinical Psychiatry* 58 Suppl. **14**, 14–31.

Postlethwaite, R. J., Garralda, M., Eminson, D., and Reynolds, J. (1996) Lessons from psychosocial studies of chronic renal failure. *Archives of Diseases in Childhood* 75, 455–9.

Pot-Mees, C. (1989) *The psychosocial effects of bone marrow transplantation in children*. Eburon, Delft.

Powls, A., Botting, N., Cooke, R. W. I., and Marlow, N. (1995) Motor impairment in children 12 to 13 years old with a birthweight of less than 1250 g. *Archives of Disease in Childhood Fetal and Neonatal Edition* 73, F62–F66.

Prendergast, M., Taylor, E., Rapoport, J. L. *et al.* (1988) The diagnosis of childhood hyperactivity: a U.S.–U.K. cross-national study of DSM-III and ICD-9. *Journal of Child Psychology and Psychiatry* 29, 289–300.

Purcell, K. and Weiss, J. (1970) Asthma. In *Symptoms of psychopathology*, ed. C. Costello, Wiley, New York, pp. 597–623.

Puzzo, A., Fiamma, G., Rubino, V. E. *et al.* (1990) Cardiovascular aspects of Martin–Bell syndrome. *Cardiologia* 35, 857–62.

Quackenbush, D., Kutcher, S., Robertson, H., Boulos, C., and Chaban, P. (1996) Premorbid and postmorbid school functioning in bipolar adolescents: description and suggested academic interventions. *Canadian Journal of Psychiatry* 41, 16–22.

Query, J. M., Reichelt, C., and Christoferson, L. A. (1990) Living with chronic illness: a retrospective study of patients shunted for hydrocephalus and their families. *Developmental Medicine and Child Neurology* 32, 119–28.

Quill, K. A. (1995) *Teaching children with autism*. Delman Publishers, New York.

Quinton, D. and Rutter, M. (1976) Early hospital admission and later disturbances of behaviour: an attempted replication of Douglas' findings. *Developmental Medicine and Child Neurology* 18, 447–59.

Quinton, D. and Rutter, M. (1985) Parenting behaviour of mothers raised 'in care'. In *Longitudinal studies in child psychology and psychiatry*, ed. A. R. Nicol, Wiley, Chichester, pp. 157–201.

Quinton, D., Rutter, M., and Gulliver, L. (1990) Continuities in psychiatric disorders from childhood to adulthood in the children of psychiatric patients. In *Straight and deviant pathways from childhood to adulthood*, ed. L. Robins and M. Rutter, Cambridge University Press, Cambridge, pp. 259–78.

Rabbett, H., Elbadri, A., Thwaites, R. *et al.* (1996) Quality of life in children with Crohn's disease. *Journal of Paediatric Gastroenterology and Nutrition* 23, 528–33.

Rachman, S. (1997) The evolution of cognitive behaviour therapy. In: *Science and practice of cognitive behaviour therapy*, ed. D. M. Clark and C. G. Fairburn, Oxford University Press, Oxford.

Radestad, I., Steineck, G., Nordin, C., and Sjogren, B. (1996) Psychological complications after stillbirth—influence of memories and immediate management: population based study. *British Medical Journal* 312, 1505–8.

Ramasamy, R., Taylor, R. L., and Ziegler, E. W. (1996) Eliminating inappropriate classroom behavior using a DRO schedule: a preliminary study. *Psychological Reports* 78, 753–4.

Ramsey, M. E., Miller, E., and Peckham, C. S. (1991) Outcome of symptomatic, confirmed cytomegalovirus infection. *Archives of Disease in Childhood* 66, 1068–9.

Rantala, H., Shari, M., Saukkonen, A., and Sorri, M. (1991) Outcome after childhood encephalitis. *Developmental Medicine and Child Neurology* 33, 858–67.

Raphael, B. (1975) The management of pathological grief. *Australian and New Zealand Journal of Psychiatry* 9, 173–80.

Rapin, I. (1996) Practitioner review: developmental language disorders: a clinical update. *Journal of Child Psychology and Psychiatry* 37, 643–55.

Rapoport, J. L. (1986) Childhood obsessive compulsive disorders. *Journal of Child Psychology and Psychiatry* 27, 289–95.

Ratcliffe, S. G. (1994) The psychological and psychiatric consequences of sex chromosome abnormalities in children based on population studies. In *Basic approaches to genetic and molecular biological developmental psychiatry*, ed. F. Poustka, Quintessenz Library of Psychiatry, pp. 99–122.

Ratcliffe, S. G. and Field, M. A. (1982) Emotional disorder in XYY children: four case reports. *Journal of Child Psychology and Psychiatry* 23, 401–6.

Ratcliffe, S. G., Butler, G., and Jones, M. (1991) EdinburghStudy of Growth and Development of Children with Sex Chromosome Abnormalities IV Birth Defects. *Original Articles Series* 26, 1–44.

Rauch, P. and Jellinek, M. S. (1988) Psychosocial development in children with cutaneous disease. In *Pediatric dermatology*, ed. L. A. Schachner and R. C. Hanson, Churchill Livingstone, New York, pp. 139–58.

Reddy, L. and Pfeiffer, S. (1997) Effectiveness of treatment foster care with children and adolescents: a review of outcome studies. *Journal of the American Academy of Child and Adolescent Psychiatry* 36, 581–8.

Reid, W. J. and Shyne, A. W. (1969) *Brief and extended casework*. Columbia University Press, New York.

Reilly, S., Skuse, D., and Poblete, X. (1996) Prevalence of feeding problems and oral motor dysfunction in children with cerebral palsy: a community study. *Journal of Pediatrics* 129, 877–82.

Reinecke, M. A., Ryan, N. E., and DuBois, D. L. (1998) Cognitive-behavioral therapy of depression and depressive symptoms during adolescence: a review and meta-analysis. *Journal of the American Academy of Child and Adolescent Psychiatry* 37, 26–34.

Reisman, J. M. (1973) *Principles of psychotherapy with children*. Wiley, New York.

Rettew, D. Swedo, S., Leonard, H., Lenane, M., and Rapoport, J. (1992) Obsessions and compulsions across time in 79 children and adolescents with obsessive compulsive disorder. *Journal of the American Academy of Child and Adolescent Psychiatry* 31, 1050–6.

Revill, S. and Blunden, R. (1979) A home training service for pre-school, developmentally handicapped children. *Behaviour Research and Therapy* 17, 207–14.

Reynell, J. (1997) *Reynell Developmental Language Scales*. NFER, Windsor.

Reynell, J. and Zinkin P. (1975) New procedures for the developmental assessment of young children with severe visual handicaps. *Child: Care, Health and Development* 1, 61–9.

Reynolds, C. A., Hewitt, J. K., Erickson, M. T. *et al.* (1996) The genetics of children's oral reading performance. *Journal of Child Psychology and Psychiatry* 37, 425–34.

Reznick, J. S., Corley, R., and Robinson, J. (1997) A longitudinal twin study of intelligence in the second year. *Monographs of the Society for Research in Child Development* 62, 1–154.

Richardson, S. A. and Royce, J. (1968) Race and physical handicap in children's preference for other children. *Child Development* 39, 467–80.

Richman, L. C. (1978) The effects of facial disfigurement on teachers' perceptions of ability in cleft palate children. *Cleft Palate Journal* 15, 115–60.

Richman, N. (1977) Is a behaviour check-list for pre-school children useful? In *Epidemiological approaches in child psychiatry*, ed. P. Graham, Academic Press, London, pp. 125–38.

Richman, N. (1981) A community survey of one to two year olds with sleep disturbances. *Journal of the American Academy of Child Psychiatry* 20, 281–91.

Richman, N. (1993) Children in situations of political violence. *Journal of Child Psychology and Psychiatry* 34, 1286–302.

Richman, N., Stevenson, J., and Graham, P. (1975) Prevalence of behaviour problems in three year old children: an epidemiological study in a London borough. *Journal of Child Psychology and Psychiatry* 16, 277–87.

Richman, N., Stevenson, J., and Graham, P. (1982) *Pre-school to school: a behavioural study*. Academic Press, London.

Richman, N., Graham, P., and Stevenson, J. (1983) Long-term effects of treatment in a pre-school day centre. *British Journal of Psychiatry* 142, 71–7.

Richman, N., Douglas, J., Hunt, H., Lansdown, R., and Levere, R. (1985) Behavioural methods in the treatment of sleep disorders—a pilot study. *Journal of Child Psychology and Psychiatry* 26, 581–90.

Richter, I., McGrath, P., Humphreys, P., Goodman, J., Firestone, P., and Keene, D. (1986) Cognitive and relaxation treatment of pediatric migraine. *Pain* 25, 195–203.

Riddle, M. A., Scahill, L., King, R. *et al.* (1992) Double-blind cross-over trial of fluoxetine and placebo in children and adolescents with obsessive–compulsive disorder. *Journal of the American Academy of Child and Adolescent Psychiatry* 31, 1050–6.

Riikonen, R. and Amnell, G. (1981) Psychiatric disorders in children with earlier infantile spasms. *Developmental Medicine and Child Neurology* 23, 747–60.

Riikonen, R. and Simell, O. (1990) Tuberous sclerosis and infantile spasms. *Developmental Medicine and Child Neurology* 32, 203–9.

Ritson, B., Chick, J., and Strang, J. (1993) Dependence on alcohol and other drugs. In *Companion to psychiatric studies*, 5th edn, ed. R. Kendall and A Zealley, Churchill Livingstone, Edinburgh, pp. 359–96.

Rivara, J. M., Jaffe, K. M., Polissar, N. L., Fay, G. C., Liaso, S., and Martin, K. M. (1996) Prediction of family functioning and change three years after traumatic brain injury in children. *Archives of Physical Medicine and Rehabilitation* 77, 754–64.

Rivinus, T. M., Jamison, D. L., and Graham, P. J. (1975) Childhood organic neurological disease presenting as psychiatric disorder. *Archives of Disease in Childhood* 50, 115–19.

Roach, E. S., Delgado, M., Anderson, L., Iannaccone, S., and Burns, D. (1996) Carbamazepine trial for Lesch–Nyhan self-mutilation. *Journal of Child Neurology* 11, 476–8.

Roberts, I. and Power, C. (1996) Does the decline in child injury mortality vary by social class? A comparison of class-specific mortality in 1981 and 1991. *British Medical Journal* 313, 784–6.

Roberts, I. B. and Pless, B. (1995) Social policy as a cause of childhood accidents. *British Medical Journal* **311**, 925–8.

Robertson, M. M. and Stern, J. S. (1997) The Gilles de la Tourette syndrome. *Critical Reviews in Neurobiology* **11**, 1–19.

Robin, A., Siegel, P., Koepke, T., Moye, A., and Tice, S. (1994) Family therapy versus individual therapy for adolescent girls with anorexia nervosis. *Journal of Developmental and Behavioral Pediatrics* **15**, 111–16.

Robins, L. N. (1978) Sturdy childhood predictors of adult antisocial behaviour: replications from longitudinal studies. *Psychological Medicine* **8**, 611–22.

Robins, L. and Rutter, M. (ed.) (1990) *Straight and deviant pathways from childhood to adulthood*. Cambridge University Press, Cambridge.

Robinson, A., Bender, B., Borelli, J., Puck, M., and Salbenblatt, J. (1983) Sex chromosome anomalies: prospective studies in children. *Behaviour Genetics* **13**, 321–9.

Roche, A., Lipman, R., Overall, J., and Hung, H. (1979) The effects of stimulant medication on the growth of hyperkinetic children. *Pediatrics* **63**, 647–50.

Rockney, R., McQuade, W., Days, A., Linn, H., and Alario, A. (1996) Encopresis treatment outcome: long-term follow-up of 45 cases. *Journal of Developmental and Behavioral Pediatrics* **17**, 380–5.

Rona, R., Chinn, S., and Burney, P. (1995) Trends in the prevalence of asthma in Scottish and English primary schoolchildren 1982–1992. *Thorax* **50**, 992–3.

Ronen, T. (1989) Assessment and evaluation of a self-control intervention package for imparting self-control skills to children and adolescents. *World Congress of Cognitive Therapy, abstracts*. Oxford.

Ronen, T., Rahav, G., and Wozner, Y. (1995) Self control and enuresis. *Journal of Cognitive Psychotherapy* **9**, 249–50.

Rosenkranz, J., Bonzel, K., Bulla, M. *et al.* (1992) Psychosocial adaptation of children and adolescents with chronic renal failure. *Pediatric Nephrology* **6**, 459–63.

Rosenthal, A. and Levine, S. V. (1971) Brief psychotherapy with children: process and therapy. *American Journal of Psychiatry* **128**, 141–5.

Rothbaum, B. A. (1992) The behavioral treatment of trichotillomania. *Behavioral Psychotherapy* **20**, 85–90.

Rovet, J. Ehrlich, R., and Sorbara, D. (1987) Intellectual outcome in chidren with fetal hypothyroidism. *Journal of Pediatrics* **110**, 700–4.

Royal College of Physicians (1992) *Smoking and the Young*. Royal College of Physicians, London.

Royal College of Physicians (1995) *Alcohol and the young*. Report of a joint Royal College of Physicians/British Paediatric Association Working Party. Royal College of Physicians, London.

Rushton, H. G. (1989) Nocturnal enuresis: epidemiology, evaluation, and currently available treatment options. *Journal of Pediatrics* **114**, 691–5.

Russ, S. W. (1998) Psychodynamically based therapies. In *Handbook of child psychopathology*, ed. T. H. Ollendick and M. Hersen, Plenum Press, New York.

Russell, G. F. M. (1979) Bulimia nervosa: an ominous variant of anorexia nervosa. *Psychological Medicine* **9**, 429–48.

Russell, G. F. M., Szmukler, G. I., Dare, C., and Eisler, I. (1987) An evaluation of family therapy in anorexia nervosa and bulimia nervosa. *Archives of General Psychiatry* **44**, 1047–56.

Rutter, M. (1967) A children's behaviour questionnaire for completion by teachers; preliminary findings. *Journal of Child Psychology and Psychiatry* **8**, 1–11.

Rutter, M. (1985) The treatment of autistic children. *Journal of Child Psychology and Psychiatry* **26**, 193–214.

Rutter, M. (1989) Annotation: child psychiatric disorders in ICD-10. *Journal of Child Psychology and Psychiatry* 30, 499–513.

Rutter, M. (1995) Clinical implications of attachment concepts: retrospect and prospect. *Journal of Child Psychology and Psychiatry* 36, 549–71.

Rutter, M. and Bartak, L. (1973) Special educational treatment of autistic children: a comparative study. II. Follow-up findings and implications for services. *Journal of Child Psychology and Psychiatry* 14, 241–70.

Rutter, M. and Garmezy, N. (1983) Developmental psychopathology. In *Handbook of child psychology*, ed. P. H. Mussen, Wiley, New York, pp. 775–911.

Rutter, M. and Giller, H. (1983) *Juvenile delinquency: trends and perspectives*. Penguin, Harmondsworth.

Rutter, M. and Madge, N. (1976) *Cycles of disadvantage*, Heinemann, London, p. 180.

Rutter, M. and Quinton, D. (1984) Parental psychiatric disorder: effects on children. *Psychological Medicine* 14, 835–80.

Rutter, M. and Smith, D. (1995) *Psychosocial disorders in young people*. Wiley, Chichester.

Rutter, M., Tizard, J., and Whitmore, K. (1970a) *Education, health and behaviour*. Longman, London.

Rutter, M., Graham, P., and Yule, W. (1970b). *A neuropsychiatric study in childhood*. Heinemann, London.

Rutter, M., Cox, A., Tupling, C., Berger, M., and Yule, W. (1975) Attainment and adjustment in two geographical areas. I. Prevalence of psychiatric disorders. *British Journal of Psychiatry* 126, 493–509.

Rutter, M., Graham, P., Chadwick, O., and Yule, W. (1976) Adolescent turmoil: fact or fiction? *Journal of Child Psychology and Psychiatry* 17, 35–56.

Rutter, M., Maughan, B., Mortimore, P., and Ouston, J. (1979) *Fifteen thousand hours*. Open Books, London.

Rutter, M., Chadwick, O., and Shaffer, D. (1983) Head injury. In *Developmental neuropsychiatry*, ed. M. Rutter, Guilford Press, New York, pp. 83–111.

Rutter, S. C. and Cole, T. R. P. (1991) Psychological characteristics of Sotos syndrome. *Developmental Medicine and Child Neurology* 33, 898–902.

Ryden, D., Nevander, L., Johnsson, P. *et al.* (1994) Family therapy in poorly controlled juvenile IDDM: effects on diabetic control, self-evaluation and behavioural symptoms. *Acta Paediatrica* 83, 285–91.

Sabbeth, B. and Leventhal, J. M. (1984) Marital adjustment to chronic childhood illness. *Pediatrics* 73, 762–8.

Sack, W. H., Seeley, J. R., and Clarke, G. N. (1997) Does PTSD transcend cultural barriers? A study from the Khymer Adolescent Refugee Project. *Journal of the American Academy of Child and Adolescent Psychiatry* 36, 49–54.

Sales, J. and Turk, J. (1991) Angelman's syndrome: is there a behavioural phenotype? Society for the Study of Behavioural Phenotypes, Annual Workshop, London: Abstracts. SSBP, Oxford.

Sanders, M., Shepherd, R., Cleghorn, G., and Woolford, H. (1994) The treatment of recurrent abdominal pain in children: a controlled comparison of cognitive behavioral family intervention and standard paediatric care. *Journal of Consulting and Clinical Psychology* 62, 306–14.

Sands, A. M. and Golub, S. (1974) Breaking the bonds of tradition: a reassessment of group treatment of latency age children. *American Journal of Psychiatry* 131, 662–5.

Sawyer, M. G., Minde, K., and Zuker, R. (1982) The burned child—scarred for life? A study of the psychosocial impact of a burn injury at different developmental stages. *Burns* 9, 205–14.

Saylor, C. F., Pallmeyer, T. P., Finch, A. J., Eason, L., Treiber, F., and Folger, C. (1987) Predictors of psychological distress in hospitalized pediatric patients. *Journal of the American Academy of Child and Adolescent Psychiatry* 26, 232–6.

Schechter, A. (1978) *Treatment aspects of drug dependence.* CRC Press, Florida.

Schlieper, A. (1985) Chronic illness and school achievement. *Developmental Medicine and Child Neurology* 27, 69–79.

Schmidt, H., Burgard, P., Pietz, J., and Rupp, A. (1996) Intelligence and professional career in young adults treated early for phenylketonuria. *European Journal of Paediatrics* 155, Suppl. 1, S97–100.

Schmidt, M., Nocks, P., Lay, B., Ewert, H.-G. *et al.* (1997) Does oligoantigenic diet influence hyperactive/conduct disordered children—a controlled trial. *European Child and Adolescent Psychiatry* 6, 88–95.

Schoeller, D., Levitsky, L., Bandini, L., Dietz, W., and Walczak, A. (1988) Energy expenditure and body composition in Prader—Willi syndrome. *Metabolism* 37, 115–20.

Schonell, F. J. and Schonell, F. E. (1950) *Diagnostic and attainment testing.* Oliver and Boyd, Edinburgh.

Schulman, J. L. (1988) Use of a coping approach in the management of children with conversion reactions. *Journal of the American Academy of Child and Adolescent Psychiatry* 27, 785–8.

Schultz, J. A. (1983) Timing of elective hypospadias repair in children. *Pediatrics* 71, 342–51.

Schwartz, J. (1994) Low-level lead exposure and children's IQ: a meta-analysis and search for a threshold. *Environmental Research* 65, 42–55.

Schweitzer, S., Shin, Y., Jakobs, C., and Brodehl, J. (1993) Long-term outcome in 134 patients with galactosaemia. *European Journal of Paediatrics* 152, 36–43.

Seligman, M. (1975) *Helplessness: on depression, development and death.* W. H. Freeman, San Francisco.

Selikowitz, M., Sunman, J., Pendergast, A., and Wright, S. (1990) Fenfluramine in Prader–Willi syndrome: a double-blind, placebo controlled trial. *Archives of Disease in Childhood* 65, 112–14.

Sell, S. H. (1987) Long-term sequelae of bacterial meningitis in children. *Pediatric Infectious Disease* 6, 775–8.

Shaffer, D. (1995) Suicide and attempted suicide. In *Child and adolescent psychiatry: modern approaches,* ed. M. Rutter, L. Hersov, and E. Taylor, Blackwells, Oxford, pp. 407–24.

Shaffer, D., Gardner, A., and Hedge, B. (1984) Behaviour and bladder disturbance of enuretic children: a rational classification of a common disorder. *Developmental Medicine and Child Neurology* 26, 781–92.

Shaffer, D., Garland, A., Gould, M., Fisher, P., and Trautman, P. (1988) Preventing teenage suicide: a critical review. *Journal of the American Academy of Child and Adolescent Psychiatry* 27, 675–87.

Shaffer, D., Schwab-Stone, M., Fisher, P. *et al.* (1993) The Diagnostic Interview Schedule for Children-Revised Version (DISC-R), I: preparation, field testing, inter-rater reliability, and acceptability. *Journal of the American Academy of Child and Adolescent Psychiatry* 32, 643–50.

Shafran, R. (1998) Cognitive behaviour therapy for childhood obsessive disorder. In *Cognitive behaviour therapy for children and families,* ed. P. J. Graham, Cambridge University Press, Cambridge, pp. 45–73.

Shannon, F. T., Fergusson, D. M., and Dimond, M. E. (1984) Early hospital admissions and subsequent behaviour problems in six year olds. *Archives of Diseases in Childhood* 59, 815–19.

Shapiro, T (1989) The psychodynamic formulation in child and adolescent psychiatry. *Journal of the American Academy of Child and Adolescent Psychiatry* **28**, 675–80.

Sharland, M., Burch, M., McKenna, W. M., and Patton, M. A. (1992) A clinical study of Noonan syndrome. *Archives of Disease in Childhood* **67**, 178–83.

Sharp, D., Hay, D. F., Pawlby, S., Schmucker, G., Allen, H., and Kumar, R. (1995) The impact of postnatal depression on boys' intellectual development. *Journal of Child Psychology and Psychiatry* **36**, 1315–36.

Sharpe, M. C. (1991) A report—chronic fatigue syndrome: guidelines for research. *Journal of the Royal Society of Medicine* **84**, 118–21.

Shaw, M. T. (1977) Accidental poisoning in children: a psychosocial study. *New Zealand Medical Journal* **85**, 269–72.

Shields, J., Varley, R., Broks, P., and Simpson, A. (1996) Social cognition in developmental language disorders and high-level autism. *Developmental Medicine and Child Neurology* **38**, 487–95.

Siebelink, B. M., Bakker, D. J., Binnic, C. D., and Kasteleijn-Nolst-Trenite, D. G. (1988) Psychological effects of sub-clinical epileptiform EEG discharges in children. II. General intelligence tests. *Epilepsy Research* **2**, 117–21.

Sieg, K. G., Gaffney, G. R., Preston, D. F., and Hellings, J. A. (1995) SPECT brain imaging abnormalities in attention deficit hyperactivity disorder. *Clinical Nuclear Medicine* **20**, 55–60.

Silberg, J., Rutter, M., Meyer, J. *et al.* (1996) Genetic and environmental influences of the covariation between hyperactivity and conduct disturbance in juvenile twins. *Journal of Child Psychology and Psychiatry* **37**, 803–16.

Silbert, A., Wolff, P. H., and Lilienthal, J. (1977) Spatial and temporal processing in patients with Turner's syndrome. *Behavioral Genetics* **7**, 11–21.

Sillanpaa, M. (1983) Changes in the prevalence of migraine and other headaches during the first seven school years. *Headache* **23**, 15–19.

Sillanpaa, M. and Anttila, P. (1996) Increasing prevalence of headache in 7-year-old children. *Headache* **36**, 466–70.

Silva, P., Williams, S., and McGee, R. (1987) A longitudinal study of children with developmental language delay at age 3. Later intelligence, reading and behaviour problems. *Developmental Medicine and Child Neurology* **29**, 630–40.

Simko, A., Hornstein, L., Soukup, S., and Bagamery, N. (1989) Fragile X syndrome: recognition in young children. *Pediatrics* **83**, 547–52.

Simonds, J. F. and Parraga, O. (1982) Prevalence of sleep disorders and sleep behaviors in children and adolescents. *Journal of the American Academy of Child Psychiatry* **21**, 383–8.

Simonoff, E., Bolton, P., and Rutter, M. (1996) Mental retardation: genetic findings, clinical implications and research agenda. *Journal of Child Psychology and Psychiatry* **37**, 259–80.

Singer, H. S., Reiss, A. L., Brown, J. E. *et al.* (1993) Volumetric MRI changes in basal ganglia of children with Tourette's syndrome. *Neurology* **43**, 950–6.

Singh, U. and Jana, U. (1994) Plasma prolactin in epilepsy and pseudoseizures. *Indian Pediatrics* **31**, 667–9.

Skuse, D. (1989) Psychosocial adversity and impaired growth: in search of causal mechanisms. In *The scope of epidemiological psychiatry: essays in honour of Michael Shepherd,*. Routledge, London, pp. 240–63

Skuse, D. H. and Burrell, S. (1982) A review of solvent abusers and their management by a child psychiatry out-patient service. *Human Toxicology* **1**, 321–9.

Skuse, D., Percy, E., and Stevenson, J. (1994) Psychosocial functioning in the Turner syndrome: a national survey. British Paediatric Association Annual Meeting, Abstracts. British Paediatric Association, London.

Skuse, D., James, R. S., Bishop, D. V. *et al.* (1997) Evidence from Turner's syndrome of an imprinted X-linked locus affecting cognitive function. *Nature* 387(6634), 705–8.

Skuse, D., Bentovim, A., Hodges, J. *et al.* (1998) Risk factors for development of sexually abusive behaviour in sexually victimised adolescent boys: cross-sectional study. *British Medical Journal* 317, 175–9.

Skynner, R. (1974) School phobia: a reappraisal. *British Journal of Medical Psychology* 47, 1–16.

Slater, E., Beard, A. W., and Clithero, E. (1963) The schizophrenia-like psychoses of epilepsy. *British Journal of Psychiatry* 109, 95–150.

Sloper, P. and Turner, S. (1993) Risk and resistance factors in the adaptation of parents of children with severe physical disability. *Journal of Child Psychology and Psychiatry* 34, 167–88.

Sluckin, W., Herbert, M., and Sluckin, A. (1983) *Maternal bonding.* Blackwell, London.

Smart, D., Sanson, A., and Prior, M. (1996) Connections between reading disability and behavior problems: testing temporal and causal hypotheses. *Journal of Abnormal Child Psychology* 24, 363–83.

Smibert, E., Anderson, V., Godber, T., and Ekert, H. (1996) Risk factors for intellectual and educational sequelae of cranial irradiation in childhood acute lymphoblastic leukaemia. *British Journal of Cancer* 73, 825–30.

Smith, D. (1995) Youth crime and conduct disorders. In *Psychosocial disorders in young people: time trends and their causes*, ed. M. Rutter and D. Smith, Wiley, Chichester, pp. 389–489.

Smith, I., Beasley, M. G., Wolff, O. H., and Ades, A. A. (1988) Behavior disturbance in 8 year old children with early treated phenylketonuria. *Journal of Pediatrics* 112, 403–8.

Smith, M. (1991) Normal family behaviour and attitudes to sexuality. In *Department of Health Yearbook of Research and Development*, HMSO, London, pp. 43–5.

Smith, M., Delves, T., Lansdown, R., Clayton, B., and Graham, P. (1983) The effects of lead exposure on urban children. *Developmental Medicine and Child Neurology, Supplement* No. 47. Heinemann/Spastics International Medical Publications, London.

Smith, P., Perrin, S., and Yule, W. (1998) Post traumatic stress disorders. In *Cognitive behaviour therapy for children and families*, ed. P. J. Graham, Cambridge University Press, Cambridge, pp. 127–42.

Smithells, R. W. and Smith, I. J. (1984) Alcohol and the fetus. *Archives of Disease in Childhood* 59, 1113–14.

Sobel, R. (1970) Psychiatric implications of accidental poisoning in childhood. *Pediatric Clinics of North America* 17, 653–85.

Sokel, B., Lansdown, R., and Kent, A. (1990) The development of a hypnotherapy service for children. *Child: Care, Health and Development* 16, 227–33.

Sollee, N. D. and Kindlon, D. J. (1987) Lateralised brain injury and behavior problems in children. *Journal of Abnormal Child Psychology* 15, 479–91.

Sonksen, P. M. (1985) A developmental approach to sensory disabilities in early childhood. *International Rehabilitation Medicine* 7, 27–32

Sonuga-Barke, E. J. S., Williams, E., Hall, M., and Saxton, T. (1996) Hyperactivity and delay aversion III: the effect on cognitive style of imposing delay after errors. *Journal of Child Psychology and Psychiatry* 37, 189–94.

Sourindrhin, I. (1985) Solvent misuse. *British Medical Journal* 290, 94–5.

Spain, B. (1974) Verbal and performance ability in pre-school spina bifida children. *Developmental Medicine and Child Neurology* 16, 773–80.

Sparrow, S., Balla, D., and Cicchetti, D. (1984) *The Vineland Adaptive Behavior Scales*. American Guidance Service, Circle Pines, MN.

Spaulding, B. R. and Morgan, S. B. (1986) Spina bifida children. Their parents: a population prone to family dysfunction? *Journal of Pediatric Psychology* 11, 359–74.

Spence, S. H. (1994) Practitioner review: cognitive therapy with children and adolescents: from theory to practice. *Journal of Child Psychology and Psychiatry* 35, 1191–228.

Spence, S. H. and Donovan, C. (1998) Interpersonal problems. In *Cognitive behaviour therapy for children and families*, ed. P. J. Graham, Cambridge University Press, Cambridge, pp. 217–45.

Spivack, G., Platt, J. J., and Shure, M. B. (1976) *The problem-solving approach to adjustment*. Jossey-Bass, San Francisco.

Spurkland, I., Bjornstad, P., Lindberg, H., and Seem E. (1993) Mental health and psychosocial functioning in adolescents with congenital heart disease. A comparison between adolescents born with severe heart defect and atrial septal defect. *Acta Paediatrica* 82, 71–6.

Sroufe, L. A. and Rutter, M. (1984) The domain of developmental psychopathology. *Child Development* 55, 17–29.

St. James Roberts, I. (1991) Infant crying patterns in the first year: normal community and clinical findings. *Journal of Child Psychology and Psychiatry* 32, 951–68.

Stark, O., Atkins, E., Wolff, O. H., and Douglas, J. W. B. (1981) Longitudinal study of obesity in the National Survey of Health and Development. *British Medical Journal* 283, 13–17.

Steffenburg, S. and Gillberg, C. (1986) Autism and autistic-like conditions in Swedish rural and urban areas: a population study. *British Journal of Psychiatry* 149, 81–7.

Steffenburg, S., Gillberg, C., Hellgren, L. *et al.* (1989) A twin study of autism in Denmark, Finland, Iceland, Norway and Sweden. *Journal of Child Psychology and Psychiatry* 30, 405–16.

Stein, A., Woolley, H., Cooper, S., and Fairburn, C. (1994) An observational study of mothers with eating disorders and their infants. *Journal of Child Psychology and Psychiatry* 35, 733–48.

Steinhausen, H. C. (1995) Children of alcoholic parents. A review. *European Child and Adolescent Psychiatry* 4, 143–52.

Stevens, J. R. (1959) The emotional activation of the electroencephalogram in patients with convulsive disorders. *Journal of Nervous and Mental Disorders* 128, 339.

Stevens, M., Cameron, A., Muir, K., Parkes, S., Reid, H., and Whitewell, H. (1991) Descriptive epidemiology of primary central nervous system tumours in children: a population-based study. *Clinical Oncology Royal College of Radiologists* 3, 323–9.

Stevens, R. J., Becker, R. C., Krumpoj, G. L., Lanz, L. J., and Tolan, C. J. (1988) Post-natal sequelae of smoking during and after pregnancy. *Journal of Reproductive and Infant Psychology* 6, 61–81.

Stevenson, J. and Richman, N. (1976) The prevalence of language delay in a population of three year old children and its association with general retardation. *Developmental Medicine and Child Neurology* 18, 431–41.

Stewart, D. A., Bailey, J. D., Netley, C. T., and Park, E. (1991) Growth, development and behavioral outcome from mid-adolescence to adulthood in subjects with chromosomal aneuploidy: the Toronto study. *Birth Defects: Original Article Series* 26, 131–88.

Stewart, M. A. and Culver, K. W. (1982) Children who set fires: the clinical picture and a follow-up. *British Journal of Psychiatry* 140, 357–63.

Stoddard, F. J., Norman, D. K., Murphy, J. M., and Beardslee, W. R. (1989) Psychiatric outcome of burned children and adolescents. *Journal of the American Academy of Child and Adolescent Psychiatry* 28, 589–95.

Stolberg, A. L. and Garrison, K. M. (1985) Evaluating a primary prevention programme for children of divorce. *American Journal of Community Psychology* 13, 111–24.

Stores, G. (1978) Schoolchildren with epilepsy at risk for learning and behaviour problems. *Developmental Medicine and Child Neurology* 20, 502–8.

Stores, G. (1985) Clinical and EEG evaluation of seizures and seizure-like disorders. *Journal of the American Academy of Child Psychiatry* 24, 10–16.

Stores, G., Zaiwalla, Z., and Bergel, L. (1991) Frontal lobe complex partial seizures in children: a form of epilepsy of particular risk of misdiagnosis. *Developmental Medicine and Child Neurology* 33, 998–1009.

Strasburger, V. C. (1995) *Adolescents and the Media*. Sage, London.

Straus, M. A., Gelles, R. J., and Steinmetz, S. K. (1980) *Behind closed doors: violence in the American family*. Anchor Doubleday, Garden City, New York.

Street, E. and Dryden, W. (1988) *Family therapy in Britain*. Open University Press, Milton Keynes.

Strober, M. and Carlson, G. (1982) Bipolar illness in adolescents with major depression: clinical, genetic and psychopharmacologic predictors in a three to four year prospective follow-up investigation. *Archives of General Psychiatry* 39, 549–55.

Stunkard, A. J., Sorensen, T., Hanis, C. *et al.* (1986) An adoption study of human obesity. *New England Journal of Medicine* 314, 193–8.

Stunkard, A. J., Craighead, L. W., and O'Brien, R. (1980) Controlled trial of behaviour therapy, pharmacotherapy and their combination in the treatment of obesity. *Lancet* ii, 1045–7.

Sturniolo, M. and Galletti, F. (1994) Idiopathic epilepsy and school achievement. *Archives of Disease in Childhood* 70, 424–8.

Su, J. C., Kemp, A. S., Varigos, G. A., and Nolan, T. (1997) Atopic eczema: its impact on the family and financial cost. *Archives of Diseases in Childhood* 76, 159–62.

Sullivan, B. J. (1979) Adjustment in diabetic adolescent girls. II. Adjustment, self-esteem and depression in diabetic adolescent girls. *Psychosomatic Medicine* 41, 127–38.

Surana, R., Quinn, F., Guiney, E., and Fitzgerald, R. (1991) Are the selection criteria for the conservative management in spina bifida still applicable? *European Journal of Paediatric Surgery*, Suppl. 1, 35–7.

Swisher, L. P. and Pinsker, E. J. (1971) The language characteristics of hyper-verbal, hydrocephalic children. *Developmental Medicine and Child Neurology* 13, 746–55.

Szajnberg, N. M., Skrinjaric, J., and Moore, A. (1989) Affect attunement, attachment, temperament and zygosity: a twin study. *Journal of the American Academy of Child and Adolescent Psychiatry* 28, 249–53.

Szatmari, P., Archer, L., Fisman, S., Streiner, D. L., and Wilson, F. (1995) Asperger's syndrome and autism: differences in behavior, cognition, and adpative functioning. *Journal of the American Academy of Child and Adolescent Psychiatry* 34, 1662–71.

Tan, A., Salgado, M., and Fahn, S. (1997) The characterization and outcome of stereotypic movements in nonautistic children. *Movement Disorders* 12, 47–52.

Tanner, J. M. and Whitehouse, R. H. (1975) Revised standards for triceps and sub-capsular skinfolds in British children. *Archives of Disease in Childhood* 50, 142–5.

Tantam, D. (1988) Asperger's syndrome: an annotation. *Journal of Child Psychology and Psychiatry* 29, 245–55.

Target, M., and Fonagy, P. (1995) The psychological treatment of child and adolescent psychiatric disorders. In *What works for whom: a critical review of psychotherapy research*, ed. A. Roth and P. Fonagy, Guilford Press, New York, pp. 263–320.

Taylor, D. C. (1982) Counselling the parents of handicapped children. *British Medical Journal* **284**, 1027–8.

Taylor, E. (1984) Diet and behaviour. *Archives of Disease in Childhood* **59**, 97–8.

Taylor, E. (1985) *The hyperactive child: a parents' guide*. Dunitz, London.

Taylor, E. (1986) Overactivity, hyperactivity and hyperkinesis: problems and prevalence. In *The overactive child*, ed. E. Taylor, McKeith, London, pp. 1–18.

Taylor, E. M. and Emery, J. L. (1988) Trends in unexpected infant death in Sheffield. *Lancet* ii, 1121–3.

Taylor, E. and Hemsley, R. (1995) Treating hyperkinetic disorders in childhood. *British Medical Journal* **310**, 1617–18.

Taylor, E., Heptinstall, H., Chadwick, O., and Danckaerts, M. (1996) Hyperactivity and conduct problems as risk factors for adolescent development. *Journal of the American Academy of Child and Adolescent Psychiatry* **35**, 1213–26.

Taylor, H. G., Michaels, R., Mazur, P. *et al.* (1984) Intellectual, psychological and achievement outcomes in children six to eight years after from hemophilus influenzal meningitis. *Pediatrics* **74**, 198–205.

Taylor, I. G. (1984) Deafness. In: J. Forfar and G. Arneil (eds) *Textbook of Paediatrics*, Churchill Livingstone, Edinburgh, pp. 1714–25.

Taylor, J., Bland, J., and Anderson, H. (1998) Misuse of illicit drugs. *British Medical Journal* **316**, 312.

Tebbutt, J., Swanston, H., Oates, R. K., and O'Toole, B. I. (1997) Five years after child sexual abuse: persisting dysfunction and problems of prediction. *Journal of the American Academy of Child and Adolescent Psychiatry* **36**, 330–9.

Tejani, A., Dobias, B., and Sambursky, J. (1982) Long-term prognosis after *H. influenzae* meningitis: prospective evaluation. *Developmental Medicine and Child Neurology* **24**, 338–43.

Telch, M. J., Killen, J. D., McAlister, A. L., Perry, C. L., and Maccoby, N. (1982) Long-term follow-up of a pilot project on smoking prevention with adolescents. *Journal of Behavioural Medicine* **5**, 1–8.

Teplin, S. W., Howard, J. A., and O'Connor, M. J. (1981) Self-concept of young children with cerebral palsy. *Developmental Medicine and Child Neurology* **23**, 730–8.

Thake, A., Todd, J., Bundey, S., and Webb, T. (1985) Is it possible to make a clinical diagnosis of the fragile X syndrome in a boy? *Archives of Disease in Childhood* **60**, 1001–7.

Thake, A., Todd, J., Webb, T., and Bundey, S. (1987) Children with the fragile X chromosome at schools for the mildly mentally retarded. *Developmental Medicine and Child Neurology* **29**, 711–19.

Thernlund, G., Dahlquist, G., Hansson, K. *et al.* (1995) Psychological stress and the onset of IDDM in children. *Diabetes-Care* **18**, 1323–9.

Theut, S. K., Pedersen, F. A., Zaslow, M. J., and Rabinovich, B. A. (1988) Pregnancy subsequent to parental loss: parental anxiety and depression. *Journal of the American Academy of Child and Adolescent Psychiatry* **27**, 289–92.

Thomas, A., Chess, S., and Birch, H. (1968) *Temperament and behavior disorders in childhood*, New York University Press, New York.

Thomas, A., Bax, M., Coombes, K., Goldson, E., Smyth, D., and Whitmore, K. (1985) *The health and social needs of physically handicapped young adults. Are they being met by the statutory services?* Supplement No. 50, No. 4. Heinemann/Spastics International Medical Publications, London.

Thompson, K. L., Bundy, K. A., and Broncheau, C. (1995) Social skills training for young adolescents: symbolic and behavioral components. *Adolescence* **30**, 724–34.

Thomson, G. O. B., Raab, G. M., Hepburn, W. S., Hunter, R., Fulton, M., and Laxen, D. P. H. (1989) Blood lead levels and children's behaviour. *Journal of Child Psychology and Psychiatry* 30, 515–28.

Till, K. (1975) *Paediatric neurosurgery*. Blackwell Scientific, Oxford.

Tillotson, S. L., Fuggle, P., Smith, I., Ades, A., and Grant, D. B. (1994) Relation between biochemical severity and intelligence in early treated hypothyroidism. *British Medical Journal* 309, 440–5.

Tizard, B. (1977) *Adoption: a second chance*. Open Books, London.

Tizard, B., Cooperman, O., Joseph, A., and Tizard, J. (1972) Environmental effects on language development: a study of children in long-stay residential nurseries. *Child Development* 43, 337–58.

Tizard, B. and Hodges, J. (1978) The effect of early institutional rearing on the development of eight year old children. *Journal of Child Psychology and Psychiatry* 19, 99–118.

Tizard, B. and Hughes, M. (1984) *Young children learning*. Fontana, London.

Tizard, B. and Phoenix, A. (1995) The identity of mixed parentage adolescents. *Journal of Child Psychology and Psychiatry* 36, 1399–410.

Tobias, A. L. and Gordon, J. B. (1980) Social consequences of obesity. *Journal of the American Dietetic Association* 76, 338–42.

Tobiasen, J. M. (1984) Psychosocial correlates of congenital facial cleft: a conceptualisation and model. *Cleft Palate* 21, 131–9.

Tobin-Richards, M. H., Boxer, A. M., and Petersen, A. (1982) The psychological significance of pubertal change: sex differences in perception of self during early adolescence. In *Girls at puberty: biological and psychological perspectives*, ed. J. Brooks-Gunn and A. Petersen, Plenum, New York, pp. 127–54.

Todd, R., Reich, W., Petti, T., Joshi, P., DePaola, J., Nurnberger, J., and Reich, T. (1996) Psychiatric diagnosis in the child and adolescent members of extended families identified through adult bipolar affective disorder probands. *Journal of the American Academy of Child and Adolescent Psychiatry* 35, 664–71.

Toedter, L. J., Lasker, J. N., and Alhadeff, J. M. (1988) The perinatal grief scale: development and initial validation. *American Journal of Orthopsychiatry* 58, 435–49.

Toone, B. K. and van der Linden, G. J. H. (1997) Attention deficit hyperactivity disorder or hyperkinetic disorder in adults. *British Journal of Psychiatry* 170, 489–91.

Topolski, T. D., Hewitt, J. K., Eaves, L. J. *et al.* (1997) Genetic and environmental influences of child reports of manifest anxiety and symptoms of separation anxiety and overanxious disorders: a community based twin study. *Behavior Genetics* 27, 15–28.

Torgerson, A. M. and Kringlen, E. (1978) Genetic aspects of temperamental differences in infants: their cause as shown through twin studies. *Journal of the American Academy of Child Psychiatry* 17, 433–44.

Trimble, M. R. (1987) Anticonvulsant drugs and cognitive function: a review of the literature. *Epilepsia* 28, 37–45.

Tröster, H. (1994) Prevalence and functions of stereotyped behaviors in nonhandicapped children in residential care. *Journal of Abnormal Child Psychology* 22, 79–97.

Truax, C. B. and Carkhuff, R. R. (1967) *Towards effective counselling and psychotherapy: training and practice*. Aldin, Chicago.

Tsiantis, J., Dragonas, T., Richardson, C., Anastopoulos, D., Masera, G., and Spinetta, J. (1996) Psychosocial problems and adjustment of children with beta-thalassemia in their family. *European Child and Adolescent Psychiatry* 5, 192–203.

Tsiantis, J., Xypolita-Tsantili, D., and Papadakou-Lagoyianni, S. (1982) Family reactions and their management in a parents' group with beta-thalassaemia. *Archives of Diseases in Childhood* 57, 860–3.

Tunali, B. and Power, T. G. (1993) Creating satisfaction: a psychological perspective on stress and coping in families of handicapped children. *Journal of Child Psychology and Psychiatry* **34**, 945–57.

Turk, J. (1992) The fragile X syndrome: on the way to a behavioural phenotype. *British Journal of Psychiatry* **160**, 24–35.

Turk, J. (1993) Cognitive approaches to the treatment of eating disorders in children. In *Childhood Onset Anorexia Nervosa and Related Eating Disorders*, ed.: B. Lask, and R. Bryant-Waugh, Lawrence Erlbaum, Hove, pp. 177–90.

Turk, J. (1996a) Working with parents of children who have severe learning disabilities. *Clinical Child Psychology and Psychiatry* **1**, 581–96.

Turk, J. (1996b) Tertiary prevention of childhood mental health problems. In *The Prevention of Mental Illness in Primary Care*, ed.. T. Kendrick, A. Tylee, and P. Feeling, Cambridge University Press, Cambridge, pp. 265–80.

Turk, J. (1997) The mental health needs of children with learning disabilities. In *Mental health in learning disabilities, Training package*, ed., G. Holt, Y. Kon, and N. Bouras, Pavilion Publications, Brighton.

Turk, J. (1998) Fragile X syndrome and attentional deficits. *Journal of Applied Research in Intellectual Disabilities* **11**, 175–91.

Turk, J. and Graham, P. (1997) Fragile X syndrome, autism and autistic features. *Autism* **1**, 175–97.

Turk, J. and Hill, P. (1995) Behavioural phenotypes in dysmorphic syndromes. *Clinical Dysmorphology* **4**, 105–15.

Turk, J. and Lask, B. (1991) Neuroleptic malignant syndrome. *Archives of Disease in Childhood* **66**, 91–2.

Turk, J. and Sales, J. (1996) Behavioural phenotypes and their relevance to child mental health professionals. *Child Psychology and Psychiatry Review* **1**, 4–11.

Turk, J., Hagerman, R. J., Barnicoat, A., and McEvoy, J. (1994) The fragile X syndrome. In *Mental health and mental retardation—recent advances and practices*, ed. N. Bouras, Cambridge University Press, Cambridge, pp. 135–53.

Turner, G., Webb, T., Wake, S., and Robinson, H. (1996) Prevalence of fragile X syndrome. *American Journal of Medical Genetics* **64**, 196–7.

Ungerer, J. A., Horgan, B., Chaiton, J., and Champion, G. D. (1988) Psychosocial functioning in children and young adults with juvenile arthritis. *Pediatrics* **81**, 195–202.

Utens, E., Verhulst, F., Meijboom, F. *et al.* (1993) Behavioural and emotional problems in children and adolescents with congenital heart disease. *Psychological Medicine* **23**, 415–24.

Utting W. (1997) *People like us: Report of the review of the safeguards for children living away from home*. Stationery Office, London.

Valleni-Basile, L., Garrison, C., Jackson, K. *et al.* (1994) Frequency of obsessive–compulsive disorder in a community sample of young adolescents. *Journal of the American Academy of Child and Adolescent Psychiatry* **33**, 782–91.

Van Bilsen, H. and Wilke, M. (1998) Drug and alcohol abuse in young people. In P. Graham (ed.) *Cognitive behaviour for children and families*. Cambridge University Press, Cambridge, pp. 246–261.

Van Eerdewegh, M. M., Clayton, P. J., and Van Eerdewegh, P. (1985) The bereaved child: variables influencing early psychopathology. *British Journal of Psychiatry* **147**, 188–94.

Van Furth, E., Van Striend, D. Martina, L., Van-Son, M., Hendrickx, J., and Van Engeland, H. (1996) Expressed emotional and the prediction of outcome in adolescent eating disorders. *International Journal of Eating Disorders* **20**, 19–31.

Vance, J., Najman, J., Thearle, M., Embelton, G., Foster, W., and Boyle, F. (1995) Psychological changes in parents eight months after the loss of an infant from stillbirth, neonatal death or sudden infant death syndrome—a longitudinal study. *Pediatrics* **96**, 933–8.

Vandvik, I. H. and Eckblad, G. (1991) Mothers of children with recent onset of rheumatic disease: association between maternal distress, psychosocial variables and the disease of the children. *Journal of Developmental Behavioral Pediatrics* **12**, 84–91.

Verhulst, F. (1995) A review of community studies. In: F. Verhulst and H. Koot (eds) *The epidemiology of child and adolescent psychiatry.* Oxford University Press, Oxford, pp. 146–77.

Verhulst, F. C. (in press) Community and epidemiological aspects. In *Anxiety disorders in children: theory, research and practice*, ed. W. K. Silverman and P. A. Treffers.

Verhulst, F. and Achenbach, T. (1995) Empirically based assessment and taxonomy of psychopathology: Cross-cultural applications. *European Child and Adolescent Psychiatry* **4**, 61–76.

Verhulst, F. C., Van der Ende, J., and Koot, H. M. (1996) *Handleiding voor de CBCL/4–18.* Afdeling Kinder- en jeudgpsychiatrie Sophia Kinderziekenhuis/Academisch Ziekenhuis/Erasmus Universiteit, Rotterdam.

Verhulst, F. C., Van der Ende, J., Ferdinand, R. F., and Kasius, M. C. (1997) The prevalence of DSM-III-R diagnoses in a national sample of Dutch adolescents. *Archives of General Psychiatry* **54**(4), 329–36.

Vernon, D. T. A., Foley, J. M., Sipowicz, R. R., and Schulman, J. L. (1965) *The psychological responses of children to hospitalization and illness.* Charles C. Thomas, Springfield, IL.

Versluis-den Bieman, H. and Verhulst, F. (1995) Self-reported and parent-reported problems in adolescent international adoptees. *Journal of Child Psychology and Psychiatry* **36**, 1411–28.

Vitiello, B. and Stoff, D. (1997) Sub-types of aggression and their relevance to child psychiatry. *Journal of the American Academy of Child and Adolescent Psychiatry* **36**, 307–15.

Vize, C. and Cooper, P. (1995) Sexual abuse in patients with eating disorders, patients with depression and normal controls. A comparative study. *British Journal of Psychiatry* **167**, 80–5.

Voeller, K. S. and Rothenburg, M. B. (1973) Psychosocial aspects of the management of seizures in children. *Journal of Pediatrics* **51**, 1072–82.

Vogler, G., DeFries, J. C., and Decker, S. N. (1985) Family history as an indicator of risk for reading disability. *Journal of Learning Disabilities* **18**, 419–21.

Volkmar, F. R. and Cohen, D. J. (1989) Disintegrative disorder or 'late onset' autism. *Journal of Child Psychology and Psychiatry* **30**, 717–24.

Vostanis, P., Harrington, R., Prendergast, M., and Farndon, P. (1994) Case reports of autism with interstitial deletion of chromosome 17 (p11.2 p11.2) and monosomy of chromosome 5 (5pter-5p15.3) *Psychiatric Genetics* **4**, 109–11.

Vostanis, P., Hayes, M., Du Feu, M., and Warren, J. (1997) Detection of behavioural and emotional problems in deaf children and adolescents: comparison of two rating scales. *Child Care Health and Development* **23**, 233–46.

Wahlstrom, J., Steffenburg, S., Hallgren, L., and Gillberg, C. (1989) Chromosome findings in twins with early onset autistic disorder. *American Journal of Medical Genetics* **32**, 19–21.

Walk, R. D. (1980) Perception. In *Developmental Psychiatry*, ed. M. Rutter, Heinemann Medical, London, pp. 177–84.

Walker, L. S., Ford, M. B., and Donald, W. D. (1987) Cystic fibrosis and family stress: effects of age and severity of illness. *Pediatrics* **79**, 239–46.

Walker, L. S., Garber, J., and Greene, J. W. (1993) Psychosocial correlates of recurrent abdominal pain, organic illness and psychiatric disorder. *Journal of Abnormal Psychology* **102**, 248–58.

Walker, L. S., Garber, J., Van Slyke, D., and Greene, J. (1995) Long-term health outcomes in children with recurrent abdominal pain. *Journal of Pediatric Psychology* **20**, 233–45.

Wallace, S. J. (1984) Febrile convulsions: their significance for later intellectual development and behaviour. *Journal of Child Psychology and Psychiatry* **25**, 15–21.

Wallace, S., Crown, J., Cox, A., and Berger, M. (1995) *Health care needs assessment: child and adolescent mental health.* Radcliffe Medical, Abingdon.

Wallander, J. L., Varni, J. W., Babani, L., Banis, H., and Wilcox, K. T. (1988) Children with chronic physical disorders. Maternal reports of their psychological adjustment. *Journal of Pediatric Psychology* **13**, 197–212.

Waller, D. and Eisenberg, L. (1980) School refusal in childhood-psychiatric-pediatric perspective. In *Out of school: modern perspectives in school refusal and truancy*, ed. L. Hersov and I. Berg, Wiley, Chichester, pp. 207–29.

Walter, G. and Rey, J. M. (1997) An epidemiological study of the use of ECT in adolescents. *Journal of the American Academy of Child and Adolescent Psychiatry* **36**, 809–15.

Wasserman, A. L. (1984) A prospective study of the impact of home monitoring on the family. *Journal of Pediatrics* **74**, 323–9.

Wasserman, G. A., Lennon, M. C., Allen, R., and Shilansky, M. (1987) Contributions to attachment in normal and physically handicapped infants. *Journal of the American Academy of Child and Adolescent Psychiatry* **26**, 9–15.

Wasson, C., Bannister, C., and Ward, G. (1992) Factors affecting the school placement of children with spina bifida. *European Journal of Pediatric Surgery* Suppl. 1, 29–34.

Webster, A., Bamford, J., Thyer, N. *et al.* (1989) The psychological, educational and auditory sequelae of early, persistent, secretory otitis media. *Journal of Child Psychology and Psychiatry* **30**, 529–46.

Webster-Stratton, C. and Hammond, M. (1997) Treating children with early-onset conduct problems: a comparison of child and parent training interventions. *Journal of Consulting and Clinical Psychology* **65**, 93–109.

Wechsler, D. (1989) *Manual for the Wechsler Pre-School and Primary Scale of Intelligence.* Psychological Corporation, New York,

Wechsler, D. (1992) *Manual for the Wechsler Intelligence Scale for Children—revised.* WISC III UK Version. Psychological Corporation, New York.

Wechsler, D. (1993) *Wechsler Objective Reading Dimensions (WORD).* Psychological Corporation, New York.

Wechsler, D. (1996) *Wechsler Objective Numerical Dimensions (WOND).* Psychological Corporation, New York.

Weinberg, N. Z. (1997) Cognitive and behavioural deficits associated with parental alcohol use. *Journal of the American Academy of Child and Adolescent Psychiatry* **36**, 1177–86.

Weissman, M. and Paykel, E. (1974) *The depressed woman: a study of social relationships.* University of Chicago Press, Chicago.

Weisz, J. R. and Weiss, B. (1993) *Effects of psychotherapy with children and adolescents.* Sage, Beverly Hills, CA.

Weldon, D. and McGeady, S. (1995) Theophylline effects on cognition, behavior and learning. *Archives of Pediatric Adolescent Medicine* **149**, 90–3.

Wellings, K., Field, J., Johnson, A., and Wadsworth, J. (1994) *Sexual behaviour in Britain.* Penguin, Harmondsworth.

Werner, E., Simonian, K., Bierman, J. E., and French, F. E. (1967) Cumulative effect of perinatal complications and deprived environment on physical, intellectual and social development of pre-school children. *Pediatrics* 39, 480–505.

Werry, J. S. and Wollersheim, J. P. (1989) Behavior therapy with children and adolescents: a twenty-year overview. *Journal of the American Academy of Child and Adolescent Psychiatry* 28, 1–18.

Werry, J., McLellan, J., and Chard, L. (1991) Childhood and adolescent schizophrenia, bipolar and schizoaffective disorders: a clinical and outcome study. *Journal of the American Academy of Child and Adolescent Psychiatry* 30, 457–65.

West, D. J. and Farrington, D. P. (1973) *Who becomes delinquent?* Heinemann Educational, London.

Whittaker, A., Johnson, J., Shaffer, D. *et al.* (1990) Uncommon troubles in young people. *Archives of General Psychiatry* 47, 487–94.

White, K., Kolman, M. L., Wexler, P., Polin, G., and Winter, R. J. (1984) Unstable diabetes and unstable families: a psychosocial evaluation of diabetic children with recurrent ketoacidosis. *Pediatrics* 73, 749–55.

Whitmore, K. and Bax, M. C. O. (1986) The school entry medical examination. *Archives of Disease in Childhood* 61, 807–17.

Wikler, L., Wasow, M., and Hatfield, E. (1981) Chronic sorrow revisited: parent vs. professional depiction of the adjustment of parents of mentally retarded children. *American Journal of Orthopsychiatry* 51, 63–70.

Wilensky, D. S., Ginsberg, G., Altman, M., Tulchinsky, T. H., Ben Yishay, F. and Auerbach, J. (1996) A community study of failure to thrive in Israel. *Archives of Disease in Childhood* 75, 145–8.

Wilkinson, P. W. (1975) Obesity in childhood. A community study in Newcastle-upon-Tyne. *Archives of Disease in Childhood* 50, 826.

Wilkinson, V. A. (1981) Juvenile chronic arthritis in adolescence: facing the reality. *International Rehabilitation Medicine* 3, 11–17.

Winchel, R. M. and Stanley, M. (1991) Self-injurious behavior: a review of the behavior and biology of self-mutilation. *American Journal of Psychiatry* 148, 306–17.

Wing, L. (1981) Asperger's syndrome: a clinical account. *Psychological Medicine* 11, 115–29.

Wing, L. (1993) The definition and prevalence of autism: a review. *European Child and Adolescent Psychiatry* 2, 61–74.

Wing, L. and Gould, J. (1979) Severe impairments of social interaction and associated abnormalities in children: epidemiology and classification. *Journal of Autism and Developmental Disorders* 9, 11–29.

Winnicott, D. W. (1953) Transitional objects and transitional phenomena. *International Journal of Psychoanalysis* 34, 87–9.

Wiseman, H. M., Guest, K., Murray, G., and Volans, G. N. (1987) Accidental poisoning in childhood: a multi-centre survey. I. General epidemiology. *Human Toxicology* 6, 293–301.

Wittkower, E. D. and Hunt, B. A. (1958) Psychological aspects of atopic dermatitis in children. *Canadian Medical Association Journal* 79, 810–17.

Wolfer, J. A. and Visintainer, M. A. (1979) Pre-hospital psychological preparation for tonsillectomy patients: effects on children's and parents' adjustment. *Pediatrics* 64, 646–55.

Wolff, P. H. and Melngailis, I. (1994) Family patterns of developmental dyslexia: clinical findings. *American Journal of Medical Genetics* 54, 122–31.

Wolff, R. P. and Wolff, L. S. (1991) Assessment and treatment of obsessive–compulsive disorder in children. *Behavior Modification* 15, 372–93.

Wolff, S. (1984) The concept of personality disorder in childhood. *Journal of Child Psychology and Psychiatry* 25, 5–13.

Wolff, S. (1991a) 'Schizoid' personality in childhood and adult life I: the vagaries of diagnostic labelling. *British Journal of Psychiatry* 159, 615–620.

Wolff, S. (1991b) 'Schizoid' personality in childhood and adult life III: the childhood picture. *British Journal of Psychiatry* 159, 629–635.

Wolff, S., Narayan, S., and Moyes, B. (1988) Personality characteristics of parents of autistic children: a controlled study. *Journal of Child Psychology and Psychiatry* 29, 143–53.

Wolff, S., Townshend, R., McGuire, R. J., and Weeks, D. J. (1991) 'Schizoid' personality in childhood and adult life II: adult adjustment and the continuity with schizotypal personality disorder. *British Journal of Psychiatry* 159, 620–9.

Wolffe, M. and Wild, J. M. (1984) The occupational success of visually handicapped adolescents in the first year after leaving school for the partially seeing. *International Journal of Rehabilitation Research* 7, 399–407.

Wolke, D. (1987) Environmental neonatology. *Archives of Disease in Childhood* 62, 987–8.

Wolke, D. (1997) The pre-term responses to the environment—long-term effects? In *Advances in perinatal medicine*, ed. F. Cockburn, Parthenon, London, pp. 305–14.

Wolkind, S. (1981) Hypertension of pregnancy. In *Pregnancy: a psychological and social study*, ed. S. Wolkind and E. Zajicek, Academic Press, London: pp. 89–106.

Wolkind, S. (1984) A child psychiatrist in court: using the contributions of developmental psychology. In *Taking a stand*, British Agencies for Adoption and Fostering, London, pp. 7–17.

Wolkind, S. and Kozaruk, A. (1983) *Children with special needs: a review of children with medical problems placed by the Adoption Resources Exchange from 1974–1977.* Report to the Department of Health and Social Security, London.

Wolkind, S. and Kruk, S. (1985) From child to parent: early separation and the adaptation to motherhood. In *Longitudinal studies in child psychology and psychiatry*, ed. A. R. Nicol, Wiley, Chichester.

Wolkind, S. and Rutter, M. (1973) Children who have been 'in care'—an epidemiological study. *Journal of Child Psychology and Psychiatry* 14, 97–105.

Wood, A., Massarano, A., Super, M., and Harrington, R. (1995) Behavioural aspects and psychiatric findings in Noonan's syndrome. *Archives of Disease in Childhood* 72, 153–155.

Wood, C. B. S. and Walker-Smith, J. A. (1981) *MacKeith's infant feeding and feeding difficulties.* Churchill Livingstone, Edinburgh.

Woodmansey, A. C. (1967) Emotion and the motions: an inquiry into the causes and perceptions of functional disorders of defaecation. *British Journal of Medical Psychology* 40, 207–23.

Woodward, S., Pope, A., Robson, W. J., and Hagan, O. (1985) Bereavement counselling after sudden infant death. *British Medical Journal* 290, 363–5.

Woolston, J. L. (1987) Obesity in infancy and early childhood. *Journal of the American Academy of Child and Adolescent Psychiatry* 26, 123–6.

World Health Organization (1980) *International classification of impairments, disabilities and handicaps; a manual of classification relating to the consequences of disease.* Geneva, WHO.

World Health Organization (1992) *The ICD-10 classification of mental and behavioural disorders: clinical descriptions and diagnostic guidelines.* World Health Organization, Geneva.

Wrate, R. M., Kolvin, I., Garside, R. F., Wolstenholme, F., Hulbert, C. M., and Leitch, I. M. (1985) Helping seriously disturbed children. In *Longitudinal studies in child psychology and psychiatry*, ed. A. R. Nicol, Wiley, Chichester, pp. 265–318.

Wright, M. and Nolan, T. (1994) Impact of cyanotic heart disease on school performance. *Archives of Disease in Childhood* **71**, 64–70.

Young Minds (1998) *Young Minds Directory 1998*. Young Minds, London.

Young, M. H., Brennen, L. C., Baker, R. D., and Baker, S. S. (1995) Functional encopresis: symptom reduction and behavioral improvement. *Journal of Developmental and Behavioral Pediatrics* **16**, 226–32.

Yude, C., Goodman, R., and McConachie, H. (1998) Peer problems of children with hemiplegia in mainstream primary schools. *Journal of Child Psychology and Psychiatry* **39**, 533–41.

Zeanah, C. H. (1989) Adaptation following perinatal loss: a critical review. *Journal of the American Academy of Child and Adolescent Psychiatry* **28**, 467–80.

Zeitlin, H. (1986) *The natural history of psychiatric disorder in childhood*. Maudsley Monographs, Oxford University Press, London.

Index

abdominal pain
  case study 437
  infants 188
  recurrent 288–91
abuse
  emotional abuse 51–4
  management 58
  Munchausen syndrome by proxy 48–50
  neglect 50–1
  outcome 59–60
  physical abuse 43–8
  sexual abuse 54–9, 253, 351–2
  see also alcohol; drugs
accidents
  Child Accident Prevention Trust
    (1989) 348
  see also injuries
adolescence 267–313
  psychological changes 268–9
  psychoses 295–304
  sexual development 269–72
adoption 471–3
adrenal cortical hyperplasia 381
adult–child continuities 314–16
adult-type psychiatric disorders 280–94
  obsessional disorders 280–3
  psychosomatic disorders 283–93
    chronic fatigue syndrome 291–3
    conversion disorder 284–8
    post-traumatic stress 293–4
    recurrent non-organic abdominal
      pain 288–91
affective disorders 299–302
age, and prevalence of psychiatric
    disorders 22
AIDS and HIV infection 350–3
alcohol consumption 394
  clinical features 311–12
  pattern 311
  pregnancy 173
  see also drug use and abuse
allergic respiratory disorders 370–5

α_2 adrenergic agonists 448
amitriptyline hydrochloride, dosage and
    characteristics 444, 449–50
amnesia 346
amphetamines 312
anaemia, thalassaemia 369–70
androgens 262
Angelman syndrome 95, 142
anorexia nervosa 273–80
  atypical syndromes 274–5
  case study 437–8
  clinical features 273–4
  treatment and outcome 278–9
antenatal care 395
anticonvulsant drugs 158, 451
antidepressant drugs 449–51
antisocial behaviour see behavioural
    problems; conduct disorder
anxiety disorders 209–20
  adolescence 215
  classification 212
  clinical features 212–15
  defined 208
  development 208–12
  general anxiety disorder 213, 218
  infants 208–9
  middle school (5–12 years) 213
  origins 210–12
  outcome 220
  phobias 214–20
  pre-school (0–5 years) 212–13
  separation anxiety disorder 209,
    213–14, 219
  specific phobias 214–20
    biological and developmental
      causes 217
    cognitive appraisal of stressful
      events 217
    experiences and life events 217
    genetic and constitutional factors 217
    learning theory 217–18
    parental behaviour 217

anxiety disorders (*continued*)
  specific phobias (*continued*)
    anxiety disorders
      social adversity 217
      social phobias 215–16, 220
      temperament 217
    treatment 218–20
anxiety and fear 208–20
anxiolytics 444
arthritis, juvenile chronic 390–1
articulation impairment (dyslalia) 75
Asperger syndrome 129–31
  clinical features 129–30
  treatment and outcome 131
assessment and diagnosis 35–42
  approaches 26–7, 97–110
  information from teachers 33
  interview with child 28–33
    fantasies 32
    observations 32–3
    screening tasks 32
    self perception 31
    stress 32
  interview with teacher 33
  interviews with parents 26–9
    building family confidence 29
    current functioning of child 27–8
    developmental history 27
    eliciting feelings and attitudes 29
    exploration of the problem 26–7
    family structure and function 27
    obtaining information 28–9
  physical examination and
    investigation 31, 33–4
  physical setting 25
  preparing the referral 25
  principles of imparting diagnosis 326–8
  procedure 24–5
  psychiatric disorders 24–35
    formulation 35
  psychological assessment 35–42
  standardized questionnaires 33
asthma 317, 370–5
  psychological factors 371–3
  treatment and outcome 374–5
atopic dermatitis 386–7
attachment disorders 11–12, 183–5
attention, normal development 110–11
attention deficit hyperactivity disorder
  (ADHD)

  assessment 116
  behavioural characteristics 112–13
  brain dysfunction 113–14
  causative variables 113–15
  genetic factors 113
  hyperkinetic syndrome 111–20
  interactional effects 115–16
  onset 112
  outcome 119–20
  prevalence 113
  treatment 116–19
autism 120–29
  assessment 125–7
  background factors 124–5
  behavioural features 121–3
  definition 120–1
  intellectual development 123
  management 127–8
  outcome 128–9
  physical conditions 123–4
  schizophrenia links 125
autosomal abnormalities 139–43

barbiturates 312
Bayley Scales, infant development 38
behaviour therapy 401–20
  case examples 417–20
  cognitive psychotherapy 414–17
  desensitization 411–12
  increasing and decreasing behaviour
    (*table*) 404
  operant methods 404–11
    (*table*) 405
  other techniques 412–14
  reinforcers 404–8
behavioural problems
  conduct disorder 235–51
  counselling 106–7
  interviews with child 31
  learning disorders 106–7
  oppositional defiant disorder (ODD)
    237–40
  see also conduct disorder
benzodiazepines 444
bereavement, depressive reaction 225
biological theories 5–6
bipolar affective disorders 299–302
  treatment and outcome 301–2
birth
  neonatal period, psychosocial

aspects 176–80
perinatal complications 175–6
puerperal psychoses 177
bladder control
management of enuresis 258–62
normal 257–8
blood disorders 364–70
body image 323
bowel control 251–7
constipation 251–4
encopresis 254–7
brain dysfunction
attention deficit hyperactivity
disorder 113–14
developmental theories and disorders 5
breastfeeding 186
British Ability Scale 39
bulimia nervosa 273–5
burns 348–9
butyrophenone 445

cannabis 310–11
carbamazepine, dosage and
characteristics 451
cardiac surgery 384–6
care, interim care and supervision
orders 474
case studies
abdominal pain 437
anorexia nervosa 437–8
behaviour therapy 417–20
cognitive psychotherapy 417–20
cystic fibrosis 428–9
family psychotherapy 436–9
headache 2
individual psychotherapy 427–30
sleep disorders 417–18
tics and Tourette syndrome 419–20
cataplexy 206
catastrophizing 416
central nervous system and muscle
disorders 149–68
cerebral palsy 96, 149–53
clinical features 149
definition 149
general intelligence 150
language disability 150
management implications 152–3
motor co-ordination abnormalities 151

perceptual abnormalities 150–1
psychiatric aspects 151–2
psychological development 149–50
cerebral tumours 161–2
clinical features 161
treatment and outcome 161–2
challenging behaviour *see* behavioural
problems; conduct disorder
Child Assessment Order 474
child health clinics 458–9
child minding 468–9
child protection 393–4, 466–79
emergency protection order (EPO) 473
prevention of injuries 348
child–adult continuities 314–16
children's homes 469
chloral hydrate 444
chlordiazepoxide 444
chlorpromazine, dosage and
characteristics 445
choreoathetosis 171
chromosomal abnormalities 138–48
see also sex chromosome abnormalities
chronic disease, psychosocial aspects 318
chronic fatigue syndrome (myalgic
encephalomyelitis) 291–3
management 292–3
classical conditioning 6, 413
classification and prevalence of psychiatric
disorders 17–24
comparison of ICD-10 and DSM–IV
systems 18–19
ICD-10 classification 19–20
cleft lip and palate 341–3
clomipramine, dosage and characteristics
207, 283, 450–1
clonidine, dosage and characteristics 68,
448
clozapin 302
cocaine 312
cognitive behaviour theories 6–8
cognitive distortions 416
cognitive psychotherapy 414–17
case studies 417–20
community paediatric team 459–60
compulsions, defined 281
conduct disorder 240–51
age and sex 245
assessment 247–8
classification 241–2

conduct disorder (*continued*)
clinical features 242–4
court reports 250
defined 240–1
delinquency 241
familial factors 245–6
interviews with child 31
management 248–50
outcome 250–1
personal factors 246–7
prevalence 244
social development and antisocial
behaviour 240–51
social and neighbourhood factors 245
see also behavioural problems
conflicts in care 477–8
confusional states (delirious states) 354
congenital heart disease 383–6
consent, treatment refusal and
consent 475–6
constipation 188, 251–4
management and outcome 253–4
Contact Order 474
continuities, child–adult disorders
314–16
conversion disorder 284–8
cot death 339–41
counselling
behavioural problems 106–7
breaking the news 101–6, 326–8
continued counselling 328–30
cot death 340
educational advice 107–8
family 431–2
genetic counselling 108, 366
learning disorders 101–6
ongoing 328–30
promotion of development 106
Tourette syndrome 67
court reports 478–9
cretinism 96, 359
cri du chat syndrome 92, 141
Crohn's disease 382
cryptorchidism 381
cystic fibrosis (mucoviscidosis)
375–8
case study 428–9
psychosocial aspects and
management 376–8
cytomegalovirus (CMV) 95, 353

deafness, screening 132
death
care of the dying child 334–7
stillborn and neonatal 338–9
sudden infant death syndrome 339–41
deficits, intelligence and learning
disorders 106–7
delirious states 302, 354
dementia 303–4
infectious diseases 355
Denver Development Screening Test
(DDST), psychological
assessment 38
depersonalization 215
depressive feelings and behaviour 223–31
adolescence 227
aetiology 228–9
assessment 229–30
bipolar affective disorders 299–302
clinical features 226–8
cognitive beliefs 225
counselling 301
definition and classification 225–6
disorders 225–31
middle childhood 227
post infection 354–5
pre school children 226–7
predisposing factors 228–9
prevalence 228
reaction to bereavement 225
treatment and outcome 230–1
ECT 302
dermatitis, atopic 386–7
desensitization, behaviour therapy
411–12
desmopressin (DDAVP) 450
developmental disorders
brain damage or dysfunction 5
intrauterine growth retardation 175
learning disorders 84–110
pervasive disorders 120–31
see also specific aspects and syndromes
developmental theories 2–12
attachment 11–12
cognitive behaviour 6–8
family 8
genetic factors 5
learning 6
life experiences 12
psychoanalytic 9–11

dexamphetamine sulphate, dosage and
      characteristics 448
diabetes mellitus 360–4
   psychological factors 361–2
   psychosocial aspects of
      management 363–4
diagnosis *see* assessment and
      diagnosis
Diagnostic and Statistical Manual of
      Mental Disorders (DSM-IV), APA
      (1994) 17–19
diazepam, dosage and characteristics 206,
      444–5
dichloralphenazone 444
dietary treatment 453–4
dieting, anorexia nervosa 274
disability
   defined 318
   see also physical disorders
disturbed children and their families
      (*table*) 456
divorce and separation 420–30, 439,
      475
Down syndrome (trisomy 21) 89–90,
      139–41
   behavioural development 140–1
   impact on family life 140
   intellectual development 139–40
   learning disorders 89–90
   management 141
   physical features 139
drug use and abuse 304–13
   alcohol and drugs, treatment 308
   cannabis 310–11
   cigarette smoking 309–10
   effects on fetus and baby 173–4
   factors involved 304–6
   interviews with child 31–2
   prevalence 305
   substance abuse (alcohol and drugs)
      306–8, 311–12
   treatment 308
   volatile substances 308–9
   withdrawal, effects on newborn 174
   see also alcohol
drugs, administered 442–52
   effects on fetus 174
   monitoring 451–2
Duchenne muscular dystrophy 167–8
dyslalia 75

dyslexia 81
dysphasia 72–3

eating disorders *see* feeding and eating
      control disorders
eczema (atopic dermatitis) 386–7
education 394, 484–5
   attainment tests 39–40
   special education 480–5
      assessment 482–4
elective mutism, speech production
      disorders 76–9
electroconvulsive therapy 302, 454
emergency protection order (EPO) 473
emotional abuse 51–4
emotional development 207–35
   children with physical disorders 324–6
   development of fear and anxiety 208–12
   disorders of mood *see* depression
   school refusal 220–3
   separation anxiety disorder 209,
      213–15, 219
   see also anxiety disorders
employment 393
encephalitis, subacute sclerosing
      panencephalitis 355
encopresis
   bowel control 254–7
   management and outcome 256–7
endocrine disorders 359–64
enuresis 257–62
   management and outcome 260–2
enzyme deficiency diseases 170–1
epilepsy 153–61
   associated behavioural and emotional
      disorders 156–8
   cause of attack 155–6
   classification (*table*) 153–4
   effects of anticonvulsant drugs 158
   impact on child, family and
      witnesses 159
   management 160–1
   psychosocial aspects 155–6
   surgery 158–9
epiloia (tuberous sclerosis) 94, 143,
      387–8
ethnicity
   and conduct disorders 245
   prevalence of psychiatric disorders 22

evidence-based psychiatry 3
extinction 406–7

failure to thrive 190–6
  aetiology 191–2
  assessment 193–4
  hospital management plan 196
  management 194–6
  outcome 196
  see also neglect
family 12–17
  care, learning disorders 101
  developmental theories and disorders
    8–9
  disturbed children and their families
    (*table*) 456
  extended families 13
  interviews 28–33
  interviews with child 31
  interviews with parents 27
  large family size 13–14
  parental care 14–15
  parental mental illness 15–16
  parental physical illness 15–16
  parental relationships 14, 320–1
  parental stimulation 15
  physical disorders, impact on
    parents 319–21
  prevalence of psychiatric disorders 23
  psychotherapy 430–9
  separation and divorce 420–30, 439,
    475
  legislation 475
  sib relationships 16–17
  single parents 13
  treatment refusal and consent,
    legislation 475–6
  unusual family structures 13
family counselling 431–2
family doctor services 457–8
family therapy, psychotherapy 430–9
feeding and eating control disorders
    186–201
  abdominal pain 188
  anorexia nervosa 273–80
  breast or bottle feeding 186–7
  constipation 188
  counselling 189–90
  crying 187–8

  diarrhoea 188
  early infancy 188–90
  failure to suck 187
  family and group approaches 200
  hospital management plan 195
  hospitalization 200
  maternal anxiety or depression 189
  obesity 197–201
    behavioural measures 200
    dietary restrictions 200
  pica 196–7
  practical help 189
  rejection of bottle or breast 187
  vomiting 188
  see also failure to thrive
fetal alcohol syndrome 173–4
fetal and infant development 172–85
  attachment
    child 181–3
    family members 180–3
  attachment disorders 183–5
    management and outcome 185
    reactive and disinhibited types
      184–5
  care in pregnancy 178–9
  effect of perinatal complications on
    psychological development 175–6
  effects of low birthweight on
    psychological development 174–5
  postnatal care 179–80
  psychological aspects 172–80
  psychosocial aspects—neonatal
    period 176–8
  smoking, alcohol and drug
    addiction 173–4
fetal infection 350–4
flooding 412
fluoxetine, dosage and characteristics 283,
    450
flupenthixol decanoate 447
fluphenazine 447
fluvoxamine 450
formulation, assessment of psychiatric
    disorders 35
foster care 470–1
fragile X syndrome 90, 146–8

gabapentin 451
galactosaemia 170, 357–8

gargoylism 171, 358
gastrointestinal disorders
  Crohn's disease 382
  peptic ulcer 382
  ulcerative colitis 382–3
gender, and prevalence of psychiatric
    disorders 22
gender identity and disorders 263–6
general practitioner 457–8
genetic counselling 108, 366
genetic disorders 356–9, 364–6, 369–70,
    375–8
  and self-injurious tendencies (*table*) 100
  see also sex chromosome abnormalities
genetic factors
  attention deficit hyperactivity
      disorder 113
  developmental theories and
      disorders 5
  learning disorders 91, 100
    genetic risk (*table*) 108
genetic risk (*table*) 108
genitourinary deformities 343–4
genitourinary disorders 378–82
  chronic renal failure 379–80
  intersex disorders 380–2
  malformations 378
  undescended testes 380
  UTIs 378–9
gifted children, intelligence and learning
    disorders 109–10
glomerulonephritis 379
glue sniffing 308–9
gonadotrophins 262
Goodenough–Harris Drawing Test 39
grief 335–6
Griffith Mental Development Scale 38
group therapy *see* psychotherapy
growth retardation, intrauterine 175
guanfacine, dosage and
    characteristics 448–9

habit disorders 64–5
haemodialysis 379
haemophilia 364–6
haemophilia 364–6
haloperidol, dosage and characteristics 58,
    249, 302, 445–6
handicap, defined 318

head injury 346–7
headache 162–5
  clinical features 163
  treatment 164–5
health services *see* mental health services
hearing
  early management of impairment 134
  normal development 132
  psychiatric disorders 134–5
  psychological development 74, 133–4
  screening for deafness 132
heart disease 383–6
  surgery 384–6
  trivial conditions 384
hermaphroditism 381
heroin 312
herpes simplex 354
Hirschsprung disease 252
historical aspects 3–5
HIV infection and AIDS 350–3
homocystinuria 92
homosexual behaviour 271–2
hospitalization 330–4, 460–1
  adverse effects 332–4
  feeding and eating control disorders 200
  in-patient units 463
  management plan, failure to thrive 196
  modifying distress 332
  short and long-term effects 331–2
housing 393
human immunodeficiency virus (HIV) 350–3
Hunter and Hurler syndromes 93, 171, 358
hydrocephalus 96
hyperbilirubinaemia 96
hyperkinetic syndrome, attention deficit
      hyperactivity disorder
      (ADHD) 111–20
hypersomnias, sleep and its disorders 206–7
hypnotherapy 452–3
hypnotics 443–4
hypochondriasis 215
hypomania, treatment 302
hypospadias 343–4
hypothyroidism 96, 359

ICD-10 classification 19–20
ileostomy 383
imipramine hydrochloride, dosage and
    characteristics 444, 449

immunisation 353
immunodeficiency disorders 389–90
  HIV infection and AIDS 389–90
impairment, defined 318
infant care
  failure to thrive 190–6
  feeding problems 186–90
infant development
  Bayley Scales 38
  see also developmental theories and
    disorders
infectious diseases 349–56
  confusional states (delirious states) 354
  congenital rubella 353
  cytomegalovirus 353
  dementia 355
  depressive states 354–5
  fetal infection 350–4
  HIV and AIDS 350–3
  learning deficits 355
  parental reactions 356
  social factors and stress 350
injuries 344–9
  accidental poisoning 347–8
  burns 348–9
  head injuries 346–7
  non-accidental injuries 43–8
  prevention 348
  self-injury 100, 171, 358–9
insulin, and diabetes mellitus 360–4
intellectual development 123
intelligence
  disorders of *see* learning disorders
  IQ (50–70) 88
  IQ classification (*table*) 86
  IQ and lead 89
  IQ less than 50 89–98
interim care and supervision orders 474
International Classification of Diseases
  (ICD-10); World Health
  Organization (1992) 17–19
interview technique, assessment of
  psychiatric disorders 28–33
intrauterine growth retardation 175

juvenile chronic arthritis 390–1

Kleine–Levin syndrome 207
Klinefelter syndrome 145

lamotrigine 451
language development 68–84
  assessment 71
  delay and learning disability 72–5
    aetiology and background factors 73
    differential diagnosis (*table*) 74–5
    management 73–4
    prognosis 74
  hearing impairment 74, 133–4
  influences 70–1
  reading and reading retardation 79–84
  theories 69–71
Laurence–Moon–Biedl syndrome 95, 198
laws and legal constrints *see* legislation
lead, and intelligence 89
learning, developmental theories 6
learning disorders 84–110
  aetiology 88–96
  causes and clinical features (*table*) 92–6
  causes of mental retardation (*fig.*) 90
  assessment 97–8
  chromosomal abnormalities 90, 92
  clinical features and prevalence 87–8
  counselling 101–9
    breaking the news 101–6
  deficits and behavioural problems
    106–7
  definition 84–5
  educational categories and IQ (*table*) 86
  family care 101
  functioning level and profile 99–100
  genetic defects 91
    risk (*table*) 108
    self-injurious tendencies (*table*) 100
  gifted children 109–10
  IQ (50–70) 88
  IQ less than (50) 89–98
  management 101–109
  physical and psychiatric problems 99
  postnatal and other causes 91
  social and emotional support 108–9
  specific syndromes
    Down syndrome 89–90
    fragile X syndrome 90
learning theories 6
legislation 473–9
  care, interim care and supervision
    orders 474
  child assessment order 474
  emergency protection order (EPO) 473

local authority accomodation 474
separation and divorce 475
treatment refusal and consent 475–6
treatment refusal and consent 475–6
wardship 475
Lesch–Nyhan syndrome 94, 171, 358–9
leukaemia 366–9
treatment and outcome 367
life experiences and events, developmental
theories and disorders 12, 23–4
lithium carbonate 451
local authority accomodation 474
logic, errors of 416
lysergic acid diethylamide (LSD) 312

maladaptive conditions 416
malformations
cleft lip and palate 341–3
genitourinary 378
malnutrition 88–9
see also failure to thrive
masturbation
adolescence 270
infancy and childhood 263–4, 266
maternal anxiety or depression 189
measles, subacute sclerosing
panencephalitis 355
meconium ileus 375
melatonin 444
menarche, age at 270
meningitis
Haemophilus infection 355
viral 355
mental health services 455–65
adoption 471–3
child health clinics 458–9
child minding 468–9
children's homes 469
community paediatric team 459–60
disturbed children and their families
(*table*) 456
family doctor 457–8
foster care 470–1
hospital care 460–1
in-patient units 463
nurseries and playgroups 469
organization 465
professional staff 464–5, 477
psychiatric clinic or out-patient
departments 461–3

school medical service 460
tiers 1–4, 456
mental illness, parental 15–16
metabolic disorders 169–71, 356–9
methylphenidate, dosage and
characteristics 207, 447–8
microcephaly 96
migrant groups, prevalence of psychiatric
disorders 22–3
mood disorders 299–302
Morquio syndrome 93
motor development 61–8
causes of delay 62–4
stereotypies and habit disorders 64–5
tics and Tourette syndrome 65–8
mucopolysaccharidoses 93, 170–1, 358
mucoviscidosis 375–8
Munchausen syndrome by proxy 48–50
muscle and CNS disorders 149–68
caused by cerebral tumours 161–2
cerebral palsy 149–53
epilepsy 153–61
muscular dystrophy (Duchenne
type) 167–8
spina bifida 165–7
mutism 76–9
myalgic encephalomyelitis (chronic fatigue
syndrome) 291–3

narcolepsy, Kleine–Levin syndrome
206–7
Neale Analysis of Reading Ability 40
neglect 50–1, 188
see also failure to thrive
neonatal care 395
neonatal death 338–9
neonatal period, psychosocial
aspects 176–80
neurodermatoses 387–9
neurofibromatosis (Von Recklinghausen
disease) 94, 388
neuroleptics 445–6
neuropeptides 444
neuropsychological deficits, reading and
reading retardation 82
night terrors and sleep walking 205–6
non-accidental injuries 43–8
Noonan syndrome 144–5
nurseries and playgroups 469

obesity 197–201
obsessional disorders 280–3, 413
obstetric units 177–8
operant conditioning 6
operant methods of treatment 404–9
oppositional defiant disorder (ODD) 237–40
  aetiology 238–9
  clinical features 237–8
organic psychotic states 302–4
  with and without dementia 303–4
out-patient departments 461–3
overweight 197–201

palate malformations 341–3
panic attacks 216, 219
parental influences *see* family
pemoline sulphate, dosage and characteristics 448
personal factors, prevalence of psychiatric disorders 23
personality disorders 313
pervasive developmental disorders 120–31
pharmacology 442–52
phenelzine 451
phenothiazines 445
phenylketonuria 92, 169–70, 356–7
phobias 214–20
phonological impairment (dyslalia) 75
physical abuse 43–8
physical disorders 317–37
  chronic disease 318
  defence mechanisms 325
  impact on the child 322–6
    defence mechanisms 325–6
    psychiatric problems 324–6
    self concept 322–4
    skill acquisition 322
  impact on parents 319–20
    attitudes to the child 321
    parental relationships 320–1
  impact on sibs 326
  intelligence and learning disorders 99
  non-neurological 338–91
  prevalence 317–18
  psychosocial management 326–30
  see also specific disorders
physical illness, parental 15–16

Piaget, Jean 6–7
pica 196–7
pimozide, dosage and characteristics 68, 445, 446
playgroups 469
poisoning, accidental 347–8
post-traumatic stress disorder 293–4
postnatal infections, mental states 354–6
postnatal period 176–80
poverty alleviation 392–3
Prader–Willi syndrome 95, 142, 198
pregnancy
  in adolescence 272–3
  psychiatric aspects 172–5, 178–9
  termination 272
prevalence of psychiatric disorders 21–4
  age, ethnicity, gender 21–2
  family and life events 23–4
  migrant groups 22–3
  personal factors 23
  secular trends 23
  social factors 22
  urbanization 22
preventive strategy 392–400
  adolescence 397–8
  management principles 398–400
  middle childhood 397
  pre-school period 395–7
  primary, secondary and tertiary 392
  public policy 392–4
  specific measures 394–8
professional staff, mental health services 464–5, 476–7
psychiatric clinic, out-patient departments 461–3
psychiatric disorders 17–42
  associated with learning disorders 99
  life experiences and events 12, 23–4
  psychological assessment 35–42
psychoanalytic theories 9–11
psychological assessment 35–42
psychoses 295–304
  adolescence and psychiatric disorders 295–304
  bipolar affective disorders 299–302
  schizophrenia 296–9
psychosocial aspects of physical disorders *see* physical disorders
psychosocial management of physical handicap *see* physical disorders

psychosomatic adult-type psychiatric
disorders 283–93
psychotherapy
family 430–9
case examples 436–9
counselling 431–2
indications and contraindications
434–5
principles 430–1
treatment 433–4
group 439–42
indications and contraindications
441–2
principles 439–41
individual 420–30
case examples 427–30
indications and contraindications 426
mechanisms of change 422–3
principles 421–2
techniques 423–5
puberty, sexual development 269–72
puerperal psychoses 177
punishment 407
pyelonephritis 379

questionnaires 33

reading and reading retardation 79–84
developmental ability 79
general backwardness 80
Neale Analysis of Reading Ability 40
neuropsychological deficits 82
clinical features and management
83–4
outcome 84
specific retardation 80
rebelliousness, adolescence 268
reinforcers 407
renal failure, chronic 379–80
renal transplantation 379
Residence Order 474
respiratory disorders 370–8
Rett syndrome 148
risperidone, dosage and characteristics 68,
445, 446–7
rituals 197–201
rubella, congenital 95, 353

safety
emergency protection order (EPO) 473
prevention of injuries 348
role of professionals 393–4
social services and child protection
466–79
Sanfilippo syndrome 93
schizophrenia 296–9
links with autism 125
treatment and outcome 299
school
influences 479–80
and interviews with child 30
medical service 460
special education 480–5
school refusal 220–3
assessment 222–3
chronic 222–3
clinical features 220–1
emotional development and disorders of
mood 220–3
outcome 223
secular trends, prevalence of psychiatric
disorders 23
selective serotonin reuptake inhibitors
(SSRLs) 302, 450
self-concept 322–4
self-hypnosis 453
self-injury
Lesch–Nyhan syndrome 171, 358–9
(*table*) genetic disorders 100
sensory development 132–8
separation anxiety disorder 209, 213–14,
219
separation and divorce 420–30, 439,
475
services *see* mental health services; social
services
sex chromosome abnormalities 143–8
fragile X syndrome 146–8
Klinefelter syndrome 145
Noonan syndrome 144–5
Rett syndrome 148
Sotos syndrome 148
Turner syndrome 143–4
XXX syndrome 92
XYY syndrome 145–6
sex-linked disorders
Duchenne muscular dystrophy 167–8
haemophilia 364–6

sexual abuse 54–9, 253, 351–2
sexual development
  adolescence 269–72
    heterosexual behaviour 270–1
    homosexual behaviour 271–2
    masturbation 270
    pregnancy 272–3
  prepubertal 262–6
    behaviour anomalies 266
    gender anomalies 264–6
    gender identity and behaviour 263
    normal 262–4
sib relationships, family influences 16–17
sickle cell disease 370
single parents, family influences 13
skin disorders 386–9
sleep
  developmental neurophysiology 201–2
  influences in early childhood 202–3
sleep disorders 201–7
  case study 417–18
  hypersomnias
    Kleine–Levin syndrome 207
    narcolepsy 206–7
  night terrors and sleep walking 205–6
  wakefulness at night 203–4
Smith–Magenis syndrome 142
smoking 309–10
  effects on fetus and baby 173
  treatment and prevention 310
social development
  and antisocial behaviour 235–51
    oppositional defiant disorder
      (ODD) 237–40
    normal 235–6
social factors, prevalence of psychiatric
    disorders 22
social phobias 215–16, 220
social services and child protection 466–79
  adoption 471–3
  child minding 468–9
  children's homes 469–70
  conflicts 477–8
  court reports 478–9
  family crises and stress 468
  foster care 470–1
  health professionals 477
  nurseries and playgroups 469
  risk factors 466–7
  social workers 476–7

social workers 476–7
sodium valproate 451
Sotos syndrome 148
special education 480–5
  assessment 482–4
speech production disorders 75–9
  elective mutism 76–9
    aetiology 77–8
    assessment 78
    clinical features 77
    definition 76–7
    outcome 79
    prevalence 78
    treatment 78
  stammering (stuttering) 76
speech *see* language development
spina bifida 96, 165–7
  developmental progress and
    intelligence 166
  implications 167
  psychiatric disorder 166–7
  psychosocial aspects 165–6
stammering (stuttering) 76
stereotypies and habit disorders, motor
    development 64–5
stillbirth and neonatal death 338–9
stimulant medication 447–8
stress
  coping behaviour 325
  defence mechanisms 325
  infection predisposition 350
  post-traumatic stress disorder 293–4
Sturge–Weber syndrome 388
subacute sclerosing panencephalitis
    355
substance abuse *see* alcohol and drugs
sudden infant death syndrome
    (cot death) 339–41
suicide and parasuicide 232–5
  characteristics of self harm 232–3
  PATHOS assessment guide 234
  treatment and outcome 234–5
sulpiride, dosage and characteristics 445,
    446
supervision orders 474
syphilis 95, 354

Tay–Sachs disease 93
testis, undescended 380

tests 36–42
  application 41
  Bayley Scales of infant development 38
  British Ability Scale 39
  construction 37–8
  educational attainment 39–40
  Goodenough–Harris Drawing Test 39
  Neale Analysis of Reading Ability 40
  risks and dangers 41
    inappropriate test used 41
    labelling 42
  overgeneralization of conclusions 41–2
    unsatisfactory test conditions 41
  specific skills 40
  Vineland Adaptive Behaviour Scale 40
  Wechsler Intelligence Scale for Children
      revised form (WISC-R)
      psychological assessment 39
  Wechsler Objective Numerical
      Dimensions test (WOND) 40
  Wechsler Objective Reading Dimensions
      (WORD) 40
  Wechsler Pre-school and Primary School
      Intelligence Scale 38–9
  Wide Range Achievement Test
      (WRAT) 40
  Word Reading Subtest of the British
      Ability Scale 39–40
thalassaemia 369–70
thioridazine 447
thyroid disorders 359–60
thyrotoxicosis 359–60
tics
  case study 419–20
  motor development 65–8
Tourette syndrome 65–8
  aetiology and prevalence 66
  assessment 66–7
  case study 419–20
  clinical features 65
  counselling 67
  treatment and outcome 67–8
toxins 89
toxoplasmosis 95
tranquillizers 445–7
treatment 400–54
  behavioural and cognitive
      psychotherapies 401–20
  diet 453–4
  drug therapy 442–52

family therapy 430–9
group therapy 439–42
hypnotherapy 452–3
individual psychotherapy 420–30
miscellaneous therapies 452–4
refusal and consent 475–6
see also psychotherapy
trifluoperazine 447
trimeprazine tartrate (Vallergan forte),
    dosage and characteristics 204,
    443–4
trisomies, other than Down's 141
tuberous sclerosis 94, 143, 387–8
Turner syndrome 143–4

ulcer, peptic 382
ulcerative colitis 382–3
urbanization, prevalence of psychiatric
    disorders 22
urinary tract infections 378–9

vigabatrin 451
Vineland Adaptive Behaviour Scale 40
vision
  impairment 136
  normal development 135–6
  psychiatric disorders 137–8
  psychological development 136–7
volatile substances
  drug misuse 308–9
volatile substances
  drug misuse (*continued*)
    treatment 309
Von Recklinghausen disease,
    neurofibromatosis 94, 388

wardship 475
Wechsler Intelligence Scale for Children
    revised form (WISC-R)
    psychological assessment 39
Wechsler Objective Numerical Dimensions
    test (WOND) 40
Wechsler Objective Reading Dimensions
    test (WORD) 40
Wechsler Pre-school and Primary School
    Intelligence Scale, psychological
    assessment 38–9

Wide Range Achievement Test
    (WRAT) 40
Williams syndrome 94
Word Reading Subtest of the British Ability
    Scale 39–40

XXX syndrome 92
XYY syndrome 145–6

Y chromosome 262